PROGRESS IN CLINICAL AND BIOLOGICAL RESEARCH

Series Editors

RECENT TITLES

Please contact publisher for information about previous titles in this series.

CHEMICALLY INDUCED CELL PROLIFERATION
CELL PROLIFERATION
Implications for Risk Assessment

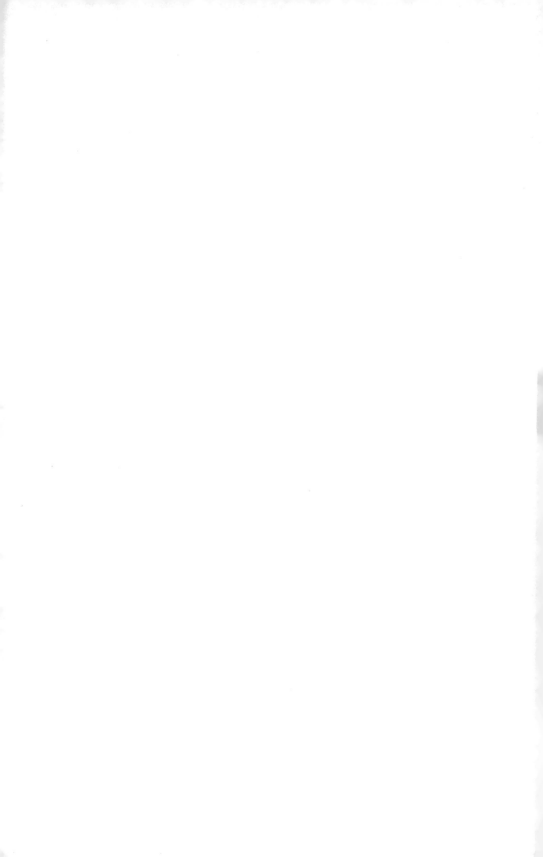

CHEMICALLY INDUCED CELL PROLIFERATION
Implications for Risk Assessment

Proceedings of the Chemically Induced Cell Proliferation Conference,
Held in Austin, Texas, November 29–December 2, 1989

Editors

Byron E. Butterworth
Chemical Industry Institute of Toxicology
Research Triangle Park, North Carolina

Thomas J. Slaga
The University of Texas
M.D. Anderson Cancer Center
Science Park–Research Division
Smithville, Texas

William Farland
Department of Health and Environmental Assessment
U.S. Environmental Protection Agency
Washington, D.C.

Michael McClain
Department of Toxicology
Hoffman-LaRoche, Inc.
Nutley, New Jersey

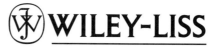

A JOHN WILEY & SONS, INC., PUBLICATION
NEW YORK • CHICHESTER • BRISBANE • TORONTO • SINGAPORE

Address all Inquiries to the Publisher
Wiley-Liss, Inc., 605 Third Avenue, New York, NY 10158–0012

Copyright © 1991 Wiley-Liss, Inc.

Printed in the United States of America

While the authors, editors, and publisher believe that drug selection and dosage and the specifications and usage of equipment and devices, as set forth in this book, are in accord with current recommendations and practice at the time of publication, they accept no legal responsibility for any errors or omissions, and make no warranty, express or implied, with respect to material contained herein. In view of ongoing research, equipment modifications, changes in governmental regulations and the constant flow of information relating to drug therapy, drug reactions and the use of equipment and devices, the reader is urged to review and evaluate the information provided in the package insert or instructions for each drug, piece of equipment or device for, among other things, any changes in the instructions or indications of dosage or usage and for added warnings and precautions.

The publication of this volume was facilitated by the authors and editors who submitted the text in a form suitable for direct reproduction without subsequent editing or proofreading by the publisher.

Library of Congress Cataloging-in-Publication Data

Chemically Induced Cell Proliferation Conference (1989 : Austin, Tex.)
    Chemically induced cell proliferation : implications for risk assessment : proceedings of the Chemically Induced Cell Proliferation Conference, held in Austin, Texas, November 29–December 2, 1989 / editors, Bryon E. Butterworth ... [et al.].
    p. cm. -- (Progress in clinical and biological research ; v. 369)
    Includes bibliographical references and index.
    ISBN 0-471-56111-8
    1. Carcinogenicity testing--Congresses. 2. Mutagenicity testing--Congresses. 3. Health risk assessment--Congresses.
I. Butterworth, Bryon E. II. Title. III. Series.
    [DNLM: 1. Cell Division--drug effects--congresses. 2. Cell Division--physiology--congresses. 3. Epithelium--cytology--congresses. 4. Neoplasms--chemically induced--congresses. 5. Regeneration--drug effects--congresses. 6. Risk--congresses. W1 PR668E v. 369 / QZ 202 C51745c 1989]
RC268.65.C54 1989
616.99'4071--dc20
DNLM/DLC
for Library of Congress
        91-15296
        CIP

Contents

REGENERATION, PROGRAMMED CELL DEATH, AND SPECIFIC METHODOLOGY

SPECIFIC EXAMPLES - I

SPECIFIC EXAMPLES - II

Contributors

Alan K. Adams, Department of Carcinogenesis, The University of Texas M.D. Anderson Cancer Center, Science Park–Research Division, Smithville, TX 78957 **[91]**

R. Siddika Ahmed, Robens Institute, University of Surrey, Guildford GU2 5XH, Surrey, England **[67]**

R.E. Albert, Department of Environmental Health, University of Cincinnati College of Medicine, Cincinnati, OH 45267 **[115]**

Gabriel G. Altmann, Department of Anatomy, The University of Western Ontario, London, Ontario, Canada, N6A 5C1 **[417]**

Bruce N. Ames, Department of Molecular and Cell Biology, University of California, Berkeley, Berkeley, CA 94720 **[1]**

Makoto Asamoto, First Department of Pathology, Nagoya City University Medical School, Nagoya 467, Aichi, Japan **[445]**

Amos Bailey, Raleigh Regional Cancer Center, Beckley, WV 25801 **[105]**

Gustav Baretton, Institute of Pathology, Medical University of Lübeck, D-2400 Lübeck, Germany **[439]**

†W. Barkley, Department of Environmental Health, University of Cincinnati College of Medicine, Cincinnati, OH 45267 **[115]**

J. Scott Brockenbrough, Department of Medicine, Division of Hematology, University of North Carolina, Chapel Hill, NC 27599 **[209]**

Janice L. Brown, Genetic Toxicology Division, Health Effects Research Laboratory, U.S. Environmental Protection Agency, Research Triangle Park, NC 27711 **[137]**

Dirk Bumann, Institute of Toxicology, Medical University of Lübeck, D-2400 Lübeck, Germany **[439]**

W. Bursch, Institut für Tumorbiologie-Krebsforschung, Universität Wien, A-1090 Vienna, Austria **[237]**

Byron E. Butterworth, Department of Experimental Pathology and Toxicology, Chemical Industry Institute of Toxicology, Research Triangle Park, NC 27709 **[253,457]**

Harold A. Campbell, Department of Oncology, McArdle Laboratory University of Wisconsin at Madison, Madison, WI 53706 **[517]**

The numbers in brackets are the opening page numbers of the contributors' articles.

† Deceased

Amador R. Cantu, Department of Carcinogenesis, The University of Texas M.D. Anderson Cancer Center, Science Park–Research Division, Smithville, TX 78957 [123]

Gail Charnley, RCG/Hagler, Bailly, Inc., Washington, DC 20024; present address: 2342 South Meade Street, Arlington, VA 22202 [291]

Chao Chen, Office of Health and Environment Assessment, U.S. Environmental Protection Agency, Washington, DC 20460 [481]

Dawn Chescoe, Microstructural Studies Unit, University of Surrey, Guildford GU2 5XH, Surrey, England [67]

Kelly H. Clifton, Department of Human Oncology, University of Wisconsin at Madison, Madison, WI 53792 [173]

T.E. Cody, Department of Environmental Health, University of Cincinnati College of Medicine, Cincinnati, OH 45267 [115]

Samuel Cohen, Departments of Pathology and Microbiology, University of Nebraska Medical Center, Omaha, NE 68198 [347]

A. Columbano, Istituto di Farmacologia e Patologia Biochemica, Faculty of Medicine, University of Cagliari, I-09124 Cagliari, Italy [217]

P. Coni, Istituto di Farmacologia e Patologia Biochemica, Faculty of Medicine, University of Cagliari, I-09124 Cagliari, Italy [217]

Lydia R. Cox, Institute of Environmental Medicine, New York University Medical Center, Tuxedo, NY 10987 [429]

M. Curto, Istituto di Farmacologia e Patologia Biochemica, Faculty of Medicine, University of Cagliari, I-09124 Cagliari, Italy [217]

Deborah E. Devor, Tumor Pathology and Pathogenesis Section, Laboratory of Comparative Carcinogenesis, National Cancer Institute, Frederick Cancer Research and Development Center, Frederick, MD 21702 [369]

Bhalchandra A. Diwan, Biological Carcinogenesis and Development Program, Program Resources, Inc./Dyncorp, National Cancer Institute, Frederick Cancer Research and Development Center, Frederick, MD 21702 [369]

Frederick E. Domann, Jr., Department of Human Oncology University of Wisconsin at Madison, Madison, WI 53792 [173]

Yvonne P. Dragan, Department of Oncology, McArdle Laboratory, University of Wisconsin at Madison, Madison, WI 53706 [517]

Leon B. Ellwein, Departments of Pathology and Microbiology, University of Nebraska Medical Center, Omaha, NE 68198 [347]

William Farland, Office of Health and Environment Assessment, U.S. Environmental Protection Agency, Washington, DC 20460 [481]

Susan M. Fischer, Department of Carcinogenesis, The University of Texas M.D. Anderson Cancer Center, Science Park–Research Division, Smithville, TX 78957 [303]

Shoji Fukushima, First Department of Pathology, Nagoya City University Medical School, Nagoya 467, Aichi, Japan [195]

Fumio Furukawa, Division of Pathology, National Institute of Hygienic Sciences, Tokyo 158, Japan [145]

Burhan I. Ghanayem, National Toxicology Program, National Institutes of Health, National Institute of Environmental Health Sciences, Research Triangle Park, NC 27709 [337]

Thomas L. Goldsworthy, Department of Experimental Pathology and Toxicology, Chemical Industry Institute of Toxicology, Research Triangle Park, NC 27709 [253]

Gay Goodman, Department of Physics, Harvard University, Cambridge, MA 02138 and Harvard University School of Public Health, Boston, MA 02115; present address: Gradient Corporation, Cambridge, MA 02138 [501]

Kevin M. Groch, Department of Human Oncology, University of Wisconsin at Madison, Madison, WI 53792 [173]

James A. Hampton, Department of Pathology, Medical College of Ohio, Toledo, OH 43699 [185]

Malgorzata Hanausek, Department of Carcinogenesis, The University of Texas M.D. Anderson Cancer Center, Science Park–Research Division, Smithville, TX 78957 [91]

James A. Hartnett, Department of Pathology, Medical College of Ohio, Toledo, OH 43699 [185]

Ryohei Hasegawa, First Department of Pathology, Nagoya City University Medical School, Nagoya 467, Aichi, Japan [195]

Yuzo Hayashi, Division of Pathology, National Institute of Hygienic Sciences, Tokyo 158, Japan [145]

Brian E. Henderson, Department of Preventive Medicine, University of Southern California School of Medicine, Los Angeles, CA 90403 [21]

John R. Henneman, Biological Carcinogenesis and Development Program, Program Resources, Inc./ DynCorp, National Cancer Institute, Frederick Cancer Research and Development Center, Frederick, MD 21702 [369]

Richard H. Hinton, Robens Institute, University of Surrey, Guildford GU2 5XH, Surrey, England [67]

Masao Hirose, First Department of Pathology, Nagoya City University Medical School, Nagoya 467, Aichi, Japan [43]

James R. Hully, Department of Oncology, McArdle Laboratory, University of Wisconsin at Madison, Madison, WI 53706 [517]

Katsumi Imaida, Division of Pathology, National Institute of Hygienic Sciences, Tokyo 158, Japan [145]

Nobuyuki Ito, First Department of Pathology, Nagoya City University Medical School, Nagoya 467, Aichi, Japan [43,445]

Randy L. Jirtle, Department of Radiology, Duke University Medical Center, Durham, NC 27710 [209]

Kevin P. Keenan, Department of Safety Assessment, Merck Sharp and Dohme Research Laboratories, West Point, PA 19486 [285]

Kirk T. Kitchin, Genetic Toxicology Division, Health Effects Research Laboratory, U.S. Environmental Protection Agency, Research Triangle Park, NC 27711 [137]

James E. Klaunig, Department of Pathology, Medical College of Ohio, Toledo, OH 43699; present address: Chemical Industry Institute of Toxicology, Research Triangle Park, NC 27709 [185,407]

A.J.P. Klein-Szanto, Department of Pathology, Fox Chase Cancer Center, Philadelphia, PA 19006 [35]

Noboru Konishi, Tumor Pathology and Pathogenesis Section, Laboratory of Comparative Carcinogenesis, National Cancer Institute, Frederick Cancer Research and Development Center, Frederick, MD 21702; present address: First Department of Pathology, Nara Medical University, Kashihara, Nara 634, Japan [369]

Arun P. Kulkarni, Toxicology Program, University of South Florida College of Public Health, Tampa, FL 33612 [137]

Yasushi Kurata, First Department of Pathology, Nagoya City University Medical School, Nagoya 467, Aichi, Japan [195]

Peeyush K. Lala, Department of Anatomy, The University of Western Ontario, London, Ontario, Canada, N6A 5C1 [417]

G.M. Ledda-Columbano, Istituto di Farmacologia e Patologia Biochemica, Faculty of Medicine, University of Cagliari, I-09124 Cagliari, Italy [217]

Martin Lipkin, Irving Weinstein Laboratory for Gastrointestinal Cancer Prevention, Gastroenterology Service, Department of Medicine, Memorial Sloan-Kettering Cancer Center, New York, NY 10021 [397]

Ronald A. Lubet, Laboratory of Comparative Carcinogenesis, National Cancer Institute, Frederick Cancer Research and Development Center, Frederick, MD 21702 [369]

E. Georg Luebeck, Department of Public Health Sciences, Fred Hutchinson Cancer Research Center, Seattle, WA 98104 [469]

Robert R. Maronpot, National Toxicology Program, National Institutes of Health, National Institute of Environmental Health Sciences, Research Triangle Park, NC 27599 [245,337]

Daniel S. Marsman, Department of Experimental Pathology and Toxicology, Chemical Industry Institute of Toxicology, Research Triangle Park, NC 27709 [389]

H.B. Matthews, National Toxicology Program, National Institutes of Health, National Institute of Environmental Health Sciences, Research Triangle Park, NC 27709 [337]

Sharon A. Meyer, Department of Radiology, Duke University Medical Center, Durham, NC 27710 [209]

George K. Michalopoulos, Department of Pathology, Duke University, Durham, NC 27710 [227]

Svein-Ole Mikalsen, Laboratory for Environmental and Occupational Cancer, Institute for Cancer Research, Norwegian Radium Hospital, N-310 Oslo, Norway [77]

Donald M. Miller, Department of Internal Medicine, University of Alabama at Birmingham, Birmingham, AL 35294 [105]

M.L. Miller, Department of Environmental Health, University of Cincinnati College of Medicine, Cincinnati, OH 45267 [115]

Thomas M. Monticello, Department of Experimental Pathology and Toxicology, Chemical Industry Institute of Toxicology, Research Triangle Park, NC 27709; present address: Pathology Associates, Inc., Durham, NC 27713 [323]

Suresh H. Moolgavkar, Department of Public Health Sciences, Fred Hutchinson Cancer Research Center, Seattle, WA 98104 [469]

Kevin T. Morgan, Department of Experimental Pathology and Toxicology, Chemical Industry Institute of Toxicology, Research Triangle Park, NC 27709 [253,323]

Rebecca J. Morris, Department of Carcinogenesis, The University of Texas M.D. Anderson Cancer Center, Science Park–Research Division, Smithville, TX 78957 [303]

Mark J. Neveu, Department of Oncology, McArdle Laboratory, University of Wisconsin at Madison, Madison, WI 53706 [517]

Kelly A. O'Brien, Department of Cell Biology, E.R. Squibb and Sons, Princeton, NJ 08543 [285]

Kumiko Ogawa, First Department of Pathology, Nagoya City University Medical School, Nagoya 467, Aichi, Japan [445]

Michael J. Olson, General Motors Research Laboratories, Warren, MI 48090 [185]

P. Pani, Istituto di Farmacologia e Patologia Biochemica, Faculty of Medicine, University of Cagliari, I-09124 Cagliari, Italy [217]

W. Parzefall, Institut für Tumorbiologie-Krebsforschung, Universität Wien, A-1090 Vienna, Austria [237]

Amy Pavone, Department of Carcinogenesis, The University of Texas M.D. Anderson Cancer Center, Science Park–Research Division, Smithville, TX 78957 [123]

G. Pichiri-Coni, Istituto di Farmacologia e Patologia Biochemica, Faculty of Medicine, University of Cagliari, I-09124 Cagliari, Italy [217]

Malcolm C. Pike, Department of Preventive Medicine, University of Southern California School of Medicine, Los Angeles, CA 90403 [21]

Henry C. Pitot, Department of Oncology, McArdle Laboratory, University of Wisconsin at Madison, Madison, WI 53706 [517]

James A. Popp, Department of Experimental Pathology and Toxicology, Chemical Industry Institute of Toxicology, Research Triangle Park, NC 27709 [253,389]

Christopher S. Potten, Department of Epithelial Biology, Paterson Institute for Cancer Research, Christie Hospital, Manchester M20 9BX, England [155]

Susan Preston-Martin, Department of Preventive Medicine, University of Southern California School of Medicine, Los Angeles, CA 90403 [21]

Kenneth S. Ramos, Department of Physiology and Pharmacology, Texas A&M University College of Veterinary Medicine, College Station, TX 77842 [429]

John J. Reiners, Jr., Department of Carcinogenesis, The University of Texas M.D. Anderson Cancer Center, Science Park - Research Division, Smithville, TX 78957 [123]

Roger Renne, Department of Pathology, Battelle Northwest, Richland, WA 99352 [323]

Edgar Rivedal, Laboratory for Environmental and Occupational Cancer, Institute for Cancer Research, Norwegian Radium Hospital, N-310 Oslo, Norway [77]

Tahir A. Rizvi, Department of Oncology, McArdle Laboratory, University of Wisconsin at Madison, Madison, WI 53706 [517]

Brad Rodu, Diagnostic Science/ Comprehensive Cancer Center, University of Alabama at Birmingham, Birmingham, AL 35294 [105]

Ronald K. Ross, Department of Preventive Medicine, University of Southern California School of Medicine, Los Angeles, CA 90403 [21]

Debra Saliba, U-Care PC, Birmingham, AL 35233 [105]

James Sanchez, University of Alabama at Birmingham, Birmingham, AL 35294; present address: 9037 Briarbrook N.E., Warren, OH 44484 [105]

Tore Sanner, Laboratory for Environmental and Occupational Cancer, Institute for Cancer Research, Norwegian Radium Hospital, N-310 Oslo, Norway [77]

Beate Schadwinkel, Institute of Toxicology, Medical University of Lübeck, D-2400 Lübeck, Germany [439]

Lydia D. Schafer, Department of Pathology, Medical College of Ohio, Toledo, OH 43699 [185]

R. Schulte-Hermann, Institut für Tumorbiologie-Krebsforschung, Universität Wien, A-1090 Vienna, Austria [237]

Ute Sherman, Department of Carcinogenesis, The University of Texas M.D. Anderson Cancer Center, Science Park - Research Division, Smithville, TX 78957 [91]

Yuenian E. Shi, Vincent T. Lombardi Cancer Research Center, Georgetown University Medical Center, Washington, DC 20007 [53]

Masa-Aki Shibata, First Department of Pathology, Nagoya City University Medical School, Nagoya 467, Aichi, Japan [195]

Tomoyuki Shirai, First Department of Pathology, Nagoya City University Medical School, Nagoya 467, Aichi, Japan [445]

Alexander Shlyakhter, Department of Physics, Harvard University, Cambridge, MA 02138 [501]

Brian G. Short, Departments of Biochemistry and Pathology, Chemical Industry Institute of Toxicology, Research Triangle Park, NC 27709; present address: Department of Experimental Pathology, SmithKline Beecham Pharmaceuticals Research and Development, King of Prussia, PA 19406 [357]

Kedar Shrestha, Department of Internal Medicine, University of Alabama at Birmingham, Birmingham, AL 35294 [105]

R. Shukla, Department of Environmental Health, University of Cincinnati College of Medicine, Cincinnati, OH 45267 [115]

Claus-Peter Siegers, Institute of Toxicology, Medical University of Lübeck, D-2400 Lübeck, Germany [439]

Joseph C. Siglin, Department of Pathology, Medical College of Ohio, Toledo, OH 43699; present address: Springborn Laboratories, Inc., Spencerville, OH 44587 [185,407]

Thomas J. Slaga, Department of Carcinogenesis, The University of Texas M.D. Anderson Cancer Center, Science Park–Research Division, Smithville, TX 78957 [303]

Peter F. Smith, Department of Safety Assessment, Merck Sharp and Dohme Research Laboratories, West Point, PA 19486 [285]

James A. Swenberg, Departments of Environmental Sciences, Engineering, and Pathology, University of North Carolina, Chapel Hill, NC 27599 [245,357]

Lois Swirsky Gold, Department of Molecular and Cell Biology, Lawrence Berkeley Laboratory, University of California, Berkeley, Berkeley, CA 94720 [1]

Michihito Takahashi, Division of Pathology, National Institute of Hygienic Sciences, Tokyo 158, Japan [145]

Satoru Takahashi, First Department of Pathology, Nagoya City University Medical School, Nagoya 467, Aichi, Japan [43]

Masae Tatematsu, First Department of Pathology, Nagoya City University Medical School, Nagoya 467, Aichi, Japan [445]

Rose Tran-Paterson, Department of Internal Medicine, University of Alabama at Birmingham, Birmingham, AL 35294 [105]

Hans-Dieter Trepkau, Institute of Toxicology, Medical University of Lübeck, D-2400 Lübeck, Germany [439]

Jerrold M. Ward, Tumor Pathology and Pathogenesis Section, Laboratory of Comparative Carcinogenesis, National Cancer Institute, Frederick Cancer Research and Development Center, Frederick, MD 21702 [369]

Christopher M. Weghorst, Tumor Pathology and Pathogenesis Section, Laboratory of Comparative Carcinogenesis, National Cancer Institute, Frederick Cancer Research and Development Center, Frederick, MD 21702 [185,369,407]

James D. Wilson, American Industrial Health Council, Washington, DC 20036; present address: Monsanto, Inc., St. Louis, MO 63167 [291]

Richard Wilson, Department of Physics, Harvard University, Cambridge, MA 02138 [501]

James D. Yager, Division of Toxicological Sciences, Department of Environmental Health Sciences, The Johns Hopkins School of Hygiene and Public Health, Baltimore, MD 21205 [53]

Sponsors

U.S. Environmental Protection Agency

The Proctor & Gamble Company

Hoffmann-LaRoche, Inc.

American Industrial Health

International Life Sciences Institute

Rohm and Haas Company

Shell Oil Company

The University of Texas M.D. Anderson Cancer Center
Science Park–Research Division

American Petroleum Institute

E.I. du Pont de Nemours & Company, Inc.

Monsanto Company

Eastman Kodak Company

Halogenated Solvents Industry Alliance

Occidental Chemical Corporation

Motor Vehicle Manufacturers Association

Preface

A better understanding of the carcinogenic process is a goal pursued by many cancer researchers, and of primary importance in this pursuit is the gaining of insight into the roles of chemically induced cell proliferation. This volume, *Chemically Induced Cell Proliferation: Implications for Risk Assessment,* presents current and much needed review and analysis of available information on cell proliferation induced by chemicals and environmental factors, thereby providing a better understanding of the mechanisms and their relative importance to human cancer risk assessment. A better understanding of these mechanisms should produce new predictive assays, improved design and interpretation for cancer bioassays, and more realistic risk assessments.

This volume is a compilation of presentations made at a conference, "Chemically Induced Cell Proliferation: Implications for Risk Assessment," held in Austin, Texas in 1989. This represents the third in a series of meetings that focused on research and contemporary issues in carcinogenesis and risk assessment. The first presentation in the volume is the keynote address by Bruce Ames, "Mitogenesis, Mutagenesis, and Animal Cancer Tests," which is followed by a section entitled "Cell Proliferation in Human Carcinogenesis." Epidemiologic evidence for the increased cell proliferation model of carcinogenesis is addressed, and a discussion of the role of chemically induced epithelial hyperplasia in the development of human cancer is presented.

The section "Basic Mechanisms of Cell Proliferation" is quite extensive and is therefore divided into two parts, both of which present possible mechanisms that bring about cell proliferation. Different models discussed are liver, skin, and pancreas, bladder, and stomach as well as cells in culture. Also discussed in this section is the role of stem cells in skin, thyroid, and intestinal cancers. The role of regeneration and programmed cell death in causing cell proliferation is also presented, as well as a discussion of specific methodologies designed for measuring different aspects of cell proliferation in rodent liver and skin.

In the sections "Specific Examples - I and II" the reader will find a detailed review of specific chemicals in well-defined models that induce cell proliferation and in turn cancer. Some of the different models addressed and related to specific chemicals inducing cell proliferation are the gastrointestinal tract, respiratory tract, kidney, bladder, and liver.

The final section, "Risk Assessment," addresses cell proliferation as a predictive assay for carcinogenicity. The role of somatic mutations and cell replication kinetics in quantitative cancer risk assessment is also discussed. In addition, the relationship between carcinogenic potency and maximum tolerated dose for mutagens and nonmutagens is presented.

This volume should be of interest to cancer research scientists, pathologists, toxicologists, pharmacologists and biochemists, as well as to cellular and molecular biologists. Those in governmental administrative and regulatory agencies dealing with environmental health hazards should also find this volume helpful.

Byron E. Butterworth
Thomas J. Slaga
William Farland
Michael McClain

Introduction

The purpose of this conference was to bring together our current knowledge on the various roles that chemically induced cell proliferation might play in the carcinogenic process. A better understanding of these mechanisms should yield new predictive assays, improved design and interpretation for cancer bioassays, and more realistic risk assessments.

Carcinogenesis is a complex process in which the functions of normal cellular growth-control genes are altered by sequential mutational events with the subsequent clonal growth of the resulting precancerous or cancerous cells. Chemical carcinogens may act by inducing mutations and/or altering cellular growth control. The observation that most mutagens are also carcinogenic is the basis for many current predictive assays and risk assessment models. there are also nonmutagenic carcinogens for which there are no predictive assays and for which conventional extrapolations to potential effects in human beings may not apply. The most obvious biological activity for many of these nongenotoxic agents is the induction of cell proliferation.

There is a misconception that only DNA-reactive compounds can affect all the changes necessary to produce tumors by themselves and be classified as so-called complete carcinogens. In fact, under the chronic lifetime maximum tolerated dose tumors (MTD) regimen typically used for cancer bioassays, nongenotoxic agents will often yield tumors as a result of those extreme conditions. Initiation events may occur as a result of increased mutational frequencies seen with sustained cell proliferation. In addition, Spontaneous foci of preneoplastic cells increase with time in tissues such as the livers of rats, owing to intrinsic factors and natural mutagenic insults, without any chemical exposure. It is probable that chemicals that increase the rate of cell turnover in that tissue, particularly in those preneoplastic cells, may shorten the time to appearance of spontaneous tumors. A strong-promoting stimulus in the two-stage mouse skin carcinogenesis model is simple abrasion of the skin with a felt wheel to remove epidermal cells, resulting in cell proliferation. Surgical removal of part of the liver (partial hepatectomy) results in regrowth of the tissue with a noncomitant increase in spontaneous tumor formation in B6C3F1 mice. Thus, some compounds appear to exhibit Carcinogenic activity as an event secondary to induced cytotoxicity and subsequent restorative cell proliferation. Other agents are directly mitogenic, stimulating growth in the target organ and possibly providing a selective growth advantage to preneoplastic cells. In fact, most carcinogens will probably exhibit both mutagenic and mitogenic activity, and it is important that both actions be considered in understanding shapes of dose-response curves.

One problem with the Ames bacterial mutagenicity assay for potential carcinogenic activity is that it fostered a simplistic view of the complex process of carcinogenesis. Chemicals are neatly classified as carcinogens/ noncarcinogens vs. mutagens/nonmutagens, with disregard for species and target organ specificity, dose-response relationships and other biological activity. The traditional concepts of initiation, promotion, and progression are difficult to define rigorously because they are so highly dependent on the specific experimental model and species under study. The terms "promotor" and "nongenotoxic carcinogen" encompass such a wide range of agents acting by different mechanisms as to be almost meaningless without more detailed information about the compound and the dose that is used. For example, risk considerations are different for the potent carcinogen 2,3,7,8-tetrachlorodibenzo-p-dioxin, which acts through a cellular receptor, and saccharin, which acts through events secondary to induced cytotoxicity and cell proliferation seen only at massive doses of the chemical, even though both may be termed nongenotoxic carcinogens. As an illustration of the complex nature of these agents, the potent skin tumor promotor 12-O-tetradecanoylphorbol-13-acetate not only induces epidermal cell proliferation, but also produces inflammation with attendant oxidative damage, induction of ornithine decarboxylase activity, and appearance of dark basal cells, all of which correlate with carcinogenic activity to some degree.

Tobacco smoking is the cause of up to 40% of the deaths from cancer. Lung cancer has risen to 49,000 deaths per year for women and 93,000 deaths per year for men. In contrast, epidemiology studies indicate no increase in cancer related to saccharin consumption. Mechanistic research clearly shows that the carcinogenic activity of this sweetener is secondary to induced cell proliferation seen only at the unrealistically high doses of the compound. Yet the word "cancer" appears as a warning on both a pack of cigarettes and a packet of saccharin, with no guidance to the average person as to their relative risks. In times of limited resources for the environment, intense economic competition, and conflicting advice to the public on personal dangers, cancer policy needs to be based on the best science available. The association of chemically induced cell proliferation with carcinogenic activity is so prevalent that it must be considered in evaluating the carcinogenic risk of chemicals to which people may be exposed. It is hoped that this compilation of excellent articles will serve both as a resource and as the basis for future work.

Byron E. Butterworth
Thomas J. Slaga
William Farland
Michael McClain

Acknowledgments

The conference "Chemically Induced Cell Proliferation: Implications for Risk Assessment," on which this volume is based, was made possible by generous contributions from both academia and private industry. The conference organizers wish to sincerely thank the Shell Oil Company, ILSI Risk Science, the Procter & Gamble Company, Dupont, the Monsanto Company, the American Petroleum Institute, the Rohm and Haas Company, and Hoffman-LaRoche, Inc. for their generous support. Also, the contributions made by the University of Texas M.D. Anderson Cancer Center, Science Park–Research Division, the Environmental Protection Agency, the American Industrial Health Council, the Halogenated Solvents Industry Alliance, the Occidental Chemical Company, Eastman Kodak Company, and the Motor Vehicle Manufacturers Association are sincerely appreciated. Special thanks are extended to the Conference Organizing Committee: Byron Butterworth, Chairman; Robert D'Amato; William Farland; Carol Henry; Andres Klein-Szanto; Michael McClain; Harvey Scribner; Thomas J. Slaga; Hugh Spitzner; and Donald Stevenson. The conference organization details were expertly directed by Karen Campbell-Engel and her staff: Mary Lou Fendley, Judy Ing, and LeNel Rice. For help in the preparation of this volume, I would especially like to thank Jean Davis, Edith K. Wilson, and Diane F. Bush of the Department of Scientific Publications at the University of Texas M.D. Anderson Cancer Center. Also special thanks to Mary Slaga, a volunteer at the Science Park–Research Division, for assistance in final manuscript preparation.

Byron E. Butterworth
Thomas J. Slaga
William Farland
Michael McClain

Chemically Induced Cell Proliferation:
Implications for Risk Assessment, pages 1-20
©1991 Wiley-Liss, Inc.

Mitogenesis, Mutagenesis, and Animal Cancer Tests

Bruce N. Ames and Lois Swirsky Gold

Carcinogens are common in rodent tests

More than half of the chemicals tested to date in chronic bioassays in both rats and mice have been found to be carcinogens at the high doses administered, the maximum tolerated dose (MTD) (1–7).[1]

Synthetic industrial chemicals account for 350 (82%) of the 427 chemicals tested in both species; approximately half (212/350) were classified as rodent carcinogens (1–7). Even though the overwhelming weight and number of the chemicals humans eat are natural, only 77 natural chemicals have been tested in both rats and mice; again, about half (37/77) are carcinogenic for rodents (1–6). The high proportion of positives does not simply result from the selection of suspicious chemical structures. Although some synthetic or natural chemicals were chosen for testing precisely because of structure or mutagenicity, most were selected because they were widely used industrially, e.g., they were high-volume chemicals, pesticides, food additives, dyes, or drugs (2). The natural world of chemicals has never been analyzed systematically. We shall explain here why the developing understanding of the mechanisms of carcinogenesis justifies the prediction that a high proportion of all chemicals—natural and synthetic—will prove to be carcinogenic to rodents if tested at the MTD. Selecting the MTD, an evolving process, is discussed by Haseman (8) and McConnell (9).

We classify a chemical as a carcinogen based on the author's positive evaluation in at least one experiment (3–6) using the criteria given by Gold et al. (2). Rodent carcinogens clearly are not all the same: Some have been tested many times in several species

---

[1]References to and analyses of individual cancer tests are in the Carcinogenic Potency Database papers (3–6). Our analyses are based on this data base, which reports only the results of chronic, long-term bioassays that can adequately detect a carcinogenic effect or lack of effect. More than 4,000 experiments met the inclusion criteria of the data base, but thousands of others did not, e.g. tests that lacked a control group, that were too short or included too few animals to detect an effect, that used routes of administration not likely to result in whole-body exposure (like skin painting or subcutaneous administration) as well as cocarcinogenesis studies and bioassays of particulate or fibrous matters.

One third of the chemicals in the database have been tested by the National Cancer Institute/National Toxicology Program using standard protocols that include testing in two species at the MTD. In contrast, about half the chemicals in the data base have been tested in only one species. Positivity rates and predictions between species have been analyzed (2).

We classified the results of an experiment as either positive or negative based on the author's opinion in the published paper, and we classified a chemical as positive if it had been evaluated as positive by the author of at least one experiment. We used the author's opinion to determine positivity because it often takes into account more information than statistical significance alone, such as historical control rates for particular sites, survival and latency, and/or dose response. Generally, this designation based on the author's opinion corresponds well with the results of statistical reanalyses regarding the significance of the dose-response effect (2).

while others have been examined at only one site in one species; some (e.g., safrole) are positive in two species, and they or their metabolites are genotoxic in animals; some (e.g., d-limonene) are only positive at one site in one species and are not genotoxic.

A high proportion of positives is also reported for rodent teratogenicity tests, which determine the potential for causing reproductive damage. Of the 2,800 chemicals tested for teratogenicity in laboratory animals, 38% were shown to cause reproductive damage in the standard, high-dose protocol (10). Thus, it is reasonable to assume that a sizable percentage of both natural and synthetic chemicals will be reproductive toxins at high doses.

Since a high proportion of both natural and synthetic test chemicals are positive, natural chemicals should be used as a reference for evaluating possible carcinogenic hazards from synthetic chemicals. In recent years, we have compared various rodent carcinogens using the HERP ratio—the human exposure:rodent potency (HERP) (1,11). It should be emphasized that as the understanding of the mechanisms of carcinogenesis improves, these comparisons can be refined, but they do not provide a direct estimate of human hazard. In this paper we do not extend the HERP comparisons because our purpose is different and space does not allow a proper analysis. HERP comparisons may, however, help describe what current animal tests can tell us about human hazard—and, if the ratio is hundreds or thousands of times smaller for certain synthetic chemicals than for many natural components of the current human diet, we may reasonably doubt that the animal evidence alone justifies expensive efforts to control the offending agent.

Natures pesticides: Mutagenicity and carcinogenicity

"Plants are not just food for animals. The world is not green. It is colored lectin, tannin, cyanide, caffeine, aflatoxin, and canavanine" [Janzen (12)].

Dietary pesticides are 99.99% natural

Nature's pesticides are one important subset of natural chemicals. Plants produce toxins to protect themselves against fungi, insects, and animal predators (12–20). Tens of thousands of these natural pesticides have been discovered, and every species of plant analyzed contains its own set of perhaps a few dozen toxins. When plants are stressed or damaged, as during a pest attack, they may greatly increase their natural pesticide levels, occasionally to levels that can be acutely toxic to humans. We estimate that Americans eat about 1.5 g per person per day of natural pesticides, which is about 10,000 times more than they eat of synthetic pesticide residues.[2]

Concentrations of natural pesticides in plants are usually measured in parts per thousand or million (12–20) rather than parts per billion (ppb), the usual concentration

---

[2]As can be seen from the references in this paper (14–21 and in legends to Table 1 and 2), a very large body of literature deals with natural toxins in plants and their role in plant defenses. The human intake of these toxins varies markedly with diet and would be higher in vegetarians. Our estimate of 1.5 g of natural pesticides per person per day is based on the content of toxins in the major plant foods, e.g. 13 g of roasted coffee per person per day contains about 765 mg of chlorogenic acid, neochlorogenic acid, caffeic acid, and caffeine (19,20, and Table 2). Phenolics from other plants are estimated to contribute another several hundred milligrams of

of synthetic pesticide residues or of water pollutants (1,22). We estimate that humans ingest roughly 5,000–10,000 different natural pesticides and their breakdown products (12-20). For example, 49 natural pesticides (and metabolites) that are ingested when eating cabbage are shown in Table 1, with indications of how few have been tested for carcinogenicity or clastogenicity. Lima beans contain a completely different array of 23 natural toxins that, in stressed plants, range in concentration from 0.2 to 33 parts per thousand fresh weight; none seems to have been tested yet for carcinogenicity or teratogenicity (16).

Many Leguminosae contain canavanine, a toxic arginine analogue, which, after being eaten by animals, is incorporated into protein in place of arginine. Feeding alfalfa sprouts (1.5% canavanine dry weight) or canavanine to monkeys causes a lupus erythematosuslike syndrome (23). In humans, lupus is characterized by a defect in the immune system that is associated with autoimmunity, antinuclear antibodies, chromosome breaks, and various types of pathology. The toxicity of nonfood plants is well known; plants are among the most commonly ingested poisonous substances among children under five years of age.

Surprisingly, few plant toxins have been tested for carcinogenicity (2-6,21). Among 1,052 chemicals tested in at least one species in chronic cancer tests, only 52 are naturally occurring plant pesticides (2-6). Among these, about half (27/52) are carcinogenic.[3]

Even though only a tiny proportion of plant toxins in our diet have been tested so far, the 27 natural pesticide rodent carcinogens are present in the following foods: anise, apples, apricots, bananas, basil, broccoli, Brussels sprouts, cabbage, cantaloupe, caraway, carrots, cauliflower, celery, cherries, cinnamon, cloves, cocoa, coffee, collard greens, comfrey herb tea, currants, dill, eggplant, endive, fennel, grapes, grapefruit

---

toxins. Flavonoids and glucosinolates account for several hundred milligrams; potato and tomato toxins may contribute another hundred, and saponins from legumes another hundred. Grains such as white flour and white rice contribute very little, but whole wheat, brown rice, and corn (maize) may contribute several hundred milligrams more. The percentage of a plant's weight that consists of toxins varies, but a small percentage of dry weight is a reasonable estimate, e.g. 1.5% of alfalfa sprouts is canavanine and 4% of coffee beans is phenolics; however, the percentage in some plant cultivars, e.g., potatoes and tomatoes, is lower.

[3]The list of 52 natural plant pesticides includes seven toxins from edible mushrooms because mushrooms are commonly considered a plant food. Fungal toxins are not included in this list, but are given below.

Plant pesticides. Carcinogens: acetaldehyde methylformylhydrazone, allyl isothiocyanate, arecoline hydrogen chloride, benzaldehyde, benzyl acetate, caffeic acid, catechol, clivorine, cycasin and methylazoxymethanol acetate mixture, estragole, ethyl acrylate, glutamyl *p*-hydrazinobenzoic acid, *p*-hydrazinobenzoic acid, lasiocarpine, *N*-methyl-*N*-formylhydrazine, *d*-limonene, α-methylbenzyl alcohol, methylhydrazine, 8-methoxypsoralen, monocrotaline, pentanal methylformalhydrazine, petasitenine, reserpine, safrole, senkirkine, sesamol, symphytine. (Cycasin as well as its metabolite methylazoxymethanol are positive in numerous tests [21] that do not meet the inclusion criteria of the database.) *Noncarcinogens:* atropine, benzyl alcohol, biphenyl, caffeine, *d*-carvone, deserpidine, disodium glycyrrhizinate, emetine dihydrogen chloride, ephedrine sulphate, eucalyptol, eugenol, beta-*N*-[γ-L(+)-glutamyl]-4-hydroxymethylphenylhydrazine, isosafrole, kaempferol, *dl*-menthol, nicotine, norharman, pilocarpine, piperidine, rotenone, rutin sulfate, sodium benzoate, vinblastine. *Uncertain: trans*-anethole, quercetin.

Among fungal toxins tested for carcinogenicity, 11/16 were positive. *Fungal toxins—carcinogens:* aflatoxin, 5-azacytidine, azaserine, citrinin, griseofulvin, luteoskyrin, mitomycin C, ochratoxin A, sterigmatocystin, streptozotocin, zearalenone. *Noncarcinogens:* erythromycin stearate, fusarenon-X, oxytetracycline hydrogen chloride, patulin, penicillin VK.

Table 1. 49 Natural Pesticides (and Metabolites) in Cabbage.[a]

Glucosinolates	4-pentenyl isothiocyanate
2-propenyl glucosinolate (sinigrin)[b]	benzyl isothiocyanate
3-methyl-thio-propyl glucosinolate	phenylethyl isothiocyanate
3-methyl-sulfinyl-propyl glucosinolate	Cyanides
3-butenyl glucosinolate	1-cyano-2,3-epithiopropane
2-hydroxy-3-butenyl glucosinolate	1-cyano-3,4-epithiobutane
4-methyl-thio-butyl glucosinolate	1-cyano-3,4-epithiopentane
4-methyl-sulfinyl-butyl glucosinolate	threo-1-cyano-2-hydroxy-3,4-epithiobutane
4-methylsulfonyl-butyl glucosinolate	erythro-1-cyano-2-hydroxy-3,4-epithiobutane
benzyl glucosinolate	2-phenylpropionitrile
2-phenyl-ethyl glucosinolate	allyl cyanide[a]
propyl glucosinolate	1-cyano-2-hydroxy-3-butene
butyl glucosinolate	1-cyano-3-methylsulfinylpropane
Indole glucosinolates and related indoles	1-cyano-4-methylsulfinylbutane
3-indolyl-methyl glucosinolate (glucobrassicin)	Alcohols
1-methoxy-3-indolylmethyl (neoglucobrassicin)	menthol
indole-3-carbinol (IC)[b]	neomenthol
indole-3-acetonitrile[b]	isomenthol
3,3'-diindolylmethane[b]	Ketones
Isothiocyanates and goitrin	carvone[a]
allyl isothiocyanate[b]	Phenols and tannins
3-methyl-thio-propyl isothiocyanate	2-methoxyphenol
3-methyl-sulfinyl-propyl isothiocyanate	3-caffoylquinic acid (chlorogenic acid)[b]
3-butenyl isothiocyanate	4-caffoylquinic acid[b]
5-vinyloxazolidine-2-thione (goitrin)	5-caffoylquinic acid (neochlorogenic acid)[b]
4-methylthiobutyl isothiocyanate	4-p-coumaroylquinic acid
4-methylsulfinylbutyl isothiocyanate	5-p-coumaroylquinic acid
4-methylsulfonylbutyl isothiocyanate	5-feruloylquinic acid

[a] Source: Hikoya Hayatsu, *Mutagens in Food: Detection and Prevention.* (Boca Raton, FL: CRC Press, 1991), 32.

[b] Discussed below; all others untested. *Clastogenicity:* Chlorogenic acid (129) and allyl isothiocyanate are positive (34). Chlorogenic acid and its metabolite caffeic acid are also mutagens (130–132), as is allyl isothiocyanate (36). *Carcinogenicity:* Allyl isothiocyanate induced papillomas of the urinary bladder in male rats (a neoplasm that is unusually rare in control rats) and was classified by the National Toxicology Program (NTP) as carcinogenic. There was no evidence of carcinogenicity in mice; however, NTP indicated "the mice probably did not receive the MTD" (3–6,133). Sinigrin (the glucosinolate, i.e., thioglycoside of allyl isothiocyanate) is cocarcinogenic for the rat pancreas (134). Carvone is negative in mice (135–138). Indole acetonitrile has been shown to form a carcinogen, nitroso indole acetonitrile, in the presence of nitrite (139). Caffeic acid is a carcinogen (140–142) and clastogen (129) and is a metabolite of its esters 3-, 4-, and 5-caffoylguinic acid (chlorogenic and neochlorogenic acid). *Metabolites:* Sinigrin gives rise to allyl isothiocyanate on eating raw cabbage (e.g., coleslaw); in cooked cabbage it is also metabolized to allyl cyanide, which is untested. Indole carbinol forms dimers and trimers on ingestion, which mimic dioxin (TCDD) (see test). *Occurrence:* see 15,18,143,144. *Toxicology:* The mitogenic effects of goitrin, which is goitrogenic, and various organic cyanides from cabbage suggest that they may be potential carcinogens (145,146). Aromatic cyanides related to those from cabbage have been shown to be mutagens and are metabolized to hydrogen cyanide and potentially mutagenic aldehydes (147).

Table 2. Concentrations of Some Natural Pesticides That Are Rodent Carcinogens.[a]

Plant food	Rodent carcinogen	Concentration (ppm)
Parsley	5- and 8-Methoxypsoralen	14
Parsnip, cooked	"	32
Celery	"	0.8
Celery, new cultivar	"	6.2
Celery, stressed	"	25
Mushroom, commercial	p-Hydrazinobenzoate	11
Mushroom, commercial	Glutamyl-p-hydrazinobenzoate	42
Cabbage	Sinigrin[b] (allyl isothiocyanate)	35–590
Collard greens	"	250–788
Cauliflower	"	12–66
Brussels sprouts	"	110–1,560
Mustard (brown)	"	16,000–72,000
Horseradish	"	4,500
Orange juice	Limonene	31
Mango	"	40
Pepper, black	"	8,000
Basil	Estragole	3,800
Fennel	"	3,000
Nutmeg	Safrole	3,000
Mace	"	10,000
Pepper, black	"	100
Pineapple	Ethyl acrylate	0.07
Sesame seeds (heated oil)	Sesamol	75
Cocoa	α-Methylbenzyl alcohol	1.3
Basil	Benzyl acetate	82
Jasmine tea	"	230
Honey	"	15
Coffee (roasted beans)	Catechol	100
Apple, carrot, celery, cherry, eggplant, endive, grapes, lettuce, pear, plum, potato	Caffeic acid	50–200
Absinthe, anise, basil, caraway, dill, marjoram, rosemary, sage, savory, tarragon, thyme	"	>1,000
Coffee (roasted beans)	"	1,800
Apricot, cherry, peach, plum	Chlorogenic acid[c] (caffeic acid)	50–500
Coffee (roasted beans)	"	21,600
Apple, apricot, broccoli, Brussels sprouts, cabbage, cherry, kale, peach, pear, plum	Neochlorogenic acid[c] (caffeic acid)	50–500
Coffee (roasted beans)	"	11,600

[a]Source: Hikoya Hayatsu, *Mutagens in Food: Detection and Prevention.* (Boca Raton, FL: CRC Press, 1991), 34.

[b]Sinigrin is a co-carcinogen (134) and is metabolized to the rodent carcinogen allyl isothiocyanate, although no adequate test has been done on sinigrin itself. The proportion converted to allyl isothiocyanate or to allyl cyanide depends on food preparation (15,143,144).

[c]Chlorogenic and neochlorogenic acid are metabolized to the carcinogens caffeic acid and catechol (a metabolite of quinic acid) but have not been tested for carcinogenicity themselves. The clastogenicity and mutagenicity of the above compounds are referenced in Table 1.

Carcinogen data are cited in references 3–6. Other carcinogens include the following: 5-methoxypsoralen (light-activated) and 8-methoxypsoralen (136) p-hydrazinobenzoate and glutamyl-p-hydrazinobenzoate (149,150), allyl isothiocyanate (3–6,133), d-limonene (137), estragole and safrole (3–6,21,151), ethyl acrylate (3–6), benzyl acetate (3–6), α-methylbenzyl

(continued on next page)

Table 2 (continued)

alcohol (138), caffeic acid (140–142), sesamol (140–142), catechol (140–142). *Concentration data:* 5-, 8-methoxypsoralen (14,152–156), *p*-hydrazinobenzoates (149,150), sinigrin (15,143,144,157), *d*-limonene (158–160), estragole and safrole (161–164), ethyl acrylate (165), benzyl acetate (166–168), α-methylbenzyl alcohol (19,20), caffeic acid, chlorogenic acid, and neochlorogenic acid (169–177) (in coffee, 28), catechol (178,179), α-methylbenzyl alcohol (19,20), and sesamol (180). *Mutagenicity and clastogenicity data:* see text. (5- and 8-Methoxypsoralen are isomeric, light-activated mutagens [14,21]; 8-methoxypsoralen was positive in an NTP gavage study (without light) and is in the data base [136]. 5-Methoxypsoralen has been tested only in a skin-painting study (with light) and is positive [148]; it is not in our data base because it is a skin-painting test.)

juice, guava, honey, honeydew melon, horseradish, kale, lentils, lettuce, mangoes, mushrooms, mustard, nutmeg, orange juice, parsley, parsnips, peaches, pears, peas, black pepper, pineapples, plums, potatoes, radishes, raspberries, rosemary, sesame seeds, tarragon, tea, tomatoes, and turnips.

The catechol-type phenolics such as tannins, and caffeic acid and its esters (chlorogenic and neochlorogenic acids), are more widespread in plant species than other natural pesticides (see Tables 1 and 2). These phenolics may have an antimicrobial role analogous to the respiratory burst of oxygen radicals from mammalian phagocytic cells. The phenolics oxidize when a plant is wounded, yielding a burst of mutagenic oxygen radicals, such as the browning of an apple when it is cut.

Caution is necessary in interpreting the implications of occurrence in the diet of natural pesticides that are rodent carcinogens. We do not argue that these dietary exposures necessarily have much relevance to human cancer. Indeed, a diet rich in fruit and vegetables is associated with lower cancer rates (24,25); this may be because some anticarcinogenic vitamins and antioxidants come from plants (24,25). What is important in our analysis is that exposures to natural rodent carcinogens may cast doubt on the relevance of far lower levels of exposures to synthetic rodent carcinogens.

Residues of synthetic pesticides

A National Research Council report dealt with the regulation of synthetic carcinogenic pesticides that are rodent carcinogens but ignored natural pesticides (26). The U.S. Food and Drug Administration (FDA) has assayed food for 200 chemicals including the synthetic pesticide residues believed to be of greatest importance and the residues of some industrial chemicals such as polychlorinated biphenyls (PCB) (22). The FDA found residues of 105 of these chemicals; the U.S. daily intake of the sum of these 105 chemicals averages about 0.09 mg per person per day, which we compare to 1.5 g of natural pesticides (i.e., 99.99% natural).[4] Other analyses of synthetic pesticide residues are similar (27). About half (0.04 mg) of this daily intake of synthetic pesticides is composed of four chemicals (22) that were not carcinogenic in rodent tests (ethylhexyl

---

[4]Figures here are based on males aged 25–30 in 1982–1984. Cancer test results are in references 10–13. The negative test on 2-ethylhexyl diphenyl phosphate is in reference 89. The latest FDA figures on actual exposures do not include every known manmade pesticide, and diets vary. Nevertheless, 0.05 mg of possibly carcinogenic pesticide residues consumed in a day seems to be a reasonable rough estimate.

diphenyl phosphate, chlorpropham, malathion, and dicloran). Thus, the intake of rodent carcinogens from synthetic residues is only about 0.05 mg a day (averaging about 0.06 ppm in plant food) even if one assumes that all the other residues are carcinogenic in rodents, an unlikely possibility.

Cooking food

The cooking of food is also a major dietary source of potential rodent carcinogens. Cooking produces about 2 g per person per day of mostly untested burned material that contains many rodent carcinogens, e.g., polycyclic hydrocarbons (28,29), heterocyclic amines (30,31), furfural (19,20), nitrosamines and nitroaromatics (1,32), as well as a plethora of mutagens (29–33). Thus, the number and amounts of carcinogenic (or total) synthetic pesticide residues seem to be minimal compared to the background of naturally occurring chemicals in the diet. Roasted coffee, for example, is known to contain 826 volatile chemicals (19,20); 21 have been tested chronically and 16 are rodent carcinogens (3–6); caffeic acid, a nonvolatile rodent carcinogen, is also present (Table 2). A typical cup of coffee contains at least 10 mg (40 ppm) of rodent carcinogens (mostly caffeic acid, catechol, furfural, hydroquinone, and hydrogen peroxide)(Table 2). The recent evidence on coffee and human health is not sufficient to show that coffee is a risk factor for cancer in humans (24,28). The same caution about the implications for humans of rodent carcinogens in the diet that were discussed above for nature's pesticides apply to coffee and the products of cooked food.

Clastogenicity and mutagenicity studies

Results from in vitro studies also indicate that the natural world should not be ignored and that positive results are commonly observed in high-dose protocols. Ishidate et al. (34), for example, reviewed experiments on the clastogenicity (ability to break chromosomes) of 951 chemicals in mammalian cell cultures. Of these 951 chemicals, we identified 72 as natural plant pesticides: 35 (48%) were positive for clastogenicity in at least one test. This was similar to results for the remaining chemicals, of which 467/879 (53%) tested positive in at least one test.

Of particular interest are the *levels* at which some of the carcinogenic plant toxins shown in Table 2 were clastogenic (34): (a) Allyl isothiocyanate was clastogenic at a concentration of 0.0005 ppm, which is about 200,000 times less than the concentration of sinigrin, its glucosinolate, in cabbage. Allyl isothiocyanate was among the most potent chemicals in the compendium (34), and has also been shown to be effective at unusually low levels in transforming (35) and mutating animal cells (36). (See also the references to cancer tests in Table 1.) (b) Safrole was clastogenic at a concentration of about 100 ppm, which is 30 times lower than the concentration in nutmeg and roughly equal to the concentration in black pepper. The rodent carcinogens safrole and estragole, and a number of related dietary natural pesticides that have not been tested in animal cancer tests, have been shown to produce DNA adducts in mice (37). (c) Caffeic acid was clastogenic at a concentration of 260 and 500 ppm, which is lower than its concentration in roasted coffee beans and close to its concentration in apples, lettuce, endive, and potato skin. Chlorogenic acid, a precursor of caffeic acid, was clastogenic at a concentration of 150 ppm, which is 100 times lower than its concentration in roasted coffee beans and similar to its concentration in apples, pears, plums, peaches, cherries, and apricots. Chlorogenic acid and its metabolite caffeic acid are also mutagens (Table 1). The genotoxic activity of coffee to mammalian cells has been demonstrated (38).

The carcinogenicity and mutagenicity of many plant pesticides were recently reviewed (21). 5- and 8-Methoxypsoralen are light-activated mutagens (14); benzyl acetate and ethyl acrylate mutate mouse lymphoma cells (36). Plant phenolics such as caffeic acid, chlorogenic acid, and tannins (esters of gallic acid) were reviewed for their mutagenicity and antimutagenicity, clastogenicity, and carcinogenicity (39).

Mechanism of carcinogenesis

It is prudent to assume that if a chemical is a carcinogen in rats and mice at the maximum tolerated dose, it may well be a carcinogen in humans *at doses close to the MTD*. However, understanding the mechanisms of carcinogenesis is critical to the attempt to predict risk to humans at low doses that are often hundreds of thousands of times below the dose at which an effect is observed in rodents. There are two major problems. First, in rodents, how can measurable carcinogenic effects at dose rates near the MTD (i.e., at doses that may cause significant cell killing and mitogenesis) be used to estimate the effects *in rodents* of dose rates so much lower that they will cause little or no cell killing— or, at any rate, cause an amount that is well within the "normal" range of cell death and replacement? Second, between species, how can carcinogenic effects in a short-lived species like the rat or mouse be used to estimate effects in a long-lived species such as the human? Cancer increases with about the fourth or fifth power of age in both short-lived rats and long-lived humans (40–43). To achieve a long lifespan, humans have evolved many types of defenses that collectively ensure that they are orders of magnitude times more resistant to spontaneous cancer at a particular age than rats (40–43). Thus, in both types of extrapolation there may be systematic factors that make the carcinogenic effects vastly less in humans than would be expected from simple extrapolation—so much so, indeed, that no quantitative extrapolation is likely to be possible in the near future from studies at or near the MTD in laboratory animals to the effects of low dose rates in human populations (40,41).

The role of mitogenesis

The study of the mechanism of carcinogenesis is a rapidly developing field that can improve regulatory policy. Both DNA damage and mitogenesis are important aspects of carcinogenesis, and increasing either substantially can cause cancer (1,44–48).

Endogenous rates of DNA damage are enormous. Mutagens are often believed to be only exogenous agents, but endogenous mutagens cause massive DNA damage (oxidative and other adducts) that can be converted to mutations during cell division. We estimated that the DNA hits per cell per day from endogenous oxidants are normally $\sim 10^5$ in the rat and $\sim 10^4$ in the human (42,43,49). This promutagenic damage is effectively but not perfectly repaired; the normal steady-state level of only 8-hydroxy-deoxyguanosine (1 of about 20 known oxidative DNA adducts) in rat DNA has been measured as $1/130,000$ bases or about 47,000 per cell (49). We have argued that this oxidative DNA damage is a major contributor to aging and the degenerative diseases associated with aging such as cancer. Thus, any agent causing chronic mitogenesis can be indirectly mutagenic (and consequently carcinogenic) because it increases the probability of endogenous promutagenic DNA damage being converted to mutations (Fig. 1). Furthermore, endogenous rates of DNA damage are so high that it may be difficult for exogenous mutagens to increase the total DNA damage significantly by low doses that do not increase mitogenesis.

Mitogenesis is itself mutagenic in numerous ways (Fig. 1). These include the following:

(a) A dividing cell is much more at risk of mutation than a quiescent cell (50). Cell division allows adducts to convert to mutations. The time interval for DNA repair during cell division is short, and adducts are converted to gaps during replication. Endogenous or exogenous damage is therefore generally increased if cells are proliferating.

(b) During cell division, single-stranded DNA is without basepairing or histones and thus is more sensitive to damage than double-stranded DNA.

(c) Cell division triggers mitotic recombination, the conversion of adducts to gaps, gene conversion, and nondisjunction, which together seem orders of magnitude more effective than an independent second mutation (51–55) in converting a heterozygous recessive gene, e.g., a tumor-suppressor gene, to homo- or hemizygosity. Heterozygotes at the human HLA-A gene are spontaneously converted to homozygotes during cell division (55). These mechanisms could account for gross chromosomal alterations that occur frequently in human tumors (55–61).

(d) Cell division allows gene duplication, which can increase expression of oncogenes that are otherwise not expressed (62).

(e) Cell division can increase the expression of the *myc* and *fos* oncogenes (63).

(f) Cell division allows 5-methyl C in DNA to be lost, which can result in dedifferentiation (64,65), thus often causing further mitogenesis.

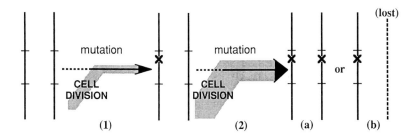

Figure 1. Mitogenesis (induced cell division) is a major multiplier of endogenous (or exogenous) DNA damage leading to mutation. The pathway to inactivating (x) both copies of a recessive tumor suppressor gene is shown (two vertical lines represent the pair of chromosomes carrying the genes). Cell division increases mutagenesis because of the following: DNA adducts converted to mutations before they are repaired (1 & 2a); mutations due to DNA replication (1 & 2a); replicating DNA is more vulnerable to damage (1 & 2a). Mitotic recombination (2a), gene conversion (2a), and nondisjunction (2b) are more frequent, and the first two give rise to the same mutation on both chromosomes. This diagram does not attempt to illustrate the complex mutational pathway to tumors.

In support of high "spontaneous" mutation rates in dividing cells is the observation that background *hprt* mutations that arise in vivo in human T lymphocytes arise preferentially in dividing T cells (66–69). The well-known mitotic instability of tumors (tumor progression) might be explained by the fact that cells in some tumors are proliferating constantly.

Suppression of intercellular communication causes mitogenesis. At near-toxic doses, some chemicals interfere with cell-cell communication in quiescent tissues (e.g., the liver, the major target site for carcinogenesis in rodents), thereby causing mitogenesis and carcinogenesis. Trosko and his associates (70,71) proposed that suppression of gap-junctional intercellular communication in contact-inhibited cells could lead to cell proliferation by cell death, cell removal, promoting chemicals, specific oncogenic products, hormones, and growth factors. In adult nondividing tissues such as the liver (2), a critical step in carcinogenesis may be lacking because mitogenesis is inhibited by intercellular communication (70–72). It is of great interest to identify chemicals causing mitogenesis at low doses relative to toxicity.

Mitogenesis from exogenous and endogenous factors may cause cancer. These include the following:

(a) Toxicity may injure tissues, resulting in replacement cell division (73–77). In an experimental cancer model, the surgical removal of part of the liver caused neighboring cells to proliferate (73–75). The incidence of liver cancer is low in humans (but not in some strains of mice) unless the liver is chronically damaged. Viruses or alcohol excess, for example, cause damage to the liver, which is a risk factor for cancer. Salt excess is a major risk factor in human stomach cancer because it causes mitogenesis (78–85). Chronic toxicity may also cause an inflammatory reaction because phagocytic cells unleash a barrage of oxidants to destroy dead cells at a wound. The oxidants produced are the same as those produced in ionizing radiation, so that chronic inflammation may be equivalent to irradiating the tissue (86). The oxidants produced as a result of inflammation may stimulate oncogenes and cell proliferation (87–90). Chronic inflammation is, as expected, a risk factor in human cancer (91–93); the carcinogenic effects of asbestos (94) and the NO_x in cigarette smoke, for example, may result primarily from inflammation, which increases both mitogenesis and mutagenesis.

(b) Chronic infection by viruses, bacteria, schistosomes, and other organisms cause cell killing and consequent cell proliferation and may be risk factors for cancer. Two examples are human virus hepatitis B, a major cause of liver cancer in the world (95,96), and human papilloma virus 16 (HPV 16), a major risk factor for cervical cancer whose main effect on cells is to increase proliferation (97). A study of transgenic mice that overproduce one protein of the hepatitis B virus, a surface antigen, showed that liver-cell injury and regenerative hyperplasia caused all of the mice to develop hepatocellular carcinomas (98).

Human T-cell leukemia virus (HTLV-1) causes constitutive expression of the T-cell IL-2 receptor (IL-2R), which may commit the cell to unremitting in vivo cell division, making the occurrence of critical mutations leading to T-cell leukemia or lymphoma more likely (99,100). Chronic *Helicobacter* (*Campylobacter*) infection is believed to be a risk factor in stomach cancer (101,102) and chronic schistosome infection a risk factor for bladder and colorectal cancer (103).

(c) Hormones may also cause mitogenesis and are major risk factors for a number of human cancers including breast cancer (103,104).

Thus, agents that cause cell proliferation are proper carcinogens and seem to be a numerous and important class of human carcinogens (103,104). The classic tumor "promoters" such as phenobarbital and tetradecanoyl phorbol acetate cause cell proliferation and are in fact complete carcinogens in animals when tested thoroughly (105). The cell division induced in the rat liver (a quiescent tissue) by certain mitogens (without cell killing) has less carcinogenic potential than that induced by toxicity (cell killing and cell replacement). A possible explanation for the mitogens' lack of effect is the death of hyperplastic tissue after the mitogenic stimulus is removed (106). Some cells normally divide more than others, and presumably this is balanced by normal defenses. Thus, cells that normally proliferate, e.g., stem cells of the small intestine, are not necessarily more susceptible to tumorigenesis. In the small intestine and other epithelial tissue, the non-stem cells that are discarded account for most of the cell division.

Animal cancer tests and mitogenesis

Mutagenicity. Analyses of animal cancer tests to date indicate that a high proportion (~40%) of chemicals that are carcinogenic in chronic tests at the MTD are not mutagenic in *Salmonella* (2,107,108). Since mitogenesis itself can be indirectly mutagenic, nonmutagens at the MTD are likely to be acting by this mechanism. If the nonmutagens that are carcinogenic in rodents at the MTD cause cancer chiefly through cytotoxic mechanisms, and if this cytotoxicity exhibits a steep upward curving (or a threshold) dose response, then for such chemicals the choice of the MTD is clearly critical for tumor induction. Other nonmutagenic carcinogens that are not active through cell killing but through mitogenesis from other causes have been discussed (46–48).

Genotoxic chemicals are even more effective at causing mitogenesis at high doses (by cell killing and cell replacement). Since they also act as mutagens, they can give a multiplicative interaction not found at low doses. However, potent mutagens like 2-acetylaminofluorene (2-AAF) have been shown to induce liver tumors in mice at moderate doses that do not increase cell division, with only the endogenous mitogenesis that primarily occurs during development (48). In rodent cancer tests, mutagens, in contrast to nonmutagens, are: a) more likely to be carcinogenic (2,107,108), b) more likely to be positive in both rats and mice (2,107,108), c) more likely to be toxic at lower doses (2), and d) more likely to cause tumors at multiple sites (108).

The dose-response relationship. Some evidence supports the idea that toxicity at or near the MTD induces mitogenesis, but below a certain dose no mitogenic effect is observed. Therefore, if animal cancer tests primarily measure the effects of mitogenesis, then the dose response would be expected to curve steeply upward (1,46–48,110–113). When doses too low to produce much mitogenesis are used, and the cell-division rate reverts to well within the normal range, no significant enhancement remains to multiply any of the chemical's other effects, leading to an upward-curving dose response for carcinogenicity, even for mutagens. This means that a 10-fold reduction in dose in a rodent experiment would produce much more than a 10-fold reduction in risk. This prediction was strongly confirmed by several recent analyses including a large-scale study on the mutagen 2-AAF (48). An extensive dose-response experiment with the well-characterized mutagens diethylnitrosamine and dimethylnitrosamine had similar results in rats (110–113). With diethylnitrosamine, at doses near the MTD, the induced ethylated adducts showed a linear dose response, and induced mitogenesis showed a threshold; the tumors induced at doses near the MTD, however, showed a clearly upward-curving dose response (110–113). Similar results were obtained with the mutagen formaldehyde (46,47,110).

Because they damage DNA, mutagens are effective at cell killing and thus also are effective at causing cell proliferation and inflammatory reactions. Thus, even though mutagens exert some effect at low doses in the absence of mitogenesis (46–48), at the MTD the carcinogenicity for both mutagens and nonmutagens is caused primarily by mitogenesis. If a chemical is nonmutagenic and its carcinogenicity is the result of cell proliferation induced by near-toxic doses, one might commonly expect a virtual threshold in the dose response (1,46–48,73–77). Mitogenesis in rodent carcinogenesis has so far not been a focus of much experimental work; experimental evidence is discussed in references 46–48, 76, and 77. In an analysis of target-organ toxicity as a factor for 53 rodent carcinogens, toxicity was not seen to have a major effect on carcinogenesis at 2 years, but the measures of target organ toxicity were largely subjective and mitogenesis was not measured (109).

Dose response in National Cancer Institute/National Toxicology Program bio-assays was examined in several studies. One analysis of the shape of dose-response curves in 344 tests indicated that, at the high doses used, a quadratic dose response is compatible with more of the data than a linear one for both mutagens and nonmutagens (Hoel and Portier, submitted for publication). Another analysis of 52 tests indicated that more than two-thirds of the carcinogenic effects would not have been detected if the high dose had been reduced from the estimated MTD to one-half the MTD (8). A third study showed that only 10% of the dose-response functions indicated a possible plateau, a leveling off of dose response. For the compounds that reached an apparent plateau at one site, the result generally was not replicated at other target sites in the same experiment, in the other sex of the same species, or in other species (114). Our explanation for the observation that a dose-response plateau is uncommon is that toxicity-induced mitogenesis is usually important (114).

Recent work suggested that cell killing also is an important factor in radiation carcinogenesis (115,116). In addition, low doses of radiation induce antioxidant defenses that protect against the mutagenic and toxic effects of larger doses of radiation or other oxidizing agents (117–121).

These considerations of mechanism suggested that, at chronic doses close to the toxic dose, any chemical, whether synthetic or natural, and whether genotoxic or nongenotoxic, is a likely rodent and human carcinogen. Not *all* chemicals would be expected to be carcinogens at high doses; the MTD may not be reached (122) or the chemical may be toxic without causing cell killing or mitogenesis.

Cancer in humans

The major preventable risk factors of cancer that have been identified thus far are tobacco, dietary imbalances (24,25,123–127), hormones (103,104), infections (95–

103), and high-dose exposures in an occupational setting (11,128), as has been discussed extensively in the literature. What is chiefly needed is serious attention to controlling the major hazards that have been reliably identified, without the focus on these major causes being diverted by a succession of highly publicized scares about factors that may well be of little or no importance as causes of human disease. Moreover, we need to make progress in identifying at least a few more major causes, and to understand better the hormonal determinants of breast cancer, the viral determinants of cervical cancer, and the dietary determinants of stomach and colon cancer. In this context, the most important contribution animal studies can offer is insight into possible mechanisms (e.g., more studies on mitogenesis) and into the complex natural world in which we live and in which life expectancy is still increasing.

Acknowledgments

We are indebted to N. B. Manley, T. Slone, R. Beier, J. Duke, J. Rine, and S. Linn for helpful discussions. This work was supported by National Cancer Institute Outstanding Investigator grant CA39910, by National Institute of Environmental Health Sciences Center grant ES01896; and contract DE-AC03-76SF00098 with the director, Office of Energy Research, Office of Health and Environmental Research, Division of the U.S. Department of Energy. This paper was adapted in part from: Ames BN, Gold LS. Dietary carcinogens, environmental pollution, and cancer: Some misconceptions. Med Oncol & Tumor Pharmacother 7:69–85, 1990; Ames BN, Gold LS. Chemical carcinogenesis: Too many rodent carcinogens. Proc Natl Acad Sci USA 87:7772–7776, 1990; Ames BN, Profet M, Gold LS. Dietary pesticides (99.99% all natural). Proc Natl Acad Sci USA 87:7777–7781, 1990; Ames BN, Profet M, Gold LS. Nature's chemicals and synthetic chemicals: Comparative toxicology. Proc Natl Acad Sci USA 87:7782–7786, 1990.

References

1. Ames BN, Magaw R, Gold LS. Ranking possible carcinogenic hazards. Science 236:271–280, 1987.
2. Gold LS, Bernstein L, Magaw R, Slone TH. Interspecies extrapolation in carcinogenesis: Prediction between rats and mice. Environ Health Perspect 81:211–219, 1989.
3. Gold LS, Sawyer CB, Magaw R, Backman GM, de Veciana M, Levinson R, Hooper NK, Haverder WR, Bernstein L, Peto R, Pike MC, Ames BN. A carcinogenic potency database of the standardized results of animal bioassays. Environ Health Perspect 58:9–319, 1984.
4. Gold LS, de Veciana M, Backman GM, Magaw R, Lopipero P, Smith M, Blumenthal M, Levinson R, Bernstein L, Ames BN. Chronological supplement to the Carcinogenic Potency Database: Standardized results of animal bioassays published through December 1982, Environ Health Perspect 67:161–200, 1986.
5. Gold LS, Slone TH, Backman GM, Magaw R, Da Costa M, Lopipero P, Blumenthal M, Ames BN. Second chronological supplement to the Carcinogenic Potency Database: Standardized results of animal bioassays published through December 1984 and by the National Toxicology Program through May 1986. Environ Health Perspect 74:237–329, 1987.
6. Gold LS, Slone TH, Backman GM, Eisenberg S, Da Costa M, Wong M, Manley NB, Rohrbach L, Ames BN. Third chronological supplement to the Carcinogenic Potency Database: Standardized results of animal bioassays published through December 1986 and by the National Toxicology Program through June 1987. Environ Health Perspect 84:215–285, 1989.
7. Gold LS, Slone TH, Bernstein L. Summary of carcinogenic potency and positivity for 492 rodent carcinogens in the carcinogenic potency database. Environ Health Perspect 79:259–272, 1989.

8. Haseman JK. Issue in carcinogenicity testing: dose selection. Fundam Appl Toxicol 5:66–78, 1985.
9. McConnell EE. The maximum tolerated dose: the debate. Journal of the American College of Toxicology 8:1115–1120, 1989.
10. Schardein JL, Schwetz BA, Kenal MF. Species sensitivities and prediction of teratogenic potential. Environ Health Perspect 61:55–67, 1985.
11. Gold LS, Backman GM, Hooper NK, Peto R. Ranking the potential carcinogenic hazards to workers from exposures to chemicals that are tumorigenic in rodents. Environ Health Perspect 76:211–219, 1987.
12. Janzen DH. Promising directions of study in tropical animal plant interactions. Annals of the Missouri Botanical Gardens 64:706–736, 1977.
13. Ames BN. Dietary carcinogens and anticarcinogens: Oxygen radicals and degenerative diseases. Science 221:1256–1264, 1983.
14. Beier RC. Natural pesticides and bioactive components in foods. In: Ware GW (ed): Reviews of Environmental Contamination and Toxicology. New York: Springer-Verlag, 1990, pp. 47–137.
15. Rosenthal GA, Janzen DH (eds): Herbivores: Their Interaction with Secondary Plant Metabolites. New York: Academic Press, 1979.
16. Green MB, Hedin PA (eds): Natural Resistance of Plants to Pests: Roles of Allelochemicals. American Chemical Society symposium 296. Washington DC: American Chemical Society, 1986, pp. 22–35.
17. VanEtten CH, Matthews DE, Matthews PS. Phytoalexin detoxification: Importance for pathogenicity and practical implications. Annu Rev Phytopathol 27:143–165, 1989.
18. Heaney RK, Fenwick GR. In: Watson DH (ed): Natural Toxicants in Food. Weinheim, Germany: VCM Verlagsgesellschaft, 1987.
19. Maarse H, Visscher CA (eds): Volatile Compounds in Foods, vol 1–7. Zeist, The Netherlands: TNO-CIVO Food Analysis Institute, 1989.
20. Stofberg J, Grundschober F. Consumption ratio and food predominance of flavoring materials. Perfumer & Flavorist 12:27, 1987.
21. Hirono I (ed): Naturally Occurring Carcinogens of Plant Origin: Toxicology, Pathology and Biochemistry, Bioactive Molecules, vol 2. Tokyo/Amsterdam: Elsevier Science, 1987.
22. Gunderson EL. FDR total diet study, April 1982–April 1984. Dietary intakes of pesticides, selected elements, and other chemicals. J Assoc Off Anal Chem 71:1200–1209, 1988.
23. Malinow MR, Bardana EJ Jr, Pirofsky B, Craig S, McLaughlin P. Systemic lupus erythematosus-like syndrome in monkeys fed alfalfa sprouts: Role of a nonprotein amino acid. Science 216:415–417, 1982.
24. National Research Council, Diet and Health. Implications for Reducing Chronic Disease Risk. Washington, DC: National Academy Press, 1989.
25. National Research Council, Diet, Nutrition, and Cancer. Implications for Reducing Chronic Disease Risk. Washington, DC: National Academy Press, 1982.
26. National Research Council, Board on Agriculture, Regulating Pesticides in Food. Washington, DC: National Academy Press, 1987.
27. Nigg HN, Beier RC, Carter O, Chaisson C, Franklin C, Lavy T, Lewis RG, Lombardo P, McCarthy JF, Maddy K, Moses M, Norris D, Peck C, Skinner K, Tardiff RG. Exposure to pesticides. In: Baker S, Wilkinson C (eds): Advances in Modern Environmental Toxicology. The Effects of Pesticides on Human Health. Princeton: Princeton Scientific Publishing, Ch. XVIII, pp. 35–130.
28. Clarke RJ, Macrae R (eds): Coffee, vol 103. New York: Elsevier Applied Science, 1988.
29. Furihata C, Matsushima T. Mutagens and carcinogens in foods. Annu Rev Nutr 6:67–94, 1986.
30. Sugimura T. Successful use of short-term tests for academic purposes: Their use in identification of new environmental carcinogens with possible risk for humans. Mutat Res 205:33–39, 1988.
31. Takayama S, Nakatsuru Y, Sato S. Carcinogenic effect of the simultaneous administration of five heterocyclic amines to F344 rats. Jpn J Cancer Res 78:1068–1072, 1987.
32. Beije B, Moller, L. 2-Nitrofluorene and related compounds: Prevalence and biological effects. Mutat Res 196:177–209, 1988.
33. Dietary Mutagens. Special issue, Environ Health Perspect 67, 1986.
34. Ishidate M Jr, Harnois MC, Sofuni T. A comparative analysis of data on the clastogenicity of 951 chemical substances tested in mammalian cell cultures. Mutat Res 195:151–213, 1988.
35. Kasamaki A, Yasuhara T, Urasawa S: Neoplastic transformation of Chinese hamster cells in vitro after treatment with flavoring agents. J Toxicol Sci 12:383–396, 1987.
36. McGregor DB, Brown A, Cattanach P, Edwards I, McBride D, Riach C, Caspary WJ. Responses of the L5178Y tk+/tk− mouse lymphoma cell forward mutation assay: III. 72 coded chemicals. Environ Mol

Mutagen 12:85–154, 1988.

37. Randerath K, Randerath E, Agrawal HP, Gupta RC, Schurdak ME, Reddy V. Postlabeling methods for carcinogen-DNA adduct analysis. Environ Health Perspect 62:57–65, 1985.

38. Tucker JD, Taylor RT, Christensen ML, Strout CL, Hanna ML. Cytogenetic response to coffee in Chinese hamster ovary AUXB1 cells and human peripheral lymphocytes. Mutagenesis 4:343–348, 1989.

39. Stich HF, Powrie WD. In: Stich HF (ed): Carcinogens and Mutagens in the Environment, vol I, Food Products. Boca Raton: CRC Press, 1982, pp. 135–145.

40. Peto R. Epidemiological reservations about risk assessment. In: Woodhead AD, Shellabarger CJ, Pond V, Hollaender A (eds): Assessment of risk from low-level exposure to radiation and chemicals, a critical overview. New York: Plenum Press, 1985.

41. Doll R, Peto R. The causes of cancer. Quantitative estimates of avoidable risks of cancer in the United States today. J Natl Cancer Inst 66:1191–1308, 1981.

42. Ames BN. Mutagenesis and carcinogenesis: Endogenous and exogenous factors. Environ Mol Mutagen 14:66–77, 1989.

43. Ames BN. Endogenous oxidative DNA damage, aging, and cancer. Free Radic Res Commun 7:121–128, 1989.

44. Pitot HC, Goldsworthy TL, Moran S, Kennan W, Glauert HP, Maronpot RR, Campbell HA. A method to quantitate the relative initiating and promoting potencies of hepatocarcinogenic agents in their dose-response relationships to altered hepatic foci. Carcinogenesis 8:1491–1499, 1987.

45. Farber E. Possible etiologic mechanisms in chemical carcinogenesis. Environ Health Perspect 75:65–70, 1987.

46. Butterworth BE, Slaga T (eds): Chemically Induced Cell Proliferation: Implications for Risk Assessment. New York: Wiley-Liss, 1990.

47. Butterworth B. Consideration of both genotoxic and nongenotoxic mechanisms in predicting carcinogenic potential. Mutat Res 239:117–132, 1990.

48. Cohen SM, Ellwein LB. Cell proliferation in carcinogenesis. Science 249:1007–1011, 1990.

49. Fraga CG, Shigenaga MK, Park J-W, Degan P, Ames BN. Oxidative damage to DNA during aging: 8-hydroxy-2^1-deoxyguanosine in rat organ DNA and urine. Proc Natl Acad Sci USA 87:4533–4537, 1990.

50. Tong C, Fazio M, Williams GM. Cell cycle-specific mutagenesis at the hypoxanthine phosphoribosyltransferase locus in adult rat liver epithelial cells. Proc Natl Acad Sci USA 77:7377–7389, 1980.

51. Schiestl RH, Gietz RD, Mehta RD, Hastings PJ. Carcinogens induce intrachromosomal recombination in yeast. Carcinogenesis 1:1445–1455, 1989.

52. Liskay RM, Stachelek JL. Evidence for intrachromosomal gene conversion in cultured mouse cells. Cell 35:157–165, 1983.

53. Fahrig R. The effect of dose and time on the induction of genetic alterations in *Saccharomyces cerevisiae* by aminoacridines in the presence and absence of visible light irradiation in comparison with the dose-effect curves of mutagens with other types of action. Mol Gen Genet 144:131–140, 1976.

54. Grodon J, Nakamura Y, German J. Molecular evidence that homologous recombination occurs in proliferating human somatic cells. Proc Natl Acad Sci USA 87:4315–4319, 1990.

55. Cavenee WK, Dryja TP, Phillips RA, Benedict WF, Godbout R, Gallie BL, Murphree AL, Strong LC, White RL. Expression of recessive alleles by chromosomal mechanisms in retinoblastoma. Nature 305:779–784, 1983.

56. Hansen MF, Cavenee WK. Genetics of cancer predisposition. Cancer Res 47:5518–5527, 1987.

57. Sasaki M, Okamoto M, Sato C, Sugio K, Soejima J, Iwama T, Ikeuchi T, Tonomura A, Miyaki M, Sasazuki T. Loss of constitutional heterozygosity in colorectal tumors from patients with familial polyposis coli and those with nonpolyposis colorectal carcinoma. Cancer Res 49:4402–4406, 1989.

58. Erisman MD, Scott JK, Astrin SM. Evidence that the familial adenomatous polyposis gene is involved in a subset of colon cancers with a complementable defect in c-*myc* regulation. Proc Natl Acad Sci USA 86:4264–4268, 1989.

59. Vogelstein B, Fearon ER, Hamilton SR, Kern SE, Preisinger AC, Leppert M, Nakamura Y, White R, Smits AMM, Bos JL. Genetic alterations during colorectal-tumor development. N Engl J Med 319:525–532, 1988.

60. Vogelstein B, Fearon ER, Kern SE, Hamilton SR, Preisinger AC, Nakamura Y, White R. Allelotype of colorectal carcinomas. Science 244:207–211, 1989.

61. Turner DR, Grist SA, Janatipour M, Morley AA. Mutations in human lymphocytes commonly involve

gene duplications and resemble those seen in cancer cells. Proc Natl Acad Sci USA 85:3189–3192, 1988.

62. Orr-Weaver TL, Spradling AC. *Drosophila* chorion gene amplification requires an upstream region regulating *s18* transcription. Mol Cell Biol 6:4624–4633, 1986.

63. Coni P, Pichiri-Coni G, Ledda-Columbano GM, Rao PM, Rajalakshmi S, Sarma DSR, Columbano A. Liver hyperplasia is not necessarily associated with increased expression of c-*fos* and c-*myc* in mRNA. Carcinogenesis 11:835–839, 1990.

64. Wilson VL, Smith RA, Ma S, Cutler RG. Genomic 5-methyldeoxycytidine decreases with age. J Biol Chem 262:9948–9951, 1987.

65. Lu L-J W, Liehr JG, Sirbasku DA, Randerath E, Randerath K. Hypomethylation of DNA in estrogen-induced and -dependent hamster kidney tumors. Carcinogenesis 9:925–929, 1988.

66. Nicklas JA, O'Neill JP, Sullivan LM, Hunter TC, Allegretta M, Chastenay BV, Libbus BL, Albertini RJ. Molecular analyses of *in vivo* hypoxanthine-guanine phosphoribosyltransferase mutations in human T-lymphocytes. II. Demonstration of a clonal amplification of *hprt* mutant T-lymphocytes *in vivo*. Environ Molec Mutagen 12:271–284, 1988.

67. Nicklas JA, Hunter TC, O'Neill JP, Albertini RJ. Molecular analyses of *in vivo hprt* mutations in human T-lymphocytes. III. Longitudinal study of *hprt* gene structural alterations and T-cell clonal origins. Mutat Res 215:147–160, 1989.

68. Albertini RJ, O'Neill JP, Nicklas JA, Allegretta M, Recio L, Skopek TR. Molecular and clonal analysis of *in vivo hprt* mutations in human cells. Proceedings of the 5th International Conference on Environmental Mutagens. New York: Alan R. Liss, 1990.

69. Allegretta M, Nicklas JA, Sriram S, Albertini RJ. T cells responsive to myelin basic protein in patients with multiple sclerosis. Science 247:718–721, 1990.

70. Trosko JE. Towards understanding carcinogenic hazards: A crisis in paradigms. J Am Coll Toxicol 89:1121–1132, 1989.

71. Trosko JE, Chang CC, Madhukar BV, Oh SY. Modulators of gap function: The scientific basis of epigenetic toxicology. In Vitro Toxicology 3:9, 1990.

72. Yamasaki H, Enomoto K, Fitzgerald DJ, Mesnil M, Katoh F, Hollstein M. Cell Differentiation, Genes and Cancer, IARC Scientific Publications No. 92. In: Kakunaga T, Sugimura T, Tomatis L, Yamasaki H (eds): Role of intercellular communication in the control of critical gene expression during multistage carcinogenesis. Lyon, France: International Agency for Research on Cancer, 1988, pp. 57–75.

73. Farber E. Clonal adaptation during carcinogenesis. Biochem Pharmacol, 39: 1837–1846, 1990.

74. Farber E, Parker S, Gruenstein M. The resistance of putative premalignant liver cell populations, hyperplastic nodules, to the acute cytotoxic effects of some hepatocarcinogens. Cancer Res 36:3879–3887, 1976.

75. Farber E. Cellular biochemistry of the stepwise development of cancer with chemicals: GHA Clowes Memorial Lecture. Cancer Res 44:5463–5474, 1984.

76. Mirsalis JC, Steinmetz KL. The role of hyperplasia in liver carcinogenesis. In: Stevenson D, Ward J, McClain M, Pitot H, Popp J, Slaga T (eds): Mouse Liver Carcinogenesis. Mechanisms and Species Comparisons. New York: Wiley-Liss, 1990.

77. Mirsalis JC, Tyson CK, Steinmetz KL, Loh EK, Hamilton CM, Bakke JP, Spalding JW. Measurement of unscheduled DNA synthesis and S-phase synthesis in rodent hepatocytes following *in vivo* treatment: Testing of 24 compounds. Environ Mol Mutagen 14:155–164, 1989.

78. Joossens JV, Geboers J. Nutrition and gastric cancer. Nutr Cancer 2:250–261, 1981.

79. Furihata C, Sato Y, Hosaka M, Matsushima T, Furukawa F, Takahashi M. NaCl induced ornithine decarboxylase and DNA synthesis in rat stomach mucosa. Biochem Biophys Res Commun 121:1027–1032, 1984.

80. Tuyns AJ. Salt and gastrointestinal cancer. Nutr Cancer 11:229–232, 1988.

81. Lu J-B, Qin Y-M. Correlation between high salt intake and mortality rates for oesophageal and gastric cancers in Henan Province, China. Int J Epidemiology 16:171–176, 1987.

82. Furihata C, Sudo K, Matsushima T. Calcium chloride inhibits stimulation of replicative DNA synthesis by sodium chloride in the pyloric mucosa of rat stomach. Carcinogenesis 10:2135–2137, 1990.

83. Coggon D, Barker DJP, Cole RB, Nelson M. Stomach cancer and food storage, J Natl Cancer Inst 81:1178–1182, 1989.

84. Charnley G, Tannenbaum SR. Flow cytometric analysis of the effect of sodium chloride on gastric cancer risk in the rat. Cancer Res 45:5608–5616, 1985.

85. Karube T, Katayama H, Takemoto K, Watanabe S. Induction of squamous metaplasia, dysplasia and carcinoma *in situ* of the mouse tracheal mucosa by inhalation of sodium chloride mist following

subcutaneous injection of 4-nitroquinoline 1-oxide. Jpn J Cancer Res 80:698–701, 1989.

86. Ward JF, Limoli CL, Calabro-Jones P, Evans JW. Radiation vs. chemical damage to DNA. In: Cerutti PA, Nygaard OF, Simic MG (eds). Anticarcinogenesis and Radiation Protection. New York: Plenum Press, 1987.

87. Crawford D, Cerutti P. Expression of oxidant stress-related genes in tumor promotion of mouse epidermal cells JB6. In: Nygaard O, Simic M, Cerutti P (eds): Anticarcinogenesis and Radiation Protection. New York: Plenum Press, 1988, pp. 183–190.

88. Chan TM, Chen E, Tatoyan A, Shargill NS, Pleta M, Hochstein P. Stimulation of tyrosine-specific protein phosphorylation in the rat liver plasma membrane by oxygen radicals. Biochem Biophys Res Commun 139:439–445, 1986.

89. Craven PA, Pfanstiel J, DeRubertis FR. Role of activation of protein kinase C in the stimulation of colonic epithelial proliferation and reactive oxygen formation by bile acids. J Clin Invest 79:532–541, 1987.

90. Sieweke MH, Stoker AW, Bissell MJ. Evaluation of the cocarcinogenic effect of wounding in Rous sarcoma virus tumorigenesis. Cancer Res 49:6419–6424, 1989.

91. Demopoulos HB, Pietronigro DD, Flamm ES, Seligman ML. The possible role of free radical reactions in carcinogenesis. J Environ Pathol Toxicol 3:273–303, 1980.

92. Templeton A. Pre-existing, non-malignant disorders associated with increased cancer risk. J Environ Pathol Toxicol 3:387–397, 1980.

93. Lewis JG, Adams DO. Inflammation, oxidative DNA damage, and carcinogenesis. Environ Health Perspect 76:19–27, 1987.

94. Petruska J, Marsh JP, Kagan E, Mossman BT. Release of superoxide by cells obtained from bronchoalveolar lavage after exposure of rats to either crocidolite or chrysotile asbestos. Am Rev Resp Dis 137:403, 1988.

95. Yeh F-S, Mo C-C, Luo S, Henderson BE, Tong MJ, Yu MC. A seriological case-control study of primary hepatocellular carcinoma in Guangxi, China. Cancer Res 45:872–873, 1985.

96. Wu TC, Tong MJ, Hwang B, Lee S-D, Hu MM. Primary hepatocellular carcinoma and hepatitis B infection during childhood. Hepatology 7:46–48, 1987.

97. Peto R, zur Hausen H (eds): Banbury Report 21. Viral Etiology of Cervical Cancer. Cold Spring Harbor: Cold Spring Harbor Laboratory, 1986.

98. Dunsford HA, Sell S, Chisari FV. Hepatocarcinogenesis due to chronic liver cell injury in hepatitis B virus transgenic mice. Cancer Res 50:3400–3407, 1990.

99. Inoue J, Seiki M, Taniguchi T, Tsuru S, Yoshida M. Induction of interleukin 2 receptor gene expression by p40^x encoded by human T-cell leukemia virus type 1. EMBO J 5:2883–2888, 1986.

100. Taniguchi T, Yamada G, Shibuya H, Maruyama M, Haradu H, Hatakeyma M, Fujita T. Regulation of the interleukin-2 system and T cell neoplasm. In: Kakunaga T, Sugimura T, Tomatis L, Yamasaki H (eds): Cell Differentiation, Genes and Cancer. Lyon, France, International Agency for Research on Cancer, vol 92, 1988, pp. 181–184.

101. Rathbone BJ, Heatley RV (eds): *Campylobacter pylori* and Gastroduodenal Disease. Oxford: Blackwell, 1989.

102. Blaser MJ (ed): Campylobacter pylori in Gastritis and Peptic Ulcer Disease. New York: Igaku-Shoin, 1989.

103. Preston-Martin S, Pike MC, Ross RK, Jones PA, Henderson BE. Increased cell division as a cause of human cancer. In: Slaga T and Butterworth B (eds): Chemically Induced Cell Proliferation, New York: Alan R. Liss, Inc., 1991.

104. Henderson BE, Ross R, Bernstein L. Estrogens as a cause of human cancer: The Richard and Hinda Rosenthal Foundation award lecture. Cancer Res 48:246–253, 1988.

105. Iversen OH (ed): Theories of Carcinogenesis. Washington: Hemisphere Publishing, 1988.

106. Columbano A, Ledda-Columbano GM, Ennas MG, Curto M, Chelo A, Pani P. Cell proliferation and promotion of liver carcinogenesis: Different effect of hepatic regeneration and mitogen-induced hyperplasia on the development of enzyme-altered foci. Carcinogenesis 11:771–776, 1990.

107. Zeiger E. Carcinogenicity of mutagens: Predictive capability of the *Salmonella* mutagenesis assay for rodent carcinogenicity. Cancer Res 27:1287–1296, 1987.

108. Ashby J, Tennant RW. Chemical structure, salmonella mutagenicity and extent of carcinogenicity as indicators of genotoxic carcinogenesis among 222 chemicals tested in rodents by the U.S. NCI/NTP. Mutat Res 204:17–115, 1988.

109. Hoel DG, Haseman JK, Hogan MD, Huff J, McConnell EE. The impact of toxicity on carcinogenicity studies—implications for risk assessment. Carcinogenesis 9:2045–2052, 1988.

110. Swenberg JA, Richardson FC, Boucheron JA, Deal FH, Belinsky SA, Charbonneau M, Short BG. High-

to low-dose extrapolation: Critical determinants involved in the dose response of carcinogenic substances. Environ Health Perspect 76:57–63, 1987.

111. Deal FH, Richardson FC, Swenberg JA. Dose response of hepatocyte replication in rats following continuous exposure to diethylnitrosamine. Cancer Res 49:6985–6988, 1989.

112. Peto R, Gray R, Brantom P, Grasso P. Effects on 4080 rats of chronic ingestion of NDEA or NDMA: An unusually detailed dose-response study. Cancer Res, in press.

113. Peto R, Gray R, Brantom P, Grasso P. Dose and time relationships for tumour induction in the liver and oesophagus of 4080 inbred rats by chronic ingestion of NDEA or NDMA. Cancer Res, in press.

114. Bernstein L, Gold LS, Ames BN, Pike MC, Hoel DG. Some tautologous aspects of the comparison of carcinogenic potency in rats and mice. Fundam Appl Toxicol 5:79–86, 1985.

115. Jones TD. A unifying concept for carcinogenic risk assessments: Comparison with radiation-induced leukemia in mice and men. Health Phys 4:533–558, 1984.

116. Little JB, Kennedy AR, McGandy RB. Effect of the dose rate on the induction of experimental lung cancer in hamsters by α radiation. Radiat Res 103:293–299, 1985.

117. Wolff S, Afzal V, Wiencke JK, Olivieri G, Michaeli A. Human lymphocytes exposed to low doses of ionizing radiation become refractory to high doses of radiation as well as to chemical mutagens that induce double-strand breaks in DNA. Int J Radiat Biol 53:39–48, 1988.

118. Yalow RS. Biologic effects of low-level radiation. In: Burns ME (ed): Low-Level Radioactive Waste Regulation: Science, Politics, and Fear. Chelsea, Michigan: Lewis Publishers, 1988, pp 239–259.

119. Wolff S, Olivieri G, Afzal V. Adaptation of human lymphocytes to radiation or chemical mutagens: Differences in cytogenetic repair. In: Natarajan AT, Obe G (eds): Chromosomal Aberrations: Basic and Applied Aspects. New York: Springer-Verlag, 1991, pp 140–150.

120. Cai L, Liu S-Z. Induction of cytogenetic adaptive response of somatic and germ cells *in vivo* and *in vitro* by low-dose x-irradiation. Int J Rad Biol 58:187-194, 1990.

121. Wolff S, Wiencke JK, Afzal V, Youngblom J, Cortes F. The adaptive response of human lymphocytes to very low doses of ionizing radiation: A case of induced chromosomal repair with the induction of specific proteins. In: Baverstock KF, Stather JW (eds): Low Dose Radiation: Biological Bases of Risk Assessment. London: Taylor & Francis, 1989.

122. Zeise L, Crouch EAC, Wilson R. A possible relationship between toxicity and carcinogenicity. J Am Coll Toxicol 5:137–151, 1986.

123. Lipkin M. Biomarkers of increased susceptibility to gastrointestinal cancer: New application to studies of cancer prevention in human subjects. Cancer Res 48:235–245, 1988.

124. Yang CS, Newmark HL. The role of micronutrient deficiency in carcinogenesis. CRC Crit Rev Oncol Hematol 7:267–287, 1987.

125. Pence BC, Buddingh F. Inhibition of dietary fat-promoted colon carcinogenesis in rats by supplemental calcium or vitamin D. Carcinogenesis 9:187–190, 1988.

126. Reddy BS, Cohen LA (eds): Diet, Nutrition, and Cancer: A Critical Evaluation, vols I and II. Boca Raton: CRC Press, 1986.

127. Joossens JV, Hill MJ, Geboers J (eds): Diet and Human Carcinogenesis. Amsterdam: Elsevier Science Publishers, 1986.

128. International Agency for Research on Cancer, IARC Monographs on the Evaluation of Carcinogenic Risks to Humans: Overall Evaluations of Carcinogenicity: An Updating of IARC Monographs vols 1-46, suppl 7, Lyon, France: International Agency for Research on Cancer, 1989.

129. Stich HF, Rosin MP, Wu CH, Powrie WD. A comparative genotoxicity study of chlorogenic acid (3-O-caffeoylquinic acid). Mutat Res 90:201–212, 1981.

130. Ariza RR, Dorado G, Barbancho M, Pueyo C. Study of the causes of direct-acting mutagenicity in coffee and tea using the Ara test in *Salmonella typhimurium*. Mutat Res 201:89–96, 1988.

131. Fung VA, Cameron TP, Hughes TJ, Kirby PE, Dunkel VC. Mutagenic activity of some coffee flavor ingredients. Mutat Res 204:219–228, 1988.

132. Hanham AF, Dunn BP, Stich HF. Clastogenic activity of caffeic acid and its relationship to hydrogen peroxide generated during autooxidation. Mutat Res 116:333–339, 1983.

133. Huff JE, Eustis SL, Haseman JK. Occurrence and relevance of chemically induced benign neoplasms in long-term carcinogenicity studies. Cancer Metastasis Rev 8:1–21, 1989.

134. Morse MA, Wang C-X, Amin SG, Hecht SS, Chung F-L. Effects of dietary sinigrin or indole-3-carbinol on O^6-methylguanine-DNA-transmethylase activity and 4-(methylnitrosamino)-1-(3-pyridyl)-1-butanone-induced DNA methylation and tumorigenicity in F344 rats. Carcinogenesis 9:1891–1895, 1988.

135. National Toxicology Program. Toxicology and Carcinogenesis Studies of d-Carvone (CAS 2244-16-8) in B6C3F1 Mice (Gavage Studies). Technical report 381, Research Triangle Park, National Toxicology Program, 1990.
136. National Toxicology Program. Toxicology and Carcinogenesis Studies of 8-Methoxypsoralen (CAS 298-81-7) in F344/N Rats (Gavage Studies). Technical report 359, Research Triangle Park: National Toxicology Program, 1989.
137. National Toxicology Program. Toxicology and Carcinogenesis Studies of d-Limonene (CAS 5989-27-5) in F344/N Rats and B6C3F1 Mice (Gavage Studies). Technical report 347, Research Triangle Park: National Toxicology Program, 1990.
138. National Toxicology Program. Toxicology and Carcinogenesis Studies of α-Methylbenzyl Alcohol (CAS 98-85-1) in F344/N Rats and B6C3F1 Mice (Gavage Studies). Technical report 369, Research Triangle Park: National Toxicology Program, 1990.
139. Wakabayashi K, Suzuki M, Sugimura T, Nagao M. Induction of tumors by 1-nitrosoindole-3-acetonitrile. Proceedings of 48th Annual Meeting of Japanese Cancer Association, October 1989, Nagoya, Japan, abstract 284, 1989.
140. Ito N, Hirose M. The role of antioxidants in chemical carcinogenesis. Jpn J Cancer Res 78:1011–1026, 1987.
141. Hirose M, Fukushima S, Shirai T, Hasegawa R, Kato T, Tanaka H, Asakawa E, Ito N. Stomach carcinogenicity of caffeic acid, sesamol and catechol in rats and mice. Jpn J Cancer Res 81:207–212, 1990.
142. Hirose M, Masuda A, Imaida K, Kagawa M, Tsuda H, Ito N. Induction of forestomach lesions in rats by oral administrations of naturally occurring antioxidants for 4 weeks. Jpn J Cancer Res 78:317–321, 1987.
143. Fenwick GR, Heaney RK, Mullin WJ. Glucosinolates and their breakdown products in food and food plants. CRC Crit Rev Food Sci Nutr 18:123–201, 1983.
144. McDanell R, McLean AEM, Hanley AB, Heaney RK, Fenwick GR. Chemical and biological properties of indole glucosinolates (glucobrassicins): a review. Food Chem Toxicol 26:59–70, 1988.
145. Nishie K, Daxenbichler ME. Toxicology of glucosinolates, related compounds (nitriles, R-goitrin, isothiocyanates) and vitamin U found in Cruciferae. Food Cosmet Toxicol 18:159–172, 1980.
146. Nishie K, Daxenbichler ME. Hepatic effects of R-goitrin in Sprague-Dawley rats. Food Chem Toxicol 20:279–280, 1982.
147. Villasenor IM, Lim-Sylianco CY, Dayrit F. Mutagens from roasted seeds of *Moringa oleifera*. Mutat Res 224:209–212, 1989.
148. International Agency for Research on Cancer. ARC Monographs on the Evaluation of Carcinogenic Risks to Humans: Some Naturally Occurring and Synthetic Food Components, Furocoumarins and Ultraviolet Radiation, vol 40. Lyon, France: International Agency for Research on Cancer, 1986.
149. McManus BM, Toth B, Patil KD. Aortic rupture and aortic smooth muscle tumors in mice: Induction by p-hydrazinobenzoic acid hydrochloride of the cultivated mushroom *Agaricus bisporus*. Lab Invest 57:78–85, 1987.
150. Toth B. Carcinogenesis by N2-[γ-L(+)-glutamyl]-4-carboxyphenylhydrazine of *Agaricus bisporus* in mice. Anticancer Res 6:917–920, 1986.
151. Miller EC, Swanson AB, Phillips DH, Fletcher TL, Liem A, Miller JA. Structure-activity studies of the carcinogenicities in the mouse and rat of some naturally occurring and synthetic alkenylbenzene derivatives related to safrole and estragole. Cancer Res 43:1124–1134, 1983.
152. Berkley SF, Hightower AW, Beier RC, Fleming DW, Brokopp CD, Ivie GW, Broome CV. Dermatitis in grocery workers associated with high natural concentrations of furanocoumarins in celery. Ann Intern Med 105:351–355, 1986.
153. Seligman PJ, Mathias CGT, O'Malley MA, Beier RC, Fehrs LJ, Serrill WS, Halperin, WE. Phytophotodermatitis from celery among grocery store workers. Arch Dermatol 123:1478–1482, 1987.
154. Beier RC, Ivie GW, Oertli EH, Holt DL. HPLC analysis of linear furocoumarins (psoralens) in healthy celery (Apium graveolens). Food Chem Toxicol 21:163–165, 1983.
155. Chaudhary SK, Ceska O, Têtu C, Warrington PJ, Ashwood-Smith MJ, Poulton GA. Oxypeucedanin, a major furocoumarin in parsley, *Petroselinum crispum*. Planta Medica 6:462–464, 1986.
156. Ivie GW, Holt DL, Ivey MC. Natural toxicants in human foods: Psoralens in raw and cooked parsnip root. Science 213:909–910, 1981.
157. Carlson DG, Daxenbichler ME, VanEtten CH, Kwolek WF, Williams PH. Glucosinolates in crucifer vegetables: Broccoli, Brussels sprouts, cauliflower, collards, kale, mustard greens, and kohlrabi. Journal of the American Society for Horticultural Science. 112:173–178, 1987.

158. Schreier P, Drawert F, Heindze I. Ueber die quantitative Zusammensetzung natuerlicher und technologisch veraenderter pflanzlicher Aromen. VII. Verhalten der Aromastoffe bei der Gefrierkonzentrierung von Orangensaft. Chem Mikrobiol Technol Lebensm 6:78–83, 1979.
159. Engel KH, Tressl R. Studies on the volatile components of two mango varieties. J Agric Food Chem 31:796–801, 1983.
160. Hasselstrom T, Hewitt EJ, Konigsbacher KS, Ritter JJ. Composition of volatile oil of black pepper, *Piper nigrum*. J Agric Food Chem 5:53–55, 1957.
161. Hecker E. Cocarcinogenesis and tumor promoters of the diterpene ester type as possible carcinogenic risk factors. J Cancer Res Clin Oncol 99:103–124, 1981.
162. Miura Y, Ogawa K, Tabata M. Changes in the essential oil components during the development of fennel plants from somatic embryoids. Planta Medica 53:95–96, 1987.
163. Archer AW. Determination of safrole and myristicin in nutmeg and mace by high-performance liquid chromatography. J Chromatogr 438:117–121, 1988.
164. Concon JM, Swerczek TW, Newburg DS. Black pepper (Piper nigrum): Evidence of carcinogenicity. Nutrition and Cancer 1:22, 1979.
165. Ohta H, Kinjo S, Osajima Y. Glass capillary gas chromatographic analysis of volatile components of canned Philippine pineapple juice. J Chromatogr 409:409–412, 1987.
166. Wootton M, Edwards RA, Faraji-Haremi R, Williams PJ. Effect of accelerated storage conditions on the chemical composition and properties of Australian honeys. 3. Changes in volatile components. J Apicultural Res 17:167–172, 1978.
167. Luo SJ, Gue WF, Fu HJ. Correlation between aroma and quality grade of Chinese jasmine tea. Dev Food Sci 17:191–199, 1988.
168. Karawya MS, Hashim FM, Hifnawy MS. Oils of *Ocimum basilicum* L. and *Ocimum rubrum* L. grown in Egypt. J Agric Food Chem 22:520–522, 1974.
169. Risch B, Herrmann K. Die Gehalte an hydroxyzimt saure Verbindungen und Catechinen in Kern- und Steinobst. Z Lebensm Unters Forsch 186:225–230, 1988.
170. Schmidtlein H, Herrmann K. Über die Phenolsäuren des gemüses. IV. Hydroxyzimtsäuren und Hydroxybenzoesäuren weiterer Ge müsearten und der Kartoffeln. Z Lebensm Unters Forsch 159:255–263, 1975.
171. Moller B, Herrmann K. Quinic acid esters of hydroxycinnamic acids in stone and pome fruit. Phytochemistry 22:477–481, 1983.
172. Mosel HD, Herrmann K. The phenolics of fruits. III. The contents of catechins and hydroxycinnamic acids in pome and stone fruits. Z Lebensm Unters Forsch 154:6–11, 1974.
173. Schafers FI, Herrmann K. Über das Vorkommen von Methyl- und Ethylestern der Hydroxyzimtsäuren und Hydroxybenzoesäuren im Gemüse. Z Lebensm Unters Forsch 175:117–121, 1982.
174. Winter M, Brandl W, Herrmann K. Determination of hydroxycinnamic acid derivatives in vegetable. Z Lebensm Unters Forsch 184:11–16, 1987.
175. Herrmann K. Übersicht über nichtessentielle Inhaltsstoffe der Ge müsearten. III. Möhren, Sellerie, Pastinaken, rote Rüben, Spinat, Salat, Endivien, Treibzichorie, Rhabarber und Artischocken Z Lebensm Unters Forsch 167:262–273, 1978.
176. Stohr H, Herrmann K. Über die Phenolsäuren des Gemüses. III. Hydroxyzimtsäuren und Hydroxybenzoesäuren des Wurzelge müses. Z Lebensm Unters Forsch 159:219–224, 1975.
177. Schuster B, Winter M, Herrmann K. 4-0-β-D-glucosides of hydroxybenzoic and hydroxycinnamic acids. Their synthesis and determination in berry fruit and vegetable. Z Naturforsch 41c:511–520, 1986.
178. Tressl R, Bahri D, Köppler H, Jensen A. Diphenole und Caramelkomponenten in Rostkaffees verschiedener Sorten. II. Z Lebensm Unters Forsch 167:111–114, 1978.
179. Rahn W, König WA. GC/MS investigations of the constituents in a diethyl ether extract of an acidified roast coffee infusion. J High Resolution Chromatogr Commun 1002:69–71, 1978.
180. Fukuda Y, Nagata M, Osawa T, Namiki M. Chemical aspects of the antioxidative activity of roasted sesame seed oil, and the effect of using the oil for frying. Agric Biol Chem 50:857–862, 1986.

Chemically Induced Cell Proliferation:
Implications for Risk Assessment, pages 21-34
©1991 Wiley-Liss, Inc.

Epidemiologic Evidence for the Increased Cell Proliferation Model of Carcinogenesis

*Susan Preston-Martin, Malcolm C. Pike, Ronald K. Ross,
and Brian E. Henderson*

Recent advances in the molecular genetics of cancer have provided a molecular basis for the concept that cell division is essential in the genesis of human cancer. The activation of oncogenes and inactivation of tumor-suppressor genes allows cancer development. The activation of oncogenes, whether by mutation, translocation, or amplification, requires cell division. Genetic errors that precede the development of a fully malignant tumor also include the loss or inactivation during mitosis of several tumor-suppressor genes whose function is to control normal cellular behavior (1–3). Most of the models currently favored suggest that the first hit is the inactivation by a mutational event of one of the two alleles of a tumor-suppressor gene present in diploid cells, followed by a reduction to homozygosity of the faulty chromosome (4). The initial mutagenic event and the loss of the wild-type allele of the tumor-suppressor gene both require cell division. Thus, for expression of the full malignant phenotype, cells are absolutely required to divide.

Epidemiologic evidence indicates that increased cell proliferation induced by external or internal stimulation is indeed a common denominator in the pathogenesis of many human cancers. "Increased" may imply division of a subset of cells that would ordinarily not be dividing or increased mitotic activity above the baseline rate. The amount of irreparable DNA damage is a function of the level of cell division. Rapid cell division may "fix" DNA-damaging events by not allowing enough time for normal repair. Cells that would ordinarily not be replicating (e.g., the Schwann cells in the nerve sheath) may at times be stimulated to divide, and when this happens, tumors (e.g., schwannomas) may develop (see below). Nondividing cells in adults, such as nerve cells and cardiomyocytes, never develop tumors.

Cell division increases the risk of errors of various kinds (5). Mutation is more likely to occur in a dividing cell because single-strand DNA is more sensitive to damaging effects than double-strand DNA. Cell division also allows mitotic recombination (e.g., nondisjunction, gene conversion), which results in changes more profound than those from a single mutation. Gene duplication that occurs during cell division may cause expression of previously unexpressed oncogenes. Cell division may also involve conversion of adducts to gaps or mutations.

Agents that may lead to increased cell proliferation and eventual neoplastic transformation include a wide variety of physical, infectious, and chemical agents (Tables 1 and 2). The cell proliferation factors listed in Table 1 are those whose primary carcinogenic action is to stimulate cell division. Those shown in Table 2 also seem likely to contribute to neoplasia by stimulating cell division, but evidence that the mechanism

Table 1. Human Cancers Associated with Agents Whose Major Action is Induction of Increased Cell Proliferation.

Factors causing cell proliferation	Cancer site
Hormones	
Estrogen	Endometrium
Estrogen and progesterone	Breast
Ovulation	Ovary
Drugs	
Oral contraceptives, anabolic steroids	Liver
Infectious agents	
Hepatitis B virus	Liver
Schistosoma hematobium	Bladder
Schistosoma japonicum	Colon
Clonorchis sinensis,	Biliary tract
Opisthorchis viverrini	
Tuberculosis	Lung
Epstein-Barr virus	Burkitt's lymphoma, AIDS lymphoma
Chemical agent	
Betel nut, lime	Oral cavity
Physical or mechanical trauma	
Asbestos	Mesothelial tissue, lung
Other chronic irritations	
Tropical ulcers	Skin

Table 2. Other Human Cancers Probably Associated with Increased Proliferation.

Factors causing cell proliferation	Cancer site
Hormones	
Testosterone	Prostate
Drugs	
Diuretics, analgesics	Kidney
Chemical agents	
Bile and pancreatic juice	Small intestine
Saturated fat	Colon
Salt	Stomach
Tobacco	Oral cavity, lung, larynx
Physical or mechanical trauma	
Hard foods (e.g., coarsely ground corn)	Stomach
Gallstones	Gall bladder
Loud noise	Acoustic nerve
Head injury	Intracranial meninges
Other chronic irritations	
Reverse smoking	Hard palate
Chronic ulcerative colitis	Colon

listed is the one critical to carcinogenesis is weaker. Other agents, including such established carcinogens as tobacco, may exert their effects partly through increasing cell division. We will present in some detail various examples of human cancers in which increased proliferation and hence increased cancer risk is caused by (1) hormones, (2) drugs, (3) infectious agents, (4) chemical agents, (5) physical or mechanical traumas, and (6) other chronic irritations.

Hormones

Increased cell proliferation caused by prolonged stimulation by steroid and polypeptide hormones is associated with the development of cancer of the breast, endometrium, and ovary, and it is probably associated with such other hormone-related cancers as prostate (6). Cancer of the endometrium and breast are the two best studied of these hormone-related cancers; evidence is strong that risk of both is related to cumulative estrogen exposure. Ovarian cancer is also well studied and presents an interesting variant of this hypothesis; the stimulus for cell proliferation is not hormonal per se, but ovulation, which is a direct result of complex hormonal changes.

Estrogen may be derived from both endogenous and exogenous sources. Endogenous sources in women include direct secretion of estrogens from the ovary, operative only during menstrual life, and peripheral conversion of adrenal-derived androgens to estrogen, primarily in fat cells. The primary exogenous source of estrogen during the reproductive years is oral contraceptives (OC), with hormone replacement therapy becoming the primary source in the postmenopausal years. Exposure to estrogens from exogenous sources may be measured directly in epidemiologic studies, either by careful interviewing or examination of medical and pharmaceutical records. Endogenous estrogen exposure often must be measured indirectly. Ovarian activity is usually measured by evaluating the onset, cessation, timing, and regularity of menstruation and the timing and frequency of pregnancy and lactation. Estrogen derived from peripheral conversion in adipose tissue is estimated primarily by evaluating various measurements of body fat.

Endometrial cancer

The endometrium proliferates in response to estrogen in the absence of progesterone. Epidemiologic evidence shows that events that increase estrogen stimulation in the absence of progesterone (unopposed estrogen) increase endometrial cancer risk, while events that decrease unopposed estrogen exposure decrease risk (7).

During the premenopausal years, unopposed estrogen stimulation, and hence endometrial proliferation, occurs during the first half of the normal menstrual cycle. Use of combination OC, which involve daily doses of estrogen and progesterone combined throughout the cycle, reduces risk because the endometrium is exposed to unopposed estrogen only during the 7 days in the 28-day cycle when no hormones are taken. In contrast, sequential OC deliver unopposed estrogen during most of the cycle and increase endometrial cancer risk. Increasing parity decreases risk because progesterone levels are high throughout pregnancy. Obesity increases risk in premenopausal women because of the associated progesterone deficiency, and it further increases risk in postmenopausal women because of the associated increase in estrogen levels. The marked increase in endometrial cancer risk with increasing duration of use of estrogen replacement therapy is further evidence that increased proliferation of endometrial tissue stimulated by increased estrogen levels increases the risk of this disease.

Breast cancer

Current evidence suggests that breast cells proliferate in response to estrogens and that the simultaneous presence of progesterone increases the rate of such cell division (8). The clearest demonstration that increased levels of these two hormones increase breast cancer risk is that early menarche and late menopause are such important risk factors for this disease. Breast cancer risk is reduced by at least 20% for each year menarche is delayed. For a fixed age at menarche, rapid establishment of regular menstrual cycles, with the associated increased hormone levels, further enhances risk. Women who stop menstruating before age 45, either naturally or through surgical intervention, have half the risk of breast cancer of women who continue to menstruate to age 55 or beyond. In premenopausal women, the association of obesity with a decrease in breast cancer can be explained by the decrease in ovulatory cycles and thus of hormone levels. After the menopause, obese women have an increased breast cancer risk because of their higher estrogen levels. Long-term OC use conveys a modest increase in breast cancer in premenopausal women, whereas long-term use of estrogen replacement therapy results in a comparable increase in risk among postmenopausal patients. In a recently published study (9), a distinctly larger increase in breast cancer was found among women who had used a progestogen along with estrogen replacement therapy than among women who used estrogen alone.

Breast cancer patients have been found to have higher estrogen levels than healthy women in control groups, and estrogen levels are higher in populations characterized by high breast cancer rates (10–12). Pregnancy is associated with very high levels of estrogen and progesterone. These hormone levels induce cell differentiation as well as cell proliferation, and the resultant effect on breast cancer risk is a short-term increase and a long-term decrease of risk. OC have only a slight effect on breast cancer risk; the reduced production of ovarian steroids caused by OC use is compensated for by the synthetic estrogen and progestogen in the OC itself.

Ovarian cancer

In humans, most ovarian cancers develop from epithelial cells on the surface of the ovary. The primary stimulus for division of these cells is ovulation. After each ovulation, these cells replicate to cover the exposed surface. According to our model, factors that prevent ovulation will protect against ovarian cancer development; a large and highly consistent body of epidemiologic literature supports this hypothesis (6). Risk of ovarian cancer declines progressively with each succeeding pregnancy. Incomplete pregnancies also convey protection. OC use protects against ovarian cancer in a duration-dependent manner. The degree of protection from these three factors is simply proportional to the duration of their associated periods of anovulation.

Prostate cancer

Testosterone is essential for the maintenance of prostate tissue, but no studies of men have related testosterone levels to the rate of cell proliferation in the prostate. Epidemiologic support for this association is weak and apparently inconsistent (13). Prostatic adenocarcinoma can be produced in rats by testosterone alone, and such treatment increases proliferation of the prostate's glandular cells that give rise to prostate cancer (14). We hypothesize that testosterone has a similar effect in men and that the increase in mitotic activity increases the risk of prostate cancer.

Drugs

Drugs, including synthetic steroid hormones, put an extra demand on the tissue that metabolizes them. With chronic use, this demand may stimulate local proliferation of cells able to process the compound. Human cancers associated with chronic drug use include kidney cancer with use of diuretics and analgesics and liver cancer associated with older-generation (high-dose) OC. The increased cell-proliferation model is a likely explanation for both of these associations, but whether long-term use of diuretics increases mitotic activity in the kidney remains to be investigated pathologically.

Benign and malignant liver tumors

In the 1960s and 1970s, when an unusual type of benign liver adenoma began occurring in young women, it was generally shown to be caused by long-term OC use. The tumors were often rapidly growing lesions that could achieve great size but regressed when OC use was discontinued (15). Subsequently, hepatocellular carcinomas have been associated with OC use, and on occasion the malignant tumor seems to develop in association with the adenoma (16,17; Table 3).

These tumors occur in women with no previous history of hepatitis or jaundice, and OC use alone appears sufficient to cause their development. Diffuse enlargement of the liver (e.g., in the lobe opposite the one in which tumors arise) was noted in early

Table 3. Duration of Oral Contraceptive Use in Young Women with Liver Cancer and Controls, Los Angeles County, 1975–1985.

Months of use	Number of cases	Number of controls	Odds ratio
0–12	3	14	1.0
13–60	6	10	2.8
61–84	3	4	3.5
≥85	7	2	16.3*

*$P < 0.05$.

OC users (15). Hepatocellular carcinoma is a rare outcome of this process. The natural estrogens delivered as hormone replacement therapy to menopausal women seem not to induce similar effects, nor do the newer-generation lower-dose OC. Anabolic steroids taken by body builders have, however, been related to the development of benign and malignant tumors of the liver (18,19).

Infectious agents

Infectious agents may cause cell deaths with subsequent cell proliferation. A number of cancers are associated with chronic infections, the most important association being that of liver cancer with hepatitis B virus (HBV).

Liver cancer and HBV

Persistent HBV infection is present in most patients who develop primary hepatocellular carcinoma (20). Chronic HBV infection, by destroying hepatocytes, produces a constant stimulus to hepatocellular regeneration. As HBV is not incorporated into hepatocyte genomes, we believe that the sustained cell proliferation it causes explains its strong association with liver cancer. Recent data suggest an independent effect of hepatitis C virus (HCV) infection in liver cancer etiology as well as a synergistic effect with HBV (Yu et al., submitted for publication).

Lung cancer

In the few studies of lung cancer patients and controls in which the subjects' histories of lung disease were investigated adequately, a marked increase was found in lung cancer risk, particularly among those with previous tuberculosis (TB) (21,22). This increase in risk was observed for both smokers and nonsmokers. Although no experimental data suggests that the tubercle bacillus is carcinogenic per se, TB provides a constant stimulus for regeneration of tissue damaged by this chronic infection. The alveolar cells that proliferate in response to chronic TB infection give rise to adenocarcinoma of the lung, which is the histologic type most common among Chinese women who are usually nonsmokers and often have a history of TB.

Lymphomas and Epstein-Barr virus (EBV)

EBV-associated Burkitt's lymphoma and autoimmune deficiency syndrome (AIDS)–related lymphoma occur in patients who are immunosuppressed as a result of chronic malaria or human immunodeficiency virus (HIV) infection (23). EBV stimulates B-cell production. In immunocompetent individuals, this production is held in check, whereas in immunosuppressed persons, this proliferation may proceed unabated.

Biliary tract, bladder and colon cancer, and parasitic infestations

Biliary tract cancers occur more commonly in persons chronically infected by liver flukes that lodge in the biliary tract and cause proliferation of epithelial cells and thickening of vessel walls where cancers arise later (24). In China and Singapore the flukes responsible are *Clonorchis sinensis* (24), in Thailand, *Opisthorchis viverini* (25). A similar response in the infested tissue also explains the high incidence of bladder cancer in Egypt where *Schistosoma haematobium* is endemic (26), and the excessive incidence of colorectal cancer in areas of China where *Schistosoma japonicum* is endemic (27). Eggs of *S. haematobium* are deposited mainly in the bladder; *S. japonicum* eggs infect the intestines. The effect of schistosomiasis on tissue lining the bladder and colon is a thickening of the stoma and proliferation of the epithelium where the cancers arise (28).

Chemical irritants

As is true for infectious agents, prolonged irritation by physical or chemical agents may cause cell death. Subsequent cell division that occurs during repair of the damaged tissue may eventually lead to a cancer at the irritated site.

Oral cavity cancer

An example of this phenomenon is oral cavity cancer that occurs among betel quid users in India and other areas in Asia and the Middle East, at the site where the quid is habitually held or where lime is applied to the buccal mucosa (29,30). The increased risk occurs even among users of betel quid that contains no tobacco. In addition to causing mechanical trauma, quids often contain lime (calcium hydroxide) whose caustic nature causes cell death and an increase in mitotic activity to replace lost cells.

Small bowel cancer

Cancer of the small bowel may also be caused by chronic irritation. We have noted that more than 25% of all adenocarcinomas of the small bowel arise in the second portion of the duodenum, a 7-cm segment comprising less than one percent of the total length of the small intestine. This segment contains the ampulla of Vater, through which bile and pancreatic juices are released into the duodenum. The carcinomas often can be mapped in close proximity to the ampulla. It seems probable that the chronic irritation from the constant influx of alkaline bile and of acidic pancreatic secretions may cause local cellular damage that stimulates localized mitotic activity in the small bowel epithelium and eventually leads to tumor development. According to our hypothesis, one would expect the level of mitotic activity in this 7-cm segment to be greater than that in other areas of the small intestine; this expectation could be supported or refuted by an autopsy study.

Colon cancer and saturated fat

The etiology of colon cancer in humans is not well understood but seems to be related to diets in which a high proportion of total calories are from saturated fat. In rodents, diets high in fats induce inflammation and superficial lysis of the colon epithelium, followed by increased mitotic activity (31). It is conceivable that these fats have a similar effect on the colon epithelium in humans and that this increase in mitotic activity raises the risk of tumor development; this hypothesis needs to be investigated pathologically.

Alcohol

Alcohol is clearly established as an etiologic agent for cancers of the oral cavity, pharynx, and esophagus (32,33). Little evidence from experimental settings suggests that alcohol is a direct carcinogen, and its irritating effect on exposed tissue explains the carcinogenic effect. In heavy drinkers, the buccal mucosa appears thin and red with multiple atrophic lesions. The most marked association between alcohol intake and cancer is seen in the upper gastrointestinal tract (oral cavity and esophagus), where cell damage is most apparent. Cancer risk at these sites is greatest among those who drink undiluted spirits (34), an effect observed even among nonsmokers (32).

Tobacco

Another established carcinogen, tobacco, is also an enormous irritant. Snuff users develop leukoplakia and eventually cancer of the buccal mucosa at the site of snuff application (35). Tobacco smoke also acts as a local irritant to the epithelial tissue lining the bronchi, lungs, larynx, pharynx, oral cavity, and esophagus where smoking-related cancers arise. Endoscopically, the linings of the upper respiratory and upper digestive tracts of a smoker appear chronically inflamed. The bronchial epithelium of heavy smokers also shows evidence of chronic irritation including cell destruction and increased mitotic activity. The increase in cancer risk with tobacco use may be partly explained by this increase in cell proliferation.

Table 4. Relationship of Acoustic Neuromas in Men to Previous Job Exposure to Extremely Loud Noise,[a,b] Los Angeles County, 1978–1985.

Long-term exposure[a]

Discordant pairs (+/–/–+)	Odds ratio	95% Confidence interval
20/8	2.5	1.1–6.6

Dose-response analysis by duration of exposure[b]

Years of exposure	Odds ratio	95% Confidence interval	P-trend
Never	1.0		0.03
<5	2.8	1.1–7.3	
5–14.99	1.9	0.7–4.9	
≥15	3.5	1.2–10.5	

[a] Had job exposure to extremely loud noise 10 or more years before year of diagnosis.
[b] Job exposure to noise determined by a blinded comparison of ocupational histories to data from National Occupational Hazards Survey.

Stomach cancer

Excessive intake of salty foods results in injury to the gastric mucosa and leads to progressive loss of surface epithelial cells (36). To replace the lost cells, surviving cells in the basal epithelium are stimulated to proliferate (37). Habitual consumption of salty foods would be expected, therefore, to cause chronic proliferation of the gastric mucosa and, based on the increased cell proliferation hypothesis, an increase in stomach cancer risk. This hypothesis is not well studied but seems to fit secular and cross-cultural comparisons of salt consumption and stomach cancer rates. In 1900, stomach cancer was the leading cause of cancer death in the United States. The decline in stomach cancer rates since then has been constant and dramatic but remains unexplained. The decline occurred in parallel with a substantial decline in per capita salt consumption in part because salt is no longer a major food preservative. In international comparisons (38), gastric cancer mortality rates correlate well ($R = 0.79$; $P < .001$) with average urinary excretion of sodium chloride.

Physical and mechanical trauma

Among the many examples of specific tumors associated with physical or mechanical trauma, one is the association of stomach cancer with eating coarse foods like ground corn, which may be explained by mechanical irritation of the stomach lining (39). We discuss several other examples below.

Gall bladder cancer

Risk of gall bladder cancer is strongly associated with a history of gallstones, and gallstones are present in 65–95% of patients who have gall bladder cancer (40). This association suggests another trauma-tumor association. We hypothesize that the association exists because stones abrade and irritate the wall of the gall bladder, causing epithelial-tissue damage and an increase in mitotic activity to replace damaged cells. This increase in cell division may at least partially explain the increase in gall bladder cancer risk.

Asbestos

Asbestos, one of the most potent occupational carcinogens yet identified, seems to be almost the sole cause of mesotheliomas (41). Asbestos fibers cause a chronic mechanical irritation of the mesothelium and a proliferative reaction, which we consider to be the cause of mesothelioma. Several years ago we observed a strong association between occupational asbestos exposure and risk of large cell lymphomas of the gastrointestinal (GI) tract (42). We speculated that this association too was a result of absorption of fibers through the GI tract mucosa, stimulating a chronic inflammatory response that included proliferation of lymphocytes. Lung cancer is also greatly increased by asbestos exposure, and it may also result from irritation and associated increased cell proliferation in lung epithelial cells.

Acoustic neuromas

We recently found that risk of developing an acoustic neuroma is related to job exposure to extremely loud noise, and, furthermore, that the strength of this association increases with the number of years of working in such jobs (43, Table 4). We proposed that these findings support the theory that mechanical trauma may contribute to tumorigenesis. Acoustic neuromas arise in the Schwann cells along the nerve sheath. Experimental studies in rodents showed that severe acoustic trauma (impulse noise) causes mechanical damage to various cells within the cochlea (44,45). In later studies in birds, the sensory hair cells in the cochlea were found to be destroyed and subsequently to regenerate following acoustic trauma (46,47). We hypothesize that a similar phenomenon takes place with Schwann cells in humans. These cells are likely to be damaged by noise trauma, and surviving cells will be stimulated to proliferate in order to replace cells that were lost. The key factor here seems to be that, after trauma, proliferation occurs in cells that would ordinarily not divide.

Meningiomas

A few noteworthy case reports suggested that head trauma may lead to the development of intracranial meningiomas. For example, in a boiler explosion, a wire 1 cm long was driven into the brain of a man who 20 years later was found to have a large meningioma with the wire at its center (48). Another man, who struck his head when he was thrown from a stretcher by a bomb explosion, developed a small lump on his head at the site of the injury. Twenty years later, the lump began gradually to increase in size, and after 5 years it was surgically removed and histologically diagnosed as a meningioma (49). Such case reports must be viewed cautiously because recall bias may create artifactual tumor-trauma relationships. However, objective data lend credibility to this association. The presence of a scar or depressed fracture at the tumor site was noted for 24 of 313 meningiomas in a clinical series (50). In two case-control studies (51,52) an excess risk of meningiomas was found both in women with histories of head trauma that was treated medically and in men who boxed competitively. A third study showed that meningioma risk increased with the number of serious head injuries, and internal evidence suggested that this finding was not attributable to differential recall (53, Table 5). We hypothesize that head trauma causes damage and subsequent repair of the meninges, and that the cell proliferation that occurs during the repair process increases the likelihood of tumor development.

We also developed a trauma hypothesis to explain the peculiar distribution of spinal meningiomas. Spinal tumors of all histologic types are rare, the most common type being spinal meningiomas that occur predominantly in postmenopausal women. We hypothesize that these tumors are caused by trauma to the spinal meninges that results from osteoporotic collapse fractures of the vertebrae, which also occur predominantly in postmenopausal women (54). The majority of spinal meningiomas arise in that portion of the thoracic spine where the majority of collapse fractures occur. Data from a case-control study currently under analysis also seem to support this hypothesis (Preston-Martin et al., in preparation).

Other chronic irritations

Among the many other examples of chronic irritation preceding neoplasia are the following three, which illustrate the development of cancers in ulcerated tissue. We hypothesize that in each of these the critical factor is the increase in mitotic activity that occurs during repair of the ulcerated tissue.

Cancers of the hard palate, skin, and colon and chronic ulceration

Reverse smoking, a habit in which the burning end of a cigarette is inserted into the mouth, causes an excess of cancers of the hard palate (55). Burns and chronic tissue ulceration precede tumor development (56). Similarly, skin cancer in Melanesians has been observed to occur in association with chronic skin ulcers, which, in the tropics, develop on the skin at the site of wounds, burns, or insect bites (57). The squamous cell carcinomas that develop in association with long-standing tropical ulcers tend to develop in the regenerating margin of the ulcer. Finally, chronic ulcerative colitis is a risk factor for cancer of the colon, with risk particularly high if the colitis began at an early age and persisted for many years (58).

Conclusion

A series of distinct genetic alterations accumulates in a cell before it becomes malignant. These changes in cellular DNA appear in some cases to activate cellular oncogenes that stimulate cell growth and other abnormal behavioral characteristics of a cancer cell. The changes also inactivate tumor-suppressor genes that normally inhibit cell growth (59). Unmasking the mutations in tumor-suppressor genes relies on the loss

Table 5. Relationship of Primary Brain Tumors in Men to Previous Severe Head Injury,[a,b] Los Angeles County, 1980–1984.

Histologic type of tumor	Discordant pairs (+/–/–/+)	Odds ratio	95% Confidence interval
Glioma	41/49	0.8	0.5–1.3
Meningioma	23/10	2.3	1.1–5.4

Dose-response analysis, meningiomas

Number of head injuries[b,c]	Odds ratio	95% Confidence interval	P-trend
0	1.0		0.03
1	1.3	0.6–2.9	
2	2.1	0.8–5.9	
3	6.2	1.2–31.7	

[a] Had serious head injury 20 or more years before year of diagnosis.
[b] Includes only injuries that led to medical visit, loss of consciousness, or dizziness.
[c] Includes all serious injuries up to 2 years before the year the case was diagnosed.

of the wild-type gene and a reduction to homozygosity of the chromosome containing the mutant allele, a process that requires cell division. Extensive changes in the cellular genome have been observed in four of the most common human cancers—lung, breast, colon, and bladder cancer (60–63).

The observation that so many genetic alterations are needed for cancer development fits the epidemiology of colon and other cancers that usually develop relatively late in life. That loss of wild-type alleles is an essential requirement for full expression of the malignant phenotype is becoming increasingly realized. Thus, the increased cell division induced by the agents discussed here may be involved not only in the genesis of mutations but also in their expression by increasing opportunities for a reduction to homozygosity. The epidemiologic data coincide, therefore, with the molecular genetics of human cancer and underline the importance of cell division to malignant transformation.

Acknowledgment

This work was supported in part by awards FRA-329 and SIG-2 from the American Cancer Society and grant 5-P30Ca14089 from the National Cancer Institute. We also acknowledge the role of the Cancer Surveillance Program in identifying cases for several of the studies cited; this program is currently supported by grant 050E-8709 from the State of California and was previously supported by grant CA17054 from the National Institutes of Health.

We thank our colleagues P. Chandrasoma and P. Jones for their input and C. Turner for preparing the manuscript.

References

1. Stanbridge EJ. Identifying tumor suppressor genes in human colorectal cancer. Science 247:12–13, 1990.
2. Fearon ER, Cho KR, Nigro JM, Kern SE, Simons JW, Ruppert JM, Hamilton SR, Preisinger AC, Thomas G, Kinzler KW, Vogelstein B. Identification of a chromosome 18q gene that is altered on colorectal cancers. Science 247:49–56, 1990.
3. Sager R. Tumor suppressor genes: The puzzle and the promise. Science 246:1406–1412, 1989.
4. Knudson AG. Mutation and cancer: Statistical study of retinoblastoma. Proc Natl Acad Sci 68:820–823, 1971.
5. Ames BN, Gold LS. Too many rodent carcinogens: Mitogenesis increases mutagenesis. Science 249:970–971, 1990.
6. Henderson BE, Ross RK, Pike MC, Casagrande JT. Endogenous hormones as a major factor in human cancer. Cancer Res 42:3232–3239, 1982.
7. Key TJA, Pike MC. The dose-effect relationship between "unopposed" estrogens and endometrial mitotic rate: Its central role in explaining and predicting endometrial cancer risk. Br J Cancer 57:205–212, 1988.
8. Key TJA, Pike MC. The role of estrogens and progestogens in the epidemiology and prevention of breast cancer. Europe J Cancer Clin Oncol 24:29–43, 1988.
9. Bergkvist L, Adami HO, Persson I, Hoover I, Schairer C. The risk of breast cancer after estrogen and estrogen-progestin replacement. N Engl J Med 321:293–297, 1989.
10. Bernstein L, Yuan JM, Ross RK, Pike MC, Lobo R, Stanczyk F, Gao YT, Henderson BE. Serum hormone levels in premenopausal Chinese women in Shanghai and white women in Los Angeles: Results from two breast cancer case-control studies. Cancer Causes and Control 1:51–58, 1990.
11. Shimizu H, Ross RK, Bernstein L, Pike MC, Henderson BE. Serum estrogen levels in postmenopausal

women: comparison of U.S. whites and Japanese in Japan. Br J Cancer, in press.

12. Key TJA, Chen J, Wang DY, Pike MC, Boreham J. Sex hormones in rural Chinese women: Comparisons with Britain and correlations with diet and breast cancer in China, Br J Cancer, in press.

13. Ross RK. Prostate. In: Schottenfeld D, Fraumeni J, Jr. (eds): Cancer Epidemiology and Prevention. Philadelphia: Oxford University Press, in press.

14. Noble RL. The development of prostatic adenocarcinoma in Nb rats following prolonged sex hormone administration. Cancer Res 37:1929–1933, 1977.

15. Edmondson HA, Reynolds TB, Henderson B, Benton B. Regression of liver cell adenomas associated with oral contraceptives. Ann Intern Med 86:180–182, 1977.

16. Henderson BE, Casagrande JT, Pike MC, Mack T, Rosario I, Duke A. The epidemiology of endometrial cancer in young women. Br J Cancer 47:749–756, 1983.

17. Neuberger J, Forman D, Doll R, Williams R. Oral contraceptives and hepatocellular carcinoma. Br Med J 292:1355–1357, 1986.

18. Johnson FL, Feagler JR, Lerner KG, Siegel M, Majerus PW, Hartmann JR, Thomas ED. Association androgenic-anabolic steroid therapy with development of hepatocellular carcinoma. Lancet 2:1273–1276, 1972.

19. Farrell GC, Joshua DE, Uren RF, Baird PJ, Perkins KW, Kronenberg H. Androgen-induced hepatoma. Lancet 1:430–432, 1975.

20. Blumberg BS, London WT. Hepatitis B virus and the prevention of primary cancer of the liver. J Natl Cancer Inst 74:267–273, 1985.

21. Zheng W, Blot WJ, Liao ML, Wang ZX, Levin LI, Zhao JJ, Fraumeni JF, Gao YT. Lung cancer and prior tuberculosis infection in Shanghai. Br J Cancer 56:501–504, 1987.

22. Wu AH, Yu MC, Thomas DC, Pike MC, Henderson BE. Personal and family history of lung disease as risk factors for adenocarcinoma of the lung. Cancer Res 48:7279–7284, 1988.

23. Henderson BE. Establishment of an association between a virus and a human cancer. J Natl Cancer Inst 81:320–321, 1989.

24. Shanmugaratnam K. Primary carcinomas of the liver and biliary tract. Br J Cancer 10:232–245, 1956.

25. Srivantanakul P, Sontipong S, Chotiwan P, Parkin DM. Liver cancer in Thailand: Temporal and geographic variations. Journal of Gastroenterology and Hepatology 3:413–420, 1988.

26. Morrison HI, Semenciw RM, Mao Y, Wigle DT. Cancer mortality among a group of fluorspar miners exposed to radon progeny. Am J Epidemiol 128:1266–1275, 1988.

27. Zhong XU, De-Long SU. Schistosoma japonicum and colorectal cancer: An epidemiological study in the People's Republic of China. Int J Cancer 34:315–318, 1984.

28. Benenson AS. Control of Communicable Diseases in Man. Washington,DC: American Public Health Association, 1985.

29. Muir CS, Krik R. Betel, tobacco and cancer of the mouth. Br J Cancer 14:598–608, 1960.

30. Jassawalla DJ, Deshpande VA. Evaluation of cancer risk in tobacco chewers or smokers: An epidemiologic assessment. Cancer 24:11–15, 1970.

31. Wargovich MJ, Eng VW, Newmark HL. Calcium inhibits the damaging and compensatory proliferative effects of fatty acids on mouse colon epithelium. Cancer Lett 23:253–258, 1984.

32. Blot WJ, McLaughlin JK, Winn DM, Austin DF, Greenberg RS, Preston-Martin S, Bernstein L, Schoenberg JB, Stemhagen A, Fraumeni JF, Jr. Smoking and drinking in relation to oral and pharyngeal cancer. Cancer Res 48:3282–3287, 1988.

33. Yu MC, Garabrant D, Peters J, Mack TM. Tobacco, alcohol, diet occupation and carcinoma of the esophagus. Cancer Res 48:3843–3848, 1988.

34. Tuyns AJ. Alcohol. In: Schottenfeld D, Fraumeni J, Jr(eds): Cancer Epidemiology and Prevention. Philadelphia: Saunders, 1982, pp. 293–303.

35. Winn WM. Tobacco chewing and snuff dipping: An association with human cancer. In: O'Neill IK, Bon Borstel RC, Miller CT, Long J, Bartsch, H (eds): N-nitroso Compounds: Occurrence, Biological Effects and Relevance to Human Cancer. Lyon: IARC Science Publications, 1984, pp. 837–849.

36. Sato T, Fukuyama T, Suzuki T, Takayanagi J. Studies on the causation of gastric cancer. 2. The relation between gastric cancer mortality rate and salted food intake in several places in Japan. Bulletin of the Institute of Public Health 8:187, 1959.

37. Furihata C, Sato Y, Hosaka M, Matsushima T, Furukawa F, Takahashi M. NaCl induced ornithine decarboxylase and DNA synthesis in rat stomach mucosa. Biochem Biophys Res Commun 121:1027, 1984.

38. Joossens JV, Geboers J. Nutrition and gastric cancer. Nutr Cancer 2:250–261, 1981.

39. Correa P. The epidemiology and pathogenesis of chronic gastritis: Three etiologic entities. Front Gastrointest 6:98, 1980.
40. Robbins SL. Environmental pathology: Asbestosis. In: Pathologic Basis of Disease. Philadelphia: Saunders, 1974, pp 513–514.
41. Selikoff IJ, Hammond EC, Churg J. Carcinogenicity of amosite asbestos. Arch Environ Health 25:183–186, 1972.
42. Ross R, Nichols P, Wright W, Lukes R, Dworsky R, Paganini-Hill A, Koss M, Henderson B. Asbestos exposure and lymphomas of the gastrointestinal tract and oral cavity. Lancet 2:1118–1120, 1982.
43. Preston-Martin S, Thomas DC, Wright WE, Henderson BE. Noise trauma in the etiology of acoustic neuromas in men in Los Angeles County, 1978–1985. Br J Cancer 59:783–786, 1989.
44. Hamernik RP, Turrentine G, Roberto M, Salvi R, Henderson D. Anatomical correlates of impulse noise-induced mechanical damage in the cochlea. Hearing Res 13:229–247, 1984.
45. Hamernik RP, Turrentine G, Wright GG. Surface morphology of the inner sulcus and related epithelial cells of the cochlea following acoustic trauma. Hearing Res 16:143–160, 1984.
46. Corwin JT, Cotanche DA. Regeneration of sensory hair cells after acoustic trauma. Science 240:1772–1774, 1988.
47. Ryals BM, Rubel EW. Hair cell regeneration after acoustic trauma in adult coturnix quail. Science 240:1774–1776, 1988.
48. Reinhardt G. Trauma-Fremdkörper-Hirngeschwulst. Munich Med Wochenschr 75:399–401, 1928.
49. Walsh J, Gye R, Connelly TJ. Meningioma: A late complication of head injury. Med J Australia 1:906–908, 1969.
50. Cushing H, Eisenhardt L. Meningiomas, Their Classification, Regional Behavior Life History and Surgical End Results. Springfield: Thomas, 1938.
51. Preston-Martin S, Paganini-Hill A, Henderson BE, Pike MC, Wood C. Case-control study of intracranial meningiomas in women in Los Angeles County. J Natl Cancer Inst 75:67–73, 1980.
52. Preston-Martin S, Yu MC, Henderson BE, Roberts C. Risk factors for meningiomas in men in Los Angeles County. J Natl Cancer Inst 70:863–866, 1983.
53. Preston-Martin S, Mack W, Henderson BE. Risk factors for gliomas and meningiomas in males in Los Angeles County. Cancer Res 49:6137–6143, 1989.
54. Saville PD. The syndrome of spinal osteoporosis. Clin Endocrinol Metab 2:177–185, 1973.
55. Ramulu C, Reddy CRRM. Carcinoma of the hard palate and its relationship to reverse smoking. Int Surg 57:636–641, 1972.
56. Bhonsle RB, Murti PR, Gupta PC, Mehta FS. Reverse dhumti smoking in Goa: An epidemiologic study of 5,449 villagers for oral precancerous lesions. Indian J Cancer 13:301–305, 1976.
57. Henderson BE, Aiken GH. Cancer in Papua New Guinea. In: National Cancer Institute Monograph 53. Second Symposium on Epidemiology and Cancer Registries in the Pacific Basin. Bethesda: U.S. Department of Health, Education, and Welfare National Institutes of Health Publication #79-1864, 1979, pp. 67–72.
58. van Heerden JA, Beart RW. Carcinoma of the colon and rectum complicating chronic ulcerative colitis. Dis Colon Rectum 23:155–159, 1980.
59. Nigro JM, Baker, Preisinger AC, Jessup, Hostetter R, Cleary K, Bigner SH, Davidson N, Baylin S, Devilee P, Glover T, Collins, Weston A, Modali R, Harris CC, Vogelstein B. Mutations in the p53 gene occur in diverse human tumor types. Nature 342:705–708, 1989.
60. Callahan R, Campbell G. Mutations in human breast cancer: An overview. J Natl Cancer Inst 81:1780, 1989.
61. Takahashi T, Nau MM, Chiba I, Birrer MJ, Rosenberg RK, Vinocour M, Levitt M, Pass H, Gazdar AF, Minna JD. p53: A frequent target for genetic abnormalities in lung cancer. Science 246:491, 1989.
62. Vogelstein B, Fearon ER, Baker SJ, Nigro JM, Kern SE, Hamilton SR, Boss J, Leppert M, Nakamura Y, White R. Genetic alterations accumulate during colorectal tumorigenesis. In: Cavenee W, Hastle N, Stanbridge E (eds): Current Communications in Molecular Biology (Recessive Oncogenes and Tumor Suppression). Cold Spring Harbor: Cold Spring Harbor Laboratory, 1989, pp 73–80.
63. Tsai YC, Nichols PW, Hiti AL, Williams Z, Skinner DG, Jones PA. Allelic losses of chromosomes 9, 11 and 17 in human bladder cancer. Cancer Res 50:44–47, 1990.

Chemically Induced Cell Proliferation:
Implications for Risk Assessment, pages 35-41
©1991 Wiley-Liss, Inc.

The Role of Chemically Induced Epithelial Hyperplasia in the Development of Human Cancer

A.J.P. Klein-Szanto

Mid-19th century pathologists like Rudolf Virchow recognized the importance of epithelial hyperplasia as a step in human tumor development: He defined hyperplasia as a growth abnormality resulting in an enlargement of an organ or tissue due to an increased number of cellular elements (1). In this century, epithelial hyperplasia has been redefined as one of the earliest alterations in the chain of events that results in cancer. In this progressive chain, a normal epithelium undergoes a dynamic series of alterations, all characterized by the common denominator of increased cell proliferation: These are known as hyperplasia, metaplasia, dysplasia, carcinoma in situ, or intra-epithelial neoplasia. The next step is invasive carcinoma. This continuum has been described as occurring in most covering epithelia such as epidermis, cervical epithelium, oral epithelium, larynx esophagus, and the bronchus (2). Although some or all of these steps can remain undetected or bypassed, it is generally accepted that in most epithelial cancers they appear sequentially as precursor lesions.

The epithelial changes can be elicited in experimental animals by numerous chemical carcinogens, as well as by ionizing and ultraviolet radiations. Investigations performed during pathological studies have also indicated that in humans, several carcinogens can induce hyperplastic lesions that precede or appear simultaneously with neoplastic lesions. Table 1 provides examples of nonhormonal agents in humans that can induce hyperplasia and have been identified as strong, weak, or putative carcinogenic stimuli. Through indirect epidemiological studies complemented by animal experimentation, most of these substances have been identified as hyperplasiogenic agents. Hormones have also been identified as the most common hyperplasiogenic stimulus related to cancer etiopathogenesis in numerous hormone-responsive organs, and will be considered in a separate chapter.

The introduction of athymic nude mice made it possible to evaluate the response of normal human tissues transplanted into these immunosuppressed animals; this facilitated the direct evaluation of normal tissue response to chemicals.

In this study we used xenotransplanted human epithelial tissues to investigate the hyperplasiogenic and carcinogenic effects of chemicals on human epidermis and human tracheobronchial epithelium.

Effect of tumor promoters on human epidermis

Several compounds are bonafide tumor promoters in the mouse model of two-stage carcinogenesis. 12-O-Tetradecanoylphorbol-13-acetate (TPA), also known as phorbol 12-myristate-13 acetate (PMA), causes skin inflammation and epidermal

Table 1. Selected Examples of Chemicals that Produce Hyperplasia in Humans.

Agent	Target tissue	Reference
Arsenicals	Epidermis	3
Anthralin	Epidermis	4
Halogenated hydrocarbons (dioxin)	Epidermis	5
Formaldehyde	Respiratory tract epithelium	6–7
Tobacco-related chemicals	Respiratory tract epithelium	8
Phenatecin	Urothelium	9
Hydantoin	Gingiva-Lymphoid Tissues	9

hyperplasia. Krueger and Shelby (10) described an increase in the labeling index (LI) of basal keratinocytes 18 hr after topical application of 10 or 100 ng TPA on human skin xenotransplanted on the backs of nude mice. This increase was dose-dependent and ranged between 50 and 80% of the basal LI values.

Other investigators have observed epidermal hyperplasia after TPA treatment in similar experimental systems (11–12). One report describes a few papillomas, probably of human derivation, that developed after multiple topical TPA applications (11). TPA also produced hyperplasia and increased LI in the forearm epidermis of a few volunteers treated with a single dose of this same skin tumor promoter (13).

Several other chemicals used in clinical dermatology for the treatment of such severe dermatoses as psoriasis are hyperplasiogenic and have been described as carcinogenic or as efficient skin tumor promoters in the murine skin model of two-stage carcinogenesis. The better known of these agents are anthralin, coal tar, and PUVA (4,14–16).

The effect of TPA on human keratinocytes in culture is controversial. Although a large body of literature indicates that phorbol esters accelerate terminal differentiation and inhibit DNA synthesis (17,18), a number of investigators have found an increased cell proliferation after TPA treatment in vitro (19,20). These differences could be attributed to different sensitivities of the keratinocyte subpopulations which might vary according to either donor age or the stage of differentiation in vitro.

Effects of chemicals on the xenotransplanted normal human respiratory epithelium

Formaldehyde (FMD) is a widely used chemical that has been identified as a putative human carcinogen in some epidemiologic studies (21,22). Although these findings remain controversial, FMD has been demonstrated to be carcinogenic in rats (23,24). Also, FMD enhanced the formation of dysplastic epithelial lesions and increased the induction of altered cell subpopulations when rats were exposed simultaneously to benzo[a]pyrene (25,26). We have developed an experimental system based on the xenotransplantation of normal respiratory epithelium, which has permitted us to study the effects of formaldehyde on tracheobronchial and nasal respiratory epithelia (6,7). The xenotransplants are produced using respiratory epithelium derived from immediate autopsies. The tissues from tracheas, bronchi, or nasal mucosa were cut into 2×2 mm pieces and explanted with the epithelium side up on a 60-mm tissue culture dish coated with a mixture of human fibronectin (10 mg/ml); collagen (30 mg/ml); and bovine serum albumin (10 mg/ml), all dissolved in MCDB 151 medium. Tissues were incubated in LHC-9 medium at 36.5°C in an atmosphere of 5% CO_2 in air. LHC-9 is a serum-free medium developed for the culture of normal human epithelial cells (27).

After 1–2 weeks of incubation, the explants were removed and the 5×10^5 epithelial cells were inoculated into de-epithelialized F344 rat tracheas. De-epithelialization was achieved by repetitive freezing (-20°C) and thawing of the tracheas over a 3-hr period.

Tracheas were transplanted into the dorsum of 4- to 6-week-old female BALB/c nude mice. Treatment consisted of exposing the transplants through a small skin incision and placing within the lumina of each transplant a hollow 16-mm silastic tube containing 0-, 0.5-, 1-, or 2-mg paraformaldehyde powder. Both ends of these silastic devices were sealed with silastic glue to avoid a massive leak of formaldehyde. After the formaldehyde-containing devices were placed intraluminally, the tracheas were sealed and the skin incision closed with surgical clips. This permits a slow, protracted release of the aldehyde and consequently a constant chronic exposure of the respiratory epithelium for 8 weeks or more. Tracheal transplants from the three dose groups were exposed during 2, 4, 8, and 16 weeks.

Before sacrifice, all animals were injected with a single pulse of tritiated thymidine. Important epithelial alterations were observed in the formaldehyde-treated transplants; a maximum effect was visible 2 weeks after exposure. While the highest dose of 2 mg produced numerous areas of epithelial erosion and inflammation in most cases, this effect was not as evident with the lower doses. All doses produced areas of hyperplastic epithelium alternating with areas of pleomorphic-atrophic epithelium. Although the differences in predominance among different epithelium types were not clearly dose-dependent, the LI showed dose dependence between 2 and 4 weeks after exposure began. The maximum mean LI was three to four times higher than normal, although in some focal hyperplastic-metaplastic lesions the LI was increased up to 20 times (Table 2). Similar changes were observed in the xenotransplanted nasal respiratory epithelium exposed to similar doses of FMD (7) (Figs. 1–4). These studies show that formaldehyde, although toxic at higher doses, is able at lower doses to elicit a proliferative response of the human respiratory epithelium that is not preceded by a massive toxic effect. This response is similar to although less severe than the one observed in rats exposed to the same aldehyde in which the chemical proved to be carcinogenic (23,24).

Table 2. Labelling Indices (LI) of Different Epithelial Lesions Present after Exposure of Human Tracheobronchial Epithelium with Formaldehyde (FMD).[1]

	FMD dose	
Epithelial type	0 mg	2 mg
Normal	0.38%	0.34%
Atrophic	0.19%	3.30%
Hyperplastic	1.08%	3.15%
Squamous metaplastic	0.11%	6.11%

The LIs shown represent the number of labeled cell/total number of cells in each lesion type. Two to three thousand cells were counted per group.
[1]Modified from ref. 6

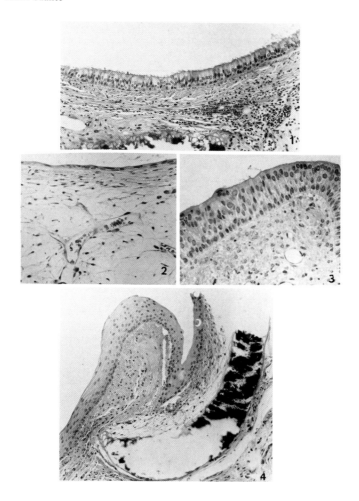

Figure 1. Human nasal mucociliary epithelium transplanted into deepithelialized rat tracheas 7 days after exposure to 0.5 mg paraformaldehyde-containing silastic device. Although the epithelium is apparently normal, note an inflammatory infiltrate in the submucosa. Hematoxylin/eosin, × 100.

Figure 2. Flat epithelium observed 2 weeks after exposure to 1 mg paraformaldehyde. This dose produced occasional areas of necrosis and epithelial regeneration that can be seen as flat cells migrating on the eroded surface. Hematoxylin/eosin, × 180.

Figure 3. Tall hyperplastic nasal epithelium devoid of cilia. Two weeks after exposure to 0.5 mg paraformaldehyde. Hematoxylin/eosin, × 200.

Figure 4. Epidermoid metaplasia of nasal epithelium 2 weeks after exposure to 0.5 mg paraformaldehyde. Hematoxylin/eosin, × 100.

Recently we have pre-exposed the human tracheobronchial epithelium to benzopyrene diolepoxide (BPDE), followed by exposure to 0.5 mg formaldehyde. No marked differences in the hyperproliferative patterns of the epithelium were noted either with or without pre-exposure to BPDE. Nevertheless, all the xenotransplants exhibited a clear-cut increased proliferation after BPDE exposure that was followed by another wave of proliferation after FMD exposure. Hyperplastic epithelia also were seen when BPDE and FMD were administered simultaneously; no obvious synergism could be detected.

Cell proliferation and the acquisition of the malignant phenotype

During the sequential changes of malignant epithelial precursor lesions, there is a gradual increase in the proliferative ability of these lesions. This is well-documented through the mitotic index and LI increases that are observed in both rodent and human preneoplastic lesions: A peak of proliferative capacity occurs in the invasive carcinomas. Table 3 shows that a clearly progressive increase in LI parallels the increased dysplasia level of the preneoplastic lesions, indicating that the progressive acquisition of malignant features is accompanied by an increased proliferative activity (28). Similar changes in humans are accompanied by the same types of changes in DNA content and cell turnover time frames (29).

In a recent experiment, we noted that benzoyl peroxide, a skin tumor promoter causes an increase in proliferative ability and enhanced invasiveness of a malignant rodent epidermal carcinoma cell line in vitro (30). Similarly, treating the immortalized human bronchial epithelial cell line BEAS-2B with TPA resulted in an increased cell proliferation as well as an enhancement of the in vitro and in vivo invasiveness (31). Cigarette smoke condensate had a similar effect (Momiki, Klein-Szanto, and Harris, in preparation).

Although the multiple and pleomorphic effects of tumor promoters are well-documented, these changes in invasiveness are attributed to an increased secretion of proteolytic enzymes, especially collagenase type IV (Table 4). The increased locomotion of the cells also enhanced by TPA and other chemicals, and the inherent capacity

Table 3. Cellular Changes in Preneoplastic Lesions of the Respiratory Tract Epithelium.*

	No. of lesions	Basal layer labeling index (%)	Suprabasal layers labeling index (%)
Normal tracheal epithelium	4	0.39 ± 0.20	–
Regular squamous metaplasia	16	16 ± 5	2.7 ± 2.6
Squamous metaplasia with moderate atypia	4	18 ± 8	6 ± 4
Squamous metaplasia with severe atyia	5	18 ± 10	9 ± 6
Carcinoma in situ	4	32 ± 6	9 ± 2
Invasive carcinoma	4	31 ± 2	10 ± 2

*Modified from ref. 30.

Table 4. Invasiveness and Labeling Index of Human Immortalized Epithelial Cell Line Induced by TPA.[1]

	Invasiveness in vitro	Collagenase type IV activity (cpm)	Labeling index (%)
No treatment	16	5732	23
TPA	564	10.004	45

[1]Modified from ref. 29.

of the cells to penetrate basement membranes, give these cells an additional advantage to metastasize. When increased cell proliferation is also induced by tumor promoters, the result is an enhanced malignant phenotype known as tumor progression.

These examples emphasize the fact that while hyperproliferative chemicals such as tumor promoters might not be very efficient in transforming a normal human cell, they could be quite effective as tumor progressors in enhancing the latent or marginal characteristics of an already malignant cell.

Acknowledgments

The research was sponsored by the National Cancer Institute (CA 44980 and CA 44981) and by a grant from the Health Effects Institute.

References

1. Virchow R. Cellular Pathology. Philadelphia: J.B. Lippincott, 1863, p. 94.
2. Henson DE and Albores Saavedra J. The pathology of incipient neoplasia. Saunders, Philadelphia, 1986.
3. USEPA—Health effect assessment for arsenic. Report No. EPA 540-1-86.1020, 1984.
4. Bock FG and Burns R. Tumor promoting properties of anthralin. J Natl Cancer Inst 30:393–398, 1963.
5. Moses M and Prioleau. Cutaneous histologic findings in chemical workers with and without chloraine with past exposure to 2,3,7,8 tetrachlorodibenzo-p-dioxin. J Am Acad Dermatol 3:497–506, 1985.
6. Ura H, Nowak P, Litwin S, Watts P, Bonfil RD, Klein-Szanto AJP. Effects of formaldehyde on normal xenotransplanted human tracheobronchial epithelium. Am J Pathol 134:99–106, 1989.
7. Klein-Szanto AJP, Ura H, Resau J. Formaldehyde-induced lesions of xenotransplanted human nasal respiratory epithelium. Toxicol Pathol 17:33–37, 1989.
8. Auerbach O, Stret AP, Hammond EC, and Garfinkel L. Changes of the bronchial epithelium in relation to cigarette smoking. N Engl J Med 265:253–257, 1961.
9. Schmahl D, Thomas C, Auer R (eds): Iatrogenic Carcinogenesis. Berlin: Springer-Verlag, 1977.
10. Krueger GG and Shelby J. Biology of human skin transplanted to the nude mouse: I. Response to agents which modify epidermal proliferation. J Invest Dermatol 76:506–510, 1981.
11. Viguera C, Nims R and Yuspas S. Maintenance of human skin on nude mice for studies of chemical carcinogenesis. Cancer Lett 6:301–310, 1979.
12. Graem N. Epidermal changes following application of 7,12-dimethylbenz[a]anthracene and 12-O-tetradecanoylphorbol-13-acetate to human skin transplanted to nude mice studied with histological species markers. Cancer Res 46:278–284, 1986.
13. Klein-Szanto AJP. Morphological evaluation of tumor promoters effects on mammalian skin. In Slaga TJ (ed): Mechanisms of Tumor Promotion, Tumor Promotion and Skin Carcinogenesis, Vol II. Boca Raton: CRC Press, 1984, pp. 41–72.
14. Mukhtar H, Das M, Bickers DR. Skin tumor initiating activity of therapeutic crude coal tar as compared to other polycyclic aromatic hydrocarbons in sencar mice. Cancer Lett 31:147–151, 1986.

15. Stern RS, Laird N, Melski J, Parrish JA, Fitzpatrick TB, Bleich HL. Cutaneous squamous-cell carcinoma in patients treated with PUVA. N Engl J Med 310:1156–61, 1984.
16. Dunnick JK, Forbes PD, Davies RE, and Iverson WO. Toxicity of 8-methoxypsoralen, 5-methoxypsoralen, 3-carbethoxypsoralen, or 5-methylisopsoralen with ultraviolet radiation in the hairless (HRA/Skh) mouse. Toxicol Appl Pharmacol 89:73–80, 1987.
17. Fischer SM, Viaje A, Mills GD, Wong EW, Weeks CE and Slaga TJ. The growth of cultured human foreskin keratinocytes is not stimulated by a tumor promoter. Carcinogenesis 5:109–112, 1984.
18. Parkinson EK. The transformation of human epidermal keratinocytes by carcinogens and viruses in vitro. In Conti C, Slaga T and Klein-Szanto A (eds): Skin Tumors: Experimental and clinical aspects. New York: Raven Press, 1989, pp. 361–361.
19. Hawley-Nelson P, Stanley JR, Schmidt J, Gullino M, Yuspa SH. The tumor promoter, 12-O-tetradecanoylphorbol-13-acetate accelerates keratinocyte differentiation and stimulates growth of an unidentified cell type in cultured human epidermis. Exp Cell Res 137:155–167, 1982.
20. Parkinson EK, Al-Yaman F., and Appleby MW. The effect of donor age on the proliferative response of human mouse kertinocytes to PMA. Carcinogenesis 8:907–912, 1987.
21. Jensen OM, Andersen SK. Lung cancer risk from formaldehyde. Lancet 1:913, 1982.
22. Blair A, Stewart P, O'Berg M, Gaffey W, Walrath J, Ward J, Bales R, Kaplan S, Cubet D. Mortality among industrial workers exposed to formaldehyde. JNCI 76:1071–1084, 1976.
23. Kerns WD, Pavkov KL, Donotrio DJ, Gralla EJ, Swenberg JA. Carcinogenicity of formaldehyde in rats and mice after long-term inhalation exposure. Cancer Res 43:4382–92, 1983.
24. Albert RE, Sellakumar AR, Laskin S, Kuschner M, Nelson M, Snyder CA. Gaseous formaldehyde and hydrogen chloride induction of nasal cancer in the rat. J Natl Cancer Inst 68:597–602, 1982.
25. Shiba M, Marchok AC, Klein-Szanto AJP, Yamaguchi Y. Pathological changes induced by formaldehyde in open-ended rat tracheal implants pre-exposed to benzo[a]pyrene. Toxicol Pathol 15:401–408, 1987.
26. Cosma GN, Marchok AC. The induction of growth-altered cell populations (tumor-initiation sites) in rat tracheal implants exposed to benzo[a]pyrene and formaldehyde. Carcinogenesis 8:1951–1953, 1987.
27. Lechner JF, Laveck MA. A serum-free method for culturing normal human bronchial epithelial cells at clonal density. Journal of Tissue Culture Methods 9:43–48, 1985.
28. Klein-Szanto AJP, Nettesheim P, Topping DC, Olson AC. Quantitative analysis of disturbed cell maturation in dysplastic lesions of the respiratory tract epithelium. Carcinogenesis 1:1007–1012, 1980.
29. Auffermann W, and Böcking A. Early detection of precancerous lesions in dysplasias of the lung by rapid DNA image cytometry. Anal Quant Cytol Histol 7:218–226, 1985.
30. Bonfil RD, Momiki S, Conti CJ, Klein-Szanto AJP. Benzoyl peroxide enhances the invasive ability of a mouse epidermal carcinoma cell line. Int J Cancer 44:165–169, 1989.
31. Bonfil RD, Momiki S, Fridman R, Reich R, Reddel R, Harris CC, Klein-Szanto A. Enhancement of the invasive ability of a transformed human bronchial epithelial cell line by 12-O-tetra-decanoyl-phorbol-13-acetate and diacylglycerol. Carcinogenesis 10:2335–2338, 1989.

Chemically Induced Cell Proliferation:
Implications for Risk Assessment, pages 43-52
©1991 Wiley-Liss, Inc.

Cellular Proliferation and Stomach Carcinogenesis Induced by Antioxidants

Nobuyuki Ito, Masao Hirose, and Satoru Takahashi

The synthetic antioxidant butylated hydroxyanisole (BHA) has been shown to induce forestomach carcinomas in rats and hamsters (1–3). It also strongly enhances forestomach carcinogenesis in rats pretreated with N-methyl-N'-nitro-N-nitroso-guanidine (MNNG) (4–7), N-methylnitrosourea (MNU) (8,9), or N,N-dibutylnitro-samine (DBN) (10). BHA rapidly induces cell proliferation in the forestomach epithelium of both rats (3) and hamsters (11), with this increase in DNA synthetic activity presumably playing an important role in the observed carcinogenic effect.

Recently, some naturally occurring antioxidants such as caffeic acid, sesamol, and catechol have been shown to also induce rapid cell proliferation in either the forestomach or glandular stomach epithelia of rats (12) and hamsters (13). These antioxidants similarly appear to exert carcinogenic potential in their target organs or enhance stomach carcinogenesis. Although some in vitro and in vivo metabolic studies of BHA have been performed (14–17), the mechanisms whereby these antioxidants induce the increased cell proliferation and/or subsequent tumors in the affected tissue remain unclear.

In this paper, we will consider the role and significance of antioxidant-induced cell proliferation for both forestomach and glandular stomach carcinogenesis in rats.

Materials and methods

Carcinogenicity studies of antioxidants

Groups of 30–50 male and female F344 rats, initially 6 weeks old (Charles River Japan, Inc., Kanagawa), were given Oriental MF powdered diet (Oriental Yeast Co., Tokyo) containing 2% BHA (purity >98%), 2% caffeic acid (purity >98%), 2% sesamol (purity >98%), or 2% p-methoxyphenol (purity >99%) for 104 weeks. BHA and catechol were obtained from Wako Pure Chemical Industries, Osaka; sesamol from Fluka Chemie, AG, Switzerland; and caffeic acid from Tokyo Kasei Kogyo Co., Tokyo. Food and water were given ad libitum. Ten or 11 male rats in each group were killed at week 4 to allow assessment of early histopathological changes. Animals that died during the experiment were necropsied; all survivors were killed under ether anesthesia and subjected to complete autopsy at the end of week 104.

Comparative assessment of forestomach lesion reversibility

Groups of 20 F344 male rats, initially 6 weeks old, were treated with the mutagens 0.1% 8-nitroquinoline (8NQ, Nakarai Chemical Ltd., Kyoto) or 0.2% 2-(2-furyl)-3-(5-

nitro-2-furyl)acrylamide (AF2, Ueno Pharmaceutical Co., Osaka) in the diet or 20 mg/kg body weight N-methyl-N'-nitro-N-nitrosoguanidine (MNNG, Tokyo Kasei Kogyo Co., Tokyo) administered intragastrically once a week or the nonmutagens 2% BHA or 2% caffeic acid in the diet for 24 weeks. Ten rats per group were killed at the end of week 24, and another 10 rats each were maintained on basal diet alone for 24 more weeks and then killed. Two groups of 10 rats were maintained as controls on the basal diet alone for 24 and 48 weeks, respectively, and then killed.

Detection of DNA adducts by the ^{32}P-postlabeling method in forestomach epithelium of rats treated with BHA

Six 6-week-old F344 male rats were treated with single daily intragastric doses of 1 g/kg body weight 3-BHA (purity >99%) in corn oil for 5 days. As a positive control, 6 Sprague-Dawley male rats were given single doses of 40 mg/kg body weight 4-nitroquinoline N-oxide (4NQO) in trioctanoine for 5 days. Control animals were administered solvent alone. All animals were decapitated 6 hr after the last administration; the forestomachs were immediately removed and epithelia were separated from muscle. DNA isolation, digestion, and ^{32}P labeling; separation of ^{32}P-labeled adducts and contact transfer to polyethyleneimine-cellulose; mapping of ^{32}P labeling; and estimation and calculation of adduct levels were performed. To separate DNA adducts associated with the treatment, two-dimensional thin-layer chromatography was conducted under three solvent systems: (A) 1.28 M lithium formate (pH 3.5), 3.0 M urea:0.21 M Tris-HCl (pH 8.0), 0.34 M LiCl, 3.0 M urea:1.70 M sodium phosphate (pH 6.1); (B) 2.14 M lithium formate (pH 3.5), 5.0 M urea:0.35 M Tris-HCl (pH 8.0), 0.57 M LiCl, 5.0 M urea:1.70 M sodium phosphate (pH 6.1); and (C) 1.8 M lithium formate (pH 3.5), 4.25 M urea:0.35 M Tris-HCl (pH 8.0), 0.57 M LiCl, 5.0 M urea:1.70 M sodium phosphate (pH 6.2).

Detection of 8-OH-deoxyguanosine (8-OH-DG) in stomach epithelia of rats treated with antioxidants

Groups of three F344 male rats, 6 weeks old, were treated for 2 weeks with 2% BHA, 2% caffeic acid, and 0.8% catechol in powdered diet or basal diet alone. Stomachs were then removed and forestomach and glandular stomach epithelia were collected using a razor blade and frozen using liquid nitrogen. The following procedures were performed according to the method of Kasai et al. (18); defrosted tissues were saturated with argon gas before homogenation in a Teflon homogenizer. DNA samples isolated from these homogenates were dissolved in 0.004 ml of 1 M sodium acetate buffer (pH 4.8), heat-denatured at 95°C for 3 min, then ice-cooled. The DNA was digested to deoxynucleosides by treatment with 0.008 ml of nuclease P1 at 37°C for 35 min and 0.008 ml of alkaline phosphatase (6.5 ml protein/ml) in 1 M Tris-HCl buffer (pH 7.15) at 37°C for 1 hr. The resulting deoxynucleoside mixture was analyzed with a high-performance liquid chromatography (HPLC) electrochemical detector (ECD) system.

Lipid hydroperoxides in rat stomach epithelia after antioxidant treatment

Groups of five F344 male rats, 6 weeks old, were treated with a powdered diet containing 2% BHA, 2% caffeic acid, 0.8% catechol, or basal diet alone for 2 weeks, then killed by exsanguination under ether anesthesia. Stomachs were removed and washed in cold saline, and the muscle layer was removed using a razor blade. Phosphate buffer adjusted to pH 7.2 was added to tissue samples which were then homogenized using a microhomogenizer. Homogenates were centrifuged at 3000 rpm for 10 min, and supernatants were processed with Determiner LPO, a commercial kit designed to detect lipid hydroperoxides (Kyowa Medics Co. Ltd., Tokyo). Values of lipid peroxides were assessed by an autoanalyzer and expressed as nanomolars per milligram protein.

Effects of diethylmaleate on BHA-induced cell proliferation and lipid peroxidation

Fifteen F344 male rats, 6 weeks old, were treated for 1 week with a powdered diet containing 0.25% diethylmaleate (DEM, purity >98%, Wako Pure Chemical Industries, Osaka), then were given 0.25% DEM plus 1% BHA for an additional 4 weeks.

Other groups of 15–17 rats each were treated with 1% BHA, 0.25% DEM, or basal diet alone for 5 weeks. Five rats in each group were killed 3 weeks after the beginning of the experiment for examination of lipid hydroxide levels in stomach epithelia. Surviving rats were killed at week 5 and processed for histopathological examination.

Effects of antioxidants on two–stage stomach carcinogenesis

Groups of 15 rats each were given a single intragastric dose of 150 mg/kg body weight of MNNG; 1 week later they began a 51-day treatment with a diet containing 1% BHA, 1% *p*-methoxyphenol, 0.8% catechol, or basal diet alone. Other groups of 10–15 animals each were treated with 1% BHA, 1% *p*-methoxyphenol, 0.8% catechol, or basal diet alone for 51 weeks without the MNNG pretreatment. All animals were killed

Table 1. Histopathological Findings in Stomach Epithelia (4 weeks).

Chemicals	Number rats	Forestomach		G_1 stomach	
		Severe hyperplasia (%)	Erosion ulceration	Submucosal growth	Erosion/ ulceration
BHA	10	10 (100)	+	0	−
Caffeic acid	10	10 (100)	++	0	−
Sesamol	11	7 (64)	+++	0	±
p-Methoxyphenol	10	10 (100)	+++	0	±
Catechol	10	1 (10)	±	6 (60)	+
Control	10	0	0	0	−

+++, marked; ++, strong; +, weak; ±, slight; −, negative

under ether anesthesia at the end of week 52, and the stomachs were processed for histopathological examination.

Carcinogenicity studies of antioxidants

Early stomach lesions induced by antioxidants

Histopathological changes induced in rat stomach epithelia after 4 weeks of antioxidant treatment are shown in Table 1. BHA, caffeic acid, and sesamol induced high incidences of severe hyperplasia (mucosal height >0.5 mm) in addition to epithelial damage as evidenced by erosion and/or ulceration. The grade of epithelial damage was higher in rats treated with sesamol than in those receiving BHA or caffeic acid. Sesamol and p-methoxyphenol induced an extensive ring-shaped erosion/ulceration along the limiting ridge in the mid region of the forestomach, while BHA and caffeic acid induced focal erosion/ulcers. Catechol induced glandular stomach submucosal growth and focal superficial erosion in 60% of animals.

Stomach carcinogenicity of antioxidants

Incidence of tumors in the stomachs of rats treated with antioxidants for up to 104 weeks is shown in Table 2 (18). The incidence of forestomach papillomas was significantly increased in both male and female rats treated with BHA, caffeic acid, and sesamol; the incidence of squamous cell carcinomas was significantly increased in both males and females treated with BHA or caffeic acid and in males treated with sesamol. In both sexes treated with catechol, the incidence of glandular stomach adenomatous hyperplasias and adenocarcinomas was clearly increased compared with controls. A carcinogenicity study of p-methoxyphenol is now in progress.

Comparative assessment of forestomach lesion reversibility

The results of the lesion reversibility study are summarized in Table 3. The incidence of hyperplasia was low in rats treated with 8NQ and AF2 for 24 weeks but increased to 100% after a further 24 weeks on the basal diet alone. Squamous cell carcinomas were found in only 25% of rats at the cessation of MNNG treatment, but a 100% incidence was evident 24 weeks later. In contrast, although severe hyperplasia was observed in 78% and 100% of animals treated, respectively, with BHA and caffeic acid for 24 weeks, in both cases it disappeared within 24 weeks after chemical administration ceased. Mild hyperplasia (epithelial height <0.1 mm) was still present, however.

Detection of DNA adducts by the ^{32}P-postlabeling method in forestomach epithelia of rats treated with BHA

Under solvent system A, four detectable but weak spots were observed in maps of the 3-BHA and control groups. When solvent system B was used, the map for 3-BHA demonstrated three weak spots; the same spots also existed in the control. Thus, no spots specifically relating to the administration of 3-BHA were detected. The relative adduct level for 3-BHA was less than 0.3 and comparable to that of the control. In contrast, four spots not observed with controls were demonstrated from the forestomach treated with 4NQO under solvent system C (20).

Detection of 8-OH-deoxyguanosine in stomach epithelia of rats treated with antioxidants

The results of the HPLC-ECD system 8-OH-dG analysis are shown in Table 4. No significant increases in the levels of 8-OH-dG were found in either the forestomach or glandular stomach epithelium in rats treated with antioxidants.

Lipid hydroperoxides in rat stomach epithelia treated with antioxidants

Levels of lipid hydroperoxides in the forestomach epithelia treated with antioxidants were 0.9 ± 0.1 nmol/mg protein for BHA, 1.2 ± 0.1 for caffeic acid, and 1.2 ± 0.1 for

Table 2. Histopathological Findings in Stomach Epithelia (104 weeks).

			Number of rats with (%)	
Chemicals	Sex	Number of rats	Squamous cell carcinoma (forestomach)	Adeno-carcinoma (G_1 stomach)
BHA	M	52	18 (34.6)***	0
	F	51	15 (29.4)***	0
Caffeic acid	M	30	17 (56.7)***	0
	F	30	15 (50)***	0
Sesamol	M	29	9 (31.0)***	0
	F	30	3 (10)	0
Catechol	M	28	0	15 (53.6)***
	F	28	0	12 (42.9)***
Control	M	30	0	0
	F	30	0	0

***$P < 0.001$ vs. control group value

Table 3. Reversibility Experiment: Histological Findings in Forestomach Epithelium.

	Treatment (week)		Number of rats	Number of rats with (%)		
Chemicals	Chemicals	Basal diet		Hyperplasia	Papilloma	Carcinoma
8NQ	24	0	10	2 (20)	0	0
	24	24	10	10 (100)	1 (10)	0
AF2	24	0	10	3 (30)	0	0
	24	24	8	8 (100)	0	0
MNNG	24	0	8	8 (100)	8 (100)	2 (25)
	24	24	6	6 (100)	6 (100)	6 (100)
BHA	24	0	9	7 (78)	0	0
	24	24	10	0	0	0
Caffeic acid	24	0	9	9 (100)	9 (11)	0
	24	24	10	0	0	0

catechol, values that were all significantly lower than those for the basal diet-alone group (1.8 ± 0.4). A decrease was particularly evident for the BHA-treated forestomach, where the level was only half that of the control value. Levels of lipid hydroperoxides in glandular stomach epithelia of rats treated with antioxidants were 3.3–3.7, and therefore were not significantly different from the control value of 3.2.

Effects of diethylmaleate on BHA-induced cell proliferation and lipid peroxidation

Data from histopathological examination and assessment of lipid hydroperoxide are presented in Table 5. Histopathologically, forestomach hyperplasia was classified as mild (<0.1 mm), moderate (0.1–0.5 mm), and severe (>0.5 mm) depending on the mucosal thickness. While treatment with BHA alone induced significant incidences of mild and moderate hyperplasia, the combination with DEM completely blocked it. Similarly, while the lipid hydroperoxide levels found in forestomach epithelia after BHA treatment were significantly lowered, those levels found in animals receiving both DEM and the antioxidant were not different from basal diet values.

Effects of antioxidants on two-stage stomach carcinogenesis

Effects of antioxidants on MNNG-initiated two-stage stomach carcinogenesis are summarized in Figure 1. Treatment with BHA significantly enhanced the development of forestomach papillomas (100% vs. 50%, $P < 0.01$) and carcinomas (100% vs. 0%, $P < 0.001$) compared with the values of the group receiving MNNG alone. All animals given BHA alone demonstrated hyperplasia, but only one papilloma and one carcinoma were

Table 4. Levels of 8-OH-dG in Stomach Epithelia of Rats Treated with Antioxidants (8-OH-dG/10^5 dG).

Chemicals	Forestomach	Glandular stomach
BHA	2.8 ± 0.9	2.7 ± 1.4
Caffeic acid	2.1 ± 0.9	2.1 ± 0.8
Catechol	3.9 ± 1.6	1.7 ± 1.4
Basal diet	4.4 ± 1.2	2.2 ± 1.0

Table 5. Histopathological Changes and Lipid Hydroperoxide Levels in Forestomach Epithelium.

Treatment	Number of rats	Number of rats with hyperplasia (%)			Lipid hydroperoxides (n mol/g protein)
		Mild	Moderate	Severe	
BHA+ DEM	10	0 ***	0 ***	0	14.4 ± 2.7***
BHA	12	12	9	3	9.2 ± 0.7
DEM	10	0	0	0	15.4 ± 0.7
Basal diet	10	0	0	0	18.1 ± 3.7

***$P < 0.001$ vs. BHA alone group

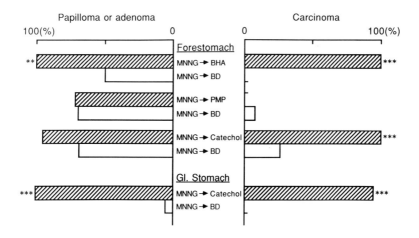

Figure 1. Incidences of tumors in two-stage stomach carcinogenesis ////// : MNNG → antioxidant; ⬜ : MNNG → basal diet; ***P < 0.001; **P < 0.01 as compared to corresponding carcinogen control group values.

found in rats treated with BHA without MNNG pretreatment (7). Although the incidence of forestomach papillomas was not significantly different in animals treated with catechol (94.7% vs. 68.4%), that of carcinomas was clearly increased (100% vs. 26.3%, P < 0.001) compared with the value for the group receiving MNNG alone. Catechol alone produced hyperplasias in 86.6% of animals (22). In contrast, p-methoxyphenol treatment did not influence the development of either forestomach papillomas or carcinomas, although p-methoxyphenol alone did induce hyperplasias in all rats (22). In the glandular stomach epithelium, catechol strongly enhanced the development of adenocarcinomas (94.7% vs. 0%, P < 0.001). After treatment with catechol alone for 51 weeks, adenomas and adenocarcinomas were observed in 100% and 20% of the animals, respectively (22).

Discussion

In addition to the well-known carcinogenic antioxidant BHA, other naturally occurring antioxidants including caffeic acid, sesamol, and catechol have now been demonstrated to induce tumors in rat forestomach or glandular stomach epithelium. None of these antioxidants have proven mutagenic as evaluated by the Ames test (23,24), and they are all characterized by epithelial damage and a strong cell proliferative response in their target tissues at early stages. However, forestomach hyperplasia induced by treatment with BHA or caffeic acid regresses after cessation of the treatment;

in clear contrast, proliferative lesions associated with the genotoxic agents 8NQ, AF2, or MNNG developed into papillomas and carcinomas without continued carcinogenic insult. Therefore, a continuously strong proliferating stimulus appears necessary for these antioxidants to induce tumors.

Concerning the mechanisms that permit these antioxidants to induce cell proliferation and carcinomas, we have already reported that BHA and its metabolites do not bind to DNA or RNA in forestomach epithelia. Lack of formation of DNA adducts in the forestomach epithelia of rats treated with BHA as evaluated by the 32P–labeling method further confirmed the nongenotoxic nature of BHA. Similarly, DNA adducts were not observed in the forestomachs or glandular stomach epithelia of rats treated with 2% caffeic acid, 2% sesamol, or 0.8% catechol for 2 weeks (unpublished data).

Recently, oxidative DNA damage has been suggested as having a close relationship to the induction of certain experimental cancers (25,26). 8-Hydroxydeoxyguanosine (8-OH-dG) is the product of DNA damage that is associated with oxidative stress through active oxygen species (18); interestingly, catechol produces significant levels of this adduct after incubation with deoxyguanosine in the presence of H_2O_2 and Fe^{3+} in an in vitro system (27). Catechol and caffeic acid are ortho-dihydroxybenzene derivatives, and BHA can be metabolized to BHA-catechol in experimental systems in vitro (17). However, the lack of any significant increase in 8-OH-dG formation in the stomach epithelia of rats after experimental administration of antioxidants does not support the presence of such mechanisms in vivo.

Lipid peroxidation has been shown to be well correlated to cytoxicity and/or promotion of carcinogenesis (28,29). The finding that lipid hydroperoxides produced by oxidative damage of lipids in forestomach epithelia were not increased but rather were lower than control levels after BHA treatment could, therefore, be anomalous. This result, however, is indicative of antioxidant action. It is interesting that simultaneous treatment with DEM, a known glutathione-depleting agent, remarkably reduced BHA-induced forestomach cell proliferation. The levels of lipid hydroperoxides were also returned to control levels by the simultaneous treatment with DEM, suggesting that DEM inhibited the antioxidant action of BHA. The most obvious conclusion is that BHA-induced forestomach hyperplasia may be partly related to its antioxidant activity.

In the two-stage stomach carcinogenesis experiment, BHA and catechol strongly promoted MNNG–initiated forestomach carcinogenesis, while p-methoxyphenol exerted a slight inhibitory influence. Since comparison of the proliferation-inducing potency of these compounds in forestomach epithelium reveals that BHA evokes the strongest response followed by p-methoxyphenol and then catechol, there appears to be no direct correlation between tumor promotion and cell division. Presumably, different metabolites might be responsible for cell proliferation and promotion as suggested by Witschi (30) or initiated cells might be killed by the cytotoxic effects of chemicals. A summary of the parallels between various parameters for antioxidants active in the rat stomach is given in Table 6.

In conclusion, regardless of the underlying mechanisms, the nongenotoxic phenolic antioxidants which are widely distributed in our environment can exert a multitude of effects on stomach epithelia. The recent finding that catechol can also promote N-methyl-N-amylnitrosamine–initiated esophageal carcinogenesis in rats further suggests possible roles in upper digestive organ carcinogenesis in man.

Table 6. Comparison of Antioxidants with Regard to Relevant Rat Stomach Parameters.

Antioxidants	Target	Cell growth	Ulceration	Reversibility	Carcinogenicity	Tumor promotion
BHA	F	+++	+	+	+	+++
Caffeic acid	F	+++	++	+	+	+
Sesamol	F	++	+++	OG	+	NE
p-Methoxyphenol	F	++	+++	OG	OG	−
Catechol	F	±	±	+	−	+++
	G	+++	++	±	+	+++

+++, marked; ++, strong; +, weak; ±, slight; −, negative; NE, not examined; OG, on going; F, forestomach; G, glandular stomach

References

1. Ito N, Fukushima S, Hagiwara A, Shibata M, Ogiso T. Carcinogenicity of butylated hydroxyanisole in F344 rats. J Natl Cancer Inst 70:343–352, 1983.
2. Ito N, Fukushima S, Tamano S, Hirose M, Hagiwara A. Dose response in butylated hydroxyanisole induction of forestomach carcinogenesis in F344 rats. J Natl Cancer Inst 77:1261–1265, 1986.
3. Masui T, Hirose M, Imaida K, Fukushima S, Tamano S, Ito N. Sequential changes of the forestomach of F344 rats, Syrian golden hamsters, and B6C3F1 mice treated with butylated hydroxyanisole. Jpn J Cancer Res 77:1083–1090, 1986.
4. Shirai T, Fukushima S, Ohshima M, Masuda A, Ito N. Effects of butylated hydroxyanisole, butylated hydroxytoluene, and NaCl on gastric carcinogenesis initiated with N-methyl-N'-nitro-N-nitrosoguanidine in F344 rats. J Natl Cancer Inst 72:1189–1198, 1984.
5. Takahashi M, Furukawa F, Toyoda K, Sato H, Hasegawa R, Hayashi Y. Effects of four antioxidants on N-methyl-N'-nitro-N-nitrosoguanidine-initiated gastric tumor development in rats. Cancer Lett 30:161–168, 1986.
6. Williams GM. Epigenetic promoting effects of butylated hydroxyanisole. Food Chem Toxicol 24:1163–1166, 1986.
7. Hirose M, Kagawa M, Ogawa K, Yamamoto A, Ito N. Antagonistic effect of diethylmaleate on the promotion of forestomach carcinogenesis by butylated hydroxyanisole (BHA) in rats pretreated with N-methyl-N'-nitro-N-nitrosoguanidine. Carcinogenesis 10:2223–2226, 1989.
8. Imaida K, Fukushima S, Shirai T, Masui T, Ogiso T, Ito N. Promoting activities of butylated hydroxyanisole, butylated hydroxytoluene and sodium ascorbate on forestomach and urinary bladder carcinogenesis initiated with methylnitrosourea in F344 male rats. Jpn J Cancer Res (Gann) 75:769–775, 1984.
9. Tsuda H, Sakata T, Shirai T, Kurata Y, Tamano S, Ito N. Modification of N-methyl-N-nitrosourea initiated carcinogenesis in the rat by subsequent treatment with antioxidants, phenobarbital and ethinyl estradiol. Cancer Lett 24:19–27, 1984.
10. Fukushima S, Sakata T, Tagawa Y, Shibata M, Hirose M, Ito N. Different modifying response of butylated hydroxyanisole, butylated hydroxytoluene, and other antioxidants in N,N-dibutylnitrosamine esophagus and forestomach carcinogenesis of rats. Cancer Res 47:2113–2116, 1987.
11. Hirose M, Masuda A, Kurata Y, Ikawa E, Mera Y, Ito N. Histologic and autoradiographic studies on the forestomach of hamsters treated with 2-tert-butylated hydroxyanisole, 3-tert-butylated hydroxyanisole, crude butylated hydroxyanisole, or butylated hydroxytoluene. J Natl Cancer Inst 76:143–149, 1986.
12. Hirose M, Masuda A, Imaida K, Kagawa M, Tsuda H, Ito N. Induction of forestomach lesions in rats by oral administrations of naturally occurring antioxidants for 4 weeks. Jpn J Cancer Res 78:317–321, 1987.
13. Hirose M, Inoue T, Asamoto M, Tagawa Y, Ito N. Comparison of the effects of 13 phenolic compounds in induction of proliferative lesions of the forestomach and increase in the labeling indices of the glandular stomach and urinary bladder of Syrian golden hamsters. Carcinogenesis 7:1285–1289, 1986.

14. Hirose M, Hagiwara A, Inoue K, Sakata T, Ito N, Kaneko H, Yoshitake A, Miyamoto J. Metabolism of 2- and 3-tert-butyl-4-hydroxyanisole (2-and 3-BHA) in the rat (I): excretion of BHA in urine, feces and expired air and distribution of BHA in the main organs. Toxicology 43:139–147, 1987.

15. Hirose M, Asamoto M, Hagiwara A, Ito N, Kaneko H, Saito K, Takamatsu Y, Yoshitake A, Miyamoto J. Metabolism of 2- and 3-tert-butyl-4-hydroxyanisole (2- and 3-BHA) in the rat (II): metabolism in forestomach and covalent binding to tissue macromolecules. Toxicology 45:13–24, 1987.

16. Hirose M, Hagiwara A, Inoue K, Ito N, Kaneko H, Saito K, Matsunaga H, Isobe N, Yoshitake A, Miyamoto J. Metabolism of 2- and 3-tert-butyl-4-hydroxyanisole in the rat (III): metabolites in the urine and feces. Toxicology 53:33–43 1988.

17. Ito N, Hirose M. Antioxidants—Carcinogenic and chemopreventive properties. Adv Cancer Res 53:247–302, 1989.

18. Kasai H, Crain PF, Kuchino Y, Nishimura S, Ootsuyama A, Tanooka H. Formation of 8-hydroxyguanine moiety in cellular DNA by agents producing oxygen radicals and evidence for its repair. Carcinogenesis 7:1849–1851, 1986.

19. Hirose M, Fukushima S, Shirai T, Hasegawa R, Kato T, Tanaka H, Asakawa E, Ito N. Stomach carcinogenicity of caffeic acid, sesamol and catechol in rats and mice. Jpn J Cancer Res 81:207–212, 1990.

20. Saito K, Yoshitake A, Miyamoto J, Hirose M, Ito N. No evidence of DNA adduct formation in forestomach of rats treated with 3-BHA and its metabolites as assessed by an enzymatic ^{32}P–postlabeling method. Cancer Lett 48:189–195, 1990.

21. Hirose M, Inoue T, Masuda A, Tsuda H, Ito N. Effects of simultaneous treatment with various chemicals on BHA–induced development of rat forestomach hyperplasia complete inhibition by diethylmaletate in a 5-week feeding study. Carcinogenesis 8:1555–1558, 1987.

22. Hirose M, Fukushima S, Kurata Y, Tsuda H, Tatematsu M, Ito, N. Modification of N-methyl- N'-nitro-N-nitrosoguanidine–induced forestomach and glandular carcinogenesis by phenolic antioxidants in rats. Cancer Res 48:5310–5315, 1988.

23. Cameron TP. National Cancer Institute, Division of Cancer Etiology, Chemical Carcinogenesis Research Information System (CCRIS), 1986.

24. Haworth S, Lawlor T, Mortelmas K, Spech W, Seiger E. Salmonella mutagenicity test results for 250 chemicals. Environmental Mutagenesis, Supplement 1:3–42, 1983.

25. Kasai H, Nishimura S, Kurokawa Y, Hayashi Y. Oral administration of the renal carcinogen, potassium bromate, specifically produces 8-hydroxydeoxyguanosine in rat target organ DNA. Carcinogenesis 8:1959–1961, 1987.

26. Fiala ES, Conaway CC, Mathis JE. Oxidative DNA and RNA damage in the livers of Sprague-Dawley rats treated with the hepatocarcinogen 2-nitropropane. Cancer Res 49:5518–5522, 1988.

27. Kasai H, Nishimura S. Hydroxylation of deoxy guanosine at the C-8 position by polyphenols and aminophenols in the presence of hydrogen peroxide and ferric ion. Jpn J Cancer Res (Gann) 75:565–566, 1984.

28. Casini AF, Pompella A, Comporti M. Glutathione depletion, lipid peroxidation, and liver necrosis following bromobenzene and iodobenzene intoxication. Toxicol Pathol 12:295–299, 1984.

29. Logani MK, Sambuco CP, Forbes PD, Davis RE. Skin-tumour–promoting activity of methyl ethyl ketone peroxide—a potent lipid–peroxidizing agent. Food and Chemical Toxicology 22:879–882, 1984.

30. Witschi MP. Separation of early diffuse alveolar cell proliferation from enhanced tumor development in mouse lung. Cancer Res 46:2675–2679, 1986.

Chemically Induced Cell Proliferation:
Implications for Risk Assessment, pages 53-65
©1991 Wiley-Liss, Inc.

Stimulation of Hepatocyte DNA Synthesis by Ethinyl Estradiol

James D. Yager and Yuenian E. Shi

Previous studies, including our own, demonstrated that the synthetic steroidal estrogens mestranol and ethinyl estradiol (EE) are strong promoters of γ-glutamyl-transpeptidase–positive (GGT⁺) foci and hepatocellular carcinomas in female rats following diethylnitrosamine initiation of hepatocarcinogenesis (1–3). These estrogens also cause the appearance of GGT⁺ foci in the livers of noninitiated rats. However, because studies failed to demonstrate any significant initiating activity or hepatogenotoxic effects of the synthetic estrogens (4,5), it is possible that the appearance of foci in non-initiated rats is due to the promotion of spontaneously initiated hepatocytes (6).

A property shared by most promoters, and perhaps all of them, is their ability to stimulate DNA synthesis. The data presented here represent a review of our studies, and those of others, on the capacity of the synthetic steroidal estrogens to stimulate liver DNA synthesis and on the mechanisms involved in this effect. The data support the hypothesis that EE is a comitogen for liver. EE appears to enhance the level of serum/plasma hepatocyte growth factor(s) but alone has only a weak ability to directly stimulate hepatocyte DNA synthesis. However, it potentiates the DNA synthetic response of hepatocytes to epidermal growth factor (EGF), suggesting that this steroidal synthetic estrogen would enhance growth stimulated by factors that work through the EGF/transforming growth factor-α (TGF-α) receptor pathway.

The materials and methods used in obtaining these data have previously been described in detail (1,7–9) and will be only briefly reviewed as needed here.

Stimulation of liver DNA synthesis

We conducted a series of in vivo experiments to determine the time course and dose-response of liver DNA synthesis in response to EE treatment. Female Sprague-Dawley rats were implanted subcutaneously with time-release tablets containing mestranol or EE. Alternatively, rats were fed diet containing phenobarbital (PB, 0.05%); this group served as a positive control for comparison with the synthetic estrogens since Peraino et al. had reported that PB stimulated liver DNA synthesis (10). Figure 1, taken from Yager et al. (7), shows the amount of liver DNA synthesis at various times after beginning treatment with EE (2.5 µg/day) or PB. It can be seen that both promoters caused a rapid 3- to 4-fold increase in [³H]thymidine incorporation (2-hr pulse) into liver DNA. However, this elevation was transient in that it only persisted for between 7 and 14 days, even though treatment with EE and PB continued. As determined at 24 hr, the increase in DNA synthesis was also caused by treatment with mestranol and, for both EE and mestranol, the stimulation was dose dependent. Thus, stimulation of liver DNA synthesis was detected in animals treated with EE at 0.1 µg/day and was maximal at 1.0–2.5 µg/day. The level of DNA synthesis induced by EE was about one-fifth to one-quarter of that induced by two-thirds surgical partial hepatectomy; however, it persisted longer than DNA synthesis following partial hepatectomy, a synthesis that is generally completed after 3 or 4 days (11). Ochs et al. (12) also investigated the effects of EE on liver DNA synthesis. They reported results similar to ours and, using auto-radiography, further showed that most of the increased DNA synthesis was due to repli-cation in hepatocytes.

It was speculated that the stimulation of DNA synthesis by EE could be accounted for by EE hepatotoxicity, which would result in a regenerative hyperplastic response. This possibility was ruled out by following the loss of [³H]thymidine from prelabeled liver DNA in controls compared with animals treated for 6 weeks with EE, mestranol, or PB. This method for the detection of hepatotoxicity is cumulative and therefore very sensitive. The results of that study (data not shown, see ref. 7) indicated that EE (1.0–5.0 µg/day), mestranol (5.0 µg/day), and PB (0.05% in diet) were not hepatotoxic.

Body, liver, and pituitary weights were determined at the end of the 6-week experimental period (7). As observed previously (1), body weight gain was significantly reduced in a dose-dependent manner by treatment with the synthetic estrogens. These treatments had no effect on liver weight, but liver weight per 100 g body weight was significantly increased in the PB, mestranol, EE at 2.5 µg/day, and EE at 5.0 µg/day groups. Perhaps most strikingly, EE treatment caused dramatic increases in pituitary weights in the control, EE at 2.5 µg/day, and EE at 5.0 µg/day groups, to 14.0 ± 0.9 µg (mean ± SEM), 36.3 ± 2.7 µg, and 25.7 ± 2.4 µg, respectively. No increases in pitu-itary weights were observed in the PB, mestranol, and EE 1.0 µg/day groups.

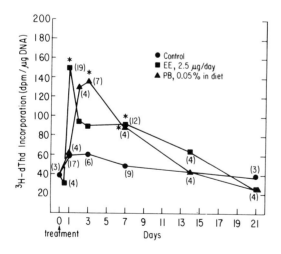

Figure 1. The time course of liver DNA synthesis following treatment with EE or PB. At time 0 the female Sprague-Dawley rats were treated by sub-cutaneous implantation of time-release tablets delivering EE at 2.5 mg/day, or fed a diet con-taining 0.05% PB. At the times indicated, the rats were injected with [³H]thymidine and killed 2 hr later. The number of rats per point is indicated in parenthe-ses and the groups determined to be significantly different from controls are indicated by aster-isks. For clarity, the SEMs are not shown, but see Yager et al. (7). *Source:* Yager et al. (7), with permission.

An important additional finding was that the stimulation of liver DNA synthesis caused by EE and mestranol was inhibited by tamoxifen (7,13). Although tamoxifen treatment did cause a slight reduction in DNA synthesis induced by PB, the effect was not statistically significant (but see below). Tamoxifen also blocked the increase in pituitary weight caused by EE treatment. As measured at 24 hr, tamoxifen itself did not stimulate liver DNA synthesis. These observations led to an experiment designed to determine whether tamoxifen could inhibit the ability of EE to promote hepato-carcinogenesis (7). The results of a 4-month study revealed that the number of GGT+ foci/cm³ and the percentage volume of liver occupied by GGT+ foci were significantly reduced in diethylnitrosamine-initiated rats treated with both EE at 5 μg/day and tamoxifen at either 15 or 50 μg/day (7,13). However, tamoxifen used alone enhanced the appearance of GGT+ lesions (7,13), indicating that by itself it is a promoter of hepatocarcinogenesis, a finding subsequently confirmed by Pitot et al. (14) and Ghia and Mereto (15). Given this finding, additional studies using more sensitive techniques to detect enhanced DNA synthesis in tamoxifen-treated rats and experiments to determine whether tamoxifen is hepatotoxic seem appropriate.

The results reviewed above provided support for the hypothesis that EE acts as a growth factor for liver. However, they did not provide information as to whether this effect was due to direct growth-stimulatory effects on hepatocytes, indirect effects mediated through an EE-induced liver growth factor, or both. Thus, we designed a series of experiments to distinguish among these possibilities.

Enhancement by ethinyl estradiol of a serum/plasma hepatocyte growth factor

Several laboratories have recently detected, purified, and characterized factors stimulatory for hepatocyte DNA synthesis from serum and plasma obtained from humans and rats (16,17). Two such factors, hepatocyte growth factor (16) and hepatopoietin A (17), are quite similar and probably belong to the same newly proposed family of hepatocyte growth factors (to be distinguished from the EGF/TGF-α family) that Zarnegar and Michalopoulos have suggested be called HepGF (17).

Our goal was to determine whether EE enhanced the levels of a factor stimulatory for hepatocyte DNA synthesis. Rat serum or plasma was fractionated on a Sephadex G-200 column, and the individual fractions were analyzed for their ability to stimulate DNA synthesis in rat hepatocytes in primary culture as described previously (8). Serum and plasma from control animals contained an "activity" of approximately 135 kD that was stimulatory for hepatocyte DNA synthesis (data not shown). Twenty-four hours after implantation of time-release tablets containing EE (2.5 μg/day), the level of this activity was increased approximately 1.6-fold. Additional characterization of the pooled Sephadex G-200 chromatographic fractions containing the activity revealed it to be heat and trypsin sensitive (8). Furthermore, determination of the effects of these pooled fractions on the specific binding of ^{125}I-labeled EGF to rat liver membranes revealed an increase in the level of competition in fractions from EE-treated compared with control animals at equal protein concentrations (8). Together, these results suggested that EE treatment had indirect effects associated with its stimulation of liver growth as indicated by the presence, in the serum and plasma, of increased levels of an activity stimulatory for hepatocyte DNA synthesis and perhaps in the EGF/TGF-α family.

Direct effects of ethinyl estradiol on DNA synthesis in cultured hepatocytes

In our studies designed to determine the effects of EE on hepatocyte DNA synthesis, the hepatocytes were obtained from the livers of female Lewis rats by collagenase perfusion and cultured on collagen-coated dishes in phenol red–free Dulbecco's modified Eagle's medium/Ham's F-12 (50:50) supplemented with insulin, selenium, and transferrin as described previously (9). The cells were allowed to attach for 4 hr; then (0 time), the medium was changed to remove unattached hepatocytes, and various agents being tested were added. Under these culture conditions, addition of EGF at 0 time stimulated hepatocyte DNA synthesis with the maximum response occurring at 48 hr at an EGF concentration of 25 ng/ml medium (4.1 nM) (9). When addition of EGF was delayed until 18 hr and EGF removed by a medium change at 30 hr (i.e., a 12-hr exposure to EGF), DNA synthesis still peaked at 48 hr but the overall response to EGF was reduced. This protocol of delayed EGF addition allows treatment of the hepatocytes with various agents before EGF treatment (9).

Figure 2 shows the stimulation of hepatocyte DNA synthesis, measured by determination of [³H]thymidine incorporation into DNA, in response to treatment with various concentrations of EE alone (open symbols). These results show that EE treatment caused a small concentration-dependent increase in DNA synthesis that reached 2.6 times the control value at an EE concentration of 15 mM.

This relatively small stimulatory effect of EE alone did not account for the larger, 4-fold stimulation of liver DNA synthesis typically observed following EE treatment in vivo (Fig. 1). Thus, we hypothesized that EE might affect the responsiveness of the hepatocytes to a growth factor known to be able to stimulate liver growth. We chose to

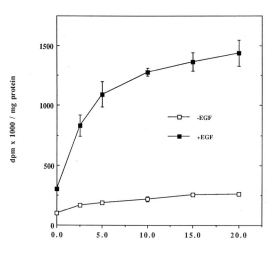

Figure 2. DNA synthesis in cultured rat hepatocytes in response to various concentrations of EE ± EGF (25 ng/ml). The protocol used was described previously (9). At 0 time the hepatocyte cultures were exposed to EE at the concentrations indicated. EGF was added 18 hr later. At 30 hr the medium was changed to basal medium and [³H]thymidine added. The cultures were harvested at 48 hr. The ordinate represents [³H]-thymidine incorporated into hepatocyte DNA. Each point is the mean ± SD of triplicate cultures. *Source:* EE + EGF data adapted from Table 3 in Shi and Yager (9), with permission.

begin with EGF. Table 1, taken from Shi and Yager (9), shows the results obtained when hepatocytes were exposed to EE (15 mM), EGF (25 ng/ml), or EE + EGF for the first 30 hr of culture. [^{3}H]Thymidine was present from 30 hr to the time of harvest at 48 hr. EE used alone caused a 2.2-fold and EGF a 10.7-fold stimulation of hepatocyte DNA synthesis. However, DNA synthesis was stimulated 32-fold over control when both agents were present together. Analysis of these data revealed the presence of a statistically significant ($P = 0.034$) interaction between EE and EGF, which was a greater response than expected based on the response to each alone.

To account for these results, we hypothesized that in some way, EE pretreatment had potentiated the responsiveness of the hepatocytes to EGF. To test this hypothesis, we employed the protocol of delayed EGF addition. The results of a time-course experiment are shown in Figure 3, taken from Shi and Yager (9). The hepatocytes were exposed to EE (15 mM) from 0–30 hr of culture, 25 ng/ml EGF from 18–30 hr of culture, or EE from 0–30 hr plus EGF from 18–30 hr. DNA synthesis was determined following a pulse of [^{3}H]thymidine 2 hr prior to harvest. The overall time course of enhanced DNA synthesis was the same in all treatment groups. At 48 hr, the fold increase over control caused by EE was 2.2; by EGF, 3.3; and by EE pretreatment followed by EGF, 8.7. These results confirmed our previous observations that indicated an interaction between EE and EGF. In addition, since the cells were treated with EE before the addition of EGF, the results provided support for our hypothesis that EE had in some way affected the hepatocytes such that their responsiveness to EGF was enhanced.

Additional studies (9) revealed that this effect of EE was dependent on the EE concentration (Fig. 2, closed symbols) with the maximum effect observed at between 10 and 15 μM, similar to the results observed for the stimulation of DNA synthesis by EE alone. Furthermore, we also found that attainment of the maximum potentiation effect of EE required that it be present continuously. If we removed EE before 9 hr, no effect on EGF responsiveness was observed (data not shown, see ref. 9). Finally, EE (15 μM) enhanced the responsiveness of the hepatocytes to EGF at all concentrations of EGF tested between 2.5 and 50 ng/ml but did not alter the point at which the response to EGF was maximum, namely, 25 ng/ml (9).

We were concerned that the effects of EE required concentrations in the micromolar range. This concern prompted a study of the metabolism of EE in the cultured

Table 1. The Effect of EE on Stimulation of Hepatocyte DNA Synthesis by EGF.

Treatment[a]	DNA synthesis[b]
Control	131 ± 10
EE	291 ± 15
EGF	1404 ± 40
EE + EGF	4196 ± 737

Source: Shi and Yager (9), with permission.

[a] The cultures were exposed to EE (15 mM) and/or EGF (25 ng/ml) for 0–30 hr and to [^{3}H]thymidine for 30–48 hr. Hepatocyte DNA synthesis was determined as described in source article (9).

[b] Mean ± SD of triplicate cultures, dpm × 10^3/mg protein. Analysis of variance indicated that results for all treated groups were significantly greater than for control and that there was a significant interaction between EE and EGF, $P = 0.034$.

hepatocytes. The results of that study (18) revealed that >95% of the EE was metabolized to sulfated and glucuronidated metabolites within the first 4 hr of its addition to the cultures. This rapid and extensive degree of metabolism may account for the relatively high concentration of hormone required to observe these effects. Alternatively, a metabolite of EE could be responsible for the effects observed. However, this possibility will require additional study.

We also examined the response of the cultured hepatocytes to PB. Figure 4 shows the effects of different concentrations of PB on DNA synthesis in cultured rat hepatocytes. PB caused a concentration-dependent increase in DNA synthesis that reached a maximum of approximately 2-fold at 1 mM. Thus, PB like EE had only a weak ability to stimulate hepatocyte DNA synthesis. However, about a 100-fold higher concentration of PB was required to achieve this effect. Next, we examined how pretreatment (0–30 hr) with EE (2 μM), PB (1 μM), or estradiol (2 μM) would affect the level of stimulation of hepatocyte DNA synthesis by EGF (18–30 hr). The results are shown in Figure 5, and Table 2 shows a comparison of the fold increases over control calculated from these data. Before EGF was added, estradiol, EE, and PB all caused a small stimulation of hepatocyte DNA synthesis. In this experiment, the effect of PB (2.9-fold stimulation) was greater than that of EE (2.0-fold stimulation): the concentration of the latter was 2 μM which does not cause a maximum response (Fig. 2). From the calculations presented in Table 2 it can be seen that in EE-pretreated cultures, a greater-than-additive response

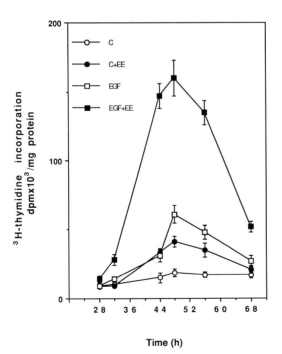

Figure 3. The time course of DNA synthesis in hepatocytes exposed to EE, to EGF, or to EE followed by EGF. The protocol was as described in Figure 2 except that the [³H]thymidine was added 2 hr before harvest at the times indicated. *Source:* Shi and Yager (9), with permission.

began to occur at an EGF concentration of 10 ng/ml (at higher EE concentrations, potentiation of the EGF responsiveness was observed at all EGF concentrations, see ref. 9). In contrast, with estradiol pretreatment, potentiation of the response to EGF was first observed at 15 ng EGF/ml and the maximum extent of potentiation was less than that observed with EE. If estrogen receptor–mediated mechanisms are involved in this effect, this result is not unexpected given that EE has an estrogenic potency approxi-

Table 2. Fold Increases a in DNA Synthesis Caused by Ethinyl Estradiol, Estradiol, and Phenobarbital in the Presence or Absence of EGF

EGF (ng/ml)	Control[b]	Ethinyl Estradiol		Estradiol		Phenobarbitol	
		A[c]	B[d]	A	B	A	B
0	-	-	2.0	-	1.7	-	2.9
5	2.3	1.7	3.8 (4.3)[a]	1.5	3.4 (4.0)	2.1	4.7 (5.2)
10	2.5	2.4	6.0 (4.5)	1.6	4.0 (4.2)	2.2	5.5 (5.4)
15	3.0	2.4	7.0 (5.0)	1.8	5.5 (4.7)	2.1	6.2 (5.9)
25	3.3	2.6	8.5 (5.3)	2.0	6.6 (5.0)	2.0	6.6 (6.2)

Note: Calculations based on data presented in Figure 5.

[a] The numbers in parentheses represent the expected fold increases if the effects of ethinyl estradiol, estradiol, and phenobarbital on DNA synthesis were simply additive with the effects of EGF alone.

[b] Actual fold increases of controls containing EGF over controls without EGF.

[c] Actual fold increases over controls containing EGF.

[d] Actual fold increases over controls without EGF.

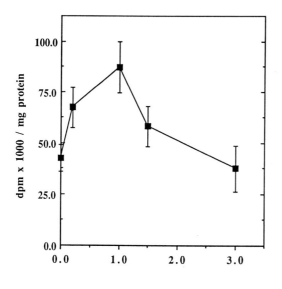

PB Concentration (mM)

Figure 4. The effect of various concentrations of PB on DNA synthesis in cultured rat hepatocytes. At 0 time the hepatocyte cultures were exposed to PB at the concentrations indicated. The cultures were harvested at 48 hr following a 2-hr pulse with [3H]thymidine. The ordinate represents [3H]-thymidine incorporated into hepatocyte DNA. Each point is the mean ± range of duplicate cultures.

mately 10 times that of estradiol. Finally, for PB pretreatment, potentiation was also first observed at 15 ng/ml EGF. However, the degree of potentiation appeared less than that caused by either of the two estrogens.

As discussed above, in vivo we found that tamoxifen significantly inhibited liver DNA synthesis stimulated by EE treatment, suggesting that the stimulatory process was mediated through estrogen receptors. In a like experiment in the cultured hepatocytes, we observed similar results (13). Tamoxifen used alone did not stimulate hepatocyte DNA synthesis and, when present at 0.25 μM and 1 μM for 30 hr, did not alter the induction of DNA synthesis by EGF (25 ng/ml, 18–30 hr). However, at 2 μM, tamoxifen had a slight inhibitory effect on hepatocyte responsiveness to EGF. In contrast, at both 0.25 and 1.0 μM, tamoxifen caused a dose-dependent inhibition of the ability of EE (2 μM) to potentiate hepatocyte responsiveness to EGF. These results supported the hypothesis that the effects of EE were estrogen receptor mediated. However, in a parallel experiment, we also observed that tamoxifen blocked the ability of PB to enhance the response to EGF (13).

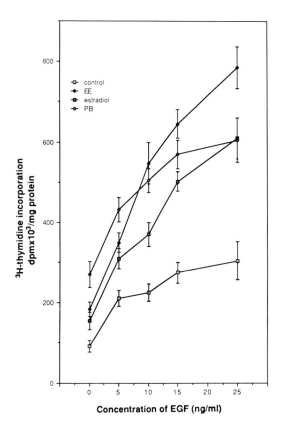

Figure 5. The effects of EE, E, and PB pretreatment on hepatocyte DNA synthesis in response to various concentrations of epidermal growth factor (EGF). At 0 time the hepatocyte cultures were exposed to EE or E (2 μM) or PB (1 μM). EGF was added 18 hr later at the concentrations indicated. At 30 hr the medium was changed to basal medium. [3H]thymidine was present from 42–44 hr, after which time the cultures were harvested. The ordinate represents [3H]thymi-dine incorporated into hepatocyte DNA. Each point in the mean ± range of duplicate cultures.

At first this result was unexpected since the effects of PB would not be expected to be mediated through the estrogen receptor. However, it then came to our attention that tamoxifen, while exerting its antiestrogenic effects through binding to the estrogen receptor, has also been shown to inhibit protein kinase C (see ref. 19 for bibliography) and to bind to a separate class of nuclear receptors in the liver (20). Sawada et al. (21) recently reported that the tumor promoter 12-O-tetradecanoylphorbol-13-acetate (TPA) enhanced the response of rat hepatocytes to EGF. Since it is known that the effects of TPA are mediated through the activation of protein kinase C (22), we conducted an experiment to determine the effects of tamoxifen on the response to TPA in the cultured hepatocytes. TPA at 0.1 µM did not stimulate DNA synthesis but dramatically enhanced the response of the hepatocytes to EGF, confirming the results of Sawada et al. (21). However, this effect of TPA was inhibited approximately 40% by 0.1 µM tamoxifen (13). Thus, on the basis of these results we cannot conclude that because the effects of EE were inhibited by tamoxifen, they are mediated through the estrogen receptor.

Effects of ethinyl estradiol on hepatocyte epidermal growth factor–receptor levels

The results presented above indicated that pretreatment of cultured hepatocytes with EE enhanced their response to EGF. To determine the mechanism of this effect, we next examined the effects of EE treatment on hepatocyte EGF-receptor levels as described previously (9). Scatchard analysis of 125I-labeled EGF equilibrium binding data after 18 hr indicated the presence of $45,145 \pm 2666$ (mean $\pm$ SD) sites per cell in control hepatocytes. Treatment with 2 µM EE for 18 hr significantly ($P < 0.001$) increased the number of 125I-EGF high affinity binding sites, to $92,665 \pm 668$ per cell. EE treatment also caused a small but significant ($P < 0.02$) decrease in binding affinity, to $2.33 \pm 0.25 \times 10$-10 from $2.97 \pm 0.12 \times 10$-10 in controls(9). In the same experiment we found that exposure to PB (1 µM) for 18 hr also caused a significant ($P < 0.005$) increase in 125I-EGF binding, to $58,801 \pm 2355$ sites per cell. 125I-EGF binding to PB-treated hepatocytes at 18 hr was significantly ($P < 0.005$) less than that to EE-treated cells, consistent with the results presented above indicating that EE was more potent in enhancing EGF responsiveness. However, the increase in 125I-EGF binding caused by PB followed an initial downregulation, observed at 3 hr. Similar results with PB have been reported by Meyer et al. (23). With EE, we did not observe any transient decrease in 125I-EGF binding (data not shown). In subsequent studies (24) we found that this increase in 125I-EGF binding reflected an increase in EGF-receptor protein that was accompanied by a decrease in the half-life of the receptor protein. Furthermore, in vivo treatment with EE also caused an increase in EGF receptors, a finding supported by the recent report of Lucier and coworkers, who have also reported on the ability of EE to promote hepatocarcinogenesis (25,26).

Comments

Our previous results and those of others have clearly demonstrated that the synthetic steroidal estrogens (1–3,7,12,25,26) and the synthetic nonsteroidal estrogen diethylstilbestrol (27) are promoters of hepatocarcinogenesis. Recently, Pitot and Campbell (28) described a method for the estimation of the relative potency of chemicals to promote hepatocarcinogenesis in the rat, based on dose/time of administration effects of promoters on the yield of preneoplastic lesions, as indicated by the percentage volume of the liver occupied by the lesions. The promotion index (PI) for 2,3,7,8-tetrachlorodibenzo-p-dioxin (TCDD) in Sprague-Dawley rats was calculated to be 28×10^6; for PB, the PI was 75 (28). Recently, Pitot also reported a PI of 93,000 for EE and a PI of 54,000, for mestranol (14). These results clearly demonstrate that the synthetic steroidal estrogens are very strong promoting agents, second only to the extremely potent TCDD.

In a recent review, Farber and Sarma (29) listed and discussed four model systems of promotion and progression in the rat liver: the chronic enzyme induction model, the resistant hepatocyte model, the choline and methionine deficiency model, and the orotic acid model. However, Schulte-Hermann and coworkers have shown that the synthetic steroidal estrogens do not cause the induction of hepatic monooxygenases (12,30) and thus these important, potent-promoting agents should not be included under the chronic enzyme induction model and need to be considered separately as a synthetic estrogen model.

The results presented above clearly demonstrate that EE, mestranol, and PB, all promoters of hepatocarcinogenesis, stimulate liver growth. In fact, this finding is not unexpected. Cell proliferation is an essential component of the carcinogenic process. It is essential for fixation of mutations responsible for initiation in the face of unrepaired DNA damage, for the clonal outgrowth of initiated cells and for the continued accumulation of mutations and chromosomal alterations associated with progression. Our results have demonstrated that the DNA synthesis caused by treatment with EE, mestranol, and PB does not reflect liver regeneration occurring as a result of their hepatotoxicity. This is in contrast to the results observed with some other agents. For example, 2-acetylaminofluorene (AAF) and 3'-methyl-4-dimethylaminoazobenzene (3'-MeDAB) are both "complete" hepatocarcinogenic agents. Both carcinogens stimulate equivalent levels of liver DNA synthesis at equal doses (31). This probably has a cocarcinogenic effect in association with the DNA damage caused by each compound and also probably acts as a promotion/progression stimulus and thus contributes to the complete carcinogenicity of both. However, the cause of the DNA synthetic response caused by each does not appear to be the same. Determinations of hepatotoxicity by measuring the loss of prelabeled [3H]thymidine from liver DNA revealed that 3'-MeDAB was quite hepatotoxic, whereas AAF at the same dose was not. Furthermore, 2-MeDAB, which is not a complete hepatocarcinogen but has been shown to be comparable to 3'-MeDAB in its genotoxicity as determined by the appearance of chromosomal abnormalities (32), was only slightly hepatotoxic and did not stimulate liver DNA synthesis (31). However, when treatment of rats with 2-MeDAB was followed by promotion with PB, many large hepatocellular carcinomas developed (33). This emphasizes the role of cell proliferation in the carcinogenic process.

Chronic feeding of a choline-deficient (CD) or choline and methionine–deficient (CMD) diet will promote hepatocarcinogenesis (29) and is associated with a persistent elevation in liver cell proliferation. Two studies have evaluated the hepatotoxicity of this promotion regimen using the prelabel loss technique (34,35). Both the CD (34) and the CMD (35) regimens caused substantial (42–60%) losses in [3H]thymidine from prelabeled liver DNA, demonstrating their hepatotoxicity. Thus, the persistent increase in liver cell proliferation accompanying treatment with these promoting regimens represents regeneration in response to their hepatotoxic effects. This is in contrast to the synthetic estrogens and PB, which stimulate cell proliferation but are not hepatotoxic. Thus, this liver proliferative response represents additive hyperplasia. However, it is important to note that the proliferative response caused by these nonhepatotoxic promoters appeared to be transient, lasting only 7–14 days. This raises the problem of how one can attribute their promoting properties causally to their ability to stimulate cell proliferation. Perhaps a low level of cell proliferation really does persist but was not detected with the 2-hr [^{3}H]thymidine pulse protocol used (7). This possibility should be addressed by reexamining liver DNA synthesis using more sensitive methods such as prolonged exposure (3–7 days) to bromodeoxyuridine and subsequent immunohisto-chemical detection of "labeled" cells. Alternatively, it could be that additive cell proliferation is transient and regulated by negative growth-regulatory factors. This would suggest that adaptation to the chronic presence of the promoter had occurred and that the clonal outgrowths of initiated cells (foci) were derived from those initiated cells no longer sensitive to such negative regulatory factors, analogous to the resistant hepatocyte model (29). Additional studies are required to determine the nature of the alterations in growth-regulatory processes in initiated cells.

The results we have presented support the hypothesis that the synthetic estrogens are comitogens for hepatocytes. Thus, while EE used alone was only able to cause a small stimulation in DNA synthesis in cultured hepatocytes, it was able to dramatically enhance the responsiveness of the cells to the stimulation of DNA synthesis by EGF. Estradiol was similar in its effects to PB, although only at concentrations almost 100 times greater than needed with EE. This is consistent with the potencies of these two agents as indicated by their calculated PIs (see above).

The results we have obtained to date support but do not prove that the effects of EE are mediated through the estrogen receptor. This support comes from the low concentrations of EE required, especially when its extensive degree of metabolism is considered (18), and the finding that the hormone must be present for at least 9 hr before its effects on EGF responsiveness are observed. The effects of EE are also blocked by tamoxifen, but this must be viewed with reservation, as described above. Future structure-activity studies will be able to definitively determine whether the effects of EE on hepatocyte EGF responsiveness are estrogen receptor–mediated.

In pursuit of the mechanisms associated with EE enhancement of EGF respon-siveness in hepatocytes, we found that EE increased the level of EGF-receptor protein through a mechanism associated with a decrease in the rate of receptor protein turnover (24). These findings indicate that EE can bring about the heterologous regulation of the EGF receptor. Other examples of this were discussed previously (9). Additional studies are required to determine the mechanism by which EE treatment results in a change in receptor protein turnover.

Clearly, cell proliferation in liver can be stimulated by various agents through a number of pathways. Since cell proliferation plays such an essential role in the carcino-genic process, it is extremely important that environmental agents to which humans are exposed be evaluated for their proliferation-inducing potential by standardized meth-odology, as was discussed during this conference. Furthermore, it is important to obtain some level of understanding of the mechanism(s) by which agents stimulate proliferation.

For example, if proliferation only occurs at high doses in response to toxicity, one would predict that at nontoxic doses, when cell proliferation is not induced, the agent would not represent a risk factor for stimulating promotion/progression. On the other hand, if the agent in question has comitogenic or mitogenic effects that occur through receptor-mediated mechanisms, one would expect these effects to be observed at very low doses and predict that exposure to low doses could represent a risk factor for stimulation of promotion/progression. Thus, a proliferation-stimulation index should be derived for agents being evaluated for "toxicity" in short-term tests. This information should then be used in the rational design of long-term tumorigenicity tests and taken into consideration in the development of risk-assessment estimates.

Acknowledgments

The studies presented were conducted while Dr. Yager was at the Dartmouth Medical School and were largely supported by NCI grant CA 36701. Additional support for equipment and services came from Norris Cotton Cancer Center Support (CORE) grant NCI CA 23108. Dr. Shi received support from a Friends of the Norris Cotton Cancer Center Predoctoral Fellowship. The authors would also like to thank Dr. J. Zurlo for intellectual contributions to the project and critical reading of the manuscript.

References

1. Yager JD, Campbell HA, Longnecker DS, Roebuck BD, Benoit MC. Enhancement of hepatocarcinogenesis in female rats by ethinyl estradiol and mestranol but not estradiol. Cancer Res 44:3862–3869, 1984.
2. Wanless IR, Medline A. Role of estrogens as promoters of hepatic neoplasia. Lab Invest 46:313–320, 1982.
3. Porter LE, Van Thiel DH, Eagon PK. Estrogens and progestins as tumor inducers. Semin Liver Dis 7:24–31, 1987.
4. Yager JD Jr, Fifield DS Jr. Lack of hepatogenotoxicity of oral contraceptive steroids. Carcinogenesis 3:625–628, 1982.
5. Schuppler J, Damme J, Schulte-Hermann R. Assay of some endogenous and synthetic sex steroids for tumour-initiating activity in rat liver using the Solt-Farber system. Carcinogenesis 4:239–241, 1983.
6. Schulte-Hermann R, Timmermann-Trosiener I, Schuppler J. Promotion of spontaneous preneoplastic cells in rat liver as a possible explanation of tumor production by nonmutagenic compounds. Cancer Res 43:839–844, 1983.
7. Yager JD, Roebuck BD, Paluszcyk TL, Memoli VA. Effects of ethinyl estradiol and tamoxifen on liver DNA turnover and new synthesis and appearance of γ glutamyl transpeptidase-positive foci in female rats. Carcinogenesis 7:2007–2014, 1986.
8. Shi YE, Yager JD. Enhancement in rats by the liver tumor promoter ethinyl estradiol of a serum factor(s) which is stimulatory for hepatocyte DNA synthesis. Biochem Biophys Res Commun 160:154–161, 1989.
9. Shi YE, Yager JD. Effects of the liver tumor promoter ethinyl estradiol on epidermal growth factor–induced DNA synthesis and epidermal growth factor receptor levels in cultured rat hepatocytes. Cancer Res 49:3574–3580, 1989.
10. Peraino C, Fry RJM, Staffeldt E. Reduction and enhancement by phenobarbital of hepatocarcinogenesis induced in the rat by 2-acetylaminofluorene. Cancer Res 31:1506–1512, 1971.
11. Hopkins HA, Campbell HA, Barbiroli B, Potter VR. Thymidine kinase and deoxyribonucleic acid metabolism in growing and regenerating livers from rats on controlled feeding schedules. Biochem J 136:955–966, 1973.

12. Ochs H, Dusterberg B, Gunzel P, Schulte-Hermann R. Effect of tumor promoting contraceptive steroids on growth and drug metabolizing enzymes in rat liver. Cancer Res 46:1224–1232, 1986.

13. Yager JD, Shi YE. Synthetic estrogens and tamoxifen as promoters of hepatocarcinogenesis. Preventive Medicine, in press, 1990.

14. Pitot HC. The role of hormones in the development of hepatocellular tumors. Preventive Medicine, in press, 1990.

15. Ghia M, Mereto E. Induction and promotion of γ-glutamyltranspeptidase–positive foci in the liver of female rats treated with ethinyl estradiol, clomiphene, tamoxifen and their associations. Cancer Let 46:195–202, 1989.

16. Nakamura T, Nawa K, Ichihara A, Kaise N, Nishino T. Purification and subunit structure of hepatocyte growth factor from rat platelets. FEBS Let 224:311–316, 1987.

17. Zarnegar R, Michalopoulos G. Purification and biological characterization of human hepatopoietin A, a polypeptide growth factor for hepatocytes. Cancer Res 49:3314–3320, 1989.

18. Standeven AM, Shi YE, Sinclair JF, Sinclair PR, Yager JD. Metabolism of the liver tumor promoter ethinyl estradiol by primary cultures of rat hepatocytes. Toxicol Appl Pharmacol 102:486–496, 1990.

19. Weiss DJ, Gurpide E. Non-genomic effects of estrogens and antiestrogens. J Steroid Biochem 31:671–676, 1988.

20. Kon OL. Antiestrogen binding sites in rat liver nuclei. Biochim Biophys Acta 843:245–252, 1985.

21. Sawada N, Staecker JL, Pitot HC. Effects of tumor-promoting agents 12-O-tetradecanoylphorbol-13-acetate and phenobarbital on DNA synthesis of rat hepatocytes in primary culture. Cancer Res 47:5665–5671, 1987.

22. Nishizuka Y. The role of protein kinase C in cell surface signal transduction and tumour promotion. Nature 308:693–698, 1984.

23. Meyer SA, Gibbs TA, Jirtle RA. Independent mechanisms for tumor promoters phenobarbital and 12-O-tetradecanoylphorbol-13-acetate in reduction of epidermal growth factor binding by rat hepatocytes. Cancer Res 49:5907–5912, 1989.

24. Shi YE, Yager JD. Regulation of rat hepatocyte epidermal growth factor receptor by the liver tumour promoter ethinyl estradiol. Carcinogenesis 11:1103–1109, 1990.

25. Vickers AEM, Nelson K, McCoy Z, Lucier GW. Changes in estrogen receptor, DNA ploidy, and estrogen metabolism in rat hepatocytes during a two-stage model for hepatocarcinogenesis using 17α-ethinylestradiol as the promoting agent. Cancer Res 49:6512–6520, 1989.

26. Campen DB, Sloop TC, Maronpoy RR, Lucier GW. Continued development of hepatic γ-glutamyl-transpeptidase–positive foci upon withdrawal of 17α-ethinylestradiol in diethylnitrosamine-initiated rats. Cancer Res 47:2328–2333, 1987.

27. Kohigashi K, Fukuda Y, Imura H. Inhibitory effect of tamoxifen on diethylstilbestrol-promoted hepatic tumorigenesis in male rats and its possible mechanism of action. Jpn J Cancer Res 79:1335–1339, 1988.

28. Pitot HC, Campbell HA. An approach to the determination of the relative potencies of chemical agents during the stages of initiation and promotion in multistage hepatocarcinogenesis in the rat. Environ Health Perspect 76:49–56, 1987.

29. Farber E, Sarma DSR. Hepatocarcinogenesis: A dynamic cellular perspective. Lab Invest 56:4–22, 1987.

30. Schulte-Hermann R, Ochs H, Parzefall W. Quantitative structure-activity studies on the effects of sixteen different steroids on growth and monooxygenases of rat liver. Cancer Res 48:2462–2468, 1988.

31. Yager JD Jr, Potter VR. A comparison of the effects of 3'-methyl-4-dimethylaminoazobenzene, 2-methyl-4-dimethylaminoazobenzene and 2-acetylaminofluorene on rat liver DNA stability and new synthesis. Cancer Res 35:1225–1234, 1975.

32. Maini MM, Stich HF. Chromosomes of tumor cells. II. Effects of various liver carcinogens on mitosis of hepatoma cells. J Natl Cancer Inst 26:1413–1427, 1961.

33. Kitagawa T, Pitot HC, Miller EC, Miller JA. Promotion by dietary phenobarbital of hepatocarcinogenesis by 2-methyl-N,N-dimethyl-4-aminoazobenzene in the rat. Cancer Res 39:112–115, 1979.

34. Giambarresi LI, Katyal SL, Lombardi B. Promotion of liver carcinogenesis in the rat by a choline-devoid diet: Role of liver cell necrosis and regeneration. Br J Cancer 46:825–829, 1982.

35. Goshal AK, Ahluwalia M, Farber E. The rapid induction of liver cell death in rats fed a choline-deficient methionine-low diet. Am J Pathol 113:309–314, 1983.

Chemically Induced Cell Proliferation:
Implications for Risk Assessment, pages 67-76
©1991 Wiley-Liss, Inc.

Hepatic Nuclear and Cytoplasmic Changes in Rats Following Withdrawal of Di(2-ethylhexyl)phthalate from the Diet

R. Siddika Ahmed, Dawn Chescoe, and Richard H. Hinton

The treatment of rats with agents that cause proliferation of peroxisomes also causes enlargement of the liver (1). In its early phase, this enlargement results from a burst of mitosis that begins soon after exposure to the compound; for example, the peak of S phase in rats treated with clofibrate by gavage occurs 24 hr after dosing (2). As in the livers of rats treated with agents that induce microsomal oxidases (3), this increase in DNA synthesis is associated not only with increased mitosis but also with an increased proportion of polyploid nuclei (4–6). The time course of the mitotic burst is dose dependent (7). Rapid at high doses, it becomes more prolonged as the dose is reduced. In rats fed high doses of di(2-ethylhexyl)phthalate (DEHP), there is no excess of mitoses over controls 7 days after commencement of treatment (7). In vitro studies show that, at a similar stage in rats treated with methyl clofenapate, the hepatocytes are unresponsive to epidermal growth factor (EGF) (C. Elcombe, personal communication).

Following withdrawal of peroxisome-proliferating agents from the diet, liver size, peroxisome number (1), and nuclear ploidy revert to normal (4–6). At the same time the liver again becomes responsive to peroxisome-proliferating agents (5,6) and to EGF (C. Elcombe, personal communication). Much less is known about the processes that lead to remodelling of the liver than about the initial response. We now report the results of time-course studies on remodelling of the liver following withdrawal of DEHP from the diet of rats. In view of the evidence for a link between changes in the liver and in specific plasma proteins (8,9), we have also examined how these alter on reversal.

Material and Methods

The male Wistar albino rats of the University of Surrey strain used in these experiments weighed approximately 200 g each when the experiments began. The rats received water ad libitum. Temperature in the animal rooms was controlled to $20 \pm 20°$, and they had a 12 hr light/12 hr dark cycle. DEHP was kindly donated by BP plc (Sully, Penarth). Equal numbers of rats were assigned to experimental and control groups. During withdrawal periods, control and experimental rats were fed the LAD2 diet (Labsure, Manea, Cambs, UK). During periods of compound administration, treated rats were fed diets containing 20,000 ppm DEHP mixed with the standard diet. In the main experiment described in this study, test rats were administered DEHP-containing diets for 7 days, returned to control diet for 7 days, and then readministered DEHP-containing diet for 7 days. Diet was changed and autopsies performed at approximately 11 A.M. Groups of 4 test and 4 control rats were killed on the last day of DEHP administration (day 0) and 1, 2, 3, 4, 7, and 14 days after return to control diet.

Samples for light microscopy were fixed in 10% neutral buffered formalin, dehydrated, wax-embedded, and 4-μm sections were cut and stained with hematoxylin and eosin. In addition, sections were cut at 4-μm thickness and stained with gallocyanin (10) for morphometric analysis of nuclear size and number. Samples for electron microscopy were fixed in 4% glutaraldehyde, counterfixed with 2% osmic acid, dehydrated, embedded, and the sections counterstained with alkaline lead citrate and uranyl acetate as described previously (11).

Morphometric analysis of nuclear size and number was carried out using a Quantimet 920 (Cambridge Instruments, Cambridge, UK). Only hepatocyte nuclei were recorded. Editing was partly automatic, with a program that eliminated nuclei with an area of less than 9.98 μm^2 or an axial ratio greater than 1.5, and partly manual. The program was set to record the number of nuclei per section and individual nuclear areas. Data on at least 300 nuclei per section were recorded. Following analysis, data from rats in each control and each experimental group were pooled to produce frequency diagrams for apparent nuclear size.

When serum was required, rats were bled by cardiac puncture after pentobarbital anesthesia (Sagatal, May and Baker, Dagenham, UK). Serum was separated by crossed immunoelectrophoresis against antirat serum (Dako, Copenhagen, Denmark) as described previously (8).

Results

In rats fed diets containing DEHP, cell number increased rapidly in the liver, the peak of mitosis occurring 3 days after the animals were first offered the DEHP-containing diets. Serum concentrations of α-1 glycoprotein associated with chemically induced liver cell division expanded in parallel with the number of mitotic figures in the liver, and by 7 days after commencement of feeding, the decline in major serum glycoproteins observed in previous experiments (8) occurred here as well.

When rats were alternately fed a diet containing DEHP for 7 days, and control diet for 7 days, hepatic cell number, nuclear ploidy, and peroxisome number cycled, being elevated in rats receiving DEHP and returning to near control levels at the end of each withdrawal period (see ref. 6 for details). Rats refed after a period of withdrawal showed a more rapid increase in liver weight than rats not previously exposed to DEHP.

In a further experiment, we observed the changes that follow return to control diet of animals subjected to two cycles of DEHP feeding. At the start of the study (day 0), the livers of DEHP-treated animals showed typical changes. Gross examination showed liver enlargement (Fig. 1). Histologic examination showed generalized loss of glycogen, electron-microscopic examination showed proliferation of peroxisomes (Fig. 2A), and morphometric analysis revealed a marked increase in polyploid nuclei (Fig. 3A). One day after the animals returned to control diet, the weight of their livers was higher than on the previous day (Fig. 1), and histologic examination showed amounts of glycogen similar to that in control animals. Morphometric analysis showed a reduced number of nuclei per unit area of liver (Fig. 4, top) but an increase in the total number of nuclei in the liver as a whole (Fig. 4, bottom). There was less difference in nuclear area between test and control rats than observed on the previous day. Electron microscopic examination showed slight autophagic activity.

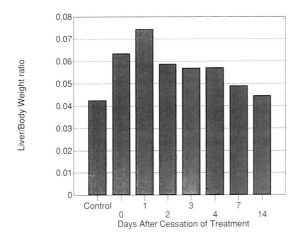

Figure 1. Changes in the liver/ body weight ratio of rats following withdrawal of DEHP from the diet. The rats had previously been fed diets containing 20,000 ppm of DEHP for 7 days, returned to control diet for 7 days, and finally been refed DEHP for another 7 days. Four rats were examined at each time point. Day 0 refers to animals examined on the final day of DEHP administration.

Although, on the first day after DEHP withdrawal from the diet, liver alterations seemed idiosyncratic, and a gradual reversion to the control state followed. Liver weight and liver cell number fell sharply on the second and third days and then more slowly, returning to control values by 14 days. The number of nuclei per unit area of liver, and hence liver cell size, returned to control values 4 days after withdrawal (Fig. 4). Similarly, the apparent differences in area of hepatocyte nuclei between test and controls animals gradually diminished with time (Fig. 3).

Electron microscopic examination showed changes in peroxisomes, autophagosomes, and the endoplasmic reticulum (Fig. 2). Visual assessment indicated a decrease in peroxisome number beginning 2 days after withdrawal of DEHP from the diet. As mentioned earlier, some autophagic activity was apparent 1 day after withdrawal. This increased over the next 2 days, peaking on day 3 after withdrawal. Some autophagosomes were still present on day 4, but by days 7 and 14 the numbers were the same as in controls. An increase in stacks of rough endoplasmic reticulum, noted 2 days after withdrawal of DEHP from the diets, expanded on days 3 and 4. At this stage, the cisternae were markedly dilated (Fig. 2C). On day 7, the stacks of rough endoplasmic reticulum were still visible but the cisternae were condensed (Fig. 2D). By day 14, the stacks had disappeared and the livers had resumed a normal appearance.

Apoptotic figures were difficult to identify with the light microscope, but the electron microscope clearly showed dying cells being sloughed into the space of Disse 3 and 4 days after DEHP was withdrawn from the diet (Fig. 5). Serum proteins were only studied 7 days after DEHP withdrawal, by which time the normal pattern had been restored.

Discussion

The development of hepatic changes in rats treated with DEHP have been described elsewhere (6). In rats previously exposed to DEHP, changes develop more rapidly than in previously unexposed animals, but neither liver weight nor peroxisomal

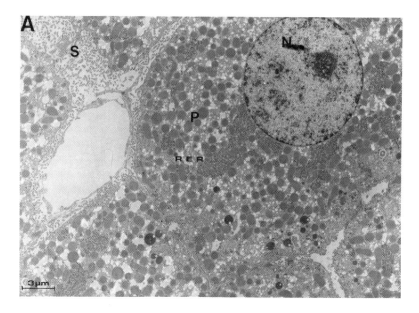

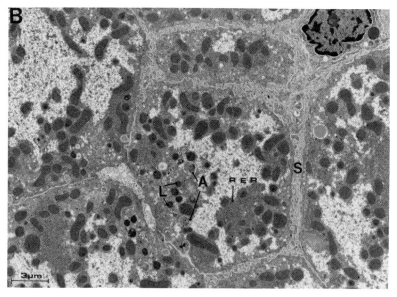

Figure 2. Electron micrographs of the livers of rats at various times after withdrawal of DEHP from the diet. Treatment schedule was as described in legend to Figure 1. Bar on micrographs represents 3 μm. (A) Day 0, shows marked proliferation of peroxisomes; (B) day 3, shows increase in autophagosomes and lysosomes; (C) day 4, shows increase in stacks of rough endoplasmic

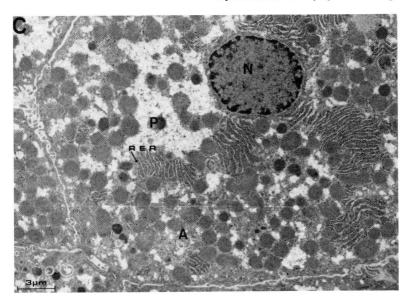

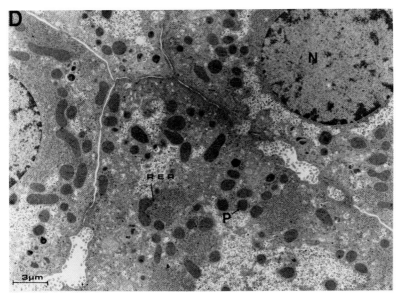

reticulum with dilated cisternae; (D) day 7, shows return to "normal" morphology, although some stacks of inactive rough endoplasmic reticulum remain. Abbreviations: A, autophagosome; N, nucleus; L, lysosome; P, peroxisome; RER, rough endoplasmic reticulum; S, sinusoid.

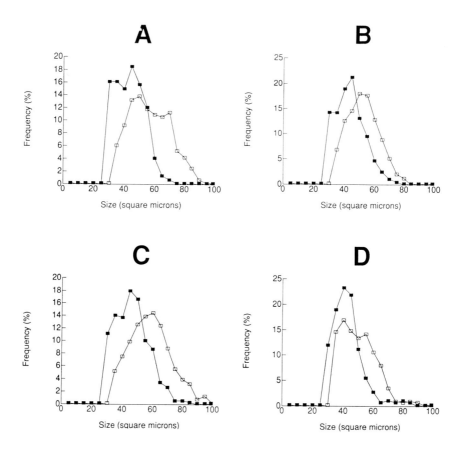

enzyme activities (6) had returned completely to control values in the seven-day withdrawal period employed in the present experiment.

Changes following withdrawal of DEHP from the diet seem to occur in at least two stages. During the first 24 hr, an increase in liver weight is accompanied by an apparent increase in liver cell size. These changes are almost certainly explicable by the observed accumulation of glycogen in the livers, for in DEHP-fed animals glycogen accounts for more than 10% of liver weight. The apparent increase in the total number of nuclei in the liver was not statistically significant, and, as the volume of the liver was estimated from its weight, the increase could have been influenced by the fact (12) that glycogen is considerably more dense than other liver components.

When the liver remodels after withdrawal of an inducing agent, there is no clear

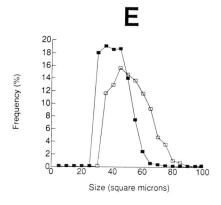

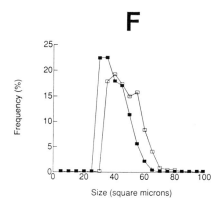

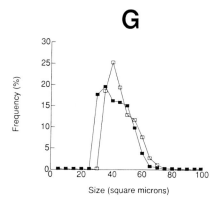

Figure 3. Changes in nuclear size of hepatocytes following withdrawal of DEHP from the diet. Previous treatment of the animals was as described in legend to Figure 1. Plots show frequency distribution of nuclear area as measured by a Quantimet 920 image analyzer set with a lower detect limit of 30 μm^2 and a step size of 5 μm^2. In each part of the figure, lines with empty symbols show mean distribution from at least 3 test animals; lines with solid symbols show results from at least 3 age-matched controls never exposed to DEHP. Different parts of figure refer to animals examined at these times after withdrawal: opposite page, (A) day 0, last day of DEHP administration; (B) day 1; (C) day 2; (D) day 3; this page, (E) day 4; (F) day 7; (G) day 14.

agreement on whether cell loss involves selective loss of cells that proliferated in the initial hyperplastic response. The available information (4) suggests that polyploid cells form by division of a specific group of precursors, so that the fall in ploidy as the liver remodels points to a specific removal of the polyploid cells. It is also possible, however, that the increase in ploidy is caused by a block in G_2 of cells that have passed through S phase immediately before the liver reached its "target" size. Withdrawal of the compound, according to this hypothesis, would lead to a round of mitosis followed by a decrease in cell number. This second model predicts, however, that ploidy would decrease faster than nuclear number. But our results showed that nuclear size falls slowly, and they support the hypothesis, although they do not prove it, that there is a specific removal of polyploid cells.

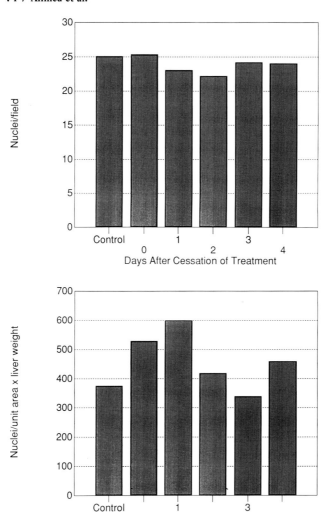

Figure 4. Top, Number of hepatocyte nuclei per unit area of liver, and bottom, number of nuclei per unit area of liver multiplied by liver weight (which provides an estimate of the total number of nuclei in the liver). Liver slides were analyzed using the Quantimet 920 as described in legend to Figure 3. Number of nuclei in at least 10 areas of liver section was counted. Results are average of at least 3 animals in the case of tests. No variation was observed among groups of control animals killed at various time points, and, accordingly, a mean value of the 3 animals examined at each time point is presented.

Morphologic studies of the liver during remodelling suggest that, as in the initial hyperplasia, changes are greatest three to four days after the change in dietary composition. At that time, we found both the greatest evidence for autophagic activity in the hepatocytes and the greatest evidence for loss of liver cells. In addition, we found at that time a marked burst of synthesis of secretory proteins, as indicated by changes in the rough endoplasmic reticulum, which coincided with restoration to normal levels of certain serum glycoproteins. Our study suggests, therefore, that in the same way that

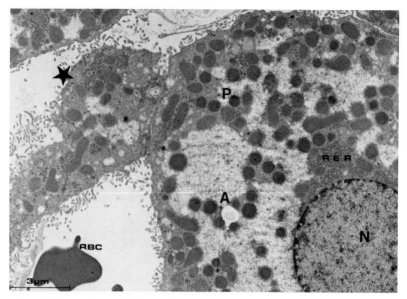

Figure 5. Electron micrograph of liver of a test animal 4 days after withdrawal of DEHP from the diet showing a cell apparently sloughing into the space of Disse. For details on previous treatment see the legend to Figure 2. Symbol: *, damaged cell apparently detaching from neighbors. Abbreviations as in Figure 2.

administration of a stimulus is followed by intracellular changes such as peroxisome proliferation in parallel with cell division, withdrawal of the stimulus brings on intracellular remodelling and removal of excess cells proceeding in parallel.

Acknowledgments

We thank Professor P. Grasso and Dr. S. C. Price for introducing us to the problem of ploidy changes during treatment with carcinogens and for many useful discussions. We also thank Mrs. J. Mullervey for preparation of material for electron microscopy. R.S.A. thanks the Science Research Council for a Graduate Studentship.

References

1. Reddy JK, Lalwani ND. Carcinogenesis by hepatic peroxisome proliferation. Evaluation of the risk of hypolipidaemic drugs and industrial plasticisers to humans. CRC Crit Rev Toxicol 12:1–58, 1984.
2. Seifert J, Mostecka H. Effect of clofibrate on DNA synthesis in rat liver and kidney. Arch Toxicol 60:131–132, 1987.
3. Schulte-Hermann R. Induction of liver growth by xenobiotic compounds and other stimuli. CRC Crit Rev Toxicol 3:97–158, 1974.
4. Styles JA, Kelly M, Elcombe CR. A cytological comparison between regeneration, hyperplasia and early neoplasms in the art. Carcinogenesis 8:391–399, 1987.

5. Ahmed RS, Price SC, Grasso P, Hinton RH. Effects of intermittent feeding of rats with di(2-ethylhexyl)phthalate. Biochem Soc Trans 17:1073–1074, 1989.
6. Ahmed RS, Price SC, Grasso P, Hinton RH. Hepatic nuclear and cytoplasmic effects following intermittent feeding of rats with DEHP. Food Chem Toxicol 28; 6:427–434, 1990.
7. Mitchell FE, Price SC, Hinton RH, Grasso P, Bridges JW. Time and dose response study on rats of the plasticiser di(2-ethylhexyl)phthalate. Toxicol Appl Pharmacol 81:371–392, 1985.
8. Hinton RH, Price SC, Mitchell FE, Mann A, Hall DE, Bridges JW. Plasma protein changes in rats treated with hypolipidaemic drugs and with phthalate esters. Hum Toxicol 4:261–271, 1985.
9. Makarananda K, Fox GA, Price SC, Hinton RH. Changes in plasma proteins in rats treated for short periods with hepatotoxins or with agents which induce cytochrome P450 isoenzymes. Hum Toxicol 6:121–126, 1987.
10. Bancroft JD, Stevens A. Theory and Practice of Histological Techniques, ed. 2. London: Churchill-Livingstone, 1982.
11. Mann AH, Price SC, Mitchell FE, Grasso P, Hinton RH, Bridges JW. Comparison of the short-term effects of di(2-ethylhexyl)phthalate, di(N-hexyl)phthalate, and di(N-octyl)phthalate in rats. Toxicol Appl Pharmacol 77:116–132.
12. Leighton F, Lopez F, Zemelman V, Morales MN, Walsen O. Cytoplasmic gradient subcellular fractionation. In Reid E (ed): Membranous Elements and the Movement of Molecules. Chichester: Ellis Horwood, 1977, pp. 197–216.

Chemically Induced Cell Proliferation:
Implications for Risk Assessment, pages 77-89
©1991 Wiley-Liss, Inc.

Hepatic Peroxisome Proliferators Induce Morphologic Transformation of Syrian Hamster Embryo Cells, But Not Peroxisomal β Oxidation

Tore Sanner, Svein-Ole Mikalsen and Edgar Rivedal

Hepatic peroxisome proliferators (HPP) are identified on the basis of their proliferative effect on peroxisomes in rodent (especially rat) liver. They are in general hepatocarcinogens in mice and rats (1–3) but have in most cases been reported to lack genotoxic activity (4–11). HPP include hypolipidemic drugs (1,12), industrial plasticizers (13,14), herbicides (15,16), and several other important substances (17,18).

Concurrently with increasing the number of peroxisomes, the HPP also induce increased activity of several enzymes, of which some are specific for the peroxisomes. Of special interest is the peroxisomal β oxidation of fatty acids, which increases fatty-acid degradating activity severalfold (up to 30–fold has been reported) (19,20). The first enzyme of peroxisomal β oxidation, the fatty acyl-CoA oxidase (FAO), generates H_2O_2 as an obligatory by-product (21). At the same time catalase, which is also peroxisome-associated, is only increased twofold or less (19,20), and the level of selenium-dependent glutathione peroxidase (cytosolic) may even decrease (22,23). Thus, the production of H_2O_2 could greatly increase during the HPP response, and the proposal is that HPP-mediated hepatocarcinogenesis is caused by oxidative stress resulting from perturbed balance of H_2O_2 production and destruction (1,24).

The oxidative stress hypothesis was supported by an increased level of lipid peroxidation found in HPP-treated rat liver (23,25), along with enhanced accumulation of lipofuscin (24). An increased steady-state level of H_2O_2 was found in liver homogenates from treated rats (26). Purified peroxisomes from HPP-treated rats caused single-strand breaks in SV40 supercoiled DNA concomitant with a 30- to 70-fold increase in H_2O_2 generation when a substrate for the peroxisomal β oxidation was provided (27). Recently, an increased level of 8-hydroxydeoxyguanosine was found in liver DNA from HPP-treated rats (28).

Cell transformation assays are generally regarded as the in vitro tests with closest resemblance to the early steps of chemical carcinogenesis in vivo. In contrast to most short-term tests, cell transformation assays may also respond to nonmutagenic agents like asbestos (29), diethylstilbestrol (30), and tumor-promoting phorbol esters (31). Di(2-ethylhexyl)phthalate (DEHP) has been found to induce morphologic transformation of Syrian hamster embryo (SHE) cells in vitro (32,33) and the HPP clofibrate and niadenate showed a promoterlike activity in the C3H/10T1/2 cell transformation assay (34). To gain further insight to the mechanism of HPP carcinogenesis, we have in the present work studied the effect of several HPP on morphologic transformation and biochemical markers in SHE cells.

Materials and methods

Chemicals

Clofibrate; 2,4-dichlorophenoxyacetic acid (2,4-D); 2,4,5-trichlorophenoxyacetic acid (2,4,5-T); digitonin; and 12-O-tetradecanoyl phorbol-13-acetate (TPA) were obtained from Sigma. DEHP was from Aldrich, mono(2-ethylhexyl)phthalate (MEHP) from Tokyo Kasei Kogyo, and $NiSO_4 \times 6 H_2O$ was purchased from Merck. Tiadenol was a gift from Dr. R. K. Berge, University of Bergen, Norway. Nickel sulphate was dissolved in water and all other chemicals in dimethylsulfoxide (DMSO).

Cell cultures and transformation assay

Primary cell cultures of SHE were prepared and cryopreserved in liquid nitrogen as described by Pienta et al. (35). Of special relevance to this study is that the embryos were eviscerated before trypsinization of the carcasses. Ampoules with cryopreserved cells were used as stock cultures for the transformation assays. The cells were grown in Dulbecco's modification of Eagle's medium (DMEM) supplemented with 14% fetal bovine serum (FBS), 2 µg/ml of insulin, and 2.2 g/l of $NaHCO_3$ at 37°C in a 10% CO_2 atmosphere. No antibiotics were used. For the transformation assay (31,32) a feeder layer of 4.5×10^4 X-irradiated cells (4500 rad) were seeded in 60-mm Petri dishes. The next day, 200 target cells were seeded on the feeder layer. Twenty-four hours later, the cells were exposed to chemicals. Five days later, the medium was removed and fresh medium with chemicals added. After a total of 7 days of exposure, the dishes were fixed in methanol and stained with Giemsa before the morphologic transformation was scored and the colonies counted. Morphologic transformation is defined as an altered colony morphology consisting of extensive crisscrossing of the cells, especially in the periphery of the colonies. Morphologic transformation is expressed as the percentage of transformed colonies relative to the total number of colonies in the same series.

For the enzyme measurements, the cells were grown in 100-mm Petri dishes for the indicated number of days. The number of cells were varied in such a way that the dishes were approximately confluent when the cells were harvested. The cells were exposed 24 hr after seeding. At harvesting, the cells were trypsinized, centrifuged, and washed twice before homogenization by sonication. The homogenates were stored at -70°C.

Enzyme assays

Catalase was measured by the titan oxysulphate method (36); peroxisomal H_2O_2-generating oxidases by the 2′,7′-dichlorofluorescin/peroxidase method (37); peroxisomal β oxidation by the radioactive method of Lazarow (38), including 1 mM KCN in the assay; the glucose-6-phosphatase assay was modified from Leighton et al. (39) using 80 mM glucose-6-phosphate in 0.1 M acetate buffer, pH 6.5; palmitoyl-CoA hydrolase was measured using 5,5′-dithio-dis-(2-nitrobenzoic acid) (40). Dihydroxy-acetonephosphate acyltransferase (41,42), acid phosphatase (43), and malate dehydrogenase (44) were measured as described.

Digitonin titration studies of the various enzymes were performed on cells directly from harvesting, without homogenization and without Triton X-100 in the assays, except when maximum activities were determined (46,47).

Protein was determined using the Bio-Rad protein assay kit, with bovine gamma globulin as standard protein.

Results

Enzyme activities in unexposed cells

The activities of several peroxisome-associated enzymes were measured in SHE cells and compared to the activities in rat hepatocytes. The specific activities (Table 1) were, in general, at least one order of magnitude lower in SHE cells than in rat hepatocytes. In particular, several of the H_2O_2-generating peroxisomal oxidases were not detectable. The activity of the peroxisomal β oxidation cycle, which is often used as a biochemical marker of peroxisome proliferation, was more than 100-fold lower in SHE cells than in rat hepatocytes (measured by the liberation of acetyl-CoA).

The peroxisomal β oxidation cycle consists of three stages: 1) FAO, which generates H_2O_2 and can be measured by peroxidase-coupled assays; 2) bifunctional enoyl-CoA hydratase/3-hydroxyacyl-CoA dehydrogenase which can be measured by NAD^+ reduction; and 3) thiolase, which can be measured by liberation of labeled acetyl-CoA (when provided with labeled fatty acyl-CoA, this can be taken as the activity of the cycle). The data in Table 1 show that the first enzyme of the cycle, FAO, had a specific activity about 10 times that of the total cycle in SHE cells. In contrast, it is assumed that FAO is the rate-limiting step of the peroxisomal β oxidation in rat liver (47).

The specific activity of catalase was very low in the SHE cells compared to rat hepatocytes, and the low catalase content in SHE cells was also confirmed by western blotting. Information on the compartmentation of different marker enzymes was obtained by digitonin titration of freshly harvested cells, a method that also indicates

Table 1. Specific enzyme activities.[a]

Enzyme	SHE cells	Rat liver
Catalase[b]	0.24	90.0
Peroxisomal β oxidation[cd]	0.025	3.80
Fatty acyl-CoA oxidase[ce]	0.30	3.25
D-amino acid oxidase[ce]	ND[f]	2.0
Glycolate acid oxidase[ce]	ND	6.0
Urate oxidase[ce]	ND	5.0
Dihydroxy acetonephosphate acyltransferase[c]	0.030	0.085

[a] In part from Mikalsen et al. (65), with permission
[b] μmol/min/mg protein
[c] nmol/min/mg protein
[d] Measured by the formation of acetyl-CoA from palmitoyl-CoA
[e] Measured by peroxidase/dichlorofluorescin assay
[f] Not detected

whether the cells have a peroxisomal compartment. The low digitonin sensitivity of catalase is consistent with sequestration in peroxisomes and shows that catalase is not a cytosolic enzyme in SHE cells (Fig. 1).

In contrast to the results mentioned above, we found that the activity of the peroxisome-associated enzyme, dihydroxyacetonephosphate acyltransferase was only slightly lower in SHE cells than in rat liver.

Morphologic cell transformation and catalase activity

In agreement with previous results in the SHE transformation assay (32,33), DEHP induced morphologic transformation (Fig. 2). Morphologic cell transformation was also induced by the HPP MEHP, the primary metabolite of DEHP (Fig. 2), clofibrate, and tiadenol (Fig. 3). These HPP also induced dose-dependent increases in catalase activity, which might indicate peroxisome proliferation.

To learn whether increased catalase activity is a general characteristic that correlates with increased frequency of morphologic cell transformation, we determined the two parameters for the tumor promoter TPA and for nickel sulphate. TPA was more potent than any of the other chemicals studied in inducing morphologic transformation, but there was no comparable increase in catalase activity (Fig. 4). Nickel sulphate also induced morphologic transformation of SHE cells without any appreciable increase in catalase activity (Fig. 4). Thus, the increase in catalase activity is not in general correlated with morphologic cell transformation.

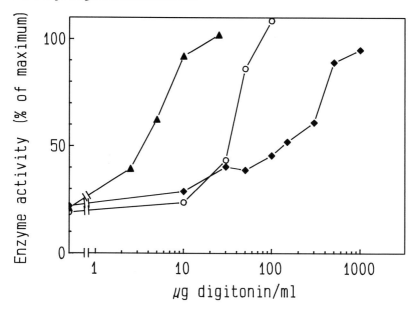

Figure 1. Digitonin latency of marker enzymes in SHE cells. (♦) Catalase, (o) acid phophatase, (▲) lactate dehydrogenase. In part from Mikalsen et al. (65), with permission.

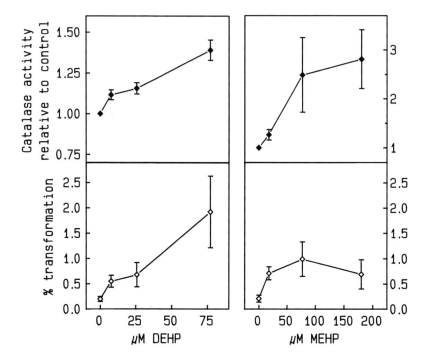

Figure 2. Effect of DEHP and MEHP on morphologic transformation (lower panels) and on relative catalase activity (upper panels). From Mikalsen et al. (66), with permission.

The two HPP, 2,4-D and 2,4,5-T, did not induce morphologic transformation of SHE cells, but 2,4,5-T did increase catalase activity in a dose-dependent manner (Fig. 5). These data suggested that an increase in catalase activity per se is unrelated to induction of morphologic transformation.

Effects on lipid-metabolizing enzymes

Since the specific activity of FAO in SHE cells was about 10-fold higher than the specific activity of the whole peroxisomal β oxidation cycle, the bifunctional enzyme or the thiolase must be the rate-limiting steps. We were not able to measure any activity of the bifunctional enzyme, either in control cells or in cells exposed to 206 μM clofibrate up to 6 days. This assay is less sensitive, however, than assays for the other enzymes in the cycle. When the cells were exposed to clofibrate (206 μM), DEHP (77 μM), or MEHP (77 μM) for 1 to 6 days, both the relative activity of FAO and of the peroxisomal β oxidation cycle, measured by liberating labeled acetyl-CoA, were between 80–180% of control (Table 2). Thus, the peroxisomal β oxidation cycle did not increase its activity, or it did so only to the same extent as catalase.

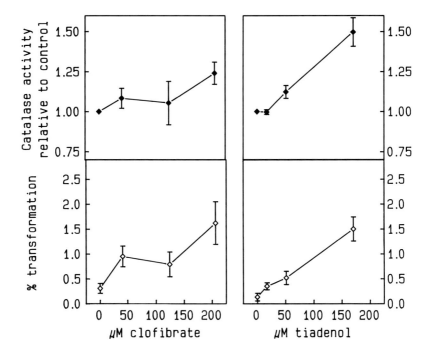

Figure 3. Effect of clofibrate and tiadenol on morphologic transformation (lower panels) and on relative catalase activity (upper panels). From Mikalsen et al. (66), with permission.

Table 2. Effects of DEHP, MEHP, and Clofibrate on the Relative Enzyme Activities in SHE Cells After 3 and 6 Days of Exposure.[a]

	Days	Peroxisomal β oxidation	FAO
Clofibrate	3	1.03 ± 0.23	1.43, 1.57
(206 µM)	6	0.94 ± 0.11	0.88, 1.68
DEHP	3	1.78 ± 0.55	1.35, 1.26
(77 µM)	6	1.74 ± 0.38	1.04, 1.77
MEHP	3	1.11, 0.71	1.06, 1.79
(77 µM)	6	1.00, 1.90	1.17, 1.32

[a]In part from Mikalsen et al. (65), with permission.

It is possible that the observed low peroxisomal β oxidation was caused by substrate depletion by palmitoyl-CoA hydrolase. Although the activity of palmitoyl-CoA hydrolase was disproportionally high in SHE cells (ratio of palmitoyl-CoA hydrolase to peroxisomal β oxidation 76:1, in rat liver 3:1), it was not found to have any adverse effect

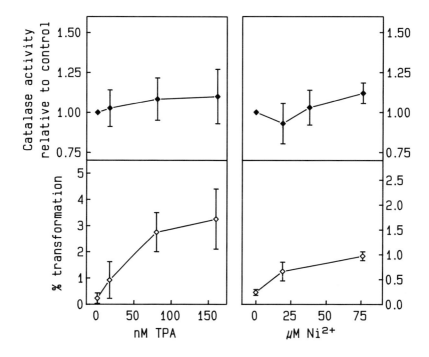

Figure 4. Effect of TPA and nickel sulphate (Ni²⁺) on morphologic transformation (lower panels) and on relative catalase activity (upper panels). From Mikalsen et al. (66), with permission.

on the peroxisomal β oxidation assay (not shown). Hydrolase was affected by HPP to the same extent as was peroxisomal β oxidation (between 90 and 170 % of control).

Marker enzymes for other organelles (not shown) did not change or changed only marginally in cells exposed to HPP (acid phosphatase, 80–105% of control; glucose-6-phosphatase, 80–110% of control). Malate dehydrogenase was slightly affected (95–170% of control), and the largest increase was found for DEHP.

In parallel with the investigations of SHE cells, we also studied rat embryo cells because rats are more sensitive to the effects of HPP than hamsters (14,48). The results in rat embryo cells were similar to those found in SHE cells. In particular, peroxisomal β oxidation did not increase more in rat embryo cells than in SHE cells (not shown).

Discussion

Several HPP were found to induce morphologic transformation of SHE cells in vitro at concentrations that may be of physiologic relevance. Thus, the therapeutic plasma concentration of clofibrate is around 50 μM (49). At that concentration, clofibrate induced an increased number of morphologically transformed colonies of SHE cells. In

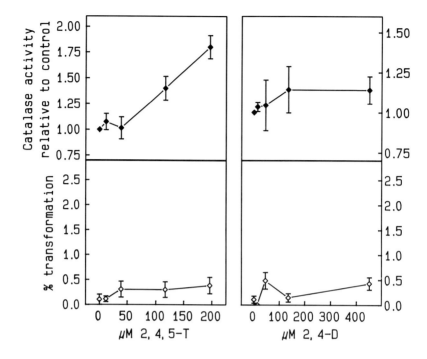

Figure 5. Effect of 2,4-D and 2,4,5-T on morphologic transformation (lower panels) and on relative catalase activity (upper panels). From Mikalsen et al. (66), with permission.

blood products stored in polyvinyl chloride plastic bags with DEHP as a plasticizer, DEHP has been found in concentrations exceeding the highest level used in the present work (50), and in the blood of transfusion patients MEHP concentrations up to 50 μM have been measured (51). Concentrations of less than 50 μM MEHP induced morphologic transformation. On the other hand, when peroxisome proliferation was studied in cultured hepatocytes (52,53), the concentrations exceeded those used in our study.

Most in vitro assays for carcinogens are based on the detection of genotoxicity. HPP generally do not yield any response in such assays (4–11). In cell transformation assays, however, several research groups have found positive results for chemicals belonging to the HPP group, although the results have not always been consistent. As can be seen in Table 3, the HPP tested in the C3H/10T1/2 transformation assay tend to be more active as promoterlike substances than as direct transforming agents. This could be due to the exposure protocol of this assay. When the complete transforming activity is tested, the cells are exposed for 24 hr, followed by a 6-week period of "recovery," which allows the transformation to be expressed. When tested for promoterlike activities, the exposure period lasts for several weeks after a 24-hr exposure to an

Table 3. Summary of results for morphological cell transformation by HPPs.

Chemical	Maximum concentration	Assay	Response	Reference
Clofibrate	206 µM	SHE[a]	++[c]	Present
	20 µM	C3H[b]	++[d]	34
DEHP	77 µM	SHE	++	Present
	768 µM	SHE	++	32
	256 µM	SHE	++	33
	2560 mM	C3H	+	54
	10 µM	C3H	-	55
MEHP	180 µM	SHE	++	Present
	100 µM	C3H	-	55
Tiadenol	170 µM	SHE	++	Present
	5 µM	C3H	-	34
Niadenate	20 µM	C3H	++[d]	34
2,4-D	450 µM	SHE	-	Present
2,4,5-T	195 mM	SHE	-	Present

[a] SHE, Syrian hamster cell transformation assay
[b] C3H, C3H/10T1/2 cell transformation assay
[c] -, negative response; +, weak positive response; ++, positive response
[d] Active only as promoterlike substance

initiating agent (e.g., 20-methylcholanthrene). In contrast, in the SHE cell transformation assay, the chemicals are present during the whole assay period of 7 days when tested for complete transforming activity. Since HPP are nonmutagenic, they might need a prolonged time period for "fixation" of the transformation. Thus, an "initiation-protocol" might not be sufficient for morphologic transformation of the C3H/10T1/2 cells.

In vivo the peroxisome proliferation might be largely liver-specific. A low level of peroxisome proliferation may take place in the kidney, small intestines, and heart (56,57), but there are no indications of peroxisome proliferation in most other extrahepatic tissues (3,57). In vitro there are biochemical indications for peroxisome proliferation in C3H/10T1/2 cells (58) and ciliary epithelial cells from bovine eye (59), and morphologic indications in keratinocytes (60). All HPP that induced morphological transformation of SHE cells also enhanced catalase activity, which could indicate peroxisome proliferation. However, the results from measurements of peroxisomal β oxidation do not support this notion, because only very modest increases were found. The finding that the other peroxisomal oxidases studied had nondetectable activities suggests that the observed morphologic transformation of SHE cells caused by HPP exposure is not an effect of peroxisome-generated oxidative stress.

In recent years, the oxidative hypothesis for HPP-induced carcinogenicity has been challenged. When rats where administered DEHP and Wy-14643 ([4-chloro-6-(2,3-xylidino)-2-pyrimidinylthio]acetic acid) at doses producing the same level of peroxisome proliferation (morphometrically and biochemically), only rats on the Wy-14,643 diet developed cancerous lesions in the liver (61). The malignant development correlated with a persistent increase in replicative DNA synthesis, consistent with previous observations (11). Ciprofibrate treatment did not, however, produce a good correlation between cell proliferation and premalignant lesions in the liver (62). Exposed to nafenopin, cultured marmoset hepatocytes showed stimulation of DNA synthesis but not peroxisomal β oxidation (63). The recent evidence for an increased level of 8-hydroxydeoxyguanosine in liver DNA from rats treated with ciprofibrate (28) seems strongly in favor of the oxidative hypothesis. However, HPP also induce proliferation of mitochondria. The total number of 8-hydroxydeoxyguanosine in mitochondrial DNA is 41,000 compared to 140,000 in nuclear DNA of an untreated rat hepatocyte (64). A mitochondrial proliferation could strongly affect the total level of 8-hydroxydeoxyguanosine in DNA without changing its level in nuclear DNA. Thus, the possibility that some HPP might induce tumors by mechanisms not involving peroxisome proliferation and oxidative stress should be considered.

Conclusions

The HPP clofibrate, DEHP, MEHP, and tiadenol induced morphologic transformation of SHE cells. Addition of these HPP to the culture medium also enhanced catalase activity by 40–60%, an enhancement similar to the increase found in rodent liver after the animals were fed HPP. Other nongenotoxic chemicals that induce morphologic transformation failed to enhance catalase activity. Catalase was shown by digitonin titration to be contained in a peroxisomelike compartment in SHE cells. Specific activities of both catalase and peroxisomal β oxidation were about 100-fold lower in SHE cells than in rat hepatocytes. Peroxisomal β oxidation did not increase or increased only very slightly when HPP were added to the culture medium. The HPP's lack of influence on peroxisomal β oxidation argues against the participation of peroxisome proliferation in the induction of morphologic transformation of SHE cells by HPP.

Acknowledgments

This work is supported by the Norwegian Cancer Society in which Svein-Ole Mikalsen is a research fellow. We thank R. K. Berge and N. Aarsaether, University of Bergen, Norway, for doing the NAD+ reduction assay of peroxisomal β oxidation.

References

1. Reddy JK, Azarnoff DL, Hignite CE. Hypolipidaemic hepatic peroxisome proliferators form a novel class of chemical carcinogens. Nature 283:397–398, 1980.
2. Reddy JK, Lalwani ND. Carcinogenesis by hepatic peroxisome proliferators: Evaluation of the risk of hypolipidemic drugs and industrial plasticizers to humans. CRC Crit Rev Toxicol 12:1–58, 1983.
3. Rao MS, Reddy JK. Peroxisome proliferation and hepatocarcinogenesis. Carcinogenesis 8:631–636, 1987.
4. Warren JR Simmon VF, Reddy JK. Properties of hypolipidemic peroxisome proliferators in the lymphocyte [3H]thymidine and Salmonella mutagenesis assay. Cancer Res 40:36–41, 1980.
5. Schmezer P, Pool BI, Klein RG, Komotowski D, Schmal D. Various short-term assays and two long-term studies with the plasticizer di(2-ethylhexyl)phthalate in the Syrian golden hamster. Carcinogenesis 9:37–43, 1988.
6. Albro PW, Corbett JT, Schroeder JL, Jordan ST. Incorporation of radioactivity form labelled di(2-ethylhexyl)phthalate into DNA of rat liver in vivo. Chem Biol Interact 44:1–16, 1983.
7. von Däniken A, Lutz WK, Jackh R, Schlätter C. Investigation of the potential for binding of di(2-

ethylhexyl)phthalate (DEHP) and di(2-ethylhexyl)adipate (DEHA) to liver DNA in vivo. Toxicol Appl Pharmacol 73:373–387, 1984.

8. Gupta RC, Goel SK, Earley K, Singh B, Reddy JK. 32P-Postlabeling analysis of peroxisome proliferator-DNA adduct formation in rat liver in vivo and hepatocytes in vitro. Carcinogenesis 6:933–936, 1985.

9. Cattley RC, Richardson K, Smith-Oliver T, Popp JA, Butterworth BE. Effect of peroxisome proliferator carcinogens on unscheduled DNA synthesis in rat hepatocytes determined by autoradiography. Cancer Lett 33:269–277, 1986.

10. Cattley RC, Smith-Oliver T, Butterworth BE, Popp JA. Failure of peroxisome proliferator WY-14,643 to induce unscheduled DNA synthesis in rat hepatocytes following in vivo treatment. Carcinogenesis 9:1179–1183, 1988.

11. Smith-Oliver T, Butterworth BE. Correlation of the carcinogenic potential of di(2-ethylhexyl)phthalate (DEHP) with induced hyperplasia rather than with genotoxic activity. Mutat Res 188:21–28, 1987.

12. Hess R, Stäubli W, Riess W. Nature of hepatomegalic effect produced by ethyl-chlorophenoxy-isobutyrate in the rat. Nature 208:856–858, 1965.

13. Warren JR, Lalwani ND, Reddy JK. Phthalate esters as peroxisome proliferator carcinogens. Environ Health Perspect 45:35–40, 1982.

14. Lake BG, Gray TJB, Foster JR, Stubberfield CR, Gangolli SD. Comparative studies on di(2-ethylhexyl)phthalate induced hepatic peroxisome proliferation in rat and hamster. Toxicol Appl Pharmacol 72:46–60, 1984.

15. Vainio H, Nickels J, Linnainmaa K. Phenoxy acid herbicides cause peroxisome proliferation in Chinese hamsters. Scand J Work Environ Health 8:70–73, 1982.

16. Vainio H, Linnainmaa K, Kähönen M, Nickels J, Hietanen E, Marniemi J, Peltonen P. Hypolipidemia and peroxisome proliferation induced by phenoxyacetic acid herbicides in rats. Biochem Pharmacol 32:2775–2779, 1983.

17. Goldsworthy TL, Popp JA. Chlorinated hydrocarbon-induced peroxisomal enzyme activity in relation to species and organ carcinogenicity. Toxicol Appl Pharmacol 1987; 88:225–233.

18. Hruban Z, Swift H, Slesers A. Ultrastructural alterations of hepatic microbodies. Lab Invest 15:1884–1901, 1966.

19. Osumi T, Hashimoto T. Enhancement of fatty acyl-CoA oxidizing activity in rat liver peroxisomes by di(2-ethylhexyl)phthalate. J Biochem 83:1361–1365, 1978.

20. Osumi T, Hashimoto T. The inducible fatty acid oxidation system in mammalian peroxisomes. Trends in Biochemical Science 9:317–319, 1984.

21. Lazarow PB, de Duve C. A fatty acyl-CoA oxidizing system in rat liver peroxisomes; enhancement by clofibrate, a hypolipidemic drug. Proc Natl Acad Sci USA 73:2043–2046, 1976.

22. Conway JG, Tomaszewski KE, Olson MJ, Cattley RC, Marsman DS, Popp JA. Relationship of oxidative damage to hepatocarcinogenicity of the peroxisome proliferators di(2-ethylhexyl)phthalate and Wy-14,643. Carcinogenesis 10:513–519, 1989.

23. Lake BG, Kozlen SL, Evans JG, Gray TJB, Young PJ, Gangolli SD. Effect of prolonged administration of clofibric acid and di(2-ethylhexyl)phthalate on hepatic enzyme activities and lipid peroxidation in the rat. Toxicology 44:213–228, 1987.

24. Reddy JK, Lalwani ND, Reddy MK, Qureshi SA. Excessive accumulation of autofluorescent lipofuscin in the liver during hepatocarcinogenesis by methyl clofenapate and other hypolipidemic peroxisome proliferators. Cancer Res 42:259–266, 1982.

25. Goel SK, Lalwani ND, Reddy JK. Peroxisome proliferation and lipid peroxidation in rat liver. Cancer Res 46:1324–1330, 1986.

26. Tomaszewski KE, Agarwal DK, Melnick RL. In vitro steady state levels of hydrogen peroxide after exposure of male F344 rats and female B6C3F1 mice to hepatic peroxisome proliferators. Carcinogenesis 7:1871–1876, 1986.

27. Fahl WE, Lalwani ND, Watanabe T, Goel SK, Reddy JK. DNA damage related to increased hydrogen peroxide generation by hypolipidemic drug-induced liver peroxisomes. Proc Natl Acad Sci USA 81:7827–7830, 1984.

28. Kasai H, Okada Y, Rao MS, Reddy JK. Formation of 8-hydroxydeoxyguanosine in liver DNA of rats following long-term exposure to a peroxisome proliferator. Cancer Res 49:2603–2605, 1989.

29. Mikalsen SO, Rivedal E, Sanner T. Morphological transformation of Syrian hamster embryo cells induced by mineral fibres and the alleged enhancement of benzo[a]pyrene. Carcinogenesis 9:891–899, 1988.

30. McLachlan JA, Wong A, Degen GH, Barrett JC. Morphological and neoplastic transformation of Syrian

hamster embryo fibroblasts by diethylstilbestrol and its analogs. Cancer Res 42:3040–3045, 1982.

31. Rivedal E, Sanner T. Promotional effects of different phorbol esters on morphological transformation of hamster embryo cells. Cancer Lett 17:1–8, 1982.

32. Sanner T, Rivedal E. Tests with the Syrian hamster embryo cell transformation assay. In: Ashby J, de Serres FJ, Draper M, Ishidate M, Margolin BH, Matter BE, Shelby MD (eds): Progress in Mutation Research, vol 5. Amsterdam: Elsevier Science Publishers, 1985, pp. 665–671.

33. Barrett JC, Lamb PW. Tests with the Syrian hamster embryo cell transformation assay. In: Ashby J, de Serres FJ, Draper M, Ishidate M, Margolin BH, Matter BE, Shelby MD (eds): Progress in Mutation Research, vol 5. Amsterdam: Elsevier Science Publishers, 1985, pp. 623–628.

34. Lillehaug JR, Aarsaether N, Berge RK, Male R. Peroxisome proliferators show tumor-promoting but no direct transforming activity in vitro. Int J Cancer 37:97–100, 1986.

35. Pienta RJ, Poiley JA, Lebherz WB. Morphological transformation of early passage golden Syrian hamster embryo cells derived from cryopreserved primary cultures as a reliable in vitro bioassay for identifying diverse carcinogens. Int J Cancer 19:642–655, 1977.

36. Baudhuin P. Isolation of rat liver peroxisomes. In: Fleischer S, Packer L (eds): Methods in Enzymology, vol. 31. New York: Academic Press, 1974, pp. 356–368.

37. Small GM, Burdett K, Connock MJ. A sensitive spectrophotometric assay for peroxisomal acyl-CoA oxidase. Biochem J 227:205–210, 1985.

38. Lazarow PB. Assay of peroxisomal β oxidation of fatty acids. In:Lowenstein JM (ed): Methods in Enzymology, vol. 72. New York: Academic Press, 1981, pp. 315–319.

39. Leighton F, Poole B, Beaufay H, Baudhuin H, Coffey JW, Fowler S, de Duve C. The large scale separation of peroxisomes, mitochondria and lysosomes from the livers of rats injected with Triton WR-1339. J Cell Biol 37:482–513, 1968.

40. Berge RK, Døssland B. Differences between microsomal and mitochondrial matrix palmitoyl-coenzyme A hydrolase, and palmitoyl-L-carnitine hydrolase from rat liver. Biochem J 181:119–125, 1979.

41. Schutgens RBH, Romeyn GJ, Wanders RJA, van den Bosch H, Schrakamp G, Heymans HSA. Deficiency of acyl-CoA:dihydroxyacetone phosphate acyltransferase in patients with Zellweger (cerebro-hepato-renal) syndrome. Biochem Biophys Res Commun 120:179–184, 1984.

42. Schutgens RBH, Romeyn GJ, Ofman R, van den Bosch H, Tager JM, Wanders RJA. Acyl-CoA dihydroxyacetone phosphate acyltransferase in human skin fibroblasts: study of its properties using a new assay method. Biochim Biophys Acta 879:286–291, 1986.

43. Barrett AJ. Lysosomal enzymes. In: Dingle JT (ed): Lysosomes, A Laboratory Handbook. Amsterdam: North-Holland Publishing, 1972, pp. 46–135.

44. Englard S, Siegel L. Mitochondrial L-malate dehydrogenase of beef heart. In: Lowenstein JM (ed): Methods in Enzymology, vol. 13. New York: Academic Press, 1969, pp. 99–106.

45. Wanders RJA, Kos M, Roest B, Meijer AJ, Schrakamp G, Heymans HSA, Tegelaers WHH, van den Bosch H, Schutgens RBH, Tager JM. Activity of peroxisomal enzymes and intracellular distribution of catalase in Zellweger syndrome. Biochem Biophys Res Commun 123:1054–1061, 1984.

46. Fukami M, Flatmark T. Studies on catalase compartmentation in digitonin-treated rat hepatocytes. Biochim Biophys Acta 889:91–94, 1986.

47. Inestrosa NC, Bronfman M, Leighton F. Detection of peroxisomal fatty acyl-coenzyme A oxidase activity. Biochem J 182:779–788, 1979.

48. Watanabe T, Horie S, Yamada J, Isaji M, Nishigaki T, Naito J, Suga T. Species differences in the effects of bezafibrate, a hypolipidemic agent, on hepatic peroxisome-associated enzymes. Biochem Pharmacol 38:367–371, 1989.

49. Olivier JL, Chachaty C, Wolf C, Salmon S, Bereziat G. Binding of spin labeled clofibrate to lipoproteins. Biochim Biophys Acta 963:515–524, 1988.

50. Rock G, Labow RS, Tocchi M. Distribution of di(2-ethylhexyl)phthalate and products in blood and blood components. Environ Health Perspect 65:309–316, 1986.

51. Sjöberg P, Gustafsson J. Exposure to plasticizers in medical care (in Swedish). Läkartidn 101:270–271, 1986.

52. Mitchell AM, Bridges JW, Elcombe CR. Factors influencing peroxisome proliferation in cultured rat hepatocytes. Arch Toxicol 55:239–246, 1984.

53. Gray TJB, Lake BG, Beamand JA, Foster JR, Gangolli SD. Peroxisome proliferation in primary cultures of rat hepatocytes. Toxicology 67:15–25, 1983.

54. Lawrence N, McGregor DB. Assays for the induction of morphological transformation in C3H/10T1/2 cells in culture with and without S9-mediated metabolic activation. In: Ashby J, de Serres FJ, Draper

M, Ishidate M, Margolin BH, Matter BE, Shelby MD (eds): Progress in Mutation Research, vol. 5. Amsterdam: Elsevier Science Publishers, 1985, pp. 651–658.

55. Sanchez JH, Abernethy DJ, Boreiko CJ. Lack of di(2-ethylhexyl)phthalate activity in the C3H/10T1/2 cell transformation system. Toxicology in Vitro 1:49–53, 1987.

56. Small GM, Burdett K, Connock MJ. Localization of carnitine acyltransferases and acyl CoA β oxidation enzymes in small intestinal microperoxisomes (peroxisomes) of normal and clofibrate treated mice. Biochem Int 7:263–272, 1983.

57. Nemali MR, Usuda N, Reddy MK, Oyasu K, Hashimoto T, Osumi T, Rao MS, Reddy JK. Comparison of constitute and inducible levels of expression of peroxisomal β oxidation and catalase genes in liver and extrahepatic tissues of rat. Cancer Res 48:5316–5324, 1988.

58. Berge RK, Lillehaug JR. Tiadenol-mediated induction of peroxisomal enzymes in cultured C3H/10T1/2CL8 cells and in chemically transformed C3H/10T1/2 MCA16 cells. Int J Cancer 36:489–494, 1985.

59. Ng MC, Shichi H. Peroxisomal palmityl CoA oxidase activity in ocular tissues and cultured ciliary epithelial cells. J Ocular Pharmacol 5:65–70, 1989.

60. Menon GK, Placzek D, Hincenbergs M, Williams ML. Lovastatin induces peroxisomes in cultured keratinocytes. J Invest Dermatol 92:480, 1989.

61. Marsman DS, Cattley RC, Conway JG, Popp JA. Relationship of hepatic peroxisome proliferation and replicative DNA synthesis to the hepatocarcinogenicity of the peroxisome proliferators di(2-ethylhexyl)phthalate and [4-chloro-6(2,3-xylidino)-2-pyrimidinylthio]acetic acid (Wy-14,643) in rats. Cancer Res 48:6739–6744, 1988.

62. Yeldani AV, Milano M, Subbarao V, Reddy JK, Rao MS. Evaluation of liver cell proliferation during ciprofibrate-induced hepatocarcinogenesis. Cancer Lett 47:21.27, 1989.

63. Bieri F, Stubli W, Waechter F, Muakkassah-Kelly S, Bentley P. Stimulation of DNA synthesis but not of peroxisomal β oxidation by nafenopin in primary cultures of marmoset hepatocytes. Cell Biol Int Rep 12:1077–1087, 1988.

64. Richter C, Park JW, Ames BN. Normal oxidative damage to mitochondrial and nuclear DNA is extensive. Proc Natl Acad Sci USA 85:6465–6467, 1988.

65. Mikalsen SO, Ruyter B, Sanner T. Effects of hepatic peroxisome proliferators and 12-O-tetradecanoyl-phorbol-13-acetate on catalase and other enzyme activities of embryonic cells in vitro. Biochem Pharmacol 39:527–535, 1990.

66. Mikalsen SO, Holen I, Sanner T. Morphological transformation and catalase activity of Syrian hamster embryo cells treated with hepatic peroxisome proliferators, 12-O-tetradecanoylphorbol-13-acetate and nickel sulphate. Cell Biol Toxicol 6:1–13, 1990.

Chemically Induced Cell Proliferation:
Implications for Risk Assessment, pages 91-103
©1991 Wiley-Liss, Inc.

Expression of a 65-kDa Tumor-Associated Protein and Persistence of Altered Hepatic Foci

Malgorzata Hanausek, Ute Sherman, and Alan K. Adams

The multistage nature of carcinogenesis, originally demonstrated in the mouse skin model (1–3), was subsequently shown to apply to hepatocarcinogenesis (4–6). In the liver system, several biochemical markers, particularly the enzyme γ-glutamyltrans-peptidase (GGT), have been used in the identification of early preneoplastic lesions or foci induced by the initiating carcinogen. The use and limitations of these markers have recently been reviewed (7). In some studies (8) 80–90% of all altered hepatic foci were scored by the GGT stain alone. However, other studies have demonstrated that some hepatic promoting agents appear to induce GGT foci within normal liver cells (9,10), while some agents may inhibit the GGT activity of altered hepatic foci (11). The administration of ethanol, the glucocorticoid hydrocortisone, and phenobarbital (PB) are known to produce increased GGT activity in the liver (10,11). Some authors have suggested that GGT is induced in proliferating liver cells such as those found in fetal livers and regenerating liver (11). Thus, the use of other markers in addition to GGT is clearly desirable in studies of hepatocarcinogenesis. Recent evidence indicates that two markers are usually needed to score more than 90% of the enzyme-altered foci, as long as one of the markers is GGT (12). The placental form of glutathione S-transferase (GST-P), an efficient marker, has recently been identified (13,14). This marker is capable of scoring more than 90% of quantifiable enzyme-altered foci in the rat liver as determined by quantitative stereology (12). However, with some promoting agents, such as those inducing proliferation of hepatic peroxisomes, additional markers are needed to score the same proportion, since many nodules promoted by these agents express GST-P or GGT (12). Thus, there is a need to develop new specific markers of malignant and premalignant alterations.

Developmental cancer markers such as differentiation proteins and oncofetal proteins (15) are useful as more than oncologic diagnostic and prognostic indicators; they also give important clues concerning the nature of the carcinogenic process. Many of these markers are organ-specific and are only expressed by a certain percentage of tumors derived from a particular cell type. Recent studies have shown (16) that certain hepatocarcinogens increased α-fetoprotein (AFP) production in rats. However, AFP is also elevated in liver regeneration (17).

An oncofetal protein that stimulates the nucleocytoplasmic transport of mRNA (18–28), and therefore is referred to as oncofetal mRNA-transport protein, exhibits certain properties that strongly favor its candidacy as a marker of premalignant and malignant alterations (29,30). Two proteins that promote nucleocytoplasmic mRNA transport in a cell-free system have also been identified: the 35-kDa protein present in normal adult cells (31) and the 65-kDa protein (p65) coexisting with the former in fetal

(19–21) and tumor cells. Small amounts of these factors are released to the circulatory system (18–30).

The 65-kDa protein has also been identified in fetal rats at 18 days of gestation (20) and in human (21) and rat (19) amniotic fluid, but not in maternal blood (19–21); it has not, however, been identified in adult rats (20,30) nor in the blood of normal human subjects or those with a variety of nonneoplastic conditions or diseases (21). It appears to also be absent from benign tumors and nonneoplastic proliferative diseases (21). A biochemical or RNA-transport assay has not detected it in the rat 1, 5, and 21 days after liver regeneration has been induced (22). In contrast, all cancer patients with confirmed active disease tested positive for the factor (21,27). It was also present in all malignant tumor-bearing rats tested (18–20,22–30). The oncofetal protein p65 is specifically induced in normal adult tissues by carcinogens but not by closely related noncarcinogens (22,25). Significantly, the 65-kDa factors appear to be immunologically identical when tested by specific polyclonal antibodies whether induced in normal rat tissues by carcinogens or produced by rat tumors or rat embryonic tissues (23). Promoting agents such as 12-O-tetradecanoylphorbol-13-acetate (TPA) or PB do not induce p65 in vivo in the rat or in cell culture (22). Nontransformed cell lines do not release detectable amounts of p65 to the culture medium (22).

In our recent study (30), four different rat and mouse hepatocellular carcinoma cell lines were tested using an antibody to rat p65. All cell lines as well as tumor tissues from two different Morris hepatomas were positive for p65. However, p65 was not detected in normal rat or mouse livers when immunoblotting analysis was conducted. The 65-kDa protein has recently been shown (29,30) to be expressed in hepatocytes of altered hepatic foci and oval cells induced using the 2-acetylaminofluorene-(AAF)-initiation/PB-promotion protocol (32). The 65-kDa protein was predominant in the cells of putative preneoplastic foci found at 24 weeks of trial in livers of rats fed AAF and PB diets; while it was highly concentrated in the foci, little or none was detected in the surrounding cells. Weak positive staining was also found in the areas of oval and ductular proliferation while no positive staining was found in control livers from rats fed only the PB diet. Immunohistochemical staining for p65 appeared to detect foci within the foci positive for GST-P. The number of p65-positive foci detected at 12–24 weeks of trial represented only about 10% of the total number of altered hepatic foci. It was suggested that p65 may detect promoter-independent altered hepatic foci (29,30).

Recent studies provide evidence for the reversible nature of a majority of chemically induced altered hepatic foci and nodules in a number of model systems of multistage hepatocarcinogenesis (33–38). Although not all of the foci and nodules regress in these systems when the promotion or selection stimulus is withdrawn, it is extremely difficult to predict whether the phenotype is of the progressively growing lesion or of those foci/nodules that regress and disappear (7).

It was previously suggested (30,31) that expression of a tumor-associated protein with a molecular weight of 65 kDa (p65) may be useful in the identification of persistent preneoplastic liver lesions. The purpose of this study was to investigate the relationship between p65 production and persistence or reversibility of altered hepatic foci initiated with a non-necrogenic dose of diethylnitrosamine (DEN) and partial hepatectomy and promoted with the choline-deficient diet. This model system is similar to another characterized by the rapid development of mostly reversible altered hepatic foci (35).

Materials and methods

Animals and treatment

Altered hepatic foci were induced in the course of DEN-initiated, choline-deficient diet-promoted hepatocarcinogenesis in the rat (39). The choline-deficient and choline-supplemented diets (40) were prepared and pelleted by Dyets, Inc., Bethlehem, PA. Female Sprague-Dawley rats weighing 150–250 g (Harlan Sprague-Dawley, Indianapolis, IN) received an initiating dose (10 mg/kg) of DEN (or vehicle alone for the controls) by gastric intubation 24 hr after a two-thirds partial hepatectomy (5). The animals were then fed regular laboratory chow for 6 weeks in order to minimize the direct effect on the postinitiation, rapid induction of p65 (26). Beginning at 6 weeks after DEN and/or partial hepatectomy, experimental and control animals were randomly assigned to different dietary groups, as shown in Table 1. Two groups of control animals, representing the base line control groups of the model system, were continually fed normal laboratory chow (Wayne Research Diets, Chicago, IL). Two groups of animals were fed the choline-deficient or choline-supplemented diets for 8 weeks continually; the third group was fed the choline-deficient diet for 4 weeks, then switched to the choline-supplemented diet for 4 weeks. All rats received their diets and drinking water ad libitum. Weight gain and food and water intake were checked periodically, and no differences were found. Beginning on week 6, four animals from each group were killed at 4- or 8-week intervals and their livers were used for immunohistochemical studies. The general scheme of experiments is outlined in Table 1.

Immunohistochemical and histopathological procedures

The livers were excised and cut into 2–3-mm-thick sections; some sections were then fixed in 10% phosphate-buffered formalin solution for routine staining with hematoxylin and eosin stain. Other sections were fixed in cold acetone for immunohistochemical examination of the protein p65 and GST-P. Either frozen or paraffin 6-μm-thick microtome sections were prepared and stained with specific antibodies. The rat p65 was purified to apparent homogeneity (30) and polyclonal antibodies were raised

Table 1. Experimental Design.[a]

Group	No. of rats	Treatment Initiation	Promotion
1	4	PH	Normal chow
2	4	PH/DEN	Normal chow
3	8	PH/DEN	CD diet
4	4	PH/DEN	CD diet/CS diet
5	8	PH/DEN	CS diet

[a]See text for details.
PH, partial hepatectomy; DEN, diethylnitrosoamine; CD, choline deficient; CS, choline supplemented.

in rabbits, as previously described (41). The p65 was visualized in the liver sections using the avidin-biotin-peroxidase complex (Vectastain ABC Kit, Vector Laboratories, Burlingame, CA). Appropriate controls with nonimmune serum were performed routinely. Antiserum to the p65 was diluted 1:200 (the dilution found to be optimal) in phosphate-buffered saline with 1% goat serum for use in the staining protocol; GST-P was visualized in paraffin liver sections by an immunohistochemical procedure described previously (42). The locations of p65 and GST-P were examined in successive serial sections. The number and size of the p65-positive and GST-P–positive foci >50 μm in diameter were measured using a computer-assisted, semiautomatic image analyzer (Olympus Optical Co., Tokyo). Four rats per group were sacrificed at times indicated and 4–8 cryostat sections per liver per marker were evaluated.

Rat liver sections that had nodules induced by the Solt-Farber selection protocol (43) were stained with polyclonal antibodies against p65 and GST-P as described above.

The results of all experiments were evaluated statistically by Student's t-test, and differences between means were regarded as significant if $P < 0.05$.

Results

p65 as a marker of new cell population

As shown in Figure 1, after 1 month of feeding the choline-deficient diet to rats initiated with a single, nonnecrogenic dose of DEN following a two-thirds partial

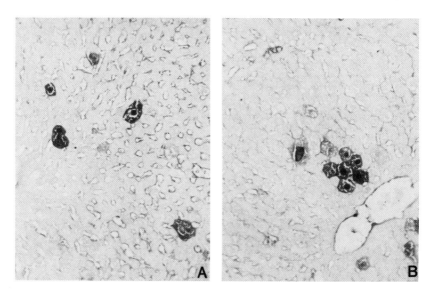

Figure 1. Immunohistochemical demonstration of single p65-positive hepatocytes (A) and minifoci (B) in sections of acetone-fixed liver tissue obtained from rats initiated with a single non-necrogenic dose of DEN following a two-thirds partial hepatectomy and promoted with the choline-deficient diet for 4 weeks. ×150.

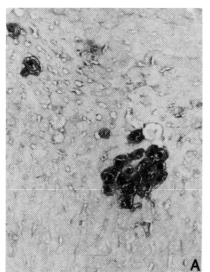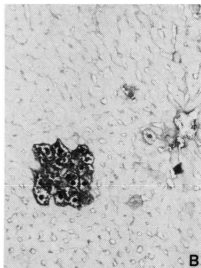

Figure 2. Immunohistochemical demonstration of minifoci (A) and foci (A and B) of p65-positive hepatocytes in the liver of rats initiated as in Figure 1 and promoted with the choline-deficient diet for 8 weeks. ×150.

hepatectomy, a number of single p65-positive hepatocytes (Fig. 2) as well as minifoci composed of 2–6 hepatocytes in cross section (Fig. 2) were apparent.

At 2 months of feeding the choline-deficient diet to rats, minifoci of p65-positive hepatocytes could still be seen (Fig. 2A) but a majority of p65-positive foci had shown a considerable increase in size (Fig. 2B). However, the foci positive for p65 were smaller than GST-P–positive foci.

Figure 3 shows immunohistochemical staining for p65 (Figs. 3A and 3C) and GST-P (Figs. 3B and 3D) of paraffin sections of livers obtained at 8 weeks of promotion from rats fed the choline-deficient diet. Staining of consecutive sections for p65 and GST-P is shown in Figures 3A and 3B, respectively. Antibodies for rat p65 appear to detect foci within those foci positive for GST-P (Figs. 3A and 3B). It was recently reported (44) that the hepatocyte nodules induced in animals on the choline-deficient diet were generally found to be positive for GST-P and GGT. Details of the p65- and GST-P–positive foci are shown under a higher magnification in Figures 3C and 3D (×900), respectively. The p65 activity appears to be clearly associated with the nuclei of the p65-positive hepatocytes; however, it is also present in the cytoplasm (Figs. 3A and 3C). GST-P is present primarily in the cytoplasm (Fig. 3D).

The distribution of the 65-kDa protein between the nucleus and cytoplasm may differ in various models of hepatocarcinogenesis. In fact, immunohistochemical staining of liver sections obtained from rats that had some nodules induced by the Solt-Farber selection protocol (43) have shown (Fig. 4) that, like GGT (data not shown), p65 was predominantly present in the nodules (Fig. 4A; ×100). The 65-kDa protein was also

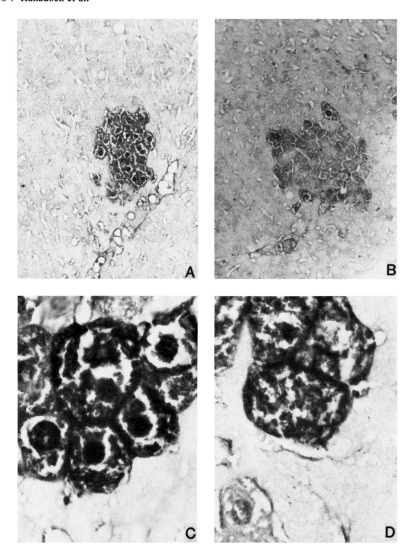

Figure 3. Immunohistochemical staining for p65 (Panels A and C) and GST-P (B,D) of paraffin sections of livers taken from rats initiated as in Figure 1 and promoted with the choline-deficient diet for 8 weeks. Consecutive sections stained for p65 and GST-P are shown in Panels A and B, respectively. ×150 (A,B); ×900 (C,D).

highly concentrated in the nodules, while little or none was detected in the surrounding liver. A p65-positive nodule from the resistant hepatocyte model is shown under a higher magnification in Figures 4B (×600) and 4C (×1000).

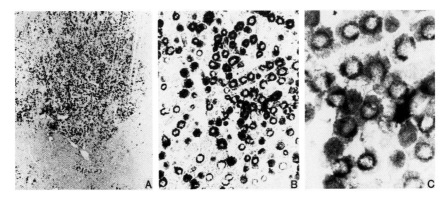

Figure 4. Immunohistochemical staining for p65 of paraffin section of the liver obtained from rats that had nodules induced by the Salt-Farber selection protocol (43). ×100 (A); ×600 (B); ×1000 (C).

As shown in Figure 4, most of the p65 activity appears to be associated with the nuclei of the p65-positive hepatocytes, and more precisely with the nuclear envelopes, with relatively little being detected in the cytoplasm. Immunohistochemical staining of the cross-sectioned nuclei seen in Figures 4B and 4C revealed that only the periphery of the nuclei, that is, the nuclear envelopes, were stained. These results affirm the putative role of p65 in the nucleocytoplasmic transport of mRNA.

Effect of withdrawal of the choline-deficient diet on the number of GST-P– and p65–positive foci

It is clear from Table 2 that the number and size of p65-positive foci were significantly smaller than those of GST-P–positive foci. As shown in Table 2 and Figure 5, withdrawal of the choline-deficient diet after 4 weeks of promotion caused a 65% reduction in the number of GST-P–positive foci detectable after an additional 4 weeks of feeding the choline-supplemented diet. The average size of GST-P–positive foci did not change significantly. However, the percent area occupied by GST-P–positive foci was reduced by 75%.

While there was no significant change in the number, size, and percent of area occupied by p65-positive foci, we found that averages for GST-P–positive foci were similar to those of GGT-positive foci induced by a similar protocol (39). The number of p65-positive foci detected at 4 and 8 weeks of promotion with the choline-deficient diet represents only about 14 and 20%, respectively, of the total number of altered hepatic foci positive for GST-P.

Thus, production of p65 during chemical hepatocarcinogenesis induced by the DEN-initiation/choline-deficient diet promotion protocol appears to be associated with the occurrence of persistent preneoplastic lesions. It remains to be determined whether antibodies to the 65-kDa protein are specific for persistent foci and nodules induced by other hepatocarcinogenesis protocols.

Table 2. Effect of Choline-deficient and Choline-supplemented Diets on GST-P–positive and p65-positive Hepatic Foci after Initiation with a Nonnecrogenic dose of DEN and Partial Hepatectomy.[a]

		Four weeks of diet feeding			Eight weeks of diet feeding		
Initiation	Dietary treatment	No. foci/cm²	Diameter (μm)	% area[b]	foci/cm²	Diameter (μm)	% area
GST-P							
PH only	Normal chow	ND	ND	ND	0.80 ± 0.01	58.3 ± 10.1	0.002 ± 0.001
PH + DEN	Normal chow	ND	ND	ND	1.08 ± 0.01	50.0 ± 11.2	0.004 ± 0.001
PH + DEN	CD	20.2 ± 0.50	220 ± 52.3	0.66 ± 0.04	19.2 ± 2.05	262.7 ± 44.0	1.04 ± 0.01
PH + DEN	CD/CS[c]	ND	ND	ND	6.80 ± 1.12[d]	186.8 ± 87.9	0.17 ± 0.06[e]
PH + DEN	CS	2.72 ± 0.07	133 ± 57.9	0.05 ± 0.01	2.75 ± 0.75	144.4 ± 60.6	0.04 ± 0.02
p65							
PH only	Normal chow	ND	ND	ND	0	0	0
PH + DEN	Normal chow	ND	ND	ND	1.00 ± 0.52	51.3 ± 19.0	0.003 ± 0.001
PH + DEN	CD	2.45 ± 0.51	203 ± 81.6	0.07 ± 0.03	3.25 ± 1.08	236.3 ± 0.06	0.09 ± 0.04
PH + DEN	CD/CS[c]	ND	ND	ND	2.99 ± 0.50	140.0 ± 54.7	0.06 ± 0.01
PH + DEN	CS	0.61 ± 0.12	107 ± 21.3	0.003 ± 0.001	1.07 ± 0.05	144.1 ± 65.8	0.01 ± 0.01

[a] See "Materials and methods," for details. ND, not determined. Each value represents the mean ± SE.

[b] Percent areas of sections occupied by GST-P or p65-positive foci

[c] 4 weeks of the CD diet followed by 4 weeks of the CS diet

[d] $P < 0.025$ against the CD (4 wk) group

[e] $P < 0.005$ against the CD (4 wk) group

Discussion

Altered hepatic foci were induced in female Sprague-Dawley rats by partial hepatectomy/DEN initiation, using the choline-deficient diet promotion protocol; foci were then quantified using specific antibodies against GST-P and p65. We found that withdrawal of the choline-deficient diet after 4 weeks of promotion caused a dramatic reduction in the number (65%) and percent area of GST-P–positive foci; however, there was no significant change in the number of p65-positive foci. Rats maintained for 10 weeks after a single intragastric dose of DEN following a two-thirds partial hepatectomy still demonstrated large numbers of single, p65-positive hepatocytes as well as minifoci. The high persistence of the lesions makes it very unlikely that the p65-positive hepatocytes were necrotizing.

It has been shown (45) that a single injection of 80 mg/kg body weight DEN generates large numbers of single GST-P–positive hepatocytes as well as minifoci that appeared to be highly persistent. It was also found (45) that DNA synthesis is not necessary for altered GST-P enzyme expression. More studies are needed to determine whether this precludes the definition of the GST-P–positive foci as "initiated" (45). In general, increasing phenotypic deviation from normal appears to be paralleled by increasing cell proliferation (46). It has not yet been determined whether p65 expression is characteristic of putative initiated cells during the early stages of hepatocarcinogenesis

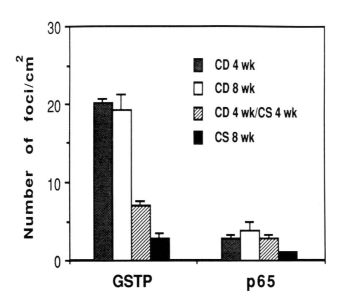

Figure 5. The effect of the choline-deficient diet and its withdrawal on the number of p65- and GSTP-positive foci in the liver of rats initiated as in Figure 1.

and whether increased DNA synthesis and cell proliferation is necessary for p65 expression.

Recent studies (38) provided evidence for the reversible nature of a majority of the partial hepatectomy/DEN-initiated altered hepatic foci promoted over the period of 16 weeks by PB, the hepatic promoting agent. These studies further support several investigations demonstrating the instability of focal lesions induced in a number of model systems of multistage hepatocarcinogenesis (7,33,47,48). We hypothesized (29,30) that p65 production during rat hepatocarcinogenesis may be associated with persistent preneoplastic lesions. The present study appears to confirm this hypothesis by showing the positive relationship between p65 production and persistence of altered hepatic foci initiated with a nonnecrogenic dose of DEN with partial hepatectomy and promoted with the choline-deficient diet. It was recently shown (49) that the carcinogenic effects of the choline-deficient diet resulted more from its strong promoting effect than from any initiating activity of the diet; withdrawal of the promoting diet caused a marked drop in the total number of altered hepatic foci. While readministration enhanced their growth, further detailed analysis of the kinetics of p65 expression in promoter-dependent lesions compared to persistent lesions should establish how the production of p65 and its release to the circulatory system depends on the occurrence of persistent foci and nodules. The 65-kDa protein was found in both the nucleus and cytoplasm of altered hepatocytes of the foci induced by the partial hepatectomy/DEN initiation and followed by the choline-deficient diet promotion protocol.

Conclusions

Considerably less p65 activity was detected in the cytoplasm of p65-positive hepatocytes of the foci induced by the AAF/PB-protocol (29,30) or, in the present study, by the Solt-Farber selection protocol. Whether a relatively higher cytoplasmic concentration of p65 in the DEN/choline-deficient diet model affects the blood level of p65 remains to be seen. The relevance of enhanced p65 expression, particularly in the nucleus, must also be examined. A marker consistently produced during the early and late stages of carcinogenesis would be very useful in following and analyzing the carcinogenic process. Our recent experiments indicate that antibodies specific against a tumor-associated protein with the molecular mass of 65 kDa (p65) are able to detect both early and late neoplastic changes during chemically induced hepatocarcinogenesis in the rat.

The 65-kDa protein was found in the cells of putative preneoplastic lesions induced in livers of rats by the partial hepatectomy/DEN-initiation/choline-deficient diet promotion hepatocarcinogenesis protocol, while little or none was present in the surrounding cells. Expression of p65 during chemical hepatocarcinogenesis induced by this protocol appears to be associated with the occurrence of persistent preneoplastic lesions.

Whether antibodies to the 65-kDa protein are specific for persistent foci and nodules induced by other hepatocarcinogenesis protocols is to be determined. Immuno-histochemical investigation revealed the generation of a single p65-positive hepatocyte. The majority of GST-P–positive altered hepatic foci induced by initiation with DEN and partial hepatectomy and promoted for 4 weeks with a choline-deficient diet disappeared upon withdrawal of that diet. There was no significant change in the number of p65-positive foci, which apparently continued to grow following withdrawal of tumor-promoting stimulus. The results gained from the investigation of the choline-deficient promoting diet pointed to the putative initiated character of the lesions. Thus, the 65-kDa protein may be a useful marker for analyzing factors relevant to both the initiation and promotion stages of hepatocarcinogenesis.

Acknowledgments

The authors wish to thank Dr. E. Farber for the gift of antisera to GST-P and paraffin sections of the livers obtained from rats that had nodules induced by the Solt-Farber selection protocol. This work was supported, in part, by a grant from The University of Texas Cancer Foundation and by grant SIG 14 from the American Cancer Society.

References

1. Berenblum I. The carcinogenic action of croton resin. Cancer Res 1:44–50, 1941.
2. Boutwell RK. Some biological aspects of skin carcinogenesis. Prog Exp Tumor Res 4:207–250, 1964.
3. Slaga TJ. Mechanisms involved in two-stage carcinogenesis in mouse skin. In Slaga TJ (ed): Mechanisms of Tumor Promotion, vol. 2. Boca Raton, FL: CRC Press, 1984, pp 1–16.
4. Peraino C, Fry RJM, Staffeldt E, Kisieleski WE. Effects of varying the exposure to phenobarbital on its enhancement of 2-acetylaminofluorene-induced hepatic tumorigenesis in the rat. Cancer Res 33:2701–2705, 1973.
5. Pitot HC, Barsness L, Goldsworthy T, Kitagawa T. Biochemical characterization of stages of hepatocarcinogenesis after a single dose of diethylnitrosoamine. Nature 271:456–458, 1978.
6. Pitot HC, Sirica HE. The stages of initiation and promotion in hepatocarcinogenesis. Biochem Biophys Acta 605:191–215, 1980.
7. Pitot HC, Glauert HP, Hanigen M. The significance of selected biochemical markers in the characterization of putative initiative cell populations in rodent liver. Cancer Lett 29:1–14, 1985.
8. Hendrich S, Campbell HA, Pitot HC. Quantitative stereological evaluation of four histochemical markers of altered foci in multistage hepatocarcinogenesis in the rat. Carcinogenesis 8:1245–1250, 1987.
9. Furukawa K, Maeura Y, Furukawa N, Williams GM. Induction by butylated hydroxytoluene of rat liver γ–glutamyl transpeptidase activity in comparison to expression in carcinogen-induced altered lesions. Chem Biol Interact 48:43–58, 1984.
10. Bone III SN, Michalopoulos GK, Jirtle RL. Ability of partial hepatectomy to induce γ-glutamyl-transpeptidase in regenerated and transplanted hepatocytes of Fischer 344 and Wistar-Furth rats. Cancer Res 45:1222–1228, 1985.
11. Hanigan MH, Pitot HC. Gamma-glutamyl transpeptidase—its role in hepatocarcinogenesis. Carcinogenesis 6:165–172, 1985.
12. Pitot HC, Campbell HA. An approach to the determination of the relative potencies of chemical agents during the stages of initiation and promotion in multistage hepatocarcinogenesis. Environ Health Perspect 76:49–56, 1987.
13. Tatematsu M, Mera Y, Ito N, Satoh K, Sato K. Relative merits of immunohistochemical demonstration of placental A, B and C forms of glutathione S-transferase and histochemical demonstration of γ-glutamyltranspeptidase as markers of altered hepatic foci during liver carcinogenesis in the rat. Carcinogenesis 6:1621–1626, 1985.
14. Rushmore TH, Sharma RN, Roomi MW, Harris L, Satoh K, Sato K, Murray RK. Identification of characteristic cytosolic peptide of rat preneoplastic hepatocyte nodules as placental glutathione S-transferase. Biochem Biophys Res Commun 143:98–103, 1987.
15. Coggin JH Jr. Oncofetal antigens. Nature 319:428, 1986.
16. Sell S, Becker F, Leffert H, Osborn K, Salman J, Lombardi B, Shinozuka H, Reddy J, Ruoslahti E, Sala-

Trepat J. Alpha-fetoprotein as a marker for early events and carcinoma development during chemical hepatocarcinogenesis. J Environ Sci Health 29:271–283, 1983.

17. Watanabe A, Miyazaki M, Taketa K. Differential mechanisms of increased α-fetoprotein production in rats following carbon tetrachloride injury and partial hepatectomy. Cancer Res 36:2171–2175, 1976.

18. Schumm DE, Webb TE. Putative transformation-dependent proteins in the blood plasma of tumor-bearing rats and cancer patients. Cancer Res 42:4964–4969, 1982.

19. Walaszek Z, Hanausek-Walaszek M, Schumm DE, Webb TE. An oncofetal 60 kilodalton protein in the plasma of tumor-bearing and carcinogen-treated rats. Cancer Lett 20:277–282, 1983.

20. Hanausek-Walaszek M, Walaszek Z, Lang RW, Webb TE. Characterization of a 60,000-dalton oncofetal protein from the plasma of tumor-bearing rats. Cancer Invest 2:433–441, 1984.

21. Schumm DE, Hanausek-Walaszek M, Walaszek Z, Webb TE. Absence of the cancer-associated factors with a molecular weight of 60,000 from the plasma of patients with a spectrum of non-neoplastic conditions. Cancer Res 44:401–406, 1984.

22. Hanausek-Walaszek M, Walaszek Z, Webb TE. Carcinogens as specific inducers of a 60-kilodalton protein in rats. Carcinogenesis 6:1725–1730, 1985.

23. Hanausek-Walaszek M, Lang R, Walaszek Z, Webb TE. Immunological identity of a 60 kd oncofetal protein induced in rats by chemical carcinogens and released by transformed cells. Biochem Biophys Res Commun 127:779–785, 1985.

24. French BT, Hanausek-Walaszek M, Walaszek Z, Schumm DE, Webb TE. Nucleocytoplasmic release of repetitive DNA transcripts in carcinogenesis correlates with a 60 kilodalton cytoplasmic protein. Cancer Lett 23:45–52, 1986.

25. Hanausek-Walaszek M, Montgomery N, Walaszek Z, Lang RW, Webb TE. Correspondence between biochemical and antigenic activity of a 60 kilodalton oncofetal protein during carcinogenesis and tumorigenesis. Cancer Lett 33:55–61, 1986.

26. Hanausek-Walaszek M, Walaszek Z, Webb TE. Use of the 60 kilodalton oncofetal protein for monitoring chemical hepatocarcinogenesis (Abstract). Fed Proc 45:698, 1986.

27. Hanausek-Walaszek M, Walaszek Z, Webb TE. A 60 kilodalton oncofetal protein as tumor marker. J Med 17:13–24, 1986.

28. Hanausek-Walaszek M, Adams AK, Del Rio M, Kriewaldt SD, Walaszek Z. Plasma oncofetal mRNA-transport protein is proportional to tumor burden in rats bearing transplantable hepatocarcinomas. Proceedings of the American Association for Cancer Res 29:167, 1988.

29. Hanausek-Walaszek M, Del Rio M, Adams AK. Immunohistochemical demonstration of mRNA-transport protein in rat liver putative preneoplastic foci. Cancer Lett 48:213–221, 1989.

30. Hanausek-Walaszek M, Del Rio M, and Adams AK. Structural and immunological identity of p65 tumor-associated factors from rat and mouse hepatocarcinomas. In Stevenson DE, McClain RM, Popp JA, Slaga TJ, Ward JM, Pitot HC (eds): Mouse Liver Carcinogenesis: Mechanisms and Comparisons. New York: Wiley-Liss, 1990, pp 109–120.

31. Moffett RB, Webb TE. Characterization of a messenger RNA-transport protein. Biochem Biophys Acta 740:231–242, 1983.

32. Peraino C, Fry RJM, Staffeldt E, Kisieleski WE. Effects of varying the exposure to phenobarbital on its enhancement of 2-acetylaminofluorene-induced hepatic tumorigenesis in the rat. Cancer Res 33:2701–2705, 1973.

33. Teebor GW, Becker FF. Regression and persistence of hyperplastic hepatic nodules induced by N-2-fluorenylacetamide and their relationship to hepatocarcinogenesis. Cancer Res 31:1–30, 1971.

34. Schulte-Hermann R, Timmermann-Trosiener I, Schuppler J. Response of liver foci in rats to hepatic tumor promoters. Toxicol Pathol 10:63–68, 1982.

35. Takahashi S, Lombardi B, Shinozuka H. Progression of carcinogen-induced foci of γ-glutamyl-transpeptidase-positive hepatocytes to hepatomas in rats fed a choline-deficient diet. Int J Cancer 29:445–450, 1982.

36. Tatematsu M, Nagamine Y, Farber E. Redifferentiation as basis for remodeling of carcinogen-induced hepatocyte nodules to normal appearing liver. Cancer Res 43:5049–5058, 1983.

37. Moore MA, Hacker HJ, Bannasch P. Phenotypic instability in focal and nodular lesions induced in a short term system in the rat liver. Carcinogenesis 4:595–603, 1983.

38. Hendrich S, Glauert HP, Pitot HC. The phenotypic stability of altered hepatic foci: Effects of withdrawal and subsequent readministration of phenobarbital. Carcinogenesis 7:2041–2045, 1986.

39. Sells MA, Kaytal SL, Sell S, Shinozuka H, Lombardi B. Induction of foci of altered γ-glutamyltranspeptidase-positive hepatocytes in carcinogen-treated rats fed a choline-deficient diet. Br J Cancer 40:274–283, 1979.

40. Shinozuka H, Lombardi B, Sell S, Immarino RM. Early histological and functional alterations of ethionine liver carcinogenesis in rats fed a choline-deficient diet. Cancer Res 38:1092–1098, 1978.

41. Coghlan L, Hanausek M. Subcutaneous immunization of rabbits with nitrocellulose paper strips impregnated with microgram quantities of protein. J Immunol Methods 129:135–138, 1990.

42. Rushmore TH, Harris L, Nagai M, Sharma RN, Hayes MA, Cameron RG, Murray RK, Farber E. Purification and characterization of P-52 (glutathione S-transferase-P or 7-7) from normal liver and putative preneoplastic liver nodules. Cancer Res 48:2805–2812, 1988.

43. Solt DB, Farber E. New principle for analysis of chemical carcinogenesis. Nature 263:701–703, 1976.

44. Goshal AK, Rushmore TH, Farber E. Initiation of carcinogenesis by a diet deficiency of choline in the absence of added carcinogens. Cancer Lett 36:289–296, 1987.

45. Moore MA, Nakagawa K, Satoh K, Ishikawa T, Sato K. Single GST-P-positive liver cells - putative initiated hepatocytes. Carcinogenesis 8:483–486, 1987.

46. Pugh TD, Goldfarb S. Quantitative histochemical and autoradiographic studies of hepatocarcinogenesis in rats fed 2-acetylaminofluorene followed by phenobarbital. Cancer Res 38:4450–4457, 1978.

47. Goldsworthy TL, Hanigan MH, Pitot HC. Models of hepatocarcinogenesis in the rat - contrasts and comparisons. Crit Rev Toxicol 9:61–89, 1985.

48. Farber E, Sarma DSR. Chemical carcinogenesis: the liver as a model. Pathology and Immunopathology Research 5:1–28, 1986.

49. Sawada N, Poirier L, Moran S, Xu YH, Pitot HC. The effect of choline and methionine deficiencies on the number and volume percentage of altered hepatic foci in the presence of or absence of diethylnitrosoamine initiation in the rat liver. Carcinogenesis 11:273–281, 1990.

Chemically Induced Cell Proliferation:
Implications for Risk Assessment, pages 105-113
©1991 Wiley-Liss, Inc.

Induced Proto-oncogene Expression Increases Susceptibility To Radiation-Induced Carcinogenesis

Amos Bailey, James Sanchez, Brad Rodu, Kedar Shrestha, Rose Tran-Paterson, Debra Saliba, and Donald M. Miller

Partial hepatectomy in rats is followed by a dramatically increased expression of c-*myc* and c-Ha-*ras* proto-oncogenes (1–5), peaking at 2 and 1 hr posthepatectomy, respectively. The increased proto-oncogene mRNA level, which is seen as early as 15 min following hepatectomy, is mediated at the transcriptional level. A similar rapid increase in proto-oncogene expression has been noted in the remaining kidneys of unilaterally nephrectomized rats (6). This is followed in 20–24 hr by an increase in the baseline level of DNA synthesis, reflecting cellular proliferation. Rosen and Cole (7) demonstrated that rats undergoing total body irradiation 3 hr after unilateral nephrectomy developed adenocarcinoma of the remaining kidneys. The coincidence between the peak of proto-oncogene expression and the increased susceptibility to radiation-induced carcinogenesis suggests that there may be a relationship between increased proto-oncogene expression and radiation sensitivity.

To investigate this relationship we have conducted a series of experiments in which rats were irradiated at various time points prior to and following unilateral nephrectomy. Following radiation, the remaining kidneys were removed immediately, and DNA was isolated and tested for the frequency of transforming oncogenes. The results of these experiments indicate that there is a direct relationship between the level of proto-oncogene expression and the susceptibility to radiation-induced carcinogenesis following unilateral nephrectomy. Our results indicate that rapidly dividing cells may be more susceptible to carcinogenesis because levels of proto-oncogene expression increased and not because of heightened DNA synthesis.

Materials and methods

Surgery

Unilateral nephrectomies were performed on female (125–150 g) Sprague-Dawley rats (Charles River Breeding Labs). Identical results were obtained in the experiments with male animals in which sham operations were performed by entering the abdominal cavity and manipulating the kidney but not removing it. At various times following unilateral nephrectomy, the animals were killed and the remaining kidneys were removed surgically. In order to determine the DNA's synthetic activity, [3H]thymidine (200 μCi/rat; specific activity 20 Ci/mmol, Amersham) was administered intraperitoneally 1 hr prior to sacrifice.

DNA and RNA analysis

Cellular DNA was isolated by proteinase K digestion and phenol extraction. The specific activity of the radiolabeled DNA was determined by measuring optical density and radioactivity of precipitated, purified DNA. Specific activity was expressed as cpm/μg DNA.

Total cellular RNA was isolated by homogenizing a 1-g section of kidney tissue in 10 ml of 6 M guanadinium isothiocyanate, followed by discontinuous cesium chloride centrifugation. RNA dot hybridization was performed essentially as described by Thomas (8). Nitrocellulose filters were hybridized to cDNA inserts which had been radiolabeled using the random hexanucleotide labeling method to a specific activity of $2-8 \times 10^8$ cpm/μg.

The hybridized filters were quantitated using laser densitometry. Northern blot analysis of total RNA was performed after electrophoresis in a 1.5% aragose formaldehyde gel. The RNA was transferred to a nitrocellulose filter (9) and hybridized as described above. The size of the c-*myc* transcript was estimated by ethidium bromide staining of phage marker DNA.

Analysis of transforming oncogenes

High molecular weight DNA was prepared using the technique of Marmur (9) as modified by Cooper and Temin (10). Renal tissue was homogenized and washed in phosphate buffer. The cells were then lysed with sodium dodecyl sulfate and digested with proteinase K. Protein was extracted with chloroform/saline/isoamyl alcohol. The DNA was further purified with RNase A and proteinase K digestion.

NIH3T3 fibroblasts were prepared for transfection by growth in minimal essential medium with 10% calf serum. The DNA sample was brought to a concentration of 10–20 mg/ml in Hepes buffered saline, 0.125 M calcium chloride was added, and DNA was allowed to precipitate. Precipitated DNA (0.5 ml) was added to each culture plate and incubated for 4 hr at 37°C. The medium was changed and 15% glycerol was added for 4 hr to enhance transformation. Transformed foci were counted at 5–15 days following transfection. DNA was isolated from the kidneys of sham laparotomy–treated rats; the nephrectomized kidneys served as control DNA samples at each step. Transformed mouse fibroblasts were assayed for the presence of the Ha-*ras* oncogene activation by polymurase chain reaction amplification and Southern blot analysis (11). DNA that had been isolated from transformed foci was used for secondary transfection experiments to confirm oncogene activation.

Results

In order to determine whether the pattern of proto-oncogene expression during compensatory hypertrophy of the kidney is similar to that of regenerating liver, we examined the level of c-*myc* and c-Ha-*ras* mRNA in the remaining kidney of rats that had undergone unilateral nephrectomy. As shown in Figure 1, the pattern of proto-oncogene expression during compensatory renal hypertrophy is almost identical to that observed during liver regeneration. There is a rapid increase in the level of c-*myc* and c-

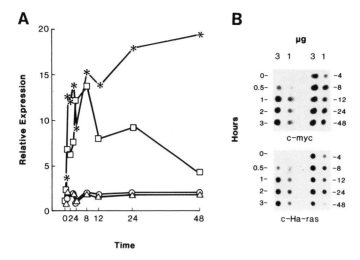

Figure 1. Effect of unilateral nephrectomy in rats on the expression of the c-*myc*, c-Ha-*ras*, c-*fos* and c-N-*ras* genes in the contralateral kidney. Unilateral nephrectomy was performed under general anesthesia (Halothane). At various times following unilateral nephrectomy, the contralateral kidney was removed. RNA was isolated as described in the text. Expression of c-*myc* and c-Ha-*ras* were assayed by dot hybridization. Autoradiograms were analyzed by densitometry and illustrated graphically as fold increase in expression over 0 hr control samples. (*) c-*myc* expression (□) c-Ha-*ras* (○) c-*fos* (△) c-N-*ras*.

Ha-*ras* mRNA, which peaks after approximately 3 hr and is followed by a more gradual increase before DNA synthesis is induced. On the other hand, there is no change in the level of c-*fos* or c-*ras* mRNA in the contralateral kidney during the 48 hr following unilateral nephrectomy.

The response of proto-oncogene expression to unilateral nephrectomy is not organ-specific, as shown in Figure 2. In this experiment, the level of c-*myc* and c-Ha-*ras* mRNA in the livers of animals that had undergone unilateral nephrectomy was determined. The pattern of proto-oncogene expression was quite similar to that observed in the kidney (see Fig. 1): There was an almost immediate increase in the level of c-*myc* and c-Ha-*ras* mRNA, although the level of c-*fos* and c-N-*ras* was unchanged. However, the absolute level of proto-oncogene expression in the liver of a nephrectomized animal is not as high as that seen in the kidney undergoing compensatory renal hypertrophy. We have previously observed a similarly rapid increase in c-*myc* and c-Ha-*ras* expression in the kidneys of rats that have undergone partial hepatectomy (12). This indicates that the proto-oncogene response to unilateral nephrectomy is not organ-specific.

We also compared the DNA synthesis levels in the kidney and liver to measure the degree of cellular proliferation 26–30 hr after unilateral nephrectomy in response to this regenerative stimulus; as indicated by the amount of [³H]thymidine incorporated, the

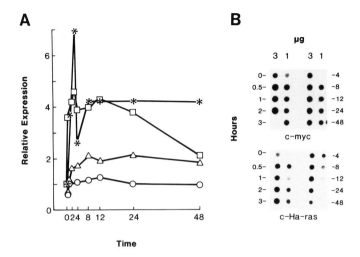

Figure 2. Effect of unilateral nephrectomy on expression of c-*myc*, c-Ha-*ras*, c-*fos*, and c-N-*ras* in liver. Livers of unilaterally nephrectomized animals were removed at various times after nephrectomy. RNA was isolated and analyzed as shown in Figure 1. (*) c-*myc* expression (□) c-Ha-*ras* (○) c-*fos* (△) c-N-*ras*.

DNA synthesis level increased 10-fold in the contralateral kidney (Fig. 3). This initial peak represents the stimulated cells' first cycle of division. In contrast, no increase in DNA synthesis was seen in the livers of animals that had undergone unilateral nephrectomy. The temporal pattern of DNA synthesis in compensatory renal hypertrophy is identical to that of liver regeneration, indicating a compensatory hyperplastic response. The increase in DNA synthesis by the contralateral kidney but not the liver of nephrectomized rats indicates that cellular proliferation is part of the compensatory hypertrophic process and is specific to the contralateral kidney.

To determine whether the susceptibility to radiation-induced carcinogenesis is altered by increased levels of proto-oncogene expression, we studied the effect that total body radiation had on inducing transforming oncogenes at various times prior to and following unilateral nephrectomy. Experimental animals received 700 rad total body radiation; after 1 hr the animals were sacrificed, the remaining kidneys and/or livers were removed, and DNA was extracted. The presence or absence of transforming oncogenes was assayed by transforming NIH3T3 cells, as previously described.

Table 1 shows the results: There was a dramatic increase in the number of transforming foci in cells transfected with DNA that had been isolated from the remaining kidney 3 hr after unilateral nephrectomy; none in those transfected with DNA from control or nephrectomized animals; and very few (<1 focus/mg DNA) in those transfected with DNA from kidneys that received irradiation alone. Representative foci, shown in Figure 4A, contained transformed cells identified according to several criteria: The ability to transform NIH3T3 cells was exhibited by DNA isolated from these foci;

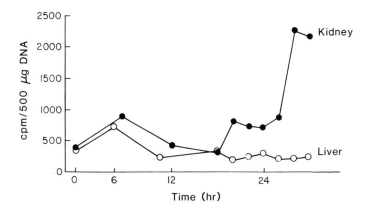

Figure 3. [3H]thymidine incorporation in liver and contralateral kidney following unilateral nephrectomy. 100 μCi [3H]thymidine was injected intraperitoneal 2 hr prior to sacrifice and DNA was isolated from liver and contralateral kidney samples of unilateral nephrectomized rats. The amount of [3H]thymidine incorporation was determined by scintillation counting. There is a l0-fold increase in [3H]thymidine incorporation in contralateral kidneys following unilateral nephrectomy but no increase in the livers or kidneys following sham laparotomy.

Table 1. Transformation of NIH3T3 Cells with DNA Isolated From Rat Kidney.

Treatment	Foci/10 cm^2
Control (untreated)	0
Nephrectomy (unirradiated)	0
Irradiated (700 rads total body, no nephrectomy)	1
Nephrectomy and irradiation (700 rads 3 hr after nephrectomy)	138
Nephrectomy and irradiation (700 rads 24 hr post-nephrectomy)	10

secondary and tertiary transformants demonstrated similar characteristics. Cells isolated from transformed foci were also able to grow in soft agar (Fig. 4B and 4C). This increase in the frequency of activated oncogenes correlates exactly with the peak of proto-oncogene expression that follows unilateral nephrectomy (see Fig. 1).

Time course experiments have shown that the frequency of transformation is only slightly increased in animals irradiated 24 hr after nephrectomy (data not shown). A similar increase in the frequency of transforming oncogenes in the liver was noted as well (data not shown). This suggests a relationship between carcinogenesis and proto-oncogene expression rather than DNA synthesis, since the livers of nephrectomized rats demonstrate increased proto-oncogene expression but no increase in DNA synthesis. In addition, the number of transforming oncogenes was observed to decrease over time following irradiation (data not shown). This suggests that either the repair of an x-ray–induced lesion or the selective death of affected cells allows protection from the radiation-induced oncogene activation.

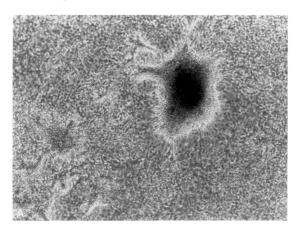

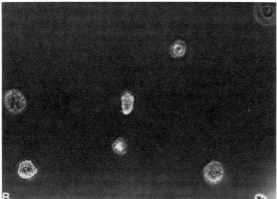

Figure 4. Transformation of NIH3T3 cells by DNA isolated from the contralateral kidneys of nephrectomized rats irradiated 3 hr after nephrectomy. (A) Representative transformed focus. (B) Soft agar colony of transformed cells. (C) Soft agar colony at higher magnification.

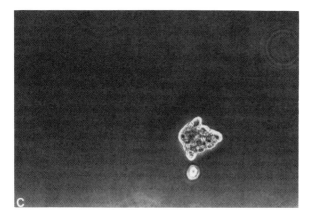

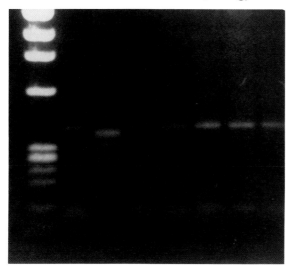

Figure 5. PCR analysis of c-Ha-*ras* gene in transformed NIH3T3 cells. High molecular weight DNA was isolated as described in "Methods." A 650-bp fragment was PCR-amplified for 35 cycles. Amplified DNA was analyzed by electrophoresis on a 2.0% agarose gel. (A) Marker DNA. (B) NIH3T3 (murine). (C) Rat liver DNA. (D) DNA from individual NIH3T3 cell lines transformed by DNA from nephrectomized irradiated rats.

Polymerase chain reaction (PCR) amplification of the transforming DNA was used to determine whether the activated proto-oncogene was c-Ha-*ras* and to detect the presence of rat c-Ha-*ras* sequences in the transformed murine NIH3T3 cells. As shown in Figure 5, this technique can distinguish rat and murine c-Ha-*ras* sequences. Titration experiments confirmed that rat c-Ha-*ras* sequences could be detected in rat mouse DNA mixtures at ratios as low as 1:100 (data not shown). However, analysis of DNA isolated from transformed cells after two transformation cycles indicated that there was no detectable rat c-Ha-*ras* sequence present in the transformed NIH3T3 cells. This suggests that the activated gene in the DNA from the irradiated animals must be a gene other than c-Ha-*ras*, a finding which is consistent with previously published results (19).

Discussion

We have demonstrated that the pattern of renal proto-oncogene expression following unilateral nephrectomy parallels that of regenerating rat liver. The almost immediate (i.e., within 15 min) dramatic increase in the level of c-*myc* and c-Ha-*ras* mRNA, followed by a second increase in transcriptional activity, suggests that compensatory renal hypertrophy is quite similar to liver regeneration. The first increase in DNA synthesis occurs at 20 hr in both cases; also, the temporal pattern of DNA synthesis during compensatory renal hypertrophy is identical to that of liver regeneration (5). The stimulation of DNA synthesis by unilateral nephrectomy indicates that compensatory renal hypertrophy involves actual cellular division and is a hyperplastic rather than a hypertrophic response.

Increased proto-oncogene expression is thought to play a role in the induction of the rapid cellular proliferation of regenerating liver or compensatory renal hypertrophy. However, the observation that hepatic proto-oncogene expression is also heightened following unilateral nephrectomy suggests that the increased expression of these genes is a response to a circulating growth factor which is not tissue-specific. It is consistent with our previous observation (12) that renal c-*myc* and c-Ha-*ras* expression also increase following partial hepatectomy. The tissue specificity of regeneration must arise at a later time and may involve other growth factors such as TGF-α, TGF-β, or both (13).

The association of increased risk of radiation-induced carcinogenesis with rapid cell division has been known for some time. In their original observation, Rosen and Cole (7) noted an 80% incidence of renal adenocarcinomas in the remaining kidney following unilateral nephrectomy and radiation at 3 hr postsurgery. Thus, the maximum susceptibility to radiation-induced carcinogenesis following unilateral nephrectomy occurs at 3 hr after nephrectomy, an interval that corresponds to the period of highest proto-oncogene expression. In order to relate their observation to the induction of transforming oncogenes at the molecular level, we have tested the ability of DNA to transform NIH3T3 cells following whole-body radiation at various times following unilateral nephrectomy. As noted in the "Results" section of this report, there is a dramatic increase in the frequency of activated proto-oncogenes in the kidneys of animals who are radiated during the peak of proto-oncogene expression. A similar increase is not observed in the kidneys of animals who are radiated prior to, or 24 hr following, unilateral nephrectomy; this suggests that the induction of proto-oncogene expression, rather than the increase in cellular proliferation, is responsible for the increased susceptibility to radiation-induced carcinogenesis. This is borne out by the fact that the liver, which demonstrates increased proto-oncogene expression but no increase in DNA synthesis, has also been noted to have an increased frequency of transforming oncogenes following unilateral nephrectomy and irradiation. It confirms the fact that proto-oncogene expression rather than DNA synthesis increases mutagenic susceptibility.

The exact identity of the transforming oncogene induced by irradiation following nephrectomy remains unclear. Members of the *ras* family have been implicated in radiation-induced thymomas in mice (14,15), or C3H/10T1/2 (16,17), or guinea pig cells chemically transformed in vitro (18). However, Borek and coworkers (19) have demonstrated quite convincingly that radiation induces an activated oncogene that is not a member of the Ha-*ras* family. Their evidence also suggests the activation of a gene other than *neu*, *trk*, or *raf*, but the restriction pattern that abrogates transformational activity suggests that the transforming oncogene must be the same in each case. Although identification of the activated oncogene is still in progress, there is a remarkable association between induced proto-oncogene expression and increased susceptibility to radiation-induced oncogene activation during compensatory renal hypertrophy. The marked increase in radiation susceptibility during periods of rapid transcription may reflect chromatin structural changes induced by growth stimuli. Taken together, our results indicate that effective anticarcinogens should be directed against proto-oncogene expression rather than cellular proliferation.

References

1. Goyette M, Petropoulos CJ, Shank PR, Fausto N. Regulated transcription of c-Ki-*ras* and c-*myc* during compensatory growth of rat liver. Molec Cell Biol 4:1493–1498, 1984.
2. Makino R, Hayashi K, Sugimura T. C-*myc* transcription is induced in rat liver at a very early stage of regeneration or by cycloheximide treatment. Nature 307:521, 1984.
3. Thompson NL, Mead JE, Braun L, Goyette M, Shank PR, Fausto N. Sequential proto-oncogene expression during rat liver regeneration. Cancer Res 46:3111–3117, 1986.
4. Campbell VW, Roesel J, Rigsby D, Sanchez J, Williams R, Nalluswami K, Miller DM. Alteration of c-*myc* expression and DNA synthesis by agents which impede liver regeneration. Oncogene Res, in press.
5. Norman JT, Bohman RE, Fischmann G, Bowen JW, McDonough A, Slamon D, Fine LG. Patterns of mRNA expression during early growth differ in kidney epithelial cells destined to undergo compensatory hypertrophy versus regenerative hyperplasia. Proc Natl Acad Sci USA 85:6768–6772, 1988.
6. Bailey A, Rigsby D, Roesel J, Alvarez R, Sanchez JD, Miller DM. C-*myc* and c-Ha-*ras* expression in response to a regenerative stimulus is not organ-specific. Oncogene Res, in press.
7. Rosen VJ Jr, Cole LJ. Accelerated induction of kidney neoplasms in mice after X radiation (690 rad) and unilateral nephrectomy. J Natl Cancer Inst 28:1031–1036, 1962.
8. Thomas PS. Hybridization of denatured RNA and small DNA fragments transferred to nitrocellulose. Proc Natl Acad Sci USA 77:5201–5205, 1980.
9. Marmur J. A procedure for the isolation of deoxyribonucleic acid from micro-organisms. J Mol Biol 3:208–218, 1961.
10. Cooper GM, Temin HM. Infectious rous sarcoma virus and reticuloendotheliosis virus DNAs. J Virol 14:1132–1141, 1974.
11. Grahan FL, van der Eb AJ. A new techinque for the assay of infectivity of human adneovirus. J of Virology 52:456–467, 1973.
12. Roesel J, Rigsby D, Bailey A, Alvarez R, Sanchez JD, Campbell VW, Miller DM. C-*myc* expression is stimulated by a circulating non-organ specific factor in regenerating liver. Oncogene Res 5:129–136, 1989.
13. Fausto N, Mead JE. Regulation of liver growth: Protooncogenes and transforming growth factors. Lab Invest 60:4–13, 1989.
14. Guerreor I, Calzada P, Mayer A, Pellicer A. A molecular approach to leukemogenesis: mouse lymphomas contain an activated c-*ras* oncogene. Proc Natl Sci USA 81:202–205, 1984.
15. Guerreor I, Villasante A, Corces V, Pellicer A. Activation of a c-K-*ras* oncogene by somatic mutation in mouse lymphomas induced by gamma radiation. Science 225:1159–1162, 1984.
16. Shih C, Shilo BZ, Goldfarb MP, Dannenberg A, Weinberg RA. Passage of phenotypes of chemically transformed cells via transfection of DNA and chromatin. Proc Natl Acad Sci USA 76:5714–5718, 1979.
17. Parada LF, Weinberg RA. Presence of a kirsten murine sarcoma virus *ras* oncogene in cells transformed by 3-methylcholanthrene. Mol Cell Biol 3:2298–2301, 1983.
18. Sukumar S, Palciani S, Doniger J, DiPaolo JA, Evans CH, Zbar B, Barbacid M. A transforming *ras* gene in tumorigenic guinea pig cell lines initiated by diverse chemical carcinogens. Science 223:1197–1199, 1984.
19. Borek C, Ong A, Mason H. Distinctive transforming genes in x-ray transformed mammalian cells. Proc Natl Acad Sci USA 84:794–798, 1987.

Chemically Induced Cell Proliferation:
Implications for Risk Assessment, pages 115-122
©1991 Wiley-Liss, Inc.

Cell Kinetics and Benzo[a]pyrene-DNA Adducts in Mouse Skin Tumorigenesis

R. E. Albert, M. L. Miller, T. E. Cody, W. Barkley, and R. Shukla

There is evidence that cell proliferation is a necessary event in the carcinogenic process. For example, tissue culture cells that are irradiated in the nonproliferative state must undergo cell replication in order to become transformed to the neoplastic state (1). It is also a generally accepted concept that DNA adducts are essential to the genotoxic action of carcinogens (2). This raises the possibility that the key measure of carcinogenic dose may be the level of DNA adducts in cells at risk for neoplastic transformation at the time of cell proliferation. Thus, the level of DNA adducts in a target tissue could be regarded as the target tissue dose and the product of the target tissue dose and the cell proliferation rate could represent the effective tumorigenic dose. If this concept were true, it might help to rationalize differences in a given tissue's tumorigenic susceptibility under conditions in which the cell proliferation rate and/or the adduct levels were altered, for example: 1) with different doses of carcinogen; 2) with such factors as dietary restriction, which tend to reduce cell proliferation rates; 3) in different strains or species; or 4) under conditions that tend to increase proliferation rates. The induction of squamous metaplasia in the bronchial epithelium, a tissue which normally has a very low rate of turnover, is one example.

We have undertaken a pilot study to determine how the level of carcinogen adducts in DNA and rate of cell proliferation both relate to tumor induction in the mouse skin using benzo[a]pyrene (B[a]P).

The results lend support to the possibility that the combination of DNA adducts and cell proliferation rate may be a measure of effective carcinogen dose.

Materials and methods

Animal handling and treatment

Female Harlan (ICR) mice, 5–6 weeks old, were quarantined for 1 week so we could observe their health. Animals were housed singly in stainless steel cages in a temperature-controlled room (23°C) regulated with a 12-hr light/dark schedule (6 A.M./6 P.M.) with food and water ad libitum. The interscapular skin of each mouse was clipped 3 days before the first B[a]P application and every 2 weeks thereafter. Mice were dosed from a pipette delivering 50 μl of B[a]P in acetone. The B[a]P-acetone solution was prepared gravimetrically and held in a brown glass vial that was kept refrigerated during storage and on ice during use to prevent evaporation of the acetone. The purity and concentration of the B[a]P stock solution was determined by high-performance liquid chromatography and ultraviolet (UV) spectrophotometry. For the cell kinetics and tumorigenesis studies, animals were treated once a week, on Monday mornings, with B[a]P. The B[a]P doses were 64-, 32-, and 16 μg. There were two control groups: one received no treatment and the other received 50 μl acetone weekly.

Tumorigenesis

The number of mice in each of the B[a]P treatment groups receiving 64-, 32-, 16-, and 0 g/week were 50, 45, 43, and 85, respectively.

The data for the groups receiving acetone only and those receiving no treatment were statistically indistinguishable, so they were combined. The mice were observed each week for 34 weeks from the start of treatment. Tumor formation was charted on a diagram of the rat's back. Tumors were determined to be present when they reached 2 mm in diameter, and their size was measured weekly. The onset of malignancy was determined by gross evidence of local invasion of the surrounding skin at the time of autopsy, and later with paraffin sections stained with hematoxylin and eosin.

Cell kinetics

Six to 20 mice per treatment group were killed at the end of each period by an overdose of Nembutal (9 mg/kg). To observe cell kinetics, a 4-mm circular punch biopsy was taken from the dorsal interscapular skin of those mice without tumors; exploratory measurements indicated that morphological changes were essentially the same throughout the B[a]P-exposed skin area. Each skin biopsy was immediately fixed in a glutaraldehyde-paraformaldehyde fixative in phosphate buffer for at least 24 hr. The specimens were cut into 1-mm strips and postfixed in OsO_4 in phosphate buffer (pH 7.4). Fixed tissue strips were dehydrated in an ethanol series, passed through propylene oxide, and embedded in Spurr resin. Skin strips were oriented in the block so that sections would be cut perpendicular to the epidermis. One-micron–thick sections on glass slides were stained with toluidine blue.

The number of basal interfollicular keratinocytes and the epidermal thickness were measured using a camera lucida mounted on a Zeiss Photomik II with a 40× objective. The number of nuclei stacked above each basal cell was counted for each consecutive basal cell in about 75 stacks per mouse; the perpendicular distance from the basement membrane to the lower keratin border was measured every 30 μm, i.e., about 24 times per section. The average of these measurements is reported as epidermal cell stacking and epidermal thickness, respectively.

For studies in which the labeling index was to be measured, mice were injected intraperitoneally with 100 μCi ^{3}H-titrium-labeled-thymidine ([^{3}H]TdR) (ICN, Irvine, CA) and killed after 1 hour. Autoradiographs were prepared by dipping 1-mm plastic sections on glass slides next to those used for light microscopy into Kodak NTB2 Nuclear Track Emulsion. Slides were incubated at 4°C for 2 weeks, developed in Kodak D-19, and stained with toluidine blue. To determine the [^{3}H]tdr labeling index, all interfollicular basal cells in each 2.5-mm strip from each mouse were examined, with a total of approximately 250 cells per strip. The background labeling of the average cell nucleus was about 0.01 grains; a cell was considered labeled if it had three or more grains per nucleus.

For mitotic indices, approximately 500 basal keratinocytes per mouse were examined, including cells from late prometaphase to early telophase, i.e., cells with condensed chromosomes and without a nuclear membrane. Pyknotic and dark cells were also counted for about 250 basal keratinocytes per mouse.

DNA adducts

In a separate experiment using a similar animal care and exposure protocol, female mice (ICR, Harlan Sprague-Dawley) 7–8 weeks old received B[a]P applications to the interscapular area of their shaved backs once every week. The weekly application levels per group were: 0- (acetone only), and 8-, 16-, 32-, and 64-µg doses B[a]P. Twenty-four hours after weekly treatments—on weeks 1, 2, and 9—15 mice from each group were sacrificed by cervical dislocation. After sacrifice, residual hair on the shaved back area was removed with a depilatory (Nair®). The back skin was removed, spread on a paper card with the epidermis up, and immediately frozen in liquid nitrogen; the epidermis was then scraped from the skin. The scrapings from 15 skins were divided between two weighed glass screw-top tubes and stored at -70°C until they were used for DNA isolation necessary in determining adduct. The DNA isolation was performed using a modified method previously described (3). Homogenates of the epidermis were extracted with chloroform:isoamyl alcohol:phenol (24:1:25) followed by diethyl ether and ethyl acetate. DNA was precipitated from the aqueous phase by adding 0.1 vol of 3 M Na acetate and 2.5 vol of ice-cold absolute ethanol. DNA content was determined by UV analysis. The DNA samples were denatured in a boiling water bath for 3 min, then chilled immediately in an ice bath. Standard adducted DNA was prepared in vitro from calf thymus DNA (Sigma) or mouse skin DNA that had been isolated from untreated skins as described above.

Analysis of BPDE adduct level in epidermal DNA was performed using a competitive ELISA test with F29, a polyclonal antibody specific for +(anti)-BPDE-DNA adducts. The polyclonal antibody was kindly provided to us by E. Kreik of the Netherlands Cancer Institute (4). The +(anti)-BPDE was obtained through the Chemical Research Resources Program of the National Cancer Institute. The procedure for preparing BPDE-DNA adducts and for determining the adduct level of the final product and the formula for calculating the percent modification of the DNA from UV spectra of the adduct-containing product, are both described by Jennette et al. (5).

Results

Cell kinetics

The results of cell kinetic studies are shown in Table 1. All measurements were made on tumor-free animals with a minimum of 4–6 animals per data point. The 64-µg–dose group was studied from the first week after B[a]P exposure began until 29 weeks later, when most of the animals had developed tumors. The controls were also studied during this time period. The evaluation of the 16- and 32-µg–dose groups began later in the study at 20, 24, and 29 weeks of B[a]P exposure. All changes in cell kinetics and morphology in the 64-µg–dose group took place during the first few weeks of

Table 1. Summary of Results of Cell Kinetic and Morphometric Studies.

			Dose	
	Acetone/control[a]	16 µg[b]	32 µg[b]	64 µb[c]
Epidermal thickness (µm)	13.1 ± 0.2[d]	19.9 ± 1.4	18.6 ± 1.0	34.9 ± 2.8
Epidermal cell stacking (No. of nuclei)	1.4 ± 0.0	1.7 ± 0.1	1.8 ± 0.1	2.3 ± 0.1
[3H]TdR labelling index (%)	4.3 ± 0.3	11.0 ± 1.4	9.2 ± 1.3	17.4 ± 2.4
Mitotic fraction (%)	0.3 ± 0.1	0.6 ± 0.1	0.5 ± 0.1	1.3 ± 0.2

[a] Average of acetone and untreated mice over entire 29 weeks
[b] Average value for 20,24,29 weeks, 96 hr after exposure
[c] Average value for 16,20,24 weeks, 96 hr after exposure
[d] ± S.E.M.

exposure and were persistent and stable thereafter. The epidermal thickness of controls averaged 13.1 µm and 1.4 nuclei per stack throughout the study period. In the 64-µg–dose group, the average epidermal thickness and number of nuclei stacked vertically increased to a plateau by the second week of exposure to 34 µm and 2.3 cells per stack, respectively (Table 1).

Epidermal thickening and vertical nuclear stacking in the 16- and 32-µg group were higher than in the controls, but were less than in the 64-µg group.

Proportionately, the increase in epidermal thickness was greater than the increase in nuclear stacking: in the 64-µg–dose group, the thickness was 2.7 times greater for the treated group than for the controls while the number of stacked nuclei increased 1.6-fold for the treated group due to the large keratinocytes that appeared early in the exposure period and were a constant skin feature in all three B[a]P dose groups, although it was less apparent in the 16- and 32-µg–dose groups.

Substantial epidermal cytotoxicity is evident from a proportional increase in dark or pyknotic keratinocytes, which developed and stabilized soon after exposure began. The numbers of dark and pyknotic cells nearly doubled in the 16- and 32-µg groups but increased approximately 10-fold in the 64-µg group.

Labeling indices increased markedly and reached a plateau within 2 weeks after exposure to B[a]P began. The percent basal keratinocytes labeled was about fourfold greater than that found in controls at the 64-µg–dose level and two- to threefold in the groups treated with 16- and 32-µg B[a]P (Table 1). The autoradiographic grain counts in the labeled cells were substantially depressed in all three dose groups by a factor of approximately 2. The mitotic index rose to a plateau during the first 2 weeks in the 64-µg–dose group to about five times higher than the controls, while the 16- and 32-µg–dose groups were only slightly increased.

All of the data shown in Table 1 was obtained from skin samples taken 96 hr after the last B[a]P exposure.

DNA adducts

Weekly topical applications of B[a]P at all dose levels resulted in measurable DNA adduct formation (see Table 2). Comparatively little formation occurred 24 hr after the first and second B[a]P application; by the fourth application, however, the adduct levels

Table 2. Effect of Level and Duration of Topical Application on BPDE-DNA Adduct Levels in Mouse Epidermis.

Days after start	Number doses	Dose (μg/week)				
		0	8	16	32	64
1	1	0.0 (.0)[a]	0.2 (.1)	0.4 (.1)	0.7 (.6)	0.5 (.9)
8	2	0.0 (.0)	0.1 (.0)	0.2 (.1)	0.6 (.0)	0.7 (.1)
22	4	0.0 (.0)	1.3 (.2)	3.7 (.3)	5.7 (.3)	6.3 (.6)
57	9	0.2 (.1)	1.5 (.3)	2.8 (.1)	5.2 (1.2)	7.5 (2.8)

[a] S.D.

increased sharply at all B[a]P doses to a level that did not change even after nine applications. At the time of the 3- and 8-week sacrifices, when an apparent plateau had been attained at all dose levels, the adduct content of the DNA was linear for those groups that had received dosages between 8- and 32-μg B[a]P (Fig. 1). Linear regression comparison of the adduct concentration and the applied B[a]P dose indicates that the increase was at the rate of 0.166 fmol adduct/g DNA per μg of B[a]P applied ($r^2 = 0.979$).

At the highest dose of 64 μg, the linearity did not hold; only 0.11 fmol adduct was formed per μg B[a]P applied weekly. At the 32- and 64-μg applications, the adduct levels in epidermal DNA did not differ significantly after four and nine treatments.

Tumorigenesis, DNA adducts and cell proliferation

Tumor formation began 12–14 weeks after B[a]P exposure began for the 64- and 32-μg–dose groups, and at 18 weeks for the 16-μg–dose group. The cumulative incidence curves for time are also consistent with a log-to-log relationship with a 6.5 slope and a 1.9 power of dose, essentially a dose-squared response. Two-thirds of the 127 tumors that formed in all the 64-μg–dose groups were identified histologically as benign papillomas.

The dose-squared response for tumor formation is not consistent with the dose response for adduct formation; the latter increases linearly to a plateau between the two higher dose groups. The tumor dose-response curve (Fig. 2) is more consistent with the upwardly curving dose-response for cell proliferation than with the adduct concentration curve. The rate of cell proliferation and tumor formation between the 16- and 32-μg–dose groups does not differ greatly. The product of the mitotic index and adduct levels is plotted against the tumor incidence at 34 weeks (Fig. 3); this was the last data point for the 64-μg–dose group because too few mice were left for further follow-up. The four points in the figure correspond to the four doses studied, i.e., control, 16-, 32- and 64 μg.

Discussion

In this study, cell kinetic changes stabilized a few weeks after B[a]P exposure began while DNA adduct levels plateaued in about one month. There was a high correlation

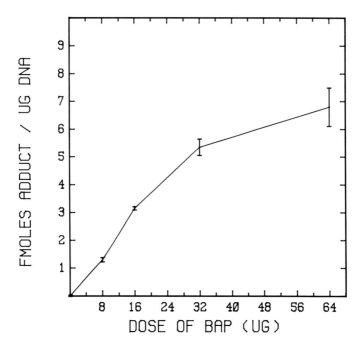

Figure 1. The dose of B[a]P is plotted against the mean level of BPDE-DNA adduct in epidermis at four and nine weekly treatments. Adduct concentrations in epidermal DNA of acetone treated controls remained at background levels throughout. Data points and standard errors are from the mean of two equivalent samples. Each sample is analyzed two to three times in triplicate.

between increased cell proliferation, as measured by net mitotic index (observed minus background), and incidence of tumors. Since there was only a minor expansion of the epidermal cell population, this cell proliferation increase must be a response to increased carcinogen-induced cell death. This is evidenced by the strong positive relationship between cell proliferation and such indicators of cytotoxicity as presence of pyknotic cells and cells with large nuclei which are probably giant cells.

Two other features of the epidermal response to chronic B[a]P treatment—appearance of excess numbers of "dark cells" and predominance of papillomas among the tumors—are both characteristic of tumor promotion. The promoting factor in this case might be the cell death caused by cytotoxic concentrations of the carcinogen. The data suggested a relationship between tumor incidence and measures of cell killing by mitosis or pyknosis; it also indicates a connection between tumor incidence and the combination of DNA adduct levels and net mitotic rates. In seeking relevant estimates of risk, it seems that the combination of adduct levels and proliferation rates has a biologic rationale; it may also have an application to conditions which may affect these

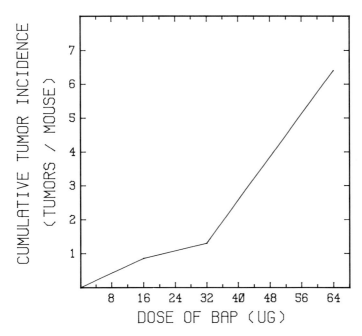

Figure 2. The dose of B[a]P is plotted against the number of tumors per mouse at 34 weeks after the beginning of weekly treatments. No tumors arose in the untreated or acetone-treated mice. A tumor was counted if its dimensions were 2 mm or greater. Grossly and histologically, papillomas predominated over carcinomas by about two to one at 64 µg.

factors independently. DNA adducts probably represent both the factors that determine the neoplastic transformation of cells and their progression to more malignant states and those that determine cell toxicity. Cell proliferation probably affects the conversion of adducts into genetic damage as well as reflects the tissue response to cell killing; it may therefore be a measure of the promoting forces that cause clonal outgrowth of neoplastic cells into tumors and, possibly, progression of such cells into more malignant states. The combination of the two factors, adduction and proliferation, may be useful in predicting tumor response under a wide variety of conditions and therefore assist in the quantitative estimation of carcinogenic risks at low levels of exposure to genotoxic environmental carcinogens.

Acknowledgments

The authors express gratitude to Nancy Knapp, Leva Wilson and Mary Jo Frost for their fine secretarial help, and to Stacey Andringa, Brenda Schumann, Kathy LaDow, and Jane Agee for technical assistance.

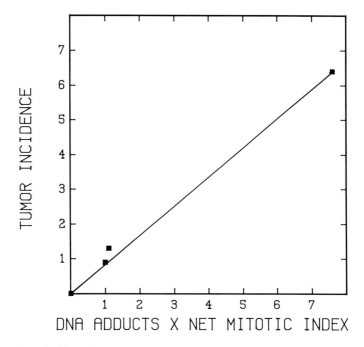

Figure 3. Tumor incidence is plotted in relation to the product of DNA adducts and net mitotic index at 0-, 16-, 32- and 64-μg B[a]P.

References

1. Borek C, Sachs L. The number of cell generations required to fix the transformed state in X-ray–induced transformation. Proc Natl Acad Sci USA, 59:83–85, 1968.
2. Miller JA. Carcinogenesis by chemicals: An overview. G.H.A. Clowes Memorial Lecture. Cancer Res 30:559–576, 1970.
3. Shugart L, Holland JM, RO Rahn. Dosimetry of PAH skin carcinogens: Covalent binding of benzo[a]pyrene to mouse skin epidermal DNA. Carcinogenesis 4:195–198, 1983.
4. Schooten, Van FJ, Kriek E, Steenwinkel MJST, Noteborn HPJM, Hillebrand MJX, Van Leeuwen FE. The binding efficiency of polyclonal and monoclonal antibodies to DNA modified with benzo[a]pyrene diol epoxide is dependent on the level of modification. Implications for quantitation of benzo[a]pyrene DNA adducts in vivo. Carcinogenesis 8:1263, 1987.
5. Jennette KW, Jeffreys AM, Blobstein SH, Beland FA, Harvey RG, Weinstein IB. Nucleoside adducts from the in vitro reaction of benzo[a]pyrene 7,8–dihydrodiol,9,10–oxide or benzo[a]pyrene 4,5–oxide with nucleic acids. Biochem 16:932–938, 1977.

Chemically Induced Cell Proliferation:
Implications for Risk Assessment, pages 123-135
©1991 Wiley-Liss, Inc.

Distribution of Constitutive and Polycyclic Aromatic Hydrocarbon-induced Cytochrome P-450 Activities in Murine Epidermal Cells That Differ in Their Stages of Differentiation

John J. Reiners, Jr., Amador R. Cantu, and Amy Pavone

Numerous studies have demonstrated that rodent epidermis can metabolize a variety of xenobiotics (1). Immunohistologic analyses with antibodies to hepatic P-450 cytochromes (2,3), and the presence of P-450–dependent monooxygenase activities in epidermal homogenates (4–7) and microsomal preparations (3,5–8), demonstrate that the P-450 cytochrome system is present in the epidermis. Furthermore, analyses of metabolite and DNA adduct stereochemistry (9,10), and the modulation of epidermal metabolism by well-characterized P-450 inhibitors (11,12), suggest that the cytochrome P-450 system makes major contributions to epidermal xenobiotic metabolism.

The epidermal component of the skin consists of several cell types including keratinocytes, Langerhans' cells, and T cells (13–15). Although the relative proportions of these cell types can vary markedly, the keratinocyte is the predominant cell type in the epidermis. There is considerable heterogeneity in the keratinocyte population due to the dynamics of skin differentiation (14). The four general keratinocyte maturation types, from least to most differentiated, are basal, spinous, granular, and squamous cells. Recent studies have demonstrated that the specific activities of several nonstructural epidermal proteins vary with the stage of differentiation. The activities of catalase (16), xanthine oxidase (17), cyclooxygenase (18) and the 5-,8-,12-, and 15-lipoxygenases (18), are all greater in differentiating keratinocytes than in basal cells.

The current study was designed to investigate whether P-450–dependent monooxygenase activities vary with the stage of murine keratinocyte (MK) differentiation. Analyses were performed in two systems. First, we used a culturing model in which MK proliferation and differentiation can be modulated as a function of medium Ca^{2+} concentration (19). Specifically, MKs proliferating in a low Ca^{2+} medium (≤ 0.05 mM) can be induced to differentiate by increasing the medium Ca^{2+} concentration to 1.2 mM. Second, we took advantage of the fact that the buoyant density of MKs decreases during terminal differentiation (20–22) and that subpopulations of MKs with differing buoyant densities can be separated on Percoll gradients (21,22).

Although analyses of the epidermal P-450 system have traditionally been hindered by low tissue activities and limited amounts of tissue, we recently reported a sensitive assay for the quantitation of monooxygenase activities in suspensions and cultures of MKs that allows activities to be expressed on a per cell basis (1,23). Using this assay and the MK differentiation systems described above, we demonstrated that the expression of constitutive P-450–dependent monooxygenase activities occurs during MK differentiation.

Materials and methods

Chemicals

We purchased d-glucose-6-phosphate, d-glucose-6-phosphate dehydrogenase, NADP⁺, 7-ethoxycoumarin, 7-hydroxycoumarin, and Percoll (Sigma Chemical Company); 7-ethoxyresorufin (Pierce Chemical Company); 7-hydroxyresorufin (Aldrich Chemical Company); Eagle's minimum essential medium (MEM) containing no Ca^{2+} (Whittaker M.A. Bioproducts); fetal bovine serum (FBS) (GIBCO); 7,12-dimethyl-benz[a]anthracene (DMBA) (Kodak Company). Benzo[a]pyrene (B[a]P) and metabolites of DMBA were acquired through the Carcinogenesis Program of the National Cancer Institute.

Preparation of keratinocytes

Epidermal cell suspensions were prepared from the dorsal skins of adult female SENCAR mice (National Cancer Institute) by the trypsin-flotation procedure (1). Cell suspensions were filtered through nylon mesh to remove large squamous sheets, and then centrifuged to pellet the cells. The pellets were suspended in MEM supplemented with growth factors, and also in 2% FBS that had been pretreated with Chelex 100 to remove Ca^{2+} (24). Cells were plated in 60-mm collagen-coated dishes (24) and grown in a humidified 5% CO_2 chamber at 37°C. Nonattached and loosely attached cells were removed 3 days after plating by washing the dishes with phosphate-buffered saline (PBS). After fresh medium was added, MK terminal differentiation was induced in some cultures by adding $CaCl_2$, thus raising the Ca^{2+} concentration in the medium to 1.2 mM.

To prepare for monooxygenase analyses, the cell pellet was resuspended in MEM and overlaid on 15 ml of 30% Percoll which had been diluted with PBS, and centrifuged for 15 min at 1500 g. This step removes debris, small squamous clumps, and a majority of the granular cells. The resulting pellet was washed once with PBS, then resuspended in P-450 buffer (1.6 mg/ml bovine serum albumin, 5 mM $MgSO_4$, 100 mM Hepes, pH 7.8) and counted. Multiple 0.75 ml samples were transferred to 35-mm tissue culture plates and stored at -70°C until analysis.

Percoll gradient separation of keratinocytes

MKs recovered after the 30% Percoll step were resuspended in 50% Percoll that had been diluted in PBS, and were separated by centrifugation into subpopulations differing in their buoyant densities (21). Gradient fractions were pooled and washed with PBS prior to suspension in P-450 buffer. Suspended MKs were counted, transferred to 35 mm tissue culture dishes, and stored at -70°C until P-450 analyses were performed.

P-450 monooxygenase assays

7-Ethoxycoumarin-O-deethylase (7-ECD) and 7-ethoxyresorufin-O-deethylase (7-ERD) activities were quantitated by measuring the production of fluorescent products. Monooxygenase assays were performed in 35- or 60-mm culture dishes containing either MK suspensions or cultures that had been subjected to a cycle of freezing and thawing. The assay protocol was reported recently (1,23). 7-ECD– and 7-ERD–specific activities were calculated from measured rates of product formation. These rates were then divided by cell number to yield a specific activity that is expressed as pmol of product per hr per 10^6 MKs.

Keratinocyte-mediated mutagenesis assay

Cocultures of MKs and Chinese hamster lung V-79 cells were established as previously described (25). The protocol for measuring mutations affecting the hypoxanthine-guanine phosphoribosyltransferase locus has been described in detail (25).

Extraction and identification of B[a]P and DMBA metabolites

The procedures used for the extraction and identification of polycyclic aromatic hydrocarbon metabolites produced by cultured MKs have been described in detail (25).

Results

Metabolism of B[a]P and DMBA

MKs cultured in a medium containing low levels of Ca^{2+} (≤ 0.04 mM) at 37°C will proliferate for several days. Raising the medium Ca^{2+} concentration to 1.2 mM by adding $CaCl_2$ induces terminal differentiation. The metabolisms of the polycyclic aromatic hydrocarbons (PAHs), DMBA, and B[a]P were markedly different in MK cultures maintained in medium containing low and high concentrations of Ca^{2+} (Table 1). Overall metabolism, as indicated by the amount of parent PAH remaining in the medium, was greater in cultures that had been Ca^{2+}–shifted 48 hr prior to adding PAH. Detailed kinetic analyses of DMBA metabolism indicated dramatic quantitative differences as early as 3 hr after PAH was added to the cultures (25).

Table 1. Effect of Ca^{2+} Concentration on PAH Metabolism in Primary Cultures of Adult MKs.

Ca^{2+}	PAH	Unchanged hydrocarbon (%)*
Low	B[a]P	40
High	B[a]P	7
Low	DMBA	50
High	DMBA	6

MK cultures were exposed to PAHs (0.25 µg/ml) for 24 hr prior to analyses of metabolites in culture medium. MKs cultured in high Ca^{2+}–containing medium were Ca^{2+} switched 48 hr prior to exposure to PAH. Data are derived from Table 1 of reference 25.
*Percentage of total PAH measured in culture medium that migrated as parent PAH by high-performance liquid chromatography analyses.

Keratinocyte-mediated mutagenesis

V-79 fibroblasts are incapable of activating the promutagen B[*a*]P to a mutagenic metabolite (26). Consequently, mutagenesis by B[*a*]P of V-79 cells cocultured with MKs requires that MKs metabolize the PAH. Treatment of cocultures with B[*a*]P at the time of the Ca^{2+} shift resulted in a dose-dependent mutagenesis (Fig. 1, top). In contrast, mutant frequencies in cocultures maintained in a low Ca^{2+}–containing medium did not differ over the range of 0.3 to 1 µM, and were less than the mutant frequencies measured in their Ca^{2+}–shifted counterparts. However, mutant frequencies in cocultures maintained in a low Ca^{2+}–containing medium were similar or greater than those measured in Ca^{2+}–shifted cultures at 3 µM or 6 µM-B[*a*]P, respectively. The basis for the dramatic increases at the higher doses of B[*a*]P are not known. However, they may be a consequence of B[*a*]P–dependent activation of the Ah receptor and subsequent induction of P-450IA1. B[*a*]P concentrations in excess of 1 µM are generally required for Ah receptor–mediated induction of cytochrome P450IA1 and the activities capable of metabolizing B[*a*]P to a mutagen (27).

The mutation data reported in Figure 1 (top) are for V-79s harvested 46 hr after the addition of B[*a*]P to the cocultures. To approximate the minimal amount of culturing time required to observe differences in mutant frequencies between cocultures maintained in a low- and high-Ca^{2+}–containing medium, we harvested V-79 cells at

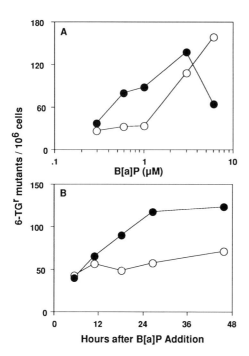

Figure 1. Dose-dependence and kinetics of B[*a*]P mutagenesis in a keratinocyte-mediated mutation assay. MKs and V-79 cells were cocultured in low Ca^{2+} (○) or high Ca^{2+} (●) containing media for either 46 hr (A) or various lengths of time (B) after the addition of B[*a*]P before being processed for mutant selection. MK differentiation was induced by Ca^{2+} switch at the time of B[*a*]P addition. The concentration of B[*a*]P used in panel B was 2 µM.

various times after adding PAH to cocultures. Mutant frequencies were similar in co-cultures maintained in either a low- or high-Ca^{2+}–containing medium for the first 11 hr following B[a]P addition (Fig. 1, bottom). Thereafter, mutant frequencies dramatically increased in the Ca^{2+}–shifted cultures. Similar results were obtained in a second study (25).

The studies reported in Table 1 and Figure 1 demonstrate that PAH metabolism is markedly different in proliferating and differentiating MKs.

Monooxygenase measurements in cultured keratinocytes

The differences in PAH metabolism between MKs cultured in media containing different levels of Ca^{2+} probably reflect variations in P-450 monooxygenase activities. To date, there have been few reports of P-450 monooxygenase measurements in cultured epidermal cells (3,5,7). For those few reports that exist, analyses were performed on homogenates or microsome fractions, and activities were calculated on the basis of extracted protein. While such analyses provide a basis for comparisons of relative activities, they may not reflect actual per cell activities. We recently reported the adaptation of fluorescence assays commonly used for measurements of monooxygenase activities in hepatic microsomes to cultured MKs and suspensions of MKs (1,23). Our assay uses cells that have been permeabilized by a cycle of freezing and thawing. Metabolism occurs in situ but the products rapidly diffuse out of the MKs. Because the cells remain intact and their numbers can be estimated, activities can be expressed on a per cell basis.

Per cell activities of the monooxygenase 7-ECD were barely measurable in MKs cultured at 37°C in a medium containing low levels of Ca^{2+} (Fig. 2, top). 7-ERD was not detectable in similar cultures (Fig. 2, bottom). However, there were dramatic increases in the activities of both monooxygenases following Ca^{2+} shift. Increases in 7-ECD per cell activities were first noted 10 hr after Ca^{2+} shift and reached a maximum 4–14 hr later; thereafter, 7-ECD–specific activities declined. Increases in 7-ERD–specific activities were detected earlier, that is, within 6 hr, but the kinetics of increase and decline generally paralleled 7-ECD activities. In general, maximum 7-ECD and 7-ERD activities were measured 12–24 hr after Ca^{2+} shift, and 7-ECD activities were increased fivefold following Ca^{2+} shift (1). In contrast, 7-ERD per cell activities were increased at least 21-fold following Ca^{2+} shift (1).

Inhibition of 7-ERD and 7-ECD induction in culture

The increases in monooxygenase activities that occurred following Ca^{2+} shift could be inhibited by adding either actinomycin D or cycloheximide to the culture medium just prior to Ca^{2+} shift (Table 2). Consequently, de novo RNA and protein synthesis are required for the increases in monooxygenase activities that occur following Ca^{2+} shift.

In vivo epidermal monooxygenase activities

The buoyant density of keratinocytes decreases as MKs differentiate (20–22). Subpopulations of MKs differing in their buoyant densities were prepared by Percoll

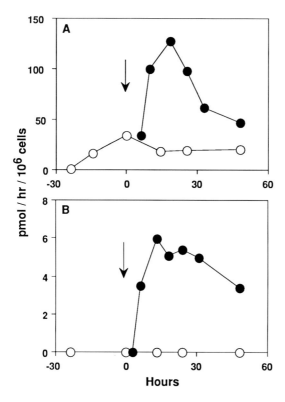

Figure 2. Kinetics of increases in 7-ECD(A) and 7-ERD(B) activities in cultured MKs following Ca^{2+} shift. MKs were cultured for 3 days in low Ca^{2+}-containing medium prior to Ca^{2+} shift (indicated by arrow). Symbols are MKs cultured in low (○) and high (●) Ca^{2+} containing medium.

gradient centrifugation (Table 3). Based upon a variety of criteria, the P_4 Percoll fraction contained basal cells; the P_3 fraction contained basal and some spinous cells; and the P_2 and P_1 fractions contained spinous cells. The P_1 fraction also contained some granular cells and nucleated squames. Gradients of monooxygenase activities ($\geq$ sevenfold) were measured in these four populations and the lowest activities were found in the P_4 basal cell fraction.

Distribution of PAH-induced in vivo 7-ERD activities

The data presented in Table 3 demonstrate that the expression of constitutive 7-ERD activity in MKs is a differentiation-related event. 7-ERD activity is a measure of the P-450IA1 gene product (28,29), and is induced by the PAH dimethylbenz[a,c]-anthracene (DB[a,c]A) (27,30). Topical treatment of SENCAR dorsal skin with 100 nmol DB[a,c]A resulted in an ~400–fold increase in 7-ERD activities in unfractionated MK suspensions within 4 hr of treatment (Table 4). Analyses of MK suspensions separated on Percoll gradients showed that the per cell activities were similar among the

Table 2. Suppression of Ca^{2+}–dependent Induction of 7-ECD and 7-ERD in Cultured Keratinocytes by Actinomycin D and Cycloheximide.

			% of Ca^{2+}-induced activity	
Ca^{2+} in Medium	Modifier	Dose (μM)	7-ECD	7-ERD
−	−	−	16.0	ND*
+	−	−	100.0	100.0
+	Act-D	0.01	39.7	43.8
+	Act-D	0.10	11.5	ND
−	−	−	16.0	ND
+	−	−	100.0	100.0
+	Chx	0.35	1.9	67.2
+	Chx	3.50	ND	ND

Adult MKs were cultured in a low Ca^{2+}-containing medium for 3 days prior to medium change and Ca^{2+} shift. Actinomycin D (Act-D) and cycloheximide (Chx) were added to the medium 10 to 15 min prior to Ca^{2+} shift. Analyses are of cultures pulled 16 hr after medium change or Ca^{2+} shift. Data are from reference 1.
*ND = Activity was not detected.

Table 3. Variation in Constitutive in Vivo 7-ECD and 7-ERD Activities as a Function of the Stage of MK Differentiation.

		pmol/hr per 10^6 cells	
Percoll fraction	Density (g/ml)	ERD	ECD
Unfractionated	−	0.71 ± 0.32	10.9 ± 2.2
P_1	≤ 1.055	1.71 ± 0.05	16.9 ± 2.9
P_2	1.055–1.062	0.57 ± 0.07	9.2 ± 4.2
P_3	1.062–1.100	0.15 ± 0.02	4.1 ± 1.5
P_4	≥ 1.100	ND*	2.6 ± 0.7

MKs isolated from untreated dorsal skin were separated on 50% Percoll gradients into four fractions. Data are mean ± SE of analyses on 2 ERD and 4 ECD preparations.
*ND = Activity was not detected.

four subpopulations; the levels of induction, however, were markedly different between the subpopulations. Whereas DB[a,c]A treatment results in an ~200–fold increase in the most differentiated P_1 fraction, there was a minimum 1850–fold increase in the P_4 basal cell population.

Discussion

Several investigators have reported that P-450–dependent monooxygenase-specific activities are higher in differentiating cells than in basal cell keratinocytes (1,3,31,32). In 1983, Coomes et al. (31) used a Percoll step gradient to prepare subpopulations of differentiated MKs and enriched basal cells (~30% basal cells). Per cell 7-ECD activity in the basal cell population was approximately one-third the activity found

Table 4. Induction and Distribution of in Vivo 7-ERD Activity as a Function of the Stage of MK Differentiation.

Percoll fraction	Density (g/ml)	pmol/hr per 10^6 cells		Fold induction
		Solvent	DB[a,c]A	
Unfractionated	–	1.3	526	404
P$_1$	≤1.055	2.6	521	200
P$_2$	1.055–1.062	0.8	544	679
P$_3$	1.062–1.100	0.3	447	1490
P$_4$	≥1.100	ND*	370	1850+

MKs were isolated from the dorsal skins of SENCAR mice 4 hr after topical treatment with 100 nmol DB[a,c]A or solvent (0.2 ml acetone). Keratinocytes were separated on 50% Percoll gradients into four fractions.
*Activity was not detected.
+Calculated using an empirically derived detection limit for 7-hydroxyresorufin as 0.2 pmol/hr per 10^6 cells for 2×10^6 cells.

in the differentiated MKs. In a later study, Pohl et al. (32) used metrizamide gradients and elutriation to enrich for MK subpopulations differing in their stages of differentiation. They measured in these cells a two- to fourfold gradient of 7-ECD activities which were normalized on the basis of DNA content. More recently, Guo et al. (3) reported a sevenfold difference in the specific activities of constitutive AHH measured in microsomes of basal and differentiated newborn rat keratinocytes. In the current study, we demonstrated a gradient of both 7-ECD and 7-ERD constitutive activities in the murine epidermis. The lowest per cell activities were measured in basal cells and were at least sevenfold less than the activities measured in the most differentiated MK preparation. It should be emphasized that the magnitude of the gradient in vivo may be considerably greater than ~sevenfold. This is because our protocol for MK fractionation eliminates a majority of the granular cells and squames prior to separation on Percoll gradients. The most differentiated fraction we assayed contained MKs in only intermediate stages of differentiation.

Topical treatment of dorsal epidermis with DB[a,c]A resulted in a several-hundred-fold increase in per cell 7-ERD activities. However, whereas there was a pronounced gradient of constitutive 7-ERD activities in murine epidermis, DB[a,c]A-induced per cell 7-ERD activities were relatively similar throughout the epidermis 4 hr after treatment with DB[a,c]A. The similarities in per cell 7-ERD activities were the consequence of different levels of induction in the various MK subpopulations. Specifically, there was an approximate 200-fold induction in the most differentiated MK Percoll population (P$_1$), and a nearly 1850-fold induction in basal cells.

An important conclusion that can be drawn from these studies is that at least some basal cells have a functioning Ah receptor that can be activated by DB[a,c]A. Our results are somewhat different from those reported by Guo et al. (3), who reported that AHH specific activities in microsomes from both basal and differentiated newborn rat epidermis were elevated threefold 24 hr after in vivo treatment with benz[a]anthracene (BA). The relative difference between the specific activities of basal versus differentiated keratinocytes was sevenfold for both constitutive and induced AHH activities. The bases for the differences between our work and that of Guo et al. (3) are unknown, but may be a consequence of either their use of microsomes and our uses of whole cells, or the times of analyses (4 hr vs. 24 hr). Treatment of the epidermis with a variety of agents often leads to the commitment of some basal cells to differentiation (21). In this regard, Knutson and Poland (33) have presented data suggesting that the Ah receptor can mediate the regulation of epidermal proliferation and differentiation in hairless mice. It is conceivable that analyses of differentiated keratinocytes 24 hr after BA treatment include some cells that were basal cells at the time of BA treatment, which became induced for AHH, and subsequently were committed to differentiation and migrated into the suprabasal layer.

MKs committed to terminal differentiation do not have the capacity to proliferate. In our studies, the Percoll-derived MK subpopulation having the lowest per cell monooxygenase activities had the greatest capacity for proliferation in vitro (22,34). The correlation noted between P-450 activities and the proliferation/differentiation status of MKs is not unique to the epidermis. As with MKs, the induction of differentiation of cultured vaginal epithelium by Ca^{2+} shift results in time-dependent changes in DMBA metabolism indicative of the induction of metabolizing enzymes (J. DiGiovanni and C. Conti, personal communication). Similarly, high levels of constitutive P-450 activities are characteristic of differentiated Clara cells, the nonciliated epithelia of bronchiolar epithelium (35).

Hepatic P-450 levels and monooxygenase activities also vary markedly with the tissue's rate of proliferation. Fetal liver, regenerating liver, hepatocellular carcinomas, and neoplastic hepatic nodules are all proliferating tissues containing a large percentage of diploid cells (36–41). White et al. (42) recently reported the separation of normal hepatocytes by fluorescence-activated flow cytometry into populations differing in their capacities to metabolize diethoxyfluorescein, a P-450 substrate. In general, the capacity for diethoxyfluorescein oxidation increased with the ploidy of the hepatocytes, i.e. tetraploid cells had greater capacity then diploid cells. Similarly, the relative content of cytochromes P-4503a and P-450c were greater in sorted tetraploid hepatocytes isolated from rats treated with phenobarbitone or methylcholanthrene, respectively (43). These findings suggest that P-450 activities should be decreased in hepatic tissues having a large percentage of diploid cells. This is exactly what has been observed. P-450s are virtually absent in the rapidly proliferating fetal liver (44,45), and are dramatically decreased on a per mg protein basis following partial hepatectomy (46,47). P-450 cytochromes and monooxygenase activities are also reduced in rapidly growing spontaneous and chemically induced hepatic nodules and hepatomas (48–50). Collectively, these studies suggest that constitutive P-450 expression in epithelial cells may be regulated as a function of the tissues' proliferation/differentiation status.

B[a]P must be metabolized in order to be tumorigenic. The entire thickness of the skin, including the basal layer, is labeled within 24 hr of topical application of radiolabeled B[a]P (51). The presence of B[a]P adducts in the basal layer agrees with our measurement of induced 7-ERD activity in the basal layer following the topical treatment with DB[a,c]A. Like DB[a,c]A, B[a]P is a good inducer of cytochrome P-450IA1, and 7-ERD reflects P450IA1 activity (29). The skin tumors that develop following the topical application of chemical carcinogens are thought to be derived from initiated stem cells. Double isotope–double emulsion autoradiographic analyses by Morris et al. (51,52) suggest that these cells may be a slow-cycling population of basal cells that sit in the center of epidermal proliferation units. These cells probably constitute only a minor percentage of the basal cell population we prepare by Percoll gradient centrifugation. Consequently, an important question is whether these cells can activate procarcinogens, or whether activation is achieved by a neighboring cell and the activated metabolite is transferred between cells. We currently are not in a position to distinguish between these two possibilities. Keratinocyte-mediated mutation assays have demonstrated that mutagenic B[a]P and DMBA metabolites generated in cultured keratinocytes can be transferred to cocultured fibroblasts (53). Recent studies by Jongen et al. (54) suggest that reactive B[a]P metabolites can be transferred between cells via gap junctions. Furthermore, studies employing both newborn (55) and adult mice (56) suggest that epithelial cells within the epidermal proliferative units communicate with each other both horizontally and vertically by gap junctions. Consequently, it is conceivable that a mutagenic/carcinogenic metabolite produced in a neighboring MK could be responsible for the initiation of a stem cell. Given the distribution of constitutive monooxygenase activities in predominantly differentiating MKs, the transfer of reactive metabolites between MKs may be particularly relevant for procarcinogens that do not induce P-450s and are metabolized by constitutive activities.

The demonstration that the constitutive monooxygenase activities of MKs vary with the stage of differentiation in vivo, and with the medium Ca^{2+} concentration in vitro, has several implications.

First, it is conceivable that constitutive P-450 expression in vivo in the epidermis may be regulated as a function of changes in Ca^{2+} concentration occurring during differentiation. There is a report suggesting the existence of an in vivo Ca^{2+} gradient in the epidermis, with little or no Ca^{2+} in the cytoplasm of the basal cells (57). Alternately, the correlation between Ca^{2+} and P-450 gradients may be coincidental. Constitutive P-450 expression in the epidermis may be a characteristic of the differentiating phenotype and independent of Ca^{2+}. We are currently attempting to resolve this issue. Second, our findings are relevant to the use of MK cultures as in vitro test systems for assaying genotoxic chemicals. Estimates of cytotoxicity, mutagenesis, and transformation may be significantly underestimated in studies with chemicals requiring metabolic activation if exposure to chemicals occurs when MKs are cultured in a low Ca^{2+}–containing medium. Third, the 67-kDa cytokeratin K1 is a very early marker of MK differentiation and is found in the spinous layer and in some basal cells that are committed to differentiation but have not yet moved to the suprabasal layer (58,59). Our Percoll studies, and an analysis of the kinetics of differentiation marker appearance in cultured MKs (1,60), suggest that the kinetics of 7-ECD and 7-ERD expression are similar to or may even precede K1 expression. Thus, constitutive monooxygenase expression is a very early marker of MK commitment to differentiation. Fourth, our data suggest that modulation of epidermal differentiation in vivo might alter epidermal xenobiotic metabolism. Modulation of differentiation might be particularly relevant to xenobiotics that are metabolized by constitutive activities, due to either an inherent inability to induce P-450s or insufficient concentration to effect an induction.

Acknowledgement

Research was supported in part by USPHS Grants CA 34469 and CA 40823.

References

1. Reiners Jr. JJ, Cantu AR, Pavone A. Modulation of constitutive cytochrome P-450 expression in vivo and in vitro in murine keratinocytes as a function of differentiation and extracellular Ca^{2+} concentration. Proc Natl Acad Sci USA 87:1825–1829, 1990.
2. Baron J, Kawabata TT, Redick JA, Knapp SA, Wick DG, Wallace RB, Jakoby WB, Guengerich FP. Localization of carcinogen-metabolizing enzymes in human and animal tissues. In Rydström J, Montelius J, Bengtsson M (eds): Extrahepatic Drug Metabolism and Chemical Carcinogenesis. Amsterdam: Elsevier Science Publishers, 1983, pp 73–87.
3. Guo Jin-feng, Brown R, Rothwell CE, Bernstein IA. Levels of cytochrome P-450-mediated aryl hydrocarbon hydroxylase (AHH) are higher in differentiated than in germinative cutaneous keratinocytes. J Invest Dermatol 94:86–93, 1990.
4. Bickers DR, Mukhtar H, Yang SK. Cutaneous metabolism of benz[*a*]pyrene: Comparative studies in C57BL/6N and DBA/2N mice and neonatal Sprague-Dawley rats. Chem Biol Interact 43:263–270, 1983.
5. Bickers DR, Marcelo CL, Dutta-Choudhury T, Mukhtar H. Studies on microsomal cytochrome P-450, monooxygenases and epoxide hydrolase in cultured keratinocytes and intact epidermis from BALB/C mice. J Pharmacol Exp Ther 223:163–168, 1982.
6. Bickers DR, Dutta-Choudhury T, Mukhtar H. Epidermis: A site of drug metabolism in neonatal rat skin. Mol Pharmacol 21:239–247, 1982.
7. Jin XP, Rothwell CE, Bernstein IA. Effects of 3-methylcholanthrene on the induction of aryl hydrocarbon hydroxylase by benz[*a*]anthracene in primary cultures of cutaneous keratinocytes from the newborn rat. J Toxicol Cutaneous Ocul Toxicol 5:63–72, 1986.
8. Ichikawa T, Hayashi S-I, Noshiro M, Takada K, Okuda K. Purification and characterization of cytochrome P-450 induced by benz[*a*]anthracene in mouse skin microsomes. Cancer Res 49:806–809, 1989.
9. Eling T, Curtis J, Battista J, Marnett LJ. Oxidation of (+)7,8-dihydroxy-7,8-dihydrobenzo[*a*]pyrene by mouse keratinocytes: Evidence for peroxyl radical and monooxygenase-dependent metabolism. Carcinogenesis 7:1957–1963, 1986.
10. DiGiovanni J, Decina PC, Prichett WP, Fisher EP, Aalfs KK. Formation and disappearance of benzo[*a*]pyrene DNA–adducts in mouse epidermis. Carcinogenesis 6:741–745, 1985.
11. Slaga TJ, Thompson S, Berry DL, DiGiovanni J, Juchau MR, Viaje A. The effects of benzoflavones on polycylic hydrocarbon metabolism and skin tumor initiation. Chem Biol Interact 17:297–312, 1977.
12. Dipple A, Pigott MA, Bigger AH, Blake DM. 7,12-Dimethylbenz[*a*]anthracene-DNA binding in mouse skin: Response of different mouse strains and effects of various modifiers of carcinogenesis. Carcinogenesis 5: 1087–1090, 1984.
13. Streilein JW. Skin-associated lymphoid tissues (SALT). J Invest Dermatol 80:122–126, 1983.
14. Potten CS. Cell replacement in epidermis (keratoporesis) via discrete units of proliferation. Int Rev Cytol 69:271–318, 1981.
15. Baxter CS, Chalfin K, Andringa A, Miller ML. Qualitative and quantitative effects on epidermal Langerhans (Ia+) and Thy-1+ dendritic cells following topical application of phobol diesters and mezerein. Carcinogenesis 9:1563–1568, 1988.
16. Reiners Jr JJ, Hale MA, Cantu AR. Distribution of catalase and its modulation by 12–O-tetradecanoylphorbol-13-acetate in murine dermis and subpopulations of keratinocytes differing in their stages of differentiation. Carcinogenesis 9:1259–1263, 1988.
17. Reiners Jr JJ, Rupp, T. Conversion of xanthine dehydrogenase to xanthine oxidase occurs during keratinocyte differentiation: Modulation by 12-O-tetradecanoylphorbol-13-acetate. J Invest Dermatol 93:132–135, 1989.
18. Cameron GS, Baldwin JK, Jasheway DW, Patrick KE, Fischer SM. Arachidonic acid metabolism varies with the state of differentiation in density gradient–separated mouse epidermal cells. J Invest Dermatol 94:292–296, 1990.

19. Hennings H, Michael D, Cheng C, Steinert P, Holbrook K, Yuspa SH. Calcium regulation of growth and differentiation of mouse epidermal cells in culture. Cell 19:245–254, 1980.
20. Sun T-T, Green H. Differentiation of epidermal keratinocytes in cell culture: formation of the cornified envelope. Cell 9:511–521, 1976.
21. Reiners Jr JJ, Slaga TJ. Effects of tumor promoters on the rate and commitment to terminal differentiation of subpopulations of murine keratinocytes. Cell 32:247–255, 1983.
22. Fischer SM, Nelson KDG, Reiners, Jr JJ, Viaje A, Pelling JC, Slaga TJ. Separation of epidermal cells by density centrifugation: A new technique for studies on normal and pathological differentiation. J Cutan Pathol 9:43–49, 1982.
23. Reiners Jr JJ, Cantu AR, Pavone A, Smith SC, Gardner CR, Laskin DL. Fluorescence assay for per cell estimation of cytochrome P-450-dependent monooxygenase activities in keratinocyte suspensions and cultures. Anal Biochem, 188:317–324, 1990.
24. Miller DR, Viaje A, Aldaz CM, Conti CJ, Slaga TJ. Terminal differentiation-resistant epidermal cells in mice undergoing two-stage carcinogenesis. Cancer Res 47:1935–1940, 1987.
25. DiGiovanni J, Gill RD, Nettikumara AN, Colby AB, Reiners Jr JJ. Effect of extracellular calcium concentration on the metabolism of polycyclic aromatic hydrocarbons by cultured keratinocytes. Cancer Res 49:5567–5574, 1989.
26. Reiners Jr JJ, Yotti LP, McKeown CK, Nesnow S, Slaga TJ. Keratinocyte cell-mediated mutagenesis assay: Correlation with in vivo tumor studies. Carcinogenesis 4:321–326, 1983.
27. Piskorska-Pliszczynska J, Keys B, Safe S, Newman MS. The cytosolic receptor binding affinities and AHH induction potencies of 20 polynuclear aromatic hydrocarbons. Toxicol Lett 34:67–74, 1986.
28. Pohl RJ, Fouts JR. A rapid method for assaying the metabolism of 7-ethoxyresorufin by microsomal subcellular fractions. Anal Biochem 107:150–155, 1980.
29. Burke MD, Thompson S, Elcombe CR, Halpert J, Haaparanta T, Mayer RT. Ethoxy-, pentoxy- and benzyloxyphenoxazones and homologues: A series of substrates to distinguish between different induced cytochrome P-450. Biochem Pharmacol 34:3337–3345, 1985.
30. Gonzalez FJ. The molecular biology of cytochrome P-450s. Pharmacol Rev 40:243–288, 1989.
31. Coomes, MW, Norling AH, Pohl RJ, Müller D, Fouts JR. Foreign compound metabolism by isolated skin cells from the hairless mouse. J Pharmacol Exp Ther 225:770–777, 1983.
32. Pohl RJ, Coomes MW, Sparks RW, Fouts JR. 7-ethoxycoumarin O-deethylation activity in viable basal and differentiated keratinocytes isolated from the skin of the hairless mouse. Drug Metab Dispos 12:25–34, 1984.
33. Knutson JC, Poland A. Response of murine epidermis to 2,3,7,8-tetrachlorodibenzo-p-dioxin: Interaction of the Ah and hr loci. Cell 30:225–234, 1982.
34. Klein-Szanto AJP, Morris P, Slaga TJ. Separation of cells from normal and abnormal epidermis. In Pretlow TG, Pretlow TP (eds): Cell Separation: Methods and Selected Applications, Vol 5. New York: Academic Press, Inc., 1987, pp 195–215.
35. Plopper CG, Weir AJ, Philpot RM, Davis CA. Pattern of cytochrome P-450 expression during Clara cell differentiation in rabbit lung. J Cell Biol 109:698 (abstract), 1989.
36. Epstein R, Gatans EA. Nuclear ploidy in mammalian parenchymal liver cells. Nature 214:1050–1051, 1967.
37. Epstein CJ. Cell size, nuclear content and the development of polyploidy in the mammalian liver. Proc Natl Acad Sci USA 57:327–334, 1967.
38. Brodsky WY, Uryvaeva IV. Cell polyploidy: Its relation to tissue growth and function. Int Rev Cytol 50:275–332, 1977.
39. Schwarze PE, Pettersen EO, Shoaib MC, Seglen PO. Emergence of a population of small, diploid hepatocytes during hepatocarcinogenesis. Carcinogenesis 5:1267–1275, 1984.
40. Saeter G, Schwarze PE, Nesland JM, Juul N, Petterson EO, Seglen PO. The polyploidizing growth pattern of normal rat liver is replaced by divisional, diploid growth in hepatocellular nodules and carcinomas. Carcinogenesis 9:939–945, 1988.
41. Sargent L, Xu Y-H, Sattler GL, Meisner L, Pitot HC. Ploidy and karyotype of hepatocytes isolated from enzyme-altered foci in two different protocols of multistage hepatocarcinogenesis in the rat. Carcinogenesis 10:387–391, 1989.
42. White INH, Green ML, Legg RF. Fluorescence-activated sorting of rat hepatocytes based on their mixed function oxidase activities towards diethoxyfluorescein. Biochem J 247:23–28, 1987.

43. White INH, Legg RF, Manson MM, Wolf CR. Characteristics of rat hepatocytes sorted by fluorescence-activated flow cytometry: Effects of mixed function oxidase inducers. Biochem Pharmacol 38:1639–1645, 1989.

44. Neims AH, Warner M, Loughnan PM, Aranda JV. Developmental aspects of the hepatic cytochrome P-450 monoxygenase system. Ann Rev Pharmacol Toxicol 16:427–445, 1976.

45. Giachelli CM, Omiecinski CJ. Developmental regulation of cytochrome P-450 genes in the rat. Mol Pharmacol 31:477–484, 1987.

46. Liddle C, Murray M, Farrell GC. Effect of liver regeneration on hepatic cytochrome P-450 isoenzymes and serum sex steroids in male rat. Gastroenterology 96:864–872, 1989.

47. Marie IJ, Dalet C, Blanchard J-M, Astre C, Szawlowski A, Aubert BS, Joyeux H, Maurel P. Inhibition of cytochrome P-450p (P450IIIA1) gene expression during liver regeneration from two-thirds hepatectomy in the rat. Biochem Pharmacol 37:3515–3521, 1988.

48. Buchmann AB, Kuhlmann W, Schwarz M, Kunz W, Wolf CR, Moll E, Friedberg T, Oesch F. Regulation and expression of four cytochrome P-450 isoenzymes, NADPH-cytochrome P-450 reductase, the glutathione transferases B and C and microsomal epoxide hydrolase in preneoplastic and neoplastic lesions of rat liver. Carcinogenesis 6:513–521, 1985.

49. Stout DL, Becker FF. Xenobiotic metabolizing enzymes in genetically and chemically initiated mouse liver tumors. Cancer Res 46:2693–2696, 1986.

50. Becker FF, Stout DL. A constitutive deficiency in the monooxygenase system of spontaneous mouse liver tumors. Carcinogenesis 5:785–788, 1984.

51. Morris RJ, Fischer SM, Slaga TJ. Evidence that a slow cycling subpopulation of adult murine epidermal cells retains carcinogen. Cancer Res 46:3061–3066, 1986.

52. Morris RJ, Fischer SM, Slaga TJ. Evidence that the centrally and peripherally located cells in the murine epidermal proliferative unit are two distinct cell populations. J Invest Dermatol 84:277–281, 1985.

53. Reiners Jr JJ, Herlick S. Cell-cell proximity is a parameter affecting the transfer of mutagenic polycyclic aromatic hydrocarbons between cells. Carcinogenesis 6:793–795, 1985.

54. Jongen WMF, van der Leede BJN, Chang CC, Troska JE. The transport of reactive intermediates in a cocultivation system: the role of intracellular communication. Carcinogenesis 8:1239–1243, 1987.

55. Kam E, Melville L, Pitts JD. Patterns of junctional communication in skin. J Invest Dermatol 87:748–753, 1986.

56. Kam E, Pitts JD. Effects of the tumor promoter 12-O-tetradecanoylphorbol-13-acetate on junctional communication in intact mouse skin: Persistance of homologous communication and increase of epidermal-dermal coupling. Carcinogenesis 9:1389–1394, 1988.

57. Menon GK, Grayson S, Elias PM. Ionic calcium reservours in mammalian epidermis: Ultrastructural localization by ion-capture cytochemistry. J Invest Dermatol 84:508–512, 1985.

58. Roop DR, Cheng CK, Titterington L, Meyers CA, Stanley JR, Steinert PM, Yuspa SH. Synthetic peptides corresponding to keratin subunits elicit highly specific antibodies. J Biol Chem 259:8037–8040, 1984.

59. Roop DR, Krieg TM, Mehrel, T, Cheng CK, Yuspa SH. Transcriptional control of high molecular weight keratin gene expression in multistage mouse skin carcinogenesis. Cancer Res 48:3245–3252, 1988.

60. Yuspa SH, Kilkenny AE, Steinert PM, Roop DR. Expression of murine epidermal differentiation markers is tightly regulated by restricted extracellular calcium concentration in vitro. J Cell Biol 109:1207–1217, 1989.

Chemically Induced Cell Proliferation:
Implications for Risk Assessment, pages 137-144
©1991 Wiley-Liss, Inc.

Ornithine Decarboxylase Induction and DNA Damage as a Predictive Assay for Potential Carcinogenicity

Kirk T. Kitchin, Janice L. Brown, and Arun P. Kulkarni

It is useful in carcinogenesis risk assessment to distinguish among initiators, promoters, and nongenotoxic carcinogens and to utilize mechanistic data when it is available. Linear models of risk assessment may be appropriate for chemicals that are carcinogenesis initiators, while threshold models of risk assessment have been proposed for promoters and nongenotoxic carcinogens. The proper risk assessment models for the regulation of carcinogenesis promoters and nongenotoxic carcinogens remains an active area of research and controversy.

Recently, the concepts of cell death, mitogenic stimulation, and increased cell proliferation have received more attention as correlates or causes of some cancers in animal bioassays. A promising two-stage mathematical model of carcinogenesis has been developed (1) in which a chemical can act as either an initiator via mutation or as a promoter by increasing rates of cell proliferation. Short-term mutagenicity tests can identify many initiators of carcinogenesis. Similarly, in a validation study of 91 compounds, the alkaline elution technique of determining in vitro DNA damage correctly identified 92% of the carcinogens tested and 85% of the noncarcinogens (2). A similar conclusion has been reached based on DNA damage studies conducted in vivo (3). It has become increasingly apparent that predictive assays are needed for promoters of carcinogenesis and nongenotoxic carcinogens (4).

Ornithine decarboxylase (ODC) induction precedes cell proliferation in many cells exposed to mitogenic or cytotoxic chemicals. Most promoters of carcinogenesis induce ODC in vivo (5–10). In this study, we selected rat hepatic ODC and DNA damage, as measured by the alkaline elution, as in vivo biochemical markers of promotion and initiation of cancer, respectively. The purpose of this research was to develop an in vivo predictive assay for cancer which: 1) provided complementary data to the Ames test, and 2) separately determines a chemical's potential to cause either promotion or initiation.

Materials and methods

Ninety-day-old female Sprague-Dawley rats (CD strain) were obtained from Charles River Laboratories and housed three per cage. The initiators and promoters selected in this study were all of the halogenated hydrocarbon class. The chemicals were obtained from standard commercial sources and orally administered to rats at doses of either 1/5 or 3/5 the rat single oral LD_{50} value (11). The first dose was given 21 hr and the second at 4 hr before sacrifice. The parameters ODC activity, glutathione content, and DNA damage respond well to a 4 hr chemical pretreatment (2,12), while the 21 hr time point is good for detecting possible changes in hepatic cytochrome P-450 content and serum alanine aminotransferase activity (13,14).

To prepare tissue samples, 1.5 g of washed, minced liver were homogenized in 6 ml of ice-cold pH 7.5 buffer containing NaCl (136 mM), KCl (5.4 mM), HEPES (20 mM), dithioerythritol (5 mM), ethylenediamine tetraacetate (EDTA) (4 mM), and pyridoxal-5'-phosphate (0.08 mM). Liver samples were homogenized with six strokes with a size C Potter-Elvehjem homogenizer (clearance 0.15–0.23 mm) operated at 300 rpm. After a 10-min settling period at 0–4°C, 75 μl of the whole liver homogenate was used for alkaline elution. The Stout and Becker (15) modification of the Kohn et al. (16) basic alkaline elution procedure to minimize protein adsorption was employed. Additional modifications of the alkaline elution technique were a 48-hr delay in the SDS-lysis step (17), addition of 0.06% Sarkosyl to the first EDTA wash, and addition of 5 mM phosphate buffer to increase the buffering capacity of the pH 12.10 eluting solution. This time-dependent sensitivity increase has been ascribed to either DNA unfolding (17) or additional DNA alkaline-labile sites and single-strand breaks (18). Alkaline elution data are expressed as the fraction of DNA eluted from the polycarbonate filter during the 14-hr elution period. A fraction of 1.00 DNA eluted means that 100% of the DNA was eluted from the filter.

In some instances, reduced glutathione depletion, cytochrome P-450 induction, and cytotoxicity have been associated with exposure of rats to chemical carcinogens. Ornithine decarboxylase activity (12), glutathione content (19,20), cytochrome P-450 content (21), and serum alanine aminotransferase activity (14) were measured by standard methods. For these four assays, we utilized the high-speed supernatant, whole homogenate, microsomes and serum, repectively. The post-mitochondrial supernatant (20 min, 20,000 g) was spun at 193,000 g for 40 min to produce the microsomal fraction and the high-speed supernatant. Statistical analysis employed analysis of variance; any significant differences were evaluated with a Student's t-test.

Results and discussion

Experimental data from studies conducted with 1,2-dibromo-3-chloropropane, 1,1-dichloro-2,2-bis(p-chlorophenyl)ethylene (p,p-DDE) and coumaphos are shown in Table 1. A dose of 35 mg/kg 1,2-dibromo-3-chloropropane (1/5 LD_{50}) increased hepatic ODC activity threefold and caused substantial DNA damage. At a dosage of 1/5 LD_{50} (175 mg/kg) p,p-DDE increased hepatic ODC activity by 6-fold and hepatic cyto-chrome P-450 by 58%. At 3/5 LD_{50} (525 mg/kg) p,p-DDE caused even more marked induction of ODC (22-fold) and cytochrome P-450 (123%). Coumaphos, a noncar-cinogen, was without biochemical effects on the five parameters examined (Table 1).

Table 2 summarizes the experimental results for 23 compounds with respect to the two key parameters in this study (DNA damage and ODC induction) (22–26) as well as the two-year cancer bioassay and Ames test results. Based on what is generally accepted by most investigators, the 23 chemicals are assigned to these categories: 1) initiators of carcinogenesis, 2) promoters and putative promoters of carcinogenesis, and 3) noncarcinogens. Although toxaphene is positive in an Ames test (37), it was classified as a putative promoter because toxaphene induced rat hepatic ODC activity and did not cause DNA damage (29).

Table 1. Effect of an Initiator, Putative Promoter, and Noncarcinogen on Five Hepatic Biochemical Parameters.

Treatment (mg/kg)	Alkaline elution (fraction of DNA eluted)	Ornithine decarboxylase (nmol CO_2/ g liver/hr)	Glutathione (μmol/g)	Cytochrome P-450 (nmol/g)	Alanine amino-transferase (IU/L)
Corn oil (14 rats)	.225 ± .014	1.81 ± .17	2.98 ± .13	3.19 ± .23	15.1 ± 1.1
1,2-dibromo-3-chloropropane (Initiator) 35 mg/kg (9 rats)	.646 ± .055[c]	6.83 ± .62[c]	3.50 ± .32	2.85 ± .29	17.1 ± 1.4
Corn oil (16 rats)	.230 ± .003	1.39 ± .25[d]	5.58 ± .22	3.59 ± .33	14.5 ± 1.3
p,p-DDE (Putative promoter)					
175 mg/kg (12 rats)	.195 ± .020	10.4 ± 1.5[b]	4.53 ± .21[b]	5.68 ± .49[b]	10.9 ± .7[a]
525 mg/kg (6 rats)	.229 ±.024	31.9 ± 5.76[b]	4.21 ± .42[b]	8.02 ± .82[b]	15.5 ± 1.8
Gum tragacanth (7 rats)	.147 ± .017	1.39 ± .25	3.93 ± .22	3.35 ± .33	12.7 ± 1.9
Coumaphos (Noncarcinogen) 3.2 mg/kg (8 rats)	.148 ± .014	1.08 ± .17	5.05 ± .48	5.59 ± .61	13.9 ± 1.3

Adult female rats were orally given two doses of *p,p*-DDE 21 and 4 hr before sacrifice. All doses were 1/5 the published oral rat LD_{50} value except for 525 mg/kg of *p,p*-DDE which was 3/5 the LD_{50}. Values are the means ± SEM for the indicated number of rats.

[a] $P < .05$

[b] $P < .01$

[c] $P < .001$

[d] 21 rather than 16 rats were used in this experiment.

DNA damage was caused by 1,2-dibromoethane, 1,2-dibromo-3-chloropropane, 1,2-dichloroethane and methylene chloride (at $3/5$ LD_{50}). It is interesting that two of the four halogenated hydrocarbons classified as initiators also induced hepatic ODC activity. For 1,2-dibromo-3-chloropropane and 1,2-dibromoethane, these data suggest that cell proliferation as well as DNA damage may jointly cause neoplasia.

Induction of hepatic ODC was found with eight of 10 halogenated hydrocarbons classified as promoters although doses higher than $1/5$ LD_{50} had to be used with hexachlorobenzene, kepone, and α-hexachlorocyclohexane (Table 2). The two halogenated compounds that did not induce rat hepatic ODC were *p,p*-DDT and TCDD. *p,p*-DDT may act via its metabolite, *p,p*-DDE, which does induce rat hepatic ODC. TCDD did not induce ODC in the female rat, but does induce ODC in mouse liver (12).

Table 2. Comparison of the Results from this Study to Cancer Bioassay and Ames Tests.

	DNA damage		ODC induction		Two-year bioassay for cancer	Ames test
	1/5 LD$_{50}$	3/5 LD$_{50}$	1/5 LD$_{50}$	3/5 LD$_{50}$		
Initiators						
1,2-dibromoethane (22)	+		+		+ (30)	+ (37)
methylene chloride (23)	−	+	−	−	+ (31)	−[a] (31)
1,2-dibromo-3-chloropropane	+		+		+ (30)	+ (37)
1,2-dichloroethane (24)	+		−		+ (30)	+ (37)
Promoters and putative promoters						
p,p-DDT (25)	−	−	−[b]	−	+ (30)	− (29)
p,p-DDE	−	−	+	+	+ (32)	− (37)
toxaphene (26)	−	−	+	+	+ (30)	+ (37)
2,3,7,8-tetrachlorodibenzo-p-dioxin (TCDD) (24)	−		−[c]		+ (30)	− (37)
mirex (24)	−		+		+ (30)	− (27)
hexachlorobenzene (26)	−	−[d]	−	+[d]	+ (30)	− (38)
kepone (26)	−	−	−	+	+ (30)	− (27)
α-hexachlorocyclohexane (26)	−	−	−	+	+ (30)	− (29)
carbon tetrachloride (23)	−	−	+	+	+ (30)	− (39)
chloroform (23)	−	+	+	+	+ (30)	− (40)
Noncarcinogens						
cyclohexylamine (26)	−	−	−	−	− (33)	− (33)
diethyldithiocarbamate (26)	−	−	+	+	− (34)	− (37)
EDTA (26)	−	−	−	−	− (34)	− (37)
caprolactam (26)	−	−	−		− (34)	− (37)
titanium(IV)oxide (26)	−	−	−		− (34)	− (37)
coumaphos	−	−	−	−	− (34)	− (37)
sucrose (26)	−	−	−		− (35)	− (35)
8-hydroxyquinoline (26)	−	−	+	+	− (34)	+ (37)
piperidine (26)	−	−	−	−	− (36)	+ (41)

[a] If sealed vessels are used, methylene chloride gives a positive Ames test.
[b] DDT is slowly metabolized to DDE which induces ODC.
[c] TCDD induces ODC in mice but not rats.
[d] A dose of 2/5 LD$_{50}$ was used for hexachlorobenzene, not 3/5 LD$_{50}$.
If data in this table is missing, the experiment was not performed or the information was not available from common published sources.

The nine noncarcinogens produced several biochemical effects at doses of 1/5 LD$_{50}$ (Table 2). However, no noncarcinogens caused DNA damage in rat liver and only two caused increased hepatic ODC activity. Concurrent induction of rat hepatic cytochrome P-450, a confirmatory biochemical marker for tumor promoters, did not occur with these two chemicals. To test the possibility that at a dose of 3/5 LD$_{50}$ many noncarcinogenic compounds would induce rat hepatic ODC activity, this higher dose level of coumaphos, EDTA, cyclohexylamine, piperidine, and caprolactam was orally administered to rats. None gave a statistically significant increase in rat hepatic ODC activity (26).

The definitions of operational characteristics for predicting carcinogenicity are defined in Table 3. The first set of 23 chemicals compiled in this study contains halogenated hydrocarbons as initiators and promoters of carcinogenesis. The second set of 16 halogenated hydrocarbons is compiled from three published sources (27–29). The third set of 73 diverse chemicals is from a National Toxicology Program (NTP) report by Tennant et al. (4).

The operational characteristics of the Ames test for these three different sets of chemicals are reported in Table 4. It should be noted that the Ames test was ineffective in indicating carcinogenicity for many halogenated hydrocarbons. The only correct classifications were made for three out of four genotoxic carcinogens, one out of ten promoters, and six out of eight noncarcinogens. The operational characteristics of the Ames test for 73 NTP chemicals (which contained few halogenated hydrocarbons) is concordance 62%, specificity 86%, positive predictivity 83%, and sensitivity 45%. We stress that these are three entirely different groups of chemicals and thus direct comparisons between the three studies cannot be made.

Overall, the operational characteristics of the in vivo test system are excellent. For example, the ranges of values for sensitivity were 44–86%, specificity 71–100% and concordance 61–95% (Table 5). The concordance of results from the in vivo biochemical system with two-year bioassays (65% at $1/5$ LD_{50}, 83% at $3/5$ LD_{50}) is far higher than the 48% concordance of the Ames test for these same 23 chemicals. At higher doses of halogenated hydrocarbons (up to $3/5$ LD_{50}), the in vivo biochemical system was an excellent predictor of carcinogenicity (Table 5).

Table 3. Definitions of Operational Characteristics.

Two-year cancer bioassay	Test system (e.g., in vivo biochemical test battery)	
	+	−
+	A	C
−	B	D

Sensitivity = % of carcinogens which test positive = A/(A + C) × 100%
Specificity = % of noncarcinogens which test negative = D/(D+B) × 100%
Positive predictivity = % of test positives that are carcinogens = A/(A + B) × 100%
Negative predictivity = % of test negatives that are noncarcinogens = D/(D + C) × 100%
Concordance = % of agreement between test system and two-year cancer bioassay results = A + D/(A + B + C + D) × 100%

Table 4. Operational Characteristics of the Ames Test for Predicting Carcinogenicity.

	Sixteen halogenated hydrocarbons (27–29)	Seventy-three National Toxicology Program chemicals (4)	Twenty-three chemicals in this study (Table 2)
Sensitivity	100% (n = 1)	45	29
Specificity	12	86	77
Positive predictivity	6	83	67
Negative predictivity	100 (n = 2)	51	41
Concordance	19	62	48

In this series of 23 compounds, the in vivo biochemical system gave better results than the Ames test for six compounds at $1/5$ LD_{50} and for nine compounds at $3/5$ LD_{50}. The six compounds were DDE, mirex, carbon tetrachloride, chloroform, piperidine, and 8-hydroxyquinoline. Hexachlorobenzene, kepone, and α-hexachlorocyclohexane were the three carcinogens that induced ODC at a dose of $3/5$ LD_{50}. For piperidine and 8-hydroxyquinoline (both noncarcinogens), the Ames test was positive, suggesting a risk as a genotoxic carcinogen. For these two noncarcinogens, in vivo studies showed that they had no genotoxicity, only ODC induction for 8-hydroxyquinoline. This suggests regulation only as a nongenotoxic promoter of carcinogenesis.

Conclusions

The in vivo biochemical assay system and the in vitro Ames test are not redundant and, in fact, give complementary experimental results. From data presented in this report it is clear that the biochemical assay system works well for halogenated hydrocarbons. In this study, the biochemical system predicted bioassay cancer results better than did the Ames test, showing a concordance of 83% versus 48%. The in vivo biochemical assay system also differentiated well between carcinogens, promoters, and noncarcinogens. Classifying chemicals by their ability either to promote or initiate cancer reduces the uncertainties of risk assessment. The question of how predictive this in vivo biochemical system is of animal carcinogenicity caused by other classes of chemical compounds will be addressed by future research.

Table 5. Operational Characteristics of the In Vivo Biochemical System for Predicting Cancer, Initiation, or Promotion.

	Dose					
	$1/5$ LD_{50}	$3/5$ LD_{50}	$1/5$ LD_{50}	$3/5$ LD_{50}	$1/5$ LD_{50}	$3/5$ LD_{50}
Predictor						
In vivo biochemical test battery parameter	DNA damage or ODC induction		DNA damage		ODC induction	
Prediction						
Bioassay or mutagenicity in short-term tests	Cancer		Initiators or mutagenicity		Promoters, preneoplastic nodules, nongenotoxic carcinogens	
Operational characteristics						
Sensitivity	57%	86%	60%	80%	44%	78%
Specificity	78%	78%	100%	100%	71%	71%
Positive predictivity	80%	86%	100%	100%	50%	64%
Negative predictivity	54%	78%	88%	94%	66%	83%
Concordance	65%	83%	91%	95%	61%	74%

The initiators and promoters were all of the halogenated hydrocarbon class.

Acknowledgments

The authors thank Kay Rigsbee and Fay Poythress of Program Resources, Inc. for their animal dosing and sacrificing and Mary Burrus for typing this manuscript.

Disclaimer

The research described in this paper has been reviewed by the Health Effects Research Laboratory, U. S. Environmental Protection Agency and approved for publication. Approval does not signify that the contents necessarily reflect the views and policies of the Agency nor does mention of trade names or commercial products constitute endorsement or recommendation for use.

References

1. Moolgavkar SH. Carcinogenesis modeling: From molecular biology to epidemiology. Annu Rev Public Health 7:151–169, 1986.
2. Sina JF, Bean CL, Dysart GR, Taylor VI, Bradley MO. Evaluation of the alkaline elution/rat hepatocyte assay as a predictor of carcinogenic/mutagenic potential. Mutat Res 113:357–391, 1983.
3. Swenberg JA, Petzold GL. The usefulness of DNA damage and repair assays for predicting carcinogenic potential of chemicals. In: Butterworth C (ed): Strategies for Short-Term Testing for Mutagens/Carcinogens. West Palm Beach, FL: CRC Press, 1979, pp. 77–86.
4. Tennant RW, Margolin BH, Shelby MD, Zeifer E, Haseman JK, Spalding J, Caspary W, Resnick M, Stasiewicz S, Anderson B, Minor R. Prediction of chemical carcinogenicity in rodents from in vitro genetic toxicity assays. Science 236:933–941, 1987.
5. O'Brien TG. The induction of ornithine decarboxylase as an early possibly obligatory event in mouse skin carcinogenesis. Cancer Res 36:2644–2653, 1976.
6. O'Brien TG, Simsiman RC, Boutwell RK. Induction of the polyamine-biosynthetic enzymes in mouse epidermis and their specificity for tumor promotion. Cancer Res 35:2426–2433, 1975.
7. Boutwell RK. Biochemical mechanism of tumor promotion. In: Slaga TJ, Sivak A, Boutwell RK (eds): Carcinogenesis, vol. 2. Mechanism of Tumor Promotion and Cocarcinogenesis. New York: Raven Press, 1978, pp. 49–58.
8. Yanagi S, Kazuyuki S, Yamamoto N. Induction by phenobarbital of ornithine decarboxylase activity in rat liver after initiation with diethylnitrosamine. Cancer Lett 12:87–91, 1981.
9. Raunio H, Pelonen O. Effect of polycyclic aromatic compounds and phorbol esters on ornithine decarboxylase and aryl hydrocarbon hydroxylase activites in mouse liver. Cancer Res 43:782–786, 1983.
10. Savage RE, Wedstrich C, Guion C, Pereira MA. Chloroform induction of ornithine decarboxylase activity in rats. Environ Health Perspect 46:157–162, 1982.
11. National Institute for Occupational Safety and Health. Registry of Toxic Effects of Chemical Substances. HEW publication no. 76-191. Washington, DC: U.S. Government Printing Office, 1976.
12. Nebert DW, Jensen NM, Perry JW, Oka T. Association between ornithine decarboxylase induction and the Ah locus in mice treated with polycyclic aromatic compounds. J Biol Chem 255:6836–6842, 1980.
13. Kitchin KT, Woods JS. 2,3,7,8-Tetrachlorodibenzo-p-dioxin induction of aryl hydrocarbon hydroxylase in female rat liver. Evidence for de novo synthesis of cytochrome P-450. Molec Pharmacol 14:890–899, 1978.
14. Plaa GL, Hewitt WR. Detection and evaluation of chemically induced liver injury. In: Hayes AW (ed): Principles and Methods of Toxicology. New York: Raven Press, pp. 407–445.
15. Stout DL, Becker FF. Fluorometric quantification of single-stranded DNA: A method applicable to the technique of alkaline elution. Anal Biochem 127:302–307, 1982.
16. Kohn KW, Ewig RAG, Erickson LC, Zwelling LA. Hanawalt PC, Freidberg EC (eds): DNA Repair: A Laboratory Manual of Research Procedures. New York: Marcel Dekker, 1981, pp. 379–401.
17. Nicolini C, Robbiano L, Pino A, Maura A, Finollo R, Brambilla G. Higher sensitivity for the detection of chemically induced DNA damage: Role of DNA unfolding in determining alkaline elution rate. Carcinogenesis 6:385–389, 1985.

18. Fornace AJ, Dobson PP, Kinsella TJ. Analysis of the effect of DNA alkylation on alkaline elution. Carcinogenesis 7:927–932, 1986.
19. Cohn VH, Lyle J. A fluorometric assay for glutathione. Anal Biochem 14:434–440, 1966.
20. Hissin PJ, Hilf R. A fluorometric method for determination of oxidized and reduced glutathione in tissues. Anal Biochem 74:214–226, 1976.
21. Omura T, Sato R. The carbon monoxide–binding pigment of liver microsomes. Evidence for its hemoprotein nature. J Biol Chem 239:2370–2378, 1964.
22. Kitchin KT, Brown JL. 1,2-Dibromoethane causes rat hepatic DNA damage at low doses. Biochem Biophys Res Commun 141:723–727, 1986.
23. Kitchin KT, Brown JL. Biochemical effects of three carcinogenic chlorinated methanes in rat liver. Teratogenesis Carcinog Mutagen 9:61–69, 1989.
24. Kulkarni A. Written report on Project No. 68-02-4175, 1988.
25. Kitchin KT, Brown JL. Biochemical effects of DDT and DDE in rat and mouse liver. Environ Res 46:39–47, 1988.
26. Kitchin KT, Brown JL. Biochemical studies of promoters of carcinogenesis in rat liver. Teratogenesis Carcinog Mutagen 9:273–285, 1989.
27. Probst GS, McMahon RE, Hill LE, Thompson CZ, Epp JK, Neal SB. Chemically induced unscheduled DNA synthesis in primary rat hepatocyte cultures: A comparison with bacterial mutagenicity using 218 compounds. Environ Mutagen 3:11–32, 1981.
28. McCann J, Choi E, Yamasaki E, Ames B. Detection of carcinogens as mutagens in the *Salmonella/* microsome test: Assay of 300 chemicals. Proc Natl Acad Sci USA 72:5135–5139, 1975.
29. Rinkus SJ, Legator MS. Chemical characterization of 465 known or suspected carcinogens and their correlation with mutagenic activity in the *Salmonella typhimurium* system. Cancer Res 39:3289–3318, 1979.
30. NTP. Fourth Annual Report on Carcinogens NTP-85-002. U.S. Department of Health and Human Services, 1985.
31. U.S. Environmental Protection Agency. Health assessment document for dichloromethane (methylene chloride). EPA/600/8-82/004F, 1985.
32. Greim H, Wolf T. Carcinogenicity of organic halogenated compounds. In: Searle CE (ed): Chemical Carcinogens, 2nd edition, ACS Monograph 182, 1984, pp. 525–575.
33. Bopp BA, Sonder RC, Kesterson JW. Toxicological aspects of cyclamate and cyclohexylamine. Crit Rev Toxicol 16:213–306, 1986.
34. Nesnow S, Argus M, Bergman H, Chu K, Frith C, Helmes T, McGaughy R, Ray V, Slaga TJ, Tennant R, Weisburger E. Chemical carcinogens: A review and analysis of the literature of selected chemicals and the establishment of the Gene-Tox Carcinogen Data Base. Mutat Res 185:1–195, 1986.
35. Trueman RW. Activity of 42 coded compounds in the Salmonella reverse mutation test. Progress in Mutation Research 1:343–350, 1981.
36. Magee PN, Montesano R, Preussmann R. *N*-Nitroso compounds and related carcinogens. In: Searle E (ed): Chemical Carcinogens, 1st Edition. Washington, D.C.: American Chemical Society, 1976, pp. 491–625.
37. Zeiger E. Carcinogenicity of mutagens: Predictive capability of the *Salmonella* mutagenesis assay for rodent carcinogenicity. Cancer Res 47:1287–1296, 1987.
38. U.S. Environmental Protection Agency. Health assessment document for chlorinated benzenes. EPA-600/8-84/015F, 1985.
39. U.S. Environmental Protection Agency. Health assessment document for carbon tetrachloride. EPA-600/8-82-001F, 1984a.
40. U.S. Environmental Protection Agency. Health assessment document for chloroform. EPA-600-8-84-004A, 1984b.
41. Bempong MN, Scully FE. Mutagenic activity of *N*-chloropiperodine. J Environ Pathol Toxicol 4:345–354, 1980.

Chemically Induced Cell Proliferation:
Implications for Risk Assessment, pages 145-154
©1991 Wiley-Liss, Inc.

Inhibitory Effects of Soybean Trypsin Inhibitor during Initiation and Promotion Phases of N-nitrosobis(2-oxopropyl)amine-induced Hamster Pancreatic Carcinogenesis

Michihito Takahashi, Katsumi Imaida, Fumio Furukawa, and Yuzo Hayashi

Feeding rats with soybean trypsin inhibitor (SBTI) is known to stimulate pancreatic cellular growth and to induce hypertrophy and hyperplasia of acinar cells and acinar cell carcinoma after long-term administration (1,2). The trophic effect of SBTI on the pancreas, however, is species-specific because such effects were not clearly observed in hamsters, mice, dogs, calves, pigs, or monkeys (3,4). Modifying effects of SBTI on pancreatic carcinogenesis have been reported in rats treated with 4-hydroxyaminoquinoline 1-oxide (HAQO) (5); growth of the preneoplastic acinar cell lesions or eosinophilic nodules were strongly stimulated by dietary supplementation. SBTI is also known to increase the levels of serum cholecystokinin (CCK) in rats (6,7), and thus, the observed enhancement of pancreatic acinar cell tumorigenesis has been considered due to this hormonal imbalance (7).

The hamster pancreatic carcinogenesis model using N-nitrosobis(2-oxopropyl)amine (BOP) is generally accepted as the most appropriate for investigation of pancreatic ductal carcinogenesis, since in terms of histological pattern and biology the induced lesions closely resemble human pancreatic carcinomas (8). Although long-term administration of CCK or raw soy flour was found not to cause enlargement of the hamster pancreas (3), SBTI did demonstrate modification potential in both initiation and promotion phases of the hamster-BOP system (9,10); in these cases, however, inhibition was observed.

The present experiments were performed to further elucidate the effects of SBTI on the initiation and/or promotion phases of hamster pancreatic ductal carcinogenesis.

Cell proliferation in the pancreas after administration of SBTI

A total of 120 male SD rats, aged 5 weeks, were used in Experiment I. Rats were divided into four groups as shown in Figure 1. Sixty rats received a single intravenous injection of HAQO dissolved in 0.005 N HCl, into the saphenous vein at a dose of 7 mg/kg body weight in 0.3 ml of solution. In Group 1 (HAQO/SBTI group), rats were then administered 5% SBTI in the diet. Group 2 (HAQO group) animals received only the HAQO injection without subsequent SBTI treatment. Group 3 (SBTI group) animals were given an equivalent amount of the acidic aqueous solution and fed 5% SBTI in the diet. Group 4 (control group) animals received the acidic aqueous solution and then the basal diet.

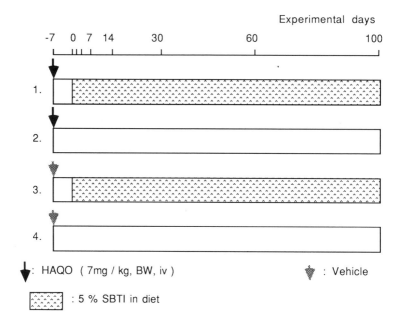

Figure 1. Design of Experiment I.

Five animals from each group were killed after 2, 4, 7, 14, 30, 60, and 100 days on SBTI diet; one hour before sacrifice, they were injected intraperitoneally with bromodeoxyuridine (BrdU) at a dose of 40 mg/kg body weight. Pancreatic tissues were removed and fixed in 10% phosphate-buffered formalin solution for routine hematoxylin and eosin staining. Immunohistochemical analysis of BrdU incorporation was performed using monoclonal mouse anti-BrdU (Amersham, England) and the Strept avidin-biotin peroxidase complex (Strept ABC) method.

Sections of splenic and gastric lobes were selected randomly, and their exocrine tissues were measured to calculate the percentage of area of tissue atrophy. In the HAQO/SBTI group, after 2 days the labeling index of the acinar cells had increased about 12-fold, dropping rapidly thereafter and returning to control values by day 30. The group that had received SBTI alone demonstrated a slightly smaller increase of about 11-fold (Fig. 2).

The comparative effects of SBTI on the pancreas of three animal species, that is, the rat, hamster, and mouse, have been investigated histopathologically and immunohistochemically (11). In rats, feeding SBTI diet for 4 weeks resulted in a significant increase of pancreatic volume in association with enlargement of acini, hypertrophy of acinar cells, and increase of intracellular zymogen granules. Such changes, however, were not observed in hamsters and mice similarly treated. Furthermore, accurate

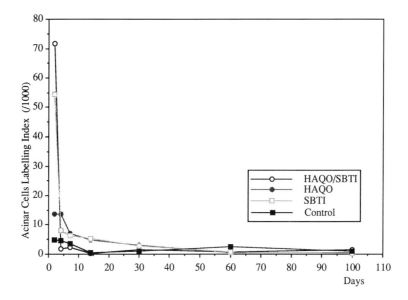

Figure 2. Sequential changes in numbers of tissue BrdU-positive acinar cells in rat pancreas.

determination of cell proliferation using the BrdU method (11) revealed labeling indices of both acinar and duct cells in SBTI-treated hamsters that were not enhanced, while those with untreated control values were enhanced (11). Thus, SBTI does not exert proliferative effects on either acinar or duct cells in the hamster.

Effects of soybean trypsin inhibitor during the initiation phase

A total of 90 female Syrian golden hamsters, 5 weeks old and weighing about 100 g, were used in Experiment II.

Hamsters were divided into three groups as shown in Figure 3. For investigation of the effects of SBTI during the initiation phase, hamsters in Group 1 were given 5 weekly subcutaneous injections of BOP at a dose of 10 mg/kg while being simultaneously treated with 5% SBTI diet. In Group 2, animals received only the subcutaneous injections of BOP. In Group 3, animals received the 5% SBTI diet for 5 weeks as given to Group 1. Animals were fed each diet ad libitum.

At week 30, all surviving animals were killed, and pancreas were excised, fixed in 10% buffered formalin, then separated into the splenic, gastric, duodenal, and pancreatic head tissues. The pancreas and the common duct were processed for histology by conventional methods and stained with hematoxylin and eosin. All pancreatic lesions were diagnosed histopathologically and counted in representative sections, as described previously (12). The results were statistically analyzed using the X2 test.

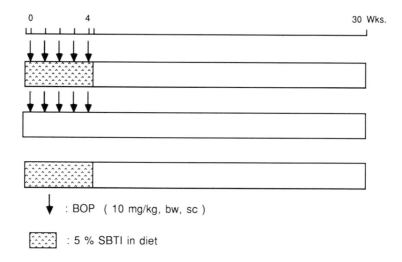

: BOP (10 mg/kg, bw, sc)

: 5 % SBTI in diet

Figure 3. Design of Experiment II.

No significant differences in body weight gains were observed between the group that received BOP and SBTI, BOP only, and the controls. As in our previous report (13), cancerous or precancerous pancreatic lesions could be histologically classified as adenocarcinomas and dysplasias. Metastasis and/or invasion were observed in the regional lymph nodes, stomach wall, liver, kidney, and peritoneum in some animals. The incidences of pancreatic lesions observed in each group of hamsters are summarized in Table 1. Although the incidences of pancreatic adenocarcinomas in the BOP and SBTI- and BOP-treated groups were not significantly different, the total numbers of pancreatic adenocarcinomas in the BOP and SBTI group, especially in the head region, were significantly decreased when compared to the BOP-only group value. Total numbers of

Table 1. Effects of SBTI Coadministration on BOP-Initiation of Pancreatic Carcinogenesis in Hamsters (Experiment II).

Group	No. of effective animals	Total no. lesions		Distribution of lesions							
				Splenic		Gastric		Duodenal		Head	
		Ca	Dys	Ca	Dys	Ca	Cys	Ca	Dys	Ca	Dys
BOP + SBTI	28	18 *	27 *	5	8 *	9	8	0	0	4 *	11
BOP	29	41	62	14	27	10	19	2	4	14	13
SBTI	30	0	0	0	0	0	0	0	0	0	0

Ca: Adenocarcinoma, Dys: Dysplastic lesion
* $P < 0.05$

dysplastic lesions in hamsters in Group 1 (receiving BOP and SBTI) were also significantly decreased. No pancreatic neoplastic lesions were observed in hamsters in control Group 3, those that were given SBTI but not BOP. The pancreas in BOP-treated animals showed invasive adenocarcinoma and atypia, and were characterized by diffuse ductal and ductular hyperplasia, periductal inflammation, and marked acinar cell destruction. In contrast, microscopic examination of the exocrine pancreas in those treated with BOP and SBTI revealed entirely normal findings.

While the mechanisms underlying the inhibitory effects remain unclear, a number of possible explanations may be considered. First, SBTI might have interfered with the cell's metabolism of BOP into active carcinogenic forms, and consequently inhibited pancreatic carcinogenesis. Second, treatment with SBTI induces high levels of pancreatic juice secretion, which might have interfered with the interactions between pancreatic tissue and BOP and/or its metabolites, preventing macromolecular binding including DNA adduct formation. In this context, it is interesting to note that secretin, which also causes high levels of pancreatic juice production, has similarly been reported to inhibit pancreatic carcinogenesis when given together with or prior to a single BOP dose (14). Third, the effects of SBTI might be due to the elimination of circulating and intracellular BOP.

Effects of soybean trypsin inhibitor during the promotion phase

A total of 90 Syrian golden hamsters were also used in Experiment III. They were divided into three groups as shown in Figure 4. In Group 1, hamsters were given 3 weekly subcutaneous injections of BOP at a dose of 10 mg/kg body weight and then were administered 5% SBTI in the diet. In Group 2, animals received subcutaneous injections of BOP only. In group 3, animals were fed 5% SBTI only. Moribund or dead animals were completely autopsied for histological examination. At week 40 of the experiment, all surviving animals were sacrificed. At autopsy, the pancreatic tissue was carefully examined macroscopically, then removed together with the duodenum and spleen, extended on filter paper, and fixed in 10% buffered formalin. It was divided into the four anatomical lobes, i.e., splenic, gastric, duodenal, and head. Tissue preparations were processed as in Experiment II.

No significant intergroup differences in mean body weight gain or mortality were observed. Incidence and distribution results for pancreatic lesions are summarized in Table 2. Most tumors occurred predominantly in the splenic and gastric lobes and were histologically diagnosed as adenocarcinomas. Several dysplastic lesions and a number of cystic changes were also found. Metastases were observed in the regional lymph nodes, stomach wall, liver, and peritoneum in some animals.

Although the incidence of pancreatic tumors was not significantly decreased in animals receiving SBTI (10.3%), as compared to the Group 2 value (17.2%), total numbers of carcinomas were significantly reduced. In tumor-bearing animals, the pattern of lesion distribution was quite comparable among the BOP-treated groups. Tumors in the SBTI-treated animals were often observed to be single and large; location of tumors tended to be the splenic lobe or the head region. The numbers of putative precursor dysplastic lesions were also significantly decreased in the BOP/SBTI-treated group.

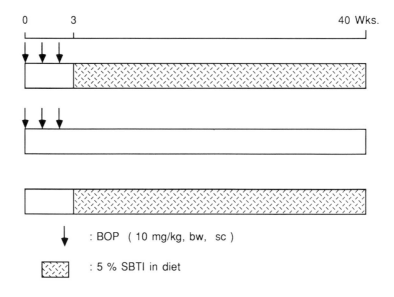

Figure 4. Design of Experiment III.

Table 2. Effects of SBTI on Development of BOP-Initiated Pancreatic Neoplastic Lesions in Hamsters (Experiment III).

Group	No. of effective animals	Total no. lesions Ca	Dys	Splenic Ca	Dys	Gastric Ca	Cys	Duodenal Ca	Dys	Head Ca	Dys
						Distribution of lesions					
BOP/SBTI	29	3	5 *	1	1	2	0	0	0	0 *	4 *
BOP	29	7	16	3	3	0	2	0	0	4	11
SBTI	30	0	0	0	0	0	0	0	0	0	0

Ca: Adenocarcinoma, Dys: Dysplastic lesion
* $P < 0.05$

Our results are therefore in line with earlier findings of inhibitory effects of CCK reported by Johnson et al. (15) and Pour et al. (9), although Anden-Sandberg et al. observed no influence (16) and Howatson and Carter found an enhancing effect (17). The discrepancies in some cases, however, may be due to variances in experimental designs and timing of the carcinogen administration. In our Experiment II, and in Pour's studies, SBTI was given simultaneously with BOP, producing results indicating that CCK level might be an important factor for initiation of pancreatic carcinogenesis in the hamster (9). Assuming that in the hamster there is a feedback mechanism for the trypsin inhibitor, the release of CCK in animals fed SBTI might account for the inhibitory effect of SBTI on BOP-induced pancreatic carcinoma.

Effects of soybean trypsin inhibitor on atrophic changes in pancreatic exocrine tissues induced by BOP

In Experiments II and III, atrophic changes of pancreatic exocrine tissues and fatty tissue infiltration were observed in hamsters treated with BOP. The ratios of exocrine atrophy in pancreatic sections were measured with the aid of an image processor (TAS Plus, West Germany). Splenic and gastric lobe sections measuring 2.4mm^2 were selected randomly, and their exocrine tissues were measured to calculate the percentage area of exocrine tissue atrophy.

The results of Experiments II and III are shown in Figures 5 and 6, respectively. In hamsters simultaneously treated with BOP and SBTI, the percent areas of intact exocrine tissues in both splenic and gastric lobes were significantly higher (87.0% and 83.5%, respectively) as compared to the BOP group values (61.1% and 61.9%), at the level of $P < 0.01$.

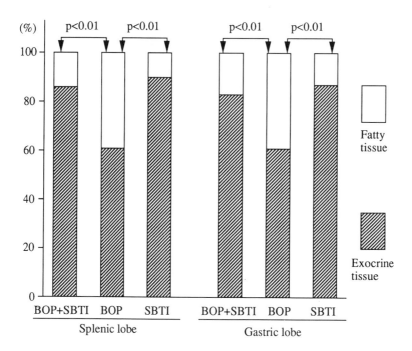

Figure 5. Percent areas of pancreatic exocrine and fatty tissues in hamsters simultaneously treated with BOP and SBTI (Experiment II).

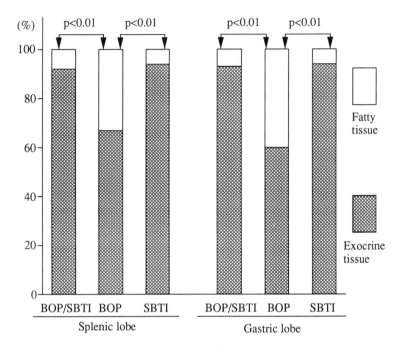

Figure 6. Percent areas of pancreatic exocrine and fatty tissues in hamsters treated with BOP followed by SBTI (Experiment III).

In Experiment III, the percent areas of intact splenic and gastric exocrine tissues were also significantly higher in the BOP/SBTI group (92.4% and 93.4%), as compared to the BOP group values (67.0% and 60.8%), at the level of $P < 0.01$.

Thus, in both experiments, atrophic pancreatic exocrine tissue changes were more severe in the BOP group than in the BOP/SBTI group; treatment with SBTI provided effective protection of acinar cells. Equivalent observations were also reported for hamsters treated with BOP followed by streptozotocin (18). These preventive effects of exocrine tissue atrophy presumably were directly associated with the inhibitory effects of BOP during the promotion phase of carcinogenesis.

Species-specific pancreatic reactions after administration of the synthetic trypsin inhibitor (Camostat) and SBTI

The effects of the synthetic trypsin inhibitor Camostat were reported to elucidate species differences among the rat, guinea pig, and hamster. Oral administration of Camostat induced a significant increase in the plasma level of CCK-like immunoreactive substance in the anesthetized rat, a small but significant increase in the anesthetized hamster, but no increase in the anesthetized guinea pig (19). It was therefore concluded that the observed species differences in hypertrophy of the pancreas, after repeated oral administrations of Camostat, may be primarily due to variations in the effectiveness of Camostat to induce endogenous CCK release and secondarily to differences in the exocrine pancreas responsiveness to secretagogues (19).

While SBTI has reported trophic effects on acinar cells (2), it also appears to induce a sensitization to the actions of chemical carcinogens. It has been proposed that SBTI acts on the pancreas indirectly by inhibiting trypsin within the lumen of the small intestine (2). Intraluminal trypsin is considered to inhibit pancreatic secretion by blocking the release of stimulant hormones such as CCK by a negative feedback mechanism in the rat (2). However, the hamster's pancreatic weight was found to not be affected by long-term SBTI administration; the hamster pancreas clearly responds quite differently to that of the rat under these conditions (3). Furthermore, since raw soy flour failed to modify the carcinogenic effects of azaserine in the mouse pancreas (20), it was apparent that significant species differences also exist with regard to this dietary influence. The varing effects of CCK on pancreatic carcinogenesis in the rat and hamster might relate to the origins of types of tumors induced in each, that is, acinar cell and ductal/ductular cell, respectively; the specific hormone action occurs only on the acinar cells. However, the lack of CCK effects on mouse pancreas with or without azaserine treatment indicates that other unknown factors might be involved (20).

Conclusion

Although SBTI promotes pancreatic acinar cell tumorigenesis in the rat, the present experiments clearly showed that it inhibits hamster pancreatic ductal carcinogenesis in both initiation and promotion phases, when administered in these respective phases together with, or following treatment with, BOP. The results thus suggest that the hamster model responds very differently to such endocrine factors as CCK. The specific mechanism that allows SBTI to inhibit pancreatic carcinogenesis in the hamster but not in the rat, however, remains to be explained.

Acknowledgments

We gratefully acknowledge the assistance of Dr. M. A. Moore in the preparation of this manuscript. This work was supported in part by a Grant-in-Aid for Cancer Research from the Ministry of Education, Science and Culture, Japan.

References

1.   McGuinnes EE, Morgan RGH, Levinson DA, Frape DL, Hopwood D, Wormsley KD. The effects of long-term feeding of soy flour on the rat pancreas. Scand J Gastroenterol 15:497–502, 1980.
2.   McGuinnes EE, Morgan RGH, Wormsley KD. Effects of soybean flour on the pancreas of rats. Environ Health Perspect 56:205–212, 1984.
3.   Liener IE, Hasdai A. The effect of the long-term feeding of raw soy flour on the pancreas of the mouse and hamster. Adv Exp Med Biol 199:189–197, 1986.
4.   Struthers BA, MacDonald JR, Dahlgren RR, Hopkins DT. Effects on the monkey, pig and rat pancreas of soy products with varying levels of trypsin inhibitor and comparison with the administration of cholecystokinin. J Nutr 113:86–97, 1983.

5. Hayashi H, Takahashi M, Furukawa F. Modifying effects of soybean trypsin inhibitor on carcinogen-induced pancreatic alterations in rats. Fifth International Congress of Toxicology, Abstracts, p.65, 1989.

6. Liddle RA, Goldfine I D, Williams JA. Bioassay of plasma cholecystokinin in rats. Gastroenterology 87:542–549, 1984.

7. Roebuk BD, Kaplita PV, Edwards BR, Praissman M. Effects of dietary fats and soybean protein on azaserine-induced pancreatic carcinogenesis and plasma cholecystokinin in rat. Cancer Res 47:1333–1338, 1987.

8. Takahashi M, Pour P, Althoff J, Donnelly T. Sequential alteration of the pancreas during carcinogenesis in Syrian golden hamsters by N-nitrosobis-(2-oxopropyl)amine. Cancer Res 37:4602–4607, 1977.

9. Pour PM, Lawson T, Helgeson S, Donnelly T, Stepan K. Effect of cholecystokinin on pancreatic carcinogenesis in the hamster model. Carcinogenesis 9:597–601, 1988.

10. Hasdai A, Liener IE. The effects of soy flour and N-nitrosobis-(2-oxopropyl)amine on the pancreas of the hamster. Drug-Nutrient Interactions 3:173–179, 1985.

11. Furukawa F, Toyoda K, Abe H, Hasegawa R, Sato H, Takahashi M, Hayashi Y. Short-term effects of feeding crude soybean trypsin inhibitor on pancreas of rat, hamster and mouse. Bulletin of Natl Inst Hyg Sci 105:46–50, 1987.

12. Takahashi M, Pour P, Althoff J, Donnelly T. The pancreas of the Syrian golden hamster (Mesocricetus auratus). I Anatomical study. Lab Anim Sci 27:336–342, 1977.

13. Takahashi M, Arai H, Kokubo T, Furukawa F, Kurata Y, Ito N. An ultrastructural study of precancerous and cancerous lesions of the pancreas in Syrian golden hamsters induced by N-nitrosobis(2-oxopropyl)amine. Gann 71:825–831, 1980.

14. Pour PM, Kazakoff K. Effect of secretin on pancreatic carcinogenesis in the hamster model. Cancer Lett 46:57–62, 1989.

15. Johnson FE, LaRegina MC, Martin SA, Bashiti HM. Cholecystokinin inhibits pancreatic carcinogenesis. Cancer Detect Prevent 6:389–402, 1983.

16. Andren-Sandberg A, Dawiskiba S, Ihse I. Studies of the effect of caerulein administration on experimental pancreatic carcinogenesis. Scand J Gastroenterol 19:122–128, 1984.

17. Howatson AG, Carter DC. Pancreatic carcinogenesis-enhancement by cholecystokinin in the hamster-nitrosamine model. Br J Cancer 51:107–114, 1985.

18. Bell RH Jr, Strayer DS. Streptozotocin prevents development of nitrosamine-induced pancreatic cancer in the Syrian hamster. J Surg Oncol 24:258–262, 1983.

19. Kanno T, Kawaguchi K, Okegawa T, Muryobayashi K, Sawada M, Yonezawa H, Kanazawa H. Species differences among rat, guinea pig, and hamster in the effectiveness of camostat to release endogenous CCK and induce pancreatic hypertrophy, and in pancreatic secretory responses to secretagogues. Biomedical Research 10:119–131, 1989.

20. Hasdai A, Liener IE. The failure of long-term feeding of raw soy flour in the presence or absence of azaserine, to induce carcinogenic changes in the mouse pancreas. Nutr Cancer 8:85–91, 1986.

Chemically Induced Cell Proliferation:
Implications for Risk Assessment, pages 155-171
©1991 Wiley-Liss, Inc.

The Role of Stem Cells in the Regeneration of Intestinal Crypts After Cytotoxic Exposure

Christopher S. Potten

Cell Replacement in the small intestine

The small intestinal mucosa consists of a single layer of polarized cells. This sheet of cells is molded during embryogenesis into a complex-shaped series of villi and crypts, forming a folding of the mucosa that causes further polarization, since the villi are the differentiated functional aspect of the tissue from which cells senesce, die, and are shed into the lumen. At the opposite pole, this cell loss is precisely balanced by cell replacement in the crypts. As a consequence, there is a constant movement of cells from the crypt to the villus. This cell migration process can be studied, and the cell velocity measured. At the top of the crypt, the cells move with a velocity of between 0.75 and 1.5 cell positions per hour (1,2). The movement of cells occurs as vertical columns, with relatively little lateral displacement (3,4).

The cells in the crypt represent one of the most rapidly proliferating systems of the body; the majority of the cells pass through two cell cycles each day. Among the 150 proliferating cells (out of about 250 total), there is a new cell division (mitosis) every 5 min.

Cellular hierarchies and stem cells

It is now generally accepted that cell replacement in the small intestine is achieved through a hierarchically organized series of cell lineages, with relatively few lineage ancestors, or stem cells, in each crypt (see reviews in 5–8). Studies on the movement of cells can be used to identify the positions in the crypt from which the cell migration/cell replacement originates (Fig. 1). In this way, somewhat uniquely, the position of the stem cells can be identified, and the properties and responses of these cells can be studied, as illustrated in Figure 2. Such approaches suggest that the stem cells are at about the 4th position from the bottom of the crypt. They are not at the absolute crypt base, as seems likely in colonic crypts, because there are as many as 30 functional Paneth cells in the small intestine. It is also possible that some or all of the stem cells may be scattered between the Paneth cells over the entire lower 4 or 5 cell positions (9). The evidence in favor of a hierarchical organization of cells in the crypt, with relatively few stem cells, comes from cell kinetic studies, in particular those involving cell migration (1,2,10,11), studies on radiation and drug clonal regeneration of the crypt (6–8,12–14), mathematical and computer modeling studies (15–17), and studies using chimeric mice and lectin binding that demonstrated the clonal origin of crypts (18), F_1 hybrids with lectin staining (19), or F_1 hybrids with X–linked enzyme markers (20); both of the latter two suggest that each crypt is ultimately dependent on a very few cells.

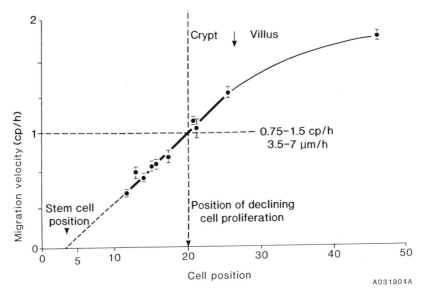

Figure 1. Cell migration velocity increases with increasing cell position from the bottom to the top of the crypt (see Fig. 2). The usual value for cells leaving the top of the proliferative compartment is 0.75–1.5 cell positions per hour or about 3.5–7.0 µm/hr. The straight line portion of the graph can be back-extrapolated to give the point in the crypt from which all the movement originates, i.e., the stem cell position. The velocity increases on the villus because several crypts feed onto each villus, which also tapers; hence columns of migrating cells therefore fuse.

Number of stem cells

The precise number of stem cells in each crypt remains somewhat unclear; the count depends on the criteria being used to identify stem cells. Radiation studies using x- or gamma rays indicate that there are 30–40 cells with clonogenic potential (13). Since this represents a double circumferential ring of cells (there being 16–18 cells in a crypt circumference), the upper ring must inevitably be displaced with time. Hence, these cells are not permanent functional stem cells but are presumably potentially functional stem cells. The cell kinetic studies (cell migration) suggest that up to one complete circumferential ring of cells (16–18 cells) is functional stem cells (7,15,17). With the complexity imposed by the distribution of Paneth cells, the overall three-dimensional structure of the crypt, and the lack of asymmetry in proliferation, it seems unlikely that the system could function with many fewer than 4 stem cells. Thus, it can be concluded that there are between 4 and 16 functional stem cells. When weak beta-irradiation or drugs are used, the results suggest that there are very few clonogenic cells (perhaps 1–6 per crypt) (8,21–23). Finally, studies on mutation incidence in the small intestine (19) or colon (20) or in chimeric mice (18) suggest that each crypt may be dependent on a very few mutable stem cells (Fig. 2).

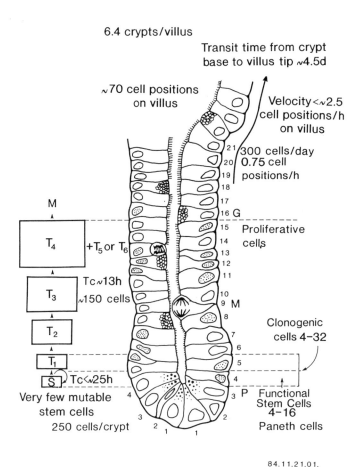

Figure 2. Diagrammatic representation of a good longitudinal crypt section showing the lumen, Paneth cells (P) at the base and, in this case, 21 cells in a vertical numbered column. Goblet cells (G) and cells in mitosis (M) can be recognized. On the left, a cell lineage with stem cells (S) and transit (T) generations that best account for the cell replacement processes. (For further details see references 6,7,15,17). The shaded nuclei represent a typical pattern for the [3H]thymidine labeling.

Duration of the stem cell cycle

Several studies have suggested that the cells at the crypt base (including the stem cells) pass through the cell cycle more slowly (Fig. 3). Some also suggest that the stem cells are particularly well synchronized with regard to circadian rhythm, that they tend to enter S and then M phases only in the early hours of the day, and that the stem cells may be responsible for the overall rhythm seen in the tissue (25,26). These circadian

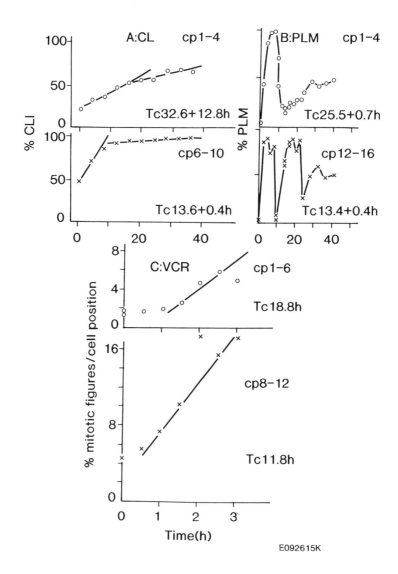

Figure 3. Results of three different cell kinetic experiments that suggest that the cell cycle at the crypt base is longer than that in the mid-crypt. (A) Continuous labeling (CL) experiment (5 μCi per mouse every 4 hr).(B) Percent labeled mitosis experiment (PLM) 2.5 μCi per mouse. (C) Stathmokinetic experiment with vincristine sulphate (VCR), 0.02 mg/mouse. The overall average cell cycle time was 25.6 hr for the crypt base and 12.9 hr for the mid-crypt.

rhythms in proliferation may account for the circadian rhythms in radiosensitivity (27). The overall conclusion would be that the stem cells have a cell cycle duration of about 25 hr; that of the transit cells is about 13 hr. However, some data conflict with this view and suggest faster cell cycle times (28,29).

Changes after exposure to cytotoxic drugs

Following most cytotoxic exposures of the intestine, the crypt shrinks in size and proliferative activity; minimum values usually are observed between 10 and 14 hr after exposure. Following this cellular depletion, which is the consequence of acute cell death and continued emigration of cells onto the villus in the temporary absence of, or reduction in, mitotic activity, there are compensatory changes in cell cycle activity and labeling and mitotic activity. These are well illustrated by the data of Al-Dewachi et al. (30), who studied the effects of hydroxyurea (HU) on the small intestine of the rat (see Fig. 4) and found that the critical compensatory proliferation (here observed 13–15 hr after treatment) is associated with cells near the base of the crypt (cell positions 2–6)— the stem cell region. Proliferation then extends into the mid- and upper-crypt regions. These studies also showed that the cell cycle for cell positions 1–4 15 hr after treatment with HU was reduced from 15.5 hr (31) in the controls to 10.9 hr (a 30% reduction) in the HU-treated rats (30). This reduction was achieved mainly by a reduction in G_1 of 49%, but S phase was also reduced (by 23%).

Similar detailed studies performed on BALB/c mouse small intestine following 400 mg/kg cytosine arbinoside (ara-C) treatment (32) failed to detect a specific regenerative response involving the stem cell region at the crypt base. However, 14 hr after treatment, labeling was elevated at cell positions 3–15. It is possible that closer sampling times would reveal a specific early response at the crypt base. Al-Dewachi et al.'s study (32) revealed a reduction in the cell cycle time at cell positions 3–4 of 23% from the control value of 14.9 hr to 11.4 hr.

Our own studies (29) using 200 mg/kg ara-C on BDF_1 mice showed that labeling was virtually eliminated from the crypt at 6 hr and that at 12 hr labeling was again observed, but primarily in the lower cell positions (cell positions 4–6) (Fig. 5).

These studies strongly suggest that regenerative changes are initiated by the stem cells and occur 10–15 hr after treatment. The regeneration may, in fact, begin earlier, but time intervals used have generally been insufficient to accurately place the first proliferative changes triggered by the cytotoxic damage. These studies also show that the cell cycle time of the stem cell is reduced. One problem with temporal studies using cytotoxic drugs is that it is difficult to know at what time the drug is present at a cytotoxic concentration at the intracellular targets and how long these concentrations persist. Partly for these reasons, we undertook a detailed temporal study of the cell positional changes following an acute dose of gamma rays (33).

Changes after small doses of radiation

The effects of very small doses (as low as 0.05 Gy) can be readily detected in the small intestinal crypts by counting the number of histologically recognizable dead or dying cells (34,35). These cells exhibit many similarities to the process called apoptosis

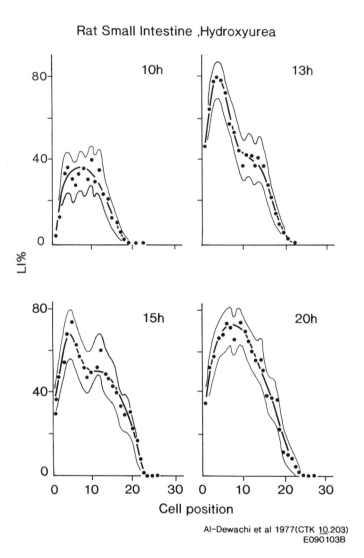

Al-Dewachi et al 1977(CTK 10.203)
E090103B

Figure 4. Labeling index versus cell position frequency plots for rat small intestine at various times after hydroxyurea treatment. Modified from Al-Dewachi et al. (30) with permission of the authors and publishers. The early dramatic response of cells at the crypt base at 13 hr can be easily seen. The upper and lower lines in each case represent the 95% confidence limits.

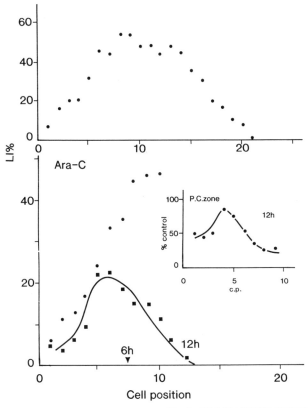

Chwalinski & Potten 1989(Am.J.Anat.186)
E090103C

Figure 5. Labeling index versus cell position studies in the small intestinal crypts of BDF₁ mice at various times after treatment with cytosine arabinoside. Modified from Chwalinski and Potten (29). Six hours after treatment, the labeling was abolished, but by 12 hr it had returned to 80% of control values at cell position 4.

(36); for convenience, that term has been adopted here (see 8,37). The number of apoptotic cells, or fragments of cells, is a sensitive indicator of radiation exposure up to a dose of about 0.5–1.0 Gy; at higher doses, it no longer appears to exhibit a dose dependence (34,35). A further characteristic of this end point is its nonrandom distribution in terms of cell position. The highest incidence of cell death after irradiation consistently is observed at the 4th or 5th cell position, i.e., in the stem cell region (38–40), suggesting that this mode of death is associated with at least some of the stem cells.

It has been observed in a number of experiments that small doses of radiation can cause immediate changes in stem cell kinetics, suggesting that the undamaged stem cells may be responding to the death of one or a few of their neighbors. This was suggested by studies on the recruitment of cells into rapid cycle, as detected by vincristine metaphase arrest, following small doses of X rays or neutrons (41–43). Other studies following 0.5 Gy irradiation have shown that cells in the crypt base are stimulated into increased levels of mitotic activity (44). Low doses of internal irradiation can be administered via agents such as tritiated thymidine [³H]TdR. Tsubouchi and Potten (44) showed that 100 µCi of [³H]TdR to a mouse, just two to four times the dose normally used for routine cell kinetic studies, stimulated an increased level of mitotic activity in the crypt base 12–16 hr after exposure. The increased levels of mitotic activity were similar to those seen after an exposure of 0.5 Gy of external gamma rays (44). Exposure to 100 µCi of [³H]TdR also resulted in a shortening of the cell cycle of the stem cells from about 25 hr to about 16 hr (24). In fact, the tritiated thymidine dose had to be reduced to 2.5 µCi per mouse before an assumed unstimulated cell cycle could be determined (24). This dose represents 1/10 or 1/20 of the usual dose for cell kinetic pulse labeling. These changes appear to be induced very rapidly, since it is the kinetics of the first cell cycle that are changed. Further evidence for the rapid and sensitive response of stem cells to radiation injury comes from an unpublished experiment [summarized in a recent review article (8)] in which the leading (upper) edge of the cell position labeling index plot was analyzed 48 hr after [³H]TdR administration. At this time, the leading labeled cells will have traversed well onto the villus. When the results are compared using 25 and 100 µCi, respectively, the leading edge following the higher dose was found to trail 16 cell positions behind that for the lower dose (Fig. 6). The most likely explanation for this is that the high dose induced some stem cell death, which resulted in one shortened cell cycle for the stem cells, during which the self-renewal probability was raised to close to 1.0. This would rapidly replace the lost stem cells but would also result in a temporary fall in output to the transit population. The data suggest that one entire transit input was lost, resulting in time in a deficiency of 16 cells (four transit generations). Similar conclusions have been reached on the self-renewal probability of spermatogonial stem cells immediately following irradiation (45), namely, that for the first postirradiation division, the self-renewal probability is changed to 1.0.

Changes after exposure to moderate doses of radiation

There have been a few detailed studies on cell proliferation changes in the crypt after irradiation (46–49). Lesher's (46) comprehensive analysis of percent labeled mitosis (PLM) studies in the duodenum of BDF₁ mice at various times after a dose of 3 Gy showed that in the crypt as a whole, the cell cycle is reduced over the period 12 hr–2 days from about 13 hr to about 10–11 hr. The results also showed that 3 Gy causes an immediate and dramatic mitotic delay. There were also some indications that S phase was shortened. These data, however, provided no information on spatial differences, i.e., hierarchy-related effects.

Cairnie (47,48) undertook a detailed study of the proliferative changes at different cell positions in the jejunum of August rats during and after continuous irradiation at 3.5 Gy/day. These studies showed that the crypts initially shrank but later were slightly enlarged. Detailed information on the behavior of stem cells (crypt base cells) is difficult to extract from these data, but it is clear that the cell cycle time for cell positions 1–6 is reduced by about 30%, from 14 hr (50) to about 10 hr.

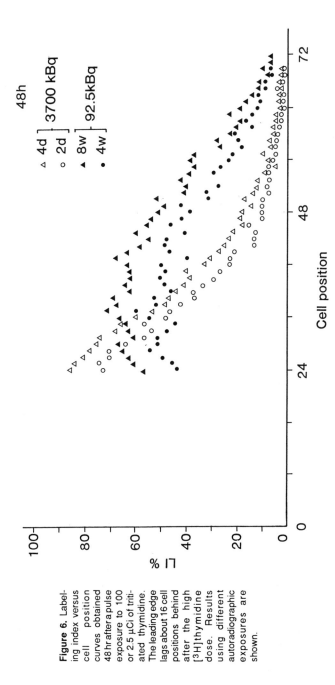

Figure 6. Labelling index versus cell position curves obtained 48 hr after a pulse exposure to 100 or 2.5 μCi of tritiated thymidine. The leading edge lags about 16 cell positions behind after the high [³H]thymidine dose. Results using different autoradiographic exposures are shown.

C121507A

We have recently undertaken a detailed temporal (34 different time points) analysis of the cell positional changes in labeling (33) and mitotic activity (unpublished) in the crypts of the ileum of BDF_1 mice after an acute exposure of 8 Gy. In Figure 7, the labeling index (LI) results have been smoothed over three cell positions in a moving average approach and have been interpolated to the nearest grid line. The following conclusions can be drawn from such an overall analysis. First, there is a dramatic reduction in the overall LI, which begins at about 3 hr and is at its minimum at 15 hr after irradiation. Most of the shrinkage in crypt size associated with these changes in LI is due to a continued near-normal rate of cell emigration from crypt to villus even though mitosis is absent or severely reduced (2). It is also likely that there is some premature maturation of cells (see Fig. 2) (i.e., T1 or T2 cells may become T3, T4, or postmitotic), as well as some acute cell death, particularly among the stem cells. Some stem cells may also undergo what amounts to premature maturation by only having a limited division potential after irradiation, i.e., becoming T1 cells. During this regressive phase, the LI never falls below about 34% of control; i.e., some cells continue to replicate their DNA at all time points after irradiation. Second, the LI increases, in the crypt as a whole from the minimum at 15 hr to reach maximum values at about 72 hr, at which time the crypt is considerably larger than those in the control animals. Third, there is a third phase of change represented by a crypt regression back toward the control crypt, which, however, was not attained within the 8 days of this experiment.

Figure 8 shows the changes in the lower cell positions on an expanded scale with one cell position highlighted (cell position 4). There appear to be fluctuations in the LI for cell position 4 over the first 48 hr; some signs of an early proliferative response are apparent at about 10–12 hr. These effects are more readily observed when the data for several cell positions are pooled (Figs. 9 and 10) and subjected to statistical analysis. These observations show that the first response in the crypt following cytotoxic insult is a wave of cell proliferation in the crypt base (cell positions 3–8), which begins at 3 hr (when there is little detectable change in the crypt except for the appearance of the small number of histologically recognizable dead (apoptotic) cells, particularly at cell positions 3–5 (34). This early proliferative burst reaches a peak at 12 hr after irradiation (when the crypt as a whole and its LI are greatly reduced). This is followed by two successive bursts of proliferation, which peak at 22–32 hr and 60–70 hr. There is some evidence of a small overshoot in labeling among the stem cells, but normal values are reestablished at about 90 hr. These three peaks could represent three successive rounds of cell division in the stem cells, in which case the interval between the first and second peak would be about 14 hr and that between the second and third peak about 34 hr. PLM analyses conducted 48 and 72 hr after 8 Gy show that the cell cycle at the crypt base at both times was reduced by about 60%, from the control value of about 25 hr (Fig. 3) (24) to about 10 hr. Besides a major reduction in G_1, there is a reduction in the length of the S phase from about 7.5 to about 5 hr (8). This appears to contradict the previous statements regarding the distances between the LI peaks in Figure 9. However, it remains unclear how the self-renewal probability and growth fraction of the stem cell population are changing during this time. Furthermore, the second peak in the stem cell LI in Figure 9 might, in fact, represent two cell cycles close together. Clonal regeneration studies (51,52) have been used to measure the number of clonogenic (stem) cells (13), and these approaches have provided data on the regeneration kinetics

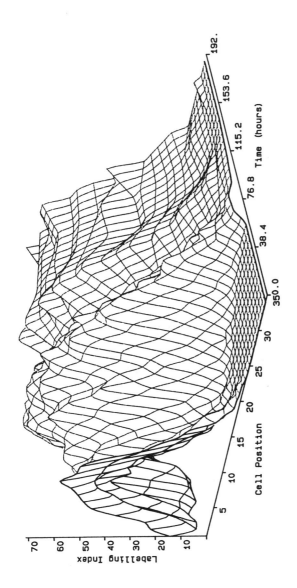

Figure 7. Three-dimensional plot of labeling index, cell position, and time after 8.0 Gy of gamma rays. The data have been smoothed over three cell positions and interpolated to the nearest grid line. Altogether, 34 time points were analyzed in detail (33). Changes that might not be significant when compared with one other LI distribution gain significance when considered in relation to the results from several time points. The initial shrinkage in LI can be seen, as can the considerable expansion in crypt size that occurs at around 72 hr. Greater detail of the earlier changes can be seen in Figure 8. Reprinted from ref. 33 with permission of the publisher.

of the clonogenic cells that indicate that they double in number over 1–4 days at a doubling time of 21 hr (13).

What these studies show is that one of the first detectable changes in the crypt is a stimulation of cell proliferation at the crypt base (in the stem cells). This occurs very

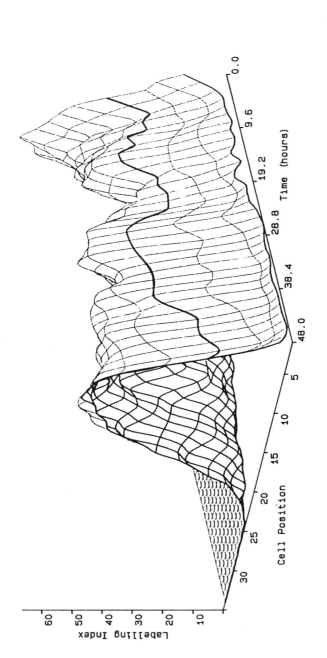

Figure 8. An expansion of the first 48 hr of the three-dimensional plot shown in Figure 7. The reverse view is shown here so that the changes at the crypt base can be more easily seen. The results for the cells at position 4 from the crypt base have been highlighted. When this is done, it shows an initial fall in LI for these cells and an early small peak at about 10 hr. There is evidence of a second peak at around 30 hr and a third, later peak (not shown). Reprinted from ref. 33 with permission of the publishers.

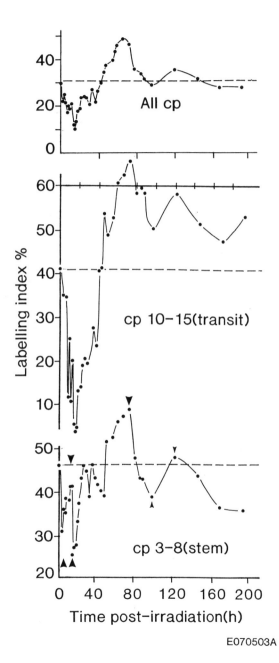

Figure 9. The changes in labeling index for the whole crypt (all cell positions, top panel), for the transit cell population (mid crypt, cell positions 10–15, middle panel) and the stem cells (lower crypt, cell positions 3–8, lower panel) with time after a dose of 8 Gy. These graphs effectively summarize the data shown in Figure 7. The important features are illustrated in the lower panel where considerable structure can be seen that is not apparent for the mid crypt and whole crypt. Bursts in labeling seen at 3–12 hr, and at 15–30 hr, and 60–72 hr. One-way analysis of variance with Duncan's or Tukey-B's multiple range test show that the peaks and troughs marked with large arrowheads are significant at the 5% level. Duncan's test alone also shows that the peaks marked with small arrowheads also are significant. See also Figure 10.

E070503A

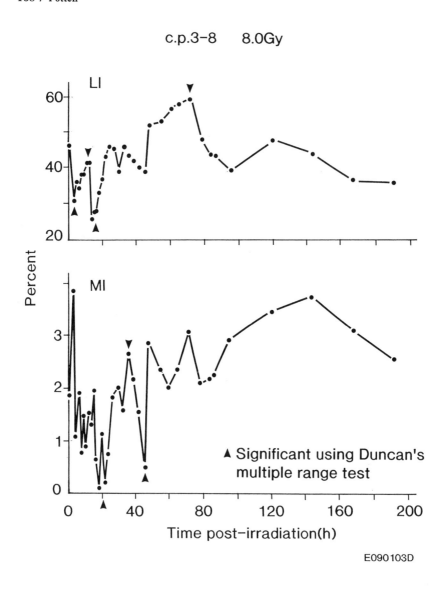

c.p.3–8   8.0Gy

E090103D

Figure 10. Changing pattern for the LI and MI for the stem cell zone of the crypt, cell positions 3–8 at various times after 8 Gy. The LI data (upper panel) are the same as shown in the lower panel in Figure 9. Similar trends to those seen in LI can be detected in the MI even though there is more scatter among the data.

rapidly after sustaining damage and is triggered either by the fall in LI seen at 3 hr or by the appearance of a few dead cells in this region of the crypt. The latter seems more likely. The stem cells are thus under a tight, extremely local control that can detect a reduction in stem cell numbers or a local stem cell death. This initiates a compensatory round of stem cell division. If the stem cell number is still deficient, as is the case after 8 Gy, further rounds of stem cell proliferation are required. A similar extremely rapid recruitment of bone marrow stem cells spleen colony-forming units (CFU-S) has also been reported (53,54) and suggests a similar extremely local control process. Indeed, in this case a stimulator can be extracted from irradiated bone marrow within 15–30 min of irradiation.

The stem cells must be delicately balanced in terms of their controls; even the deletion of a single stem cell may be enough to push them all into a round of cell division, as is suggested by the data summarized earlier. After a major cytotoxic exposure such as to 8 Gy of radiation, the entire repopulation of the crypt could be determined solely by the repopulation kinetics of the stem cells, i.e., by their cell cycle time, which can be measured directly, and their self-renewal probabilities, which can only be deduced.

Conclusions

We can conclude from these observations that the stem cells play a vital role in the crypts following cytotoxic insult (specifically a radiation exposure). We hypothesize that they are delicately balanced in terms of their cell proliferation control processes, which appear to be extremely local in nature. Minor damage, such as the death of a single stem cell out of the possible 4–16 in a normal crypt, is immediately detected by the remaining stem cells, possibly because of a stimulatory factor released during apoptotic cell death. The stem cells respond by an immediate reduction in their cell cycle duration, possibly by a rapid entry of cells from G_1 into a shortened S phase and a change in their self-renewal probability, which for this first postinsult cell cycle is from the steady-state value of 0.5 to a value close to 1.0. If the damage is minor, the next stem cell cycle may be normal in duration and self-renewal probability. If the stem cell numbers are still deficient, further rapid cell cycles may be needed, but the self-renewal probability cannot be maintained at close to 1.0 for these subsequent cell cycles. If it were, a severe deficiency in differentiated cells would result. In the second and subsequent stem cell cycles, the cell cycle may continue to be short, at about 9–10 hr, but the self-renewal probability is now more likely to be about 0.6. Four or five days after the severe initial damage, the stem cell numbers may overshoot. As a consequence, the total cellularity may overshoot more extensively, since each extra stem cell would be capable of generating an extra transit cell lineage of probably 16 cells. Some stem cells after cytotoxic exposure may also prematurely senesce (enter the transit population without cell division) rather than die through apoptosis.

Acknowledgements

This work has been supported by the Cancer Research Campaign (UK). The work summarized here has involved collaboration with others, notably Drs. J. Hendry, K. Ijiri, S. Tsubouchi, S. Chwalinski, and P. Kaurand would have been impossible without the valuable technical help of S. Tickle, P. Taylor, G. Owen, Y. Taylor, H. Moffat, and C. Chadwick.

References

1. Kaur P, Potten CS. Circadian variation in migration velocity in small intestinal epithelium. Cell Tissue Kinet 19:591–600, 1986.
2. Kaur P, Potten CS. Cell migration velocities in the crypts after cytotoxic insult are not dependent on mitotic activity. Cell Tissue Kinet 19:601–610, 1986.
3. Schmidt GH, Wilkinson MM, Ponder BAJ. Cell migration pathway in the intestinal epithelium: An in situ marker system using mouse aggregation chimeras. Cell 40:425–429, 1985.
4. Wilson TJG, Ponder BAJ, Wright NA. Use of a mouse chimaeric model to study cell migration patterns in the small intestinal epithelium. Cell Tissue Kinet 18:333–344, 1985.
5. Wright NA, Alison M. The Biology of Epithelial Cell Populations. Oxford: Clarendon Press, 1984, pp. 539–1247.
6. Potten CS, Hendry JH, Moore JV, Chwalinski S. Cytotoxic effects in gastrointestinal epithelium (as exemplified by small intestine). In: Potten CS, Hendry JH (eds): Insult to Tissue: Effects on Cell Lineages. Edinburgh: Churchill-Livingstone, 1983, pp. 105–152.
7. Potten CS, Hendry JH. Stem cells in murine small intestine. In: Potten CS (ed): Stem Cells: Their Identification and Characterisation. Edinburgh: Churchill-Livingstone, 1983, pp. 155–199.
8. Potten CS. The response of the murine small intestine to acute irradiation: A comprehensive study of BDF_1 mice. Int J Radiat Biol, in press.
9. Bjerknes M, Cheng H. The stem-cell zone of the small intestinal epithelium. I. Evidence from Paneth cells in the adult mouse. Am J Anat 160:51–63, 1981.
10. Cheng H, Leblond CP. Origin, differentiation and renewal of the four main epithelial cell types in the mouse small intestine. V. Unitarian theory of the origin of the four epithelial cell types. Am J Anat 141:537–561, 1974.
11. Leblond CP, Cheng H. Identification of stem cells in the small intestine of the mouse. In: Cairnie AB, Lala PK, Osmond DG (eds): Stem cells of renewing cell populations. New York: Academic Press, pp. 7–31, 1990.
12. Potten CS, Hendry JH. Differential regeneration of intestinal proliferative cells and crytogenic cells after regeneration Int J Radiat Biol 27:413–424, 1975.
13. Potten CS, Taylor Y, Hendry JH. The doubling time of regenerating clonogenic cells in the crypts of the irradiated mouse small intestine. Int J Radiol 54:1041–1051, 1988.
14. Inoue M, Imada M, Fukushima Y, Matsuura N, Shiozaki H, Mori T, Kitamura Y, Fujita H. Macroscopic intestinal colonies of mice as a tool for studying differentiation of multipotential intestinal stem cells. Am J Pathol 132:49–58, 1988.
15. Loeffler M, Stein R, Wichmann HE, Potten CS, Kaur P, Chwalinski S. Intestinal cell proliferation I. A comprehensive model of steady state proliferation in the crypt. Cell Tissue Kinet 19:627–645, 1986.
16. Loeffler M, Potten CS, Paulus U, Glatzer J, Chwalinski S. Intestinal crypt proliferation. II. Computer modelling of mitotic index data provides further evidence for lateral and vertical cell migration in the absence of mitotic activity. Cell Tissue Kinet 21: 247–258, 1988.
17. Potten CS, Loeffler M. A comprehensive model of the crypts of the small intestine of the mouse provides insight into the mechanisms of cell migration and the proliferative hierarchy. J Theoret Biol 127:381–391, 1987.
18. Ponder BAJ, Schmidt GH, Wilkinson MM, Wood MJ, Monk M, Reid A. Derivation of mouse intestinal crypts from single progenitor cells. Nature 313:689–691, 1985.
19. Winton DJ, Blount MA, Ponder BAJ. A clonal marker induced by mutation in mouse intestinal epithelium. Nature 333:463–466, 1988.
20. Griffiths DFR, Davies SJ, Williams D, Williams GT, Williams ED. Demonstration of somatic mutation and colonic crypt clonality by X-linked enzyme histochemistry. Nature 333: 461–463, 1988.
21. Moore JV. Ablation of murine jejunal crypts by alkylating agents. Br J Cancer 39:175–181, 1979.
22. Moore JV. Clonogenic response of cells of murine intestinal crypts to 12 cytotoxic drugs. Cancer Chemother Pharmacol 15:11–15, 1985.
23. Hendry JH, Potten CS, Ghafoor A, Moore JV, Roberts SA, Williams PC. The response of murine intestinal crypts to short-range promethium-147 beta-irradiation: Deductions concerning clonogenic cell numbers and positions. Radiat Res 118:364–374, 1989.
24. Potten CS. Cell cycles in cell hierarchies. Int J Radiat Biol 49:257–278, 1986.
25. Hendry JH, Moore JV, Potten CS. The proliferative status of microcolony-forming cells in mouse small intestine. Cell Tissue Kinet 17:41–47, 1984.

26. Potten CS, Al-Barwari SE, Hume WJ, Searle J. Circadian rhythms of presumptive stem cells in three different epithelia of the mouse. Cell Tissue Kinet 10:557–568, 1977.
27. Hendry JH. Diurnal variations in radiosensitivity of mouse intestine. Br J Radiol 48:312–314, 1975.
28. Boarder TA, Blackett NM. The proliferative status of intestinal epithelial clonogenic cells: Sensitivity to S phase specific cytotoxic agents. Cell Tissue Kinet 9:589–596, 1976.
29. Chwalinski S, Potten CS. Crypt base columnar cells in ileum of BDF1 male mice—their numbers and some features of their proliferation. Am J Anat 186:397–406, 1989.
30. Al-Dewachi HS, Wright NA, Appleton DR, Watson AJ. The effect of a single injection of hydroxyurea on cell population kinetics in the small bowel mucosa of the rat. Cell Tissue Kinet 10:203–213, 1977.
31. Al-Dewachi HS, Wright NA, Appleton DR, Watson AJ. The cell cycle time in the rat jejunal mucosa. Cell Tissue Kinet 7:587–594, 1974.
32. Al-Dewachi HS, Wright NA, Appleton DR, Watson AJ. The effect of a single injection of cytosine arabinoside on cell population kinetics in the mouse jejunal crypt. Virchows Arch [B] 34:299–309, 1980.
33. Potten CS, Owen G, Roberts SA. The temporal and spatial changes in cell proliferation within the irradiated crypts of the murine small intestine. Int J Radiat Biol 57:185–199, 1989.
34. Potten CS. Extreme sensitivity of some intestinal crypt cells to X and gamma irradiation. Nature 269:518–521, 1977.
35. Hendry JH, Potten CS, Chadwick C, Bianchi M. Cell death (apoptosis) in the mouse small intestine after low doses: Effects of dose-rate, 14.7 MeV neutrons, and 600 MeV (maximum energy) neutrons. Int J Radiat Biol 42:611–620, 1982.
36. Kerr JFR, Wyllie AH, Currie AR. Apoptosis: A basic biological phenomenon with wide-ranging implications in tissue kinetics. Br J Cancer 26:239–257, 1972.
37. Potten CS. Stem cells in gastrointestinal mucosa. In: Scolnick EM, Levine AJ (eds): Tumor Viruses and Differentiation. New York: Alan R. Liss, 1983. pp 381–398.
38. Ijiri K, Potten CS. Response of intestinal cells of differing topographical and hierarchical status to ten cytotoxic drugs and five sources of radiation. Br J Cancer 47:175–185, 1983.
39. Ijiri K, Potten CS. Further studies on the response of intestinal crypt cells of differing hierarchical status to 18 different cytotoxic agents. Br J Cancer 55:113–123, 1987.
40. Ijiri K, Potten CS. Cell death in cell hierarchies in adult mammalian tissues. In: Potten CS (ed): Perspectives on Mammalian Cell Death. Oxford: Oxford University Press, 1987, pp. 326–356.
41. Hanson WR, Henninger DL, Fry RJM, Sallese AR. The response of small intestinal stem cells in the mouse to drug and irradiation treatment. In: Appleton DR, Sunter JP, Watson AJ, (eds): Cell Proliferation in the Gastrointestinal Tract. Tunbridge Wells: Pitman Medical, 1980, pp. 198–212.

Chemically Induced Cell Proliferation:
Implications for Risk Assessment, pages 173-183
©1991 Wiley-Liss, Inc.

Thyroid Clonogen Biology and Carcinogenesis

Kelly H. Clifton, Kevin M. Groch, and Frederick E. Domann, Jr.

Understanding the biology of normal cells—from which cancers arise—is essential for a full comprehension of the carcinogenic process. Over a decade has passed since we began investigations of the cellular origins of radiogenic and hormonal cancers in the rat mammary and thyroid glands. Our approach was based on the known hormonal control of thyroid and mammary proliferation, differentiation, and function; on the susceptibility of these organs to radiogenic cancer; and on the cancer-promoting effects of mitogenic hormones. The hypophysial thyroid-stimulating hormone (TSH) is the primary stimulant of iodine concentration, thyroid hormone synthesis and release, and thyroid cell proliferation. Virtually any condition that induces a sustained increase in TSH titers promotes the neoplastic process in initiated thyroid cells (1).

It is not likely that all cells in an organ are susceptible to malignant initiation; therefore, analyses of whole tissues following exposure to a carcinogen may not reflect events in the critical target cells. Cells that are necessary for tissue repopulation and repair following injury constitute the most likely cancer-susceptible subpopulation. We found that when thyroid tissue is enzymatically monodispersed, and the cells are transplanted into thyroidectomized syngeneic hosts, functioning glandular thyroid structures or follicular units develop in the graft sites in response to the elevated TSH levels (2). A terminal dilution transplantation assay was developed in which follicular units served as the end point to estimate the concentration of follicular unit–forming cells following radiation exposure and/or a variety of physiological conditions (3). The assay is based on the assumption that if the titer of TSH is elevated, most or all competent cells will respond with follicular unit formation. The cumulative data from our studies are most consistent with the conclusion that follicular units are clonal in origin (4), and that about 1% of monodispersed cells from young rat thyroids are clonogenic.

The assay has also been used to estimate the frequency of radiogenic malignant initiation per surviving transplanted thyroid clonogen. In these carcinogenesis studies, thyroidectomized rats were grafted with unirradiated or irradiated thyroid cells and were maintained on an iodine-deficient diet to sustain chronically elevated TSH titers. The results show that initiation of neoplasia is a common event at the clonogenic cell level (5,6).

This presentation summarizes the older studies and reviews some recent findings on thyroid clonogen biology and carcinogenesis.

Methodology

The terminal dilution transplantation assay procedure has been described (3). Briefly, thyroid glands are aseptically removed from donor rats, pooled, minced, and dispersed by treatment with collagenase followed by pronase and DNase. The suspension is then filtered through a 53 μm pore filter and the concentration of morphologically intact, predominantly monodispersed cells is determined microscopically with a hemocytometer. A series of 6–8 appropriate serial dilutions containing known numbers of morphologically intact cells are then prepared. Aliquots of each dilution are injected into 3–5 sites in the interscapular and inguinal subcutaneous white fat pads of each syngeneic recipient rat for a total of 15–25 graft sites per cell concentration. Four weeks after transplantation, the graft sites are removed, fixed, stained, and examined for the presence of follicular units. In routine assays, both donors and recipients have usually been 5-week-old F344 male rats (Harlan Sprague Dawley, Madison, WI); the recipients are usually thyroidectomized 1–2 days before transplantation to induce elevated TSH levels. Rats are killed by ether overdose.

The fractions of graft sites with one or more follicular units in each cell dose group are computer-fit against the mean numbers of cells grafted per site in each group according to a modification of the transplantation model described by Porter et al. (7). A computer program estimates the slope of the cell dose–follicular unit response relationship and the clonogenic fraction by a maximum likelihood iterative procedure and calculates the follicular dose level value at 50% (FD50) (3). The FD50 value is the mean number of monodispersed cells required to produce one or more follicular units in 50% of the graft sites, and is inversely proportional to the clonogenic fraction.

In studies of the radiation dose–clonogen survival relationship and of postirradiation intracellular repair (8), the thyroid cells were irradiated with gamma- or x-rays in situ before removal for transplantation assay or in vitro after monodispersion. The surviving fraction of clonogens was calculated by dividing the FD50 value of unirradiated cells by the FD50 value of cells that had been exposed to a given radiation dose. The clonogen survival data were analyzed according to the multitarget–single hit model (9):

$$S = 1 - [1 - \exp(-D/D_0)]^n$$

in which S is the surviving fraction, D is the radiation dose, D_0 is the inverse of the terminal slope of the survival curve, and n is the "extrapolation number", i.e., the value at the point of intercept of the terminal slope extrapolated to the ordinate.

The same transplantation procedure was employed in estimating the frequency of radiogenic neoplastic initiation (5,6). In the latter, the series of cell doses per graft site were chosen on the basis of the results of the radiation dose–clonogen survival data from FD50 assays. The end point, however, was the formation of overt neoplasms.

Three regimens have been used to induce sustained high titers of TSH. In the carcinogenesis studies, the thyroid graft recipient rats were thyroidectomized and maintained throughout life on an iodine-deficient diet. This was done to minimize the synthesis of the iodine-containing thyroid hormones thyroxine (T4) and triiodothyronine (T3) by follicular units that developed in the graft sites (1). T4 and T3 deficiency leads to an increase in TSH secretion through feedback regulation. A second regimen was to administer the goitrogenic agent aminotriazole (ATA) in the drinking water. ATA is an inhibitor of thyroid peroxidase, an enzyme which plays an essential role in the organification of iodine during T3 and T4 synthesis (1). ATA was used in studies of cell population kinetics and hormone secretion during goitrogenesis. A third regimen, also used in the latter studies, was a combination of potassium perchlorate in the drinking water and an iodine-deficient diet. The complex perchlorate ion inhibits the uptake of iodide across the thyroid cell membrane (1) thus effectively blocking T4 and T3 synthesis and inducing an increase in TSH titers. Serum titers of TSH, T4, and T3 hormones were determined by radioimmunoassay as necessary.

Results and discussion

In thyroidectomized recipients maintained on a normal diet, the follicular units that developed in sites grafted with low cell numbers were frequently individual thyroid follicles lined with cuboidal epithelium surrounding a colloid-filled lumen. In sites with larger cell numbers, follicles often occurred in clusters. Morphological studies during their development show that follicular units were formed by cell proliferation (10); there was no evidence of thyroid cell reaggregation (4). Follicular units concentrated radio-iodine (2), and could secrete T4 in thyroidectomized graft recipients on normal diets (11). In standard 4-week assays, the follicular units that developed in thyroidectomized recipients on an iodine-deficient diet resembled follicles in intact animals given such diets: They were colloid-deficient and featured hypertrophic follicular epithelia (10). The FD50 value in the latter animals was, however, unaltered from that in thyroidectomized recipients on normal diet (11). In short, follicular units responded like normal thyroid follicles in situ.

When thyroid cells were irradiated in situ in donor animal glands and removed immediately for FD50 assay, or were exposed after removal and dispersion for assay, the radiation dose–clonogen survival response data were not significantly different; the data were well fit by the multitarget-single hit model (8). Over the dose range of 0-16 Gy, the D_0 value was ~2.0 Gy, and the extrapolation number n was ~3 (Fig. 1). The n value is assumed to represent a complex of intracellular processes related to the number of radiation-sensitive sites, the capacity to accumulate damage, and the titers of radio-protective agents. The clonogens were irradiated in the donor glands in situ and after 24 hours were removed and dispersed for FD50 assay. The D_0 value was not significantly changed from ~2.0 Gy, but the n value was increased to ~10; i.e., during the 24-hr interval after exposure, extensive repair of potentially lethal damage had occurred (Fig. 1). This type of repair was first observed in mammary clonogens when similarly irradiated in situ and assayed several hours later, and was termed in situ repair (12). This phenomenon has also been observed in irradiated liver clonogens (13) and may be characteristic of other epithelia. The potentially lethal damage repair seen in such epithelia is considerably greater than that seen in most mammalian cells in monolayer culture.

The radiation dose–clonogen survival data were used in the design of experiments aimed at determining the frequency of initiation per irradiated clonogenic cell. In the first of these experiments, the frequencies of carcinomas were determined in grafts of thyroid cells. The graft inocula were adjusted to contain ~26, 52, 103, 206, or 411 viable 5 Gy irradiated or unirradiated clonogens per graft site in thyroidectomized recipients maintained on an iodine-deficient diet.

There were two major findings (5). First, as expected, more carcinomas developed in the sites grafted with irradiated cells than in those that received an equivalent number of unirradiated cells. In irradiated cell grafts, the cancer incidence increased with cell dose; in the grafts of unirradiated cells, there was no obvious cell dose effect on the cancer incidence. Second, over the 16-fold range of irradiated cell doses, the cancer incidence increased only 4-fold; i.e., the processes of tumor promotion–progression were more efficient in the grafts of small clonogen numbers than in those with larger numbers.

The latter finding suggested the existence of cell number–dependent interactions that suppressed promotion-progression. Hence, in the second experiment, similarly irradiated thyroid cells were grafted to similarly treated recipient rats. The inocula

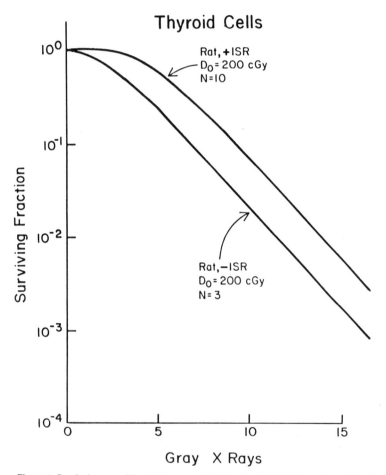

Figure 1. Survival curves of thyroid clonogens following irradiation in situ as determined by FD50 transplantation assays (8). Lower curve: Cells removed and prepared for transplantation assay immediately after exposure. Upper curve: Cells removed for transplantation 24 hr after irradiation. The increase in survival shown in the delayed assay curve is due to repair of potentially lethal damage.

contained ~11–~720 viable 5 Gy-irradiated clonogens alone or admixed with suspensions containing ~1200–2500 unirradiated clonogens per transplant site (6). The final carcinoma incidences increased from 34% in grafts of ~11 irradiated clonogens alone to 78% in grafts of ~720 irradiated clonogens. When adjusted for cancer incidence in unirradiated clonogen grafts, the cancer frequency in grafts of ~11 clonogens per site was one carcinoma per ~75 clonogenic cells (4), or a risk of ~1.3×10^{-2} radiogenic initiating events per clonogen.

Final carcinoma incidences per grafted irradiated clonogen decreased progressively as the number of irradiated clonogens per graft site was increased (Fig. 2). Furthermore, the addition of unirradiated clonogens to the graft inocula further suppressed the final cancer incidences by factors of 0.16–0.35 (Fig. 2). These effects on the efficiency of malignant promotion–progression could result a) from a grafted cell number–related hormonal feedback effect on TSH secretion, b) from local cell interactions which suppress the process, or c) both. The titers of TSH, T3, and T4 were thus measured in sera from thyroidectomized rats grafted with ~2, 10, 50, or 250 clonogens and

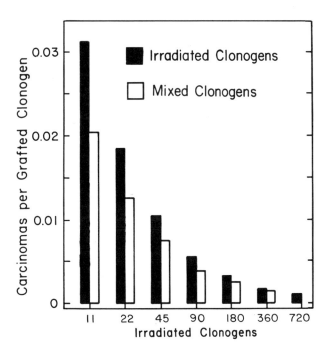

Figure 2. Final cancer incidence as a function of the number of 5 Gy-irradiated thyroid clonogens grafted per site (6). Solid bars: Grafts of the indicated numbers of surviving irradiated clonogens alone. Open bars: Grafts of the indicated numbers of surviving irradiated clonogens mixed with unirradiated thyroid cells.

maintained for 10 weeks on an iodine-deficient diet (<50 ng I/g).Despite the deficiency in iodide, rats grafted with the larger clonogen numbers had T3 and T4 titers that resembled those in intact rats on normal diet (Fig. 3). Conversely, TSH levels were progressively reduced with increasing grafted clonogen numbers, reaching normal levels in rats that had received the highest cell dose (Fig. 3). In the carcinogenesis experiments, the neoplasm-promoting effects of elevated TSH would thus be higher for a longer period of time in those animals grafted with small clonogen numbers than in those with large clonogen numbers. A major portion of the grafted cell number–related suppression of neoplastic promotion–progression can be attributed to reestablishment of the regulation of TSH levels by T3 and T4 from the follicular units formed in the graft sites despite the limited iodine intake. There may be local effects of large cell numbers on promotion-progression as well (see below).

Treatment of rats with a goitrogenic agent such as ATA or perchlorate leads to rapid hyperplasia and goitrous hypertrophy followed by a plateau in goiter size and cellularity (1). We have investigated serum hormone titers and clonogen population kinetics during treatment with these two agents to determine whether the plateau phase is attributable to changes in these cells and their responsiveness to TSH. In ATA-treated rats, TSH titers rapidly increased to several times the normal level and remained elevated throughout 12 weeks of treatment. Goitrous growth occurred during the first 6 weeks of treatment; thereafter, no significant increase in total thyroid DNA was observed (Fig. 4). In contrast to the total cell population, the size of the subpopulation of clonogenic cells remained near normal during the first 6 weeks of treatment. The total clonogen population then increased rapidly during the plateau phase to several times the normal number (Fig. 4), although the clonogen concentration remained less than in the normal gland as indicated by a greater FD50. The subpopulation of clonogens thus responds to physiologic conditions differently than does the total epithelial cell population.

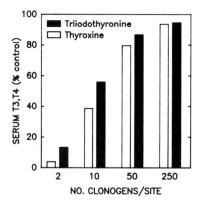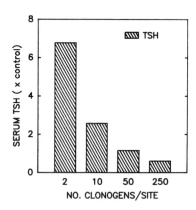

Figure 3. Serum hormone levels 10 weeks after thyroidectomy and grafting of the indicated numbers of thyroid clonogens in rats maintained on an iodine deficient diet, i.e. less than 50 ng I per gram.

In rats on perchlorate plus an iodine-deficient diet, TSH titers were comparable to those in ATA-treated animals (Fig. 5); the plateau phase was reached after the same period of treatment. However, the plateau phase–goiters of perchlorate-treated rats were less than half as large as those in ATA-treated rats (Fig. 6) and the clonogen concentration was significantly smaller as shown by the greater FD50 (Fig. 5).

It was important to determine whether clonogens derived from goiters respond differently than do normal thyroid clonogens when grafted in recipients with elevated TSH levels. Thyroidectomized recipient rats were grafted with cells from normal glands or from early plateau phase goiters of donors treated for 6 weeks with ATA or perchlorate. The total grafted cell numbers were chosen to contain ~10, 80, or 640 clonogens from one of the three donor groups per recipient. Eight weeks later, the serum T4 titers in the recipient rats were measured: Similar patterns of increase in T4 levels with increasing total grafted cell dose were observed in rats that had received cells from either normal- or goitrogen-treated donors; however, many more total cells were required from the goiters (Fig. 7, top). When T4 levels were plotted against the number of clonogens per graft, however, the differences caused by donor treatment disappeared;

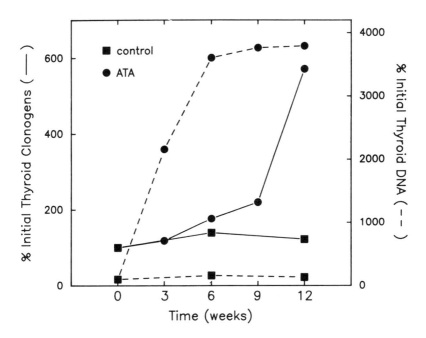

Figure 4. Changes in total thyroid DNA (broken lines) and total thyroid clonogen numbers (solid lines) in glands of untreated rats (solid squares) and in rats treated with the goitrogen ATA (solid circles).

T4 titers were dependent on the numbers of grafted clonogens, not on the total numbers of grafted cells (Fig. 7, bottom). We conclude that the plateau-phase goiters induced by either ATA or perchlorate contain a subpopulation of cells that are as capable of responding to elevated TSH levels with clonal proliferation and hormone secretion as are the clonogenic cells of the normal thyroid. Goiter growth stasis during the plateau phase cannot be attributed to the absence of such TSH-responsive cells. Furthermore, if graft inocula contain the same number of clonogenic cells, the total number of cells injected may differ by nearly two orders of magnitude without affecting development of functional follicular units from the clonogens.

A large experiment, now in progress, was designed to investigate tumorigenesis in grafts of ~3, 10, 30, or 90 unirradiated or 5 Gy irradiated surviving "test" clonogens under similar hormonal conditions. Each graft recipient received one inoculum of each of the four cell concentrations. Any effect of T3 and T4 secretion by the grafts of larger clonogen numbers on the TSH levels, and thus on neoplastic promotion-progression, was equalized in all graft recipients. To test whether there were local effects of unirradiated cells on promotion-progression of initiated cells, other groups of recipients received either four graft inocula in which test clonogens were mixed with 350 unirradiated clonogens in each inoculum, or in which the test cells were inoculated alone and a total of 1400 (4 × 350) unirradiated cells were grafted in a fifth site.

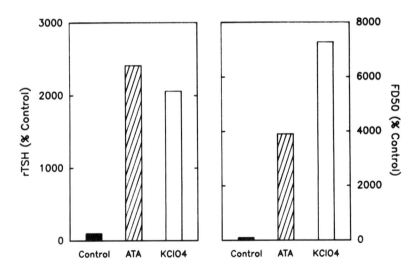

Figure 5. Comparison of the effects of 6 weeks of treatment with the goitrogenic regimens ATA or perchlorate plus iodine-deficient diet on serum TSH levels, and on FD50 values of thyroid cells prepared for transplantation assay from treated rats.

The results to date again show an increase in tumors with increasing irradiated clonogen numbers per graft site and support the conclusion that one effect of the addition of unirradiated clonogens to the test inocula is mediated through suppression of TSH. It is not yet clear whether there are local cell interactions as well that influence neoplastic promotion-progression; the data thus far do not exclude that possibility.

Conclusions

Thyroid cancer arises from a subpopulation of clonogenic epithelial cells in which radiogenic neoplastic initiation is a common event. We have speculated that initiation is a generic term that includes any intracellular events, genetic or epigenetic, that increase the probability of progression of a cell or its progeny to cancer (6). This includes any event that increases the probability of a mutation in a growth-regulating gene in the future, as well as mutations in such genes directly induced by the treatment. In the former, the probability of a mutational event occurring later is further increased by promotion.

Hypophysial TSH plays an essential role in goitrogenesis and in promotion-progression of overt cancer from initiated thyroid clonogens. However, other factors are necessary in limiting goiter size. It is not yet clear to what extent local cell-to-cell interactions may alter the promotion-progression of initiated thyroid cells.

It is important to note that regulation of the cancer progenitor cell subpopulation of clonogens differs from regulation of the total thyroid epithelial cell population. We

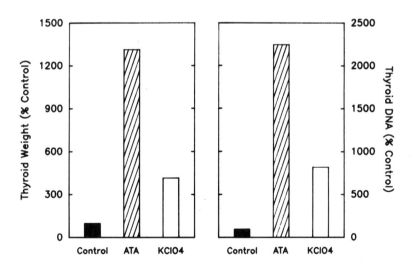

Figure 6. Comparison of the effects of 6 weeks of treatment with the goitrogenic regimens ATA or perchlorate plus iodine-deficient diet on thyroid weight and on total thyroid DNA.

suggest that this is likely true in other tissues. A greater understanding of the physiologic control of cancer precursor cell subpopulations is requisite for an understanding of the malignant process.

Acknowledgments

The authors are indebted to Ms. Joan Mitchen, Ms. Jennifer Willet and Ms. Jane Barnes for excellent technical assistance and to Ms. Peggy Ziebarth for aid with the manuscript. This project is supported by Department of Energy Grant DE FG02 87ER60507 to Kelly H. Clifton, who also receives partial salary support from National Cancer Institute Grant P30 CA14520 to the University of Wisconsin Clinical Cancer Center.

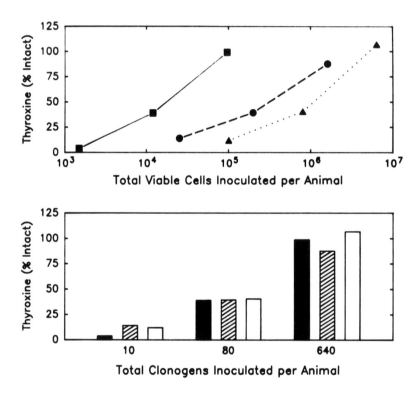

Figure 7. *Upper:* Serum thyroxine levels in thyroidectomized rats 8 weeks after grafting of the indicated numbers of total thyroid cells from normal thyroid glands (solid squares), ATA-induced goiters (solid circles), and perchlorate-iodine–deficient diet-induced goiters (solid triangles).

Lower: Serum thyroxine levels in the same rats as above plotted against the grafted thyroid clonogen numbers from normal thyroids (solid bars), ATA-induced goiters (hatched bars) and perchlorate-iodine deficient diet-induced goiters (open bars).

References

1. Dumont JE, Malone JF, Van Herle AJ. Irradiation and Thyroid Disease: Dosimetric, Clinical and Carcinogenic Aspects (EUR 6713 ER). Luxemborg: Commission of the European Communities, 1980.
2. Clifton KH, DeMott RK, Mulcahy RT, Gould MN. Thyroid gland formation from inocula of monodispersed cells: Early results on quantitation, function, neoplasia and radiation effects. Int J Radiat Oncol Biol Phys 4:987–990, 1978.
3. Clifton KH, Gould MN. Clonogen transplantation assay of mammary and thyroid epithelial cells. In Potten CS, Hendry JH (eds): Cell Clones: Manual of Mammalian Cell Techniques. Edinburgh: Churcill Livingstone, 1985, pp 128–138.
4. Clifton KH. The clonogenic cells of the rat mammary and thyroid glands: Their biology, frequency of initiation and promotion/progression to cancer. In Moolgavkar S, Thomsen D (eds): Mathematical Modeling: Statistical Issues in Cancer Risk Assessment. New York: Birkhauser Boston Inc., 1989, in press.
5. Mulcahy RT, Gould MN, Clifton KH. Radiogenic initiation of thyroid cancer: A common cellular event. Int J Radiat Biol 45:419–426, 1984.
6. Watanabe H, Tanner MA, Domann FE, Gould MN, Clifton KH. Inhibition of carcinoma formation and of vascular invasion in grafts of radiation-initiated thyroid clonogens by unirradiated thyroid cells. Carcinogenesis 9:1329–1335, 1988.
7. Porter EH, Hewitt HB, Blake ER. The transplantation kinetics of tumor cells. Br J Cancer 27:55–62, 1973.
8. Mulcahy RT, Gould MN, Clifton KH. The survival of thyroid cells: In vivo irradiation and in situ repair. Radiat Res 84:523–528, 1980.
9. Elkind MM, Sutton H. Radiation response of mammalian cells grown in culture. I. Repair of x-ray damage in surviving Chinese hamster cells. Radiat Res 13:556–593, 1960.
10. Mulcahy RT, DeMott RK, Clifton KH. Transplantation of monodispersed rat thyroid cells: Hormonal effects on follicular unit development and morphology. Proc Soc Exp Biol Med 163:100–110, 1980.
11. Mulcahy RT, Rose DP, Mitchen JM, Clifton KH. Hormonal effects on the quantitative transplantation of monodispersed rat thyroid cells. Endocrinology 106:1769–1775, 1980.
12. Gould MN, Clifton KH. Evidence for a unique in situ component of the repair of radiation damage. Radiat Res 77:149–155, 1979.
13. Jirtle RL, Michalopoulos G. A clonal assay in vivo for parenchymal hepatocytes. In Potten CS, Hendry JH (eds): Cell Clones: Manual of Mammalian Cell Techniques. Edinburgh: Churchill Livingstone, 1985, pp. 139–151.

Chemically Induced Cell Proliferation:
Implications for Risk Assessment, pages 185-194
©1991 Wiley-Liss, Inc.

Correlation between Species and Tissue Sensitivity to Chemical Carcinogenesis in Rodents and the Induction of DNA Synthesis

James E. Klaunig, Joseph C. Siglin, Lydia D. Schafer, James A. Hartnett, Christopher M. Weghorst, Michael J. Olson, and James A. Hampton

A number of chemical carcinogens that are not mutagenic and do not appear to directly damage nuclear DNA will induce hepatocellular cancer in rodents when chronically administered. While the mechanism(s) by which these compounds function in the induction and development of hepatocellular cancer is unknown, exposure to these "nongenotoxic" carcinogens produces a number of changes in rodent liver, including: increased target cell division and cell proliferation, induction of mixed function oxidative enzyme activity, and inhibition of gap junctional intercellular com-munication between adjacent cells. The ability to induce DNA synthesis and cell prolif-eration appears to be a common characteristic of many nongenotoxic carcinogens. However, the role that cell proliferation plays in the induction of tumorigenesis by chemical carcinogens remains to be resolved. Both hepatic and renal tumors induced in rodents by chemical carcinogens has been shown to be species, organ, and gender specific. For example, trichloroethylene (TCE) is a hepatic carcinogen in mice but not in rats (1). Treatment of rodents with unleaded gasoline produced hepatic tumors in female mice (not male mice) and renal tumors in male rat kidneys (but not female rat kidneys) (1,2). The barbiturate phenobarbital (PB) has been shown to induce only hepatic tumors in both male and female rats and mice (3–8), while another barbiturate, sodium barbital (BB), is a liver carcinogen in both rats and mice and also a renal carcinogen in rats (9). In this study, we examined the species, organ, and gender specificity of cell proliferation induced in rats and mice by PB, BB, TCE, and unleaded gasoline and attempted to correlate these findings with these compounds' known organ site, gender, and species-specific carcinogenicity. If the induction of cell proliferation by nongenotoxic carcinogens is important in the tumorigenesis process, then we might expect to see a selectivity for each nongenotoxic carcinogen that mimics the site specificity of tumor formation.

Materials and methods

Chemicals. PB and barbituric acid (BA) were obtained from Sigma Chemical Co, St. Louis, MO; TCE was purchased from Aldrich Chemical Co., Milwaukee, WI; and research-grade unleaded gasoline was obtained from the General Motors Biosciences Department, Warren, MI. These chemicals were obtained in the highest available purities (99%+).

Animals. Six- to eight-week-old male and female B6C3F1 mice and male and female F344 rats were obtained from Charles River Laboratories, Inc. (Kingston, NY).

All rodents received Certified Purina Rodent Chow (Ralston Purina Co., St Louis, MO) and fresh drinking water ad libitum. After a 2-week period of acclimation, animals were treated as described below. All animals were housed and treated at the Medical College of Ohio in Toledo.

Experimental treatments

Male and female B6C3F1 mice and F344 rats were treated for 3, 7, and 14 days (3 animals per group) with either TCE, unleaded gasoline, PB, or BB. TCE (500 mg/kg body weight) and unleaded gasoline (500 mg/kg body weight) were administered in corn oil by daily gavage. PB (500 mg/L) and BB (500 mg/L) were administered daily in drinking water. Controls included both untreated male and female rats and mice, and male and female rats and mice receiving corn oil by gavage only (5 ml corn oil/kg body weight). These concentrations have been shown to induce renal and/or hepatic tumors in rodents when administered chronically (10). Seven days prior to sampling (or 3 days prior, in the case of the 3-day exposure) rats and mice were subcutaneously implanted with a single osmotic minipump (Alza Corp., Palo Alto, CA) containing tritiated thymidine (60 Ci/mmole; 0.5 µCi delivered per hour per animal). All animals were killed by carbon dioxide asphyxiation after treatment ended, and body weights, liver weights, and kidney weights were determined. Livers and kidneys were removed, grossly examined for lesions, sliced into 2–4-mm-thick slices, fixed in 10% phosphate-buffered formalin, embedded in paraffin, and sectioned. Sections for light microscopic examination were stained with hematoxylin and eosin. Sections for autoradiographic examination were deparaffinized, dipped in Kodak NBT-2 liquid emulsion, incubated at 4°C for 5 weeks, developed in dektol (Kodak), and counterstained with hematoxylin and eosin. DNA synthesis was measured in treated and control tissues by counting both the number of cells in DNA synthesis (labeled nuclei) and the total number of cells per field. The percentage of labeled cells was calculated by dividing the number of positive-stained cells by the total. DNA synthesis was determined in hepatocytes and in the proximal tubule cells. Labeling indices were determined for a minimum of 10 random areas (500 cells each) for each organ and animal examined. Values were analyzed statistically using chi square and two-way ANOVA (11).

Results

The effect of continuous PB treatment on the mouse and rat hepatocyte labeling index is shown in Figures 1 and 2, respectively. PB induced an increase in DNA synthesis over untreated control levels in both male and female mice after 3, 7, and 14 days of exposure. Male mouse hepatocytes showed a greater response than did female mouse liver cells. PB also induced DNA synthesis in female and male rat hepatocytes after 3, 7, and 14 days of treatment, but had no effect on the renal proximal tubule DNA labeling index in either male or female rats or mice at any of the exposure intervals examined (data not shown).

BB also induced hepatocyte DNA synthesis in male and female mouse livers and in male and female rat livers in a duration-dependent manner (Figs. 3 and 4). Male rats and mice both displayed a greater increase in the DNA labeling index compared to their

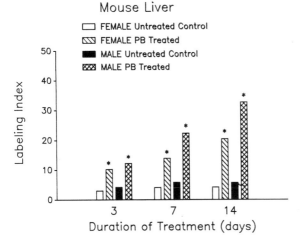

Figure 1. The effect of PB (500 mg/l in the drinking water) on the hepatocyte labeling index in male and female B6C3F1 mice after 3, 7, and 14 days of continuous treatment.

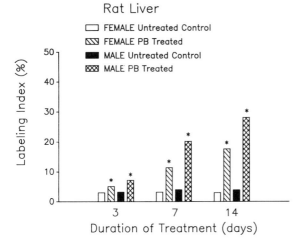

Figure 2. The effect of PB (500 mg/l in the drinking water) on the hepatocyte labeling index in male and female F344 rat livers after 3, 7, and 14 days of continuous treatment.

female counterparts. Sodium barbital failed to induce DNA synthesis in the renal tubules in either the male or female mouse (Fig. 5) or in the female rat (Fig. 6). Sodium barbital did, however, induce a significant increase in the renal labeling index in male rats after 7 and 14 days of treatment (Fig. 6).

Exposure to unleaded gasoline produced a significant increase in hepatocyte DNA synthesis in the female mouse liver after 7 and 14 days of treatment compared to the corn oil-only–treated controls (Fig. 7). Unleaded gasoline had no effect on hepatocyte DNA synthesis in the male mouse liver (Fig. 7) or on the female and male rat liver

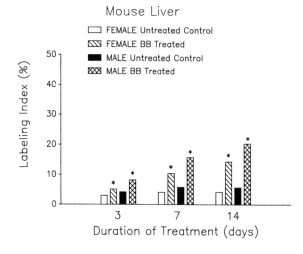

Figure 3. Hepatocyte labeling index after continuous treatment with BB (500 mg/l in the drinking water) to male and female B6C3F1 mouse liver for 3, 7, and 14 days of treatment.

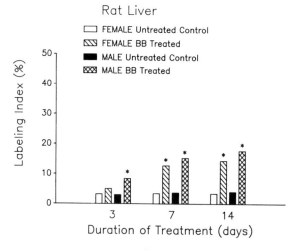

Figure 4. The effect of continuous treatment with BB (500 mg/l in the drinking water) for 3, 7, and 14 days on the labeling index of male and female F344 rats.

(Fig. 8). In male and female mouse renal cells, no induction of DNA synthesis was observed during the treatment period (Fig. 9). Similarly, unleaded gasoline had no effect on DNA synthesis in female rat renal cells, but did induce an exposure-dependent increase in male rat renal cells (Fig. 10). Male and female rats (Fig. 11) and female mice (Fig. 12) exposed to TCE for up to 14 days showed no significant difference in hepatocyte DNA synthesis. TCE did induce an increase in DNA labeling after 7 and 14 days of treatment in male mouse hepatocytes (Fig. 12) and in male rat renal cells after 14 days of exposure (Fig. 13), but had no effect on female rat or mouse renal DNA synthesis (Figs. 13–14).

Mouse Kidney

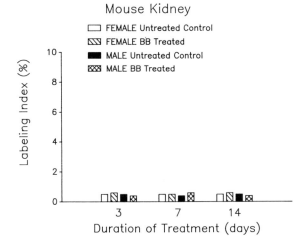

Figure 5. The effect of continuous BB treatment (500 mg/l in the drinking water) for 3, 7, and 14 days on murine kidney proximal tubule cell proliferation.

Rat Kidney

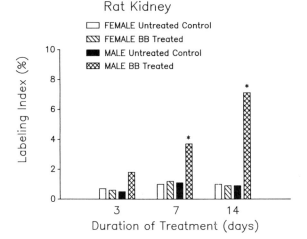

Figure 6. The effect of continuous BB treatment (500 mg/l in the drinking water) for 3, 7, and 14 days on male and female rat kidney proximal tubule cell proliferation.

Discussion

A common effect of many of the nongenotoxic chemical carcinogens is the induction of increased rates of both DNA synthesis and cell proliferation in normal rodent tissue following short-term exposure. In this study, we investigated whether a correlation existed between the induction of cell proliferation in the target tissue—the tissue where tumors arise following chronic exposure to the chemical compound—and the induction of cancer. In rodents, the induction of chemical carcinogenesis with nongenotoxic specific carcinogens displays clearly species, gender, and organ site specificity.

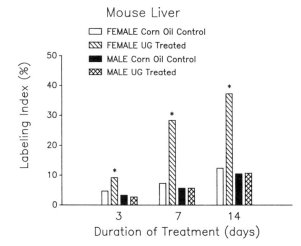

Figure 7. Labeling index in male and female B6C3F1 mouse liver after daily gavage treatment for 3, 7, and 14 days with unleaded gasoline (UG) (500 mg/kg body weight).

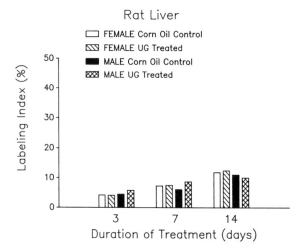

Figure 8. Effect of treatment via daily gavage with unleaded gasoline (UG) (500 mg/kg body weight) on labeling index in male and female rat liver after 3, 7, and 14 days of treatment.

The present study has confirmed that the induction of DNA synthesis following short-term treatment with four nongenotoxic carcinogens—unleaded gasoline, BB, PB, or TCE—follows this organ, gender, and species specificity of tumor induction. The mechanism by which these compounds induce cancer and the role that the induction of cell proliferation/DNA synthesis has in this process remains unresolved, but two possible mechanisms can be considered.

In one scenario, the induction of rapid cell proliferation may increase the spontaneous mutation rate of these rapidly dividing cells. These newly initiated cells may

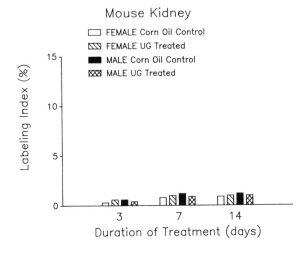

Figure 9. Daily gavage treatment with unleaded gasoline (UG) (500 mg/kg body weight) for 3, 7, and 14 days on male and female B6C3F1 mouse kidney proximal tubule cell proliferation.

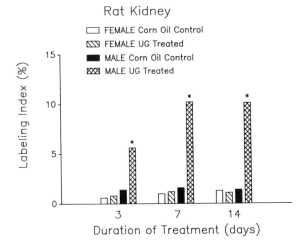

Figure 10. DNA labeling index in male and female rat proximal tubule cells following daily gavage (500 mg/kg body weight) treatment with unleaded gasoline (UG) for 3, 7, and 14 days.

then advance onto neoplasia either through intrinsic promotion or through promotion by continued treatment with nongenotoxic compounds. The possibility that cancer is a disease involving mutation and DNA modification, and the already-observed presence of spontaneous tumors in rodents, both suggest that selective organs in certain strains of rodents are very susceptible to mutation. Arguments against this possibility are that the induction of DNA synthesis and cell proliferation only occurs in normal livers for a short duration, then continual treatment with the nongenotoxic compound will produce no increase in DNA synthesis or cell proliferation (i.e., a refractoriness to the

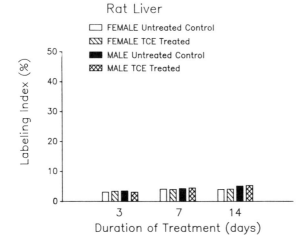

Figure 11. DNA labeling index in F344 male and female rat liver following daily gavage treatment for 3, 7, and 14 days with TCE (500 mg/kg body weight).

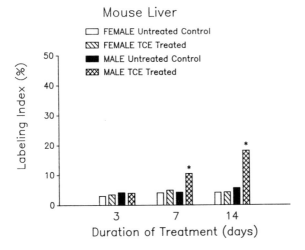

Figure 12. DNA labeling index in male and female B6C3F1 mouse liver following daily gavage treatment for 3, 7, and 14 days with TCE (500 mg/kg body weight).

cell proliferative effects of these compounds in the normal tissue is seen). The paradox is that long-term treatment with these nongenotoxic carcinogens is required to induce cancer while the induction of cell proliferation is seen only for a short period of time.

A second hypothesis is that these nongenotoxic carcinogens are selectively inducing the proliferation of previously initiated cells present in the target tissue, and thus act as tumor promoters. This hypothesis is supported by the fact that following chronic treatment with these nongenotoxic carcinogens, normal cells become refractory to the cell proliferative effects of these agents, while cell proliferation and DNA synthesis in preneoplastic foci (clones of initiated cells) are selectively maintained at increased

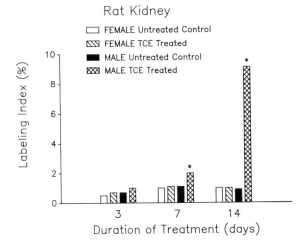

Figure 13. Labeling index in male and female F344 rat kidney proximal tubule cells following treatment via daily gavage for 3, 7, and 14 days with TCE (500 mg/kg body weight).

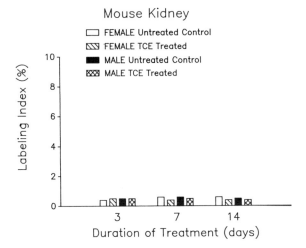

Figure 14. Effect of daily gavage treatment of male and female B6C3F1 mice with TCE (500 mg/kg body weight) for 3, 7, and 14 days on kidney proximal tubule labeling index.

levels as long as the chemical is administered. Since tumor promoters by definition selectively induce initiated cells to clonally expand, these nongenotoxic compounds appear to be acting as tumor promoters. Initiated cells are already present in the cells of some rodent species as is evident by the formation of spontaneous tumors. Also, treatment with nongenotoxic carcinogens results in an increase in both the tumor incidence and multiplicity over that which occurs spontaneously, another characteristic of tumor promoters. And finally, the production of tumors by these nongenotoxic chemical carcinogens requires long-term chronic exposure, another hallmark of tumor promotion.

References

1. Carcinogenesis bioassay of trichloroethylene. Case #79-01-6, NCI, CG, TR-2, DHEW Publ. No. (NIH) 76-802, National Cancer Institute, 1976.
2. MacFarland H, Ulrich C, Holdsworth C, Kitchen D, Halliwell W, Blum S. A chronic inhalation study with unleaded gasoline vapor. J Amer Cell Tox 3:231–247, 1984.
3. Peraino C, Fry RJM, Staffeldt E. Reduction and enhancement by phenobarbital of hepatocarcinogenesis induced in rat by 2-acetylaminofluorene. Cancer Res 31:1506–1512, 1971.
4. Peraino C, Fry RJM, Staffeldt E, Kisieleski WE. Effects of varying the exposure to phenobarbital on its enhancement of 2-acetylaminofluorene-induced hepatic tumorigenesis in the rat. Cancer Res 33:2701–2705, 1973.
5. Peraino C, Fry RJM, Staffeldt E. Enhancement of spontaneous hepatic tumorigenesis in C3H mice by dietary phenobarbital. J Natl Cancer Inst 5:1349–1350, 1973.
6. Peraino C, Staffeld EF, Haugen DA, Lombard LS, Stevens FJ, Fry RJM. Effect of varying the dietary concentration of phenobarbital on its enhancement of 2-acetylaminofluorene-induced hepatic tumorgenesis. Cancer Res 40:3268–3273, 1980.
7. Pereira MA, Klaunig JE, Herren-Freund SL, Ruch FJ. Effect of phenobarbital on the development of liver tumors in juvenile and adult mice. J Natl Cancer Inst 77:449–452, 1986.
8. Pereira MA, Herren-Freud SL, Long RE. Dose-response relationship of phenobarbital promotion of diethylnitrosamine initiated tumors in rat liver. Cancer Lett 32:305–311, 1968.
9. Diwan BA, Rice JM, Ohshima M, Ward JM, Dove LF. Comparative tumor promoting activities of phenobarbital, amobarbital, barbital sodium, and barbituric acid on livers and other organs of male F344/NCr rats following initiation with N-nitrosodiethylamine. J Natl Cancer Inst 74:325–336, 1985.
10 Diwan BA, Rice JM, Ohshima M, Ward JM. Interstrain differences in susceptibility to liver carcinogenesis initiated by N-nitrosodiethylamine and its promotion by phenobarbital in C57Bl/6NCr, C3H/HeNCrmtv- and DBA/2NCr mice. Carcinogenesis 7:215–220, 1986.
11. Gad S, Weil CS. Statistics and Experimental Design for Toxicologists. Telford Press: New Jersey, 1986.

Chemically Induced Cell Proliferation:
Implications for Risk Assessment, pages 195-208
©1991 Wiley-Liss, Inc.

The Roles of L-Ascorbic Acid, Urinary pH, and Na or K Ion Concentration in Rat Bladder Epithelial Cell Proliferation with Special Reference to Tumor Promotion

*Shoji Fukushima, Masa-Aki Shibata, Yasushi Kurata,
and Ryohei Hasegawa*

Two-stage bladder carcinogenesis has been extensively studied in rats and consequently many bladder tumor promoters have been identified. They can be classified into several types according to the evoked urinary response (1): For example, the first-class promoters, including sodium or potassium salts of carbonate, sodium salts of L-ascorbic acid (AsA), or saccharin, increase urinary pH and Na^+ or K^+ concentration (2–4); the second-class promoters, exemplified by diphenyl and uracil, induce urolithiasis (5–7); in contrast, those in the third class, including the antioxidants butylated hydroxyanisole (BHA), butylated hydroxytoluene, and ethoxyquin, do not generally alter urinary components (7–9). As demonstrated previously about the first-class promoters, despite the inactivity of the parent compounds, sodium L-ascorbate (AsA-Na) and sodium citrate could exert significant enhancing activity in rat bladder carcinogenesis (2,10–12). Subsequently, it was shown that administration of $NaHCO_3$ or K_2CO_3, especially in combination with AsA, but not $MgCO_3$ or $CaCO_3$, can similarly enhance bladder carcinogenesis (2,3). Moreover, the promoting activity of AsA-Na is correlated with increased urinary pH, whereas the administration of AsA concurrently with NH_4Cl, which causes a drop in the pH of the urine, is associated with a reduction in promoting activity (2). These results therefore suggest crucial roles for the urinary concentrations of sodium and potassium ions and pH in the modulation of bladder carcinogenesis.

Scanning electron microscopy studies have suggested that the appearance of pleomorphic microvilli on the luminal surfaces of bladder epithelial cells indicates a change from reversible to irreversible hyperplasia induced by bladder carcinogens (4,13,14); this lesion has been interpreted by some investigators as a preneoplastic marker. However, it was subsequently discovered that pleomorphic microvilli found on bladder epithelium were not specific to neoplasia; these lesions are therefore now regarded as simply indicative of epithelial proliferation (15,16). The pleomorphic microvilli observed by scanning electron microscopy are, however, not seen in normal rat bladders at any age. Further studies have indicated that bladder tumor promoters induce an elevation in DNA synthesis in the bladder epithelium and produce distinct morphological alterations observable on the luminal surface when viewed by scanning electron microscopy (7,17–22).

Elevated levels of prostaglandins, especially prostaglandin E_2, have been found in various malignant tumor tissues (23–26) as well as in human bladder epithelial cells following application of tumor promoters (27,28). The bladder epithelium of rats and rabbits has substantial prostaglandin synthetic activity (29,30); a previous study suggested that metabolism of N-[4-(5-nitro-2-furyl)-2-thiazolyl]formamide by prostaglandin synthetase may be involved in the activation of carcinogens necessary to induce bladder cancer (24). Moreover, all prostaglandins including E_2 stimulate the formation of cAMP in a number of tissues and cells including bladder epithelium (31–34). This metabolite is also known to be an important regulator of cellular growth and differentiation. For example, analogues of cAMP cause effects on growth properties and morphological characteristics of cultured neoplastic cells (35). However, the exact relationship between intracellular cAMP levels and growth control remains unclear.

The purpose of the present experimentation was to investigate changes in urinary composition, level of DNA synthesis, and degree of morphological alteration in the bladder epithelium induced by various treatments, some of which have been shown in other studies to have tumor-promoting effects. In addition, investigations were performed to assess the differences between AsA and AsA-Na with respect to prostaglandin E_2, cAMP, and AsA content of bladder tissue and proliferation in vivo. A comparison with the effects of BHA, a class III promoter (8), was included to further clarify the relevance of these parameters to the promotion process. A long-term sequential analysis of proliferation-related parameters was also performed.

Materials and methods

Test chemicals. AsA-Na, $NaHCO_3$, NH_4Cl, K_2CO_3, $MgCO_3$, and $CaCO_3$ were purchased from Wako Pure Chemical Industries, Osaka, Japan. AsA was obtained from Tanabe Seiyaku Co. Ltd, Osaka, Japan.

Animals. A total of 434 male 6-week-old F344 rats (Charles River Japan, Inc., Atsugi, Japan) were used. They were housed in plastic cages on hardwood chip bedding in an environmentally controlled room, maintained at $22 \pm 2°C$ and artificially illuminated for 12 hr each day.

Experiment 1

Groups of 17 or 12 rats were given 1 of 9 treatments. They received powdered basal diet (Oriental MF, Oriental Yeast Company, Tokyo, Japan) with no additional chemical (control) or supplementation with one of the following: 3% $NaHCO_3$; 3% K_2CO_3; 3% $MgCO_3$; 3% $CaCO_3$; 5% AsA; 5% AsA + 3% $NaHCO_3$; 5% AsA + 3% K_2CO_3; 5% AsA + 3% $MgCO_3$; 5% AsA + 3% $CaCO_3$. The rats were observed daily, and body weights and food and water consumption were measured weekly.

Urinalysis. During week 4, fresh urine specimens were obtained from rats of each group by forced micturition at 8:00 A.M. For pH determination (using a pH meter, model F-8DP, Hitachi-Horiba, Tokyo, Japan), the portion voided first was excluded because of possible contamination with bacteria and foreign matter from the external genitalia. AsA in the fresh urine was analyzed semiquantitatively with urine-testing strips (Stix, Ames Division Miles Laboratories, Inc., Elkhart, IN). Acetic acid solution (5 µl) was added to the urine samples before testing for AsA because a urinary pH >7.5 causes an abnormal reaction in the ascorbic acid reagent area.

Urine samples were also collected from rats placed in individual metabolic cages over a 4-hr period (9 A.M.–1 P.M.) without food or water. The urine volume was measured by weighing and its osmolality determined by freezing-point depression using Osmett A (Precision System Inc., MA). Aliquots were then used to measure sodium, chloride, potassium, calcium, magnesium, and phosphorus concentrations. The remainders of the samples were centrifuged and examined microscopically for sediment.

DNA synthesis. At week 8, 5 rats from each of the groups were injected intraperitoneally with 100 mg 5-bromo-2'-deoxyuridine (BrdU)/kg body weight for examination of flash labeling. BrdU (Sigma Chemical Corp., St Louis, MO) and dimethyl sulfoxide and saline (1:3,v/v) were used as solvents. One hour later, the rats were killed by exsanguination under diethyl ether anesthesia. The bladders were ligated at the neck, inflated by intraluminal injection of 10% phosphate-buffered formalin, removed quickly, and immersed in the fixative. After 2 hr fixation, they were bisected sagitally and cut longitudinally into 6 strips. The strips were preserved again in fixative overnight, rinsed in running tap water for 12 hr, then embedded in paraffin and sectioned. Immunohistochemical staining for BrdU incorporation was performed by the avidin-biotin-peroxidase complex immunohistochemical method (36) with anti-BrdU monoclonal antibody (Becton Dickinson Immunocytometry System, Mountain View, CA). Numbers of labeled cells per 1,000 cells were counted under the light microscope and labeling indices were expressed as percentage values.

Morphological investigation. The bladders from the remaining rats killed at week 8 (5 rats/group) were inflated with 2% glutaraldehyde in 0.1 M cacodylate buffer and divided in half longitudinally. One half was stained with hematoxylin and eosin for light microscopy, and the other half was processed for scanning electron microscopy (Hitachi S-450, Hitachi Co., Ltd., Japan) as previously described (18).

Experiment 2

Rats were divided into 4 groups of 11 rats each. They were given powdered basal diet alone (control) or diet containing 5% AsA-Na, 1% NH$_4$Cl, or 5% AsA-Na + 1% NH$_4$Cl. All surviving rats in each group were killed at week 8.

Urinalysis. During week 8, the volume, pH, and osmolality values of the urine were measured and urinary levels of electrolytes, total ascorbic acid, and sediment were determined as in Experiment 1.

DNA synthesis. Five rats in each group were killed for examination of BrdU flash labeling of the bladder epithelium as in Experiment 1. In addition, since normal bladder epithelium in rats has a very low labeling index, continuous labeling techniques were used for detecting slowly proliferating cells and for excluding diurnal differences in cell turnover. Alzet miniosmotic pumps (Alza Co., Palo Alto, CA) containing BrdU solution (0.25 ml, 10% BrdU) were inserted into the intraperitoneal cavities of 3 rats in each group for 4 days. BrdU-treated rats were killed and labeling was assessed in formalin-fixed tissue sections as for Experiment 1.

Morphological investigation. The remaining rats (3 per group) were killed and examined for morphological alterations of the bladder epithelium by light microscopy and scanning electron microscopy.

Experiment 3

Rats were divided into 4 groups of 60 rats each. They were respectively given powdered basal diet (Oriental MF, Oriental Yeast Co., Tokyo, Japan) containing 5% AsA, 5% AsA-Na, 2% BHA, or no added chemical for up to 36 weeks.

DNA synthesis. Five rats in each of the groups were killed for examination of BrdU flash labeling of the bladder epithelium as performed in Experiment 1 at weeks 2, 4, 8, 16, and 36.

Measurement of prostaglandin E_2. Minced half-bladder samples were immersed in 0.25 ml of ice-cold 1 M phosphate buffer, pH 6.8, 1.5 ml methanol, and 0.05 ml [^{3}H]prostaglandin E_2 (4000 disintegrations per minute/0.1 ml). Since prostaglandin E_2 is also generated during the extraction process (37), 0.1 ml of 0.05 M indomethacin in methanol was added to each sample. Following homogenization and centrifugation at 3000 r.p.m. for 10 min, the samples were extracted with chloroform and methanol (1:1, v/v) and applied to silicic acid columns. The prostaglandin E_2–containing fraction obtained columns serially with solvent (benzene:ethyl acetate:methanol,60:40:2) (38). The collected fractions containing prostaglandin E_2 were dried at 40°C under a stream of nitrogen and the residue dissolved in 0.01 M Tris-HCl buffer, pH 7.4, containing 0.9% NaCl and 0.1% gelatin. Aliquots of this buffered solution were measured for prostaglandin E_2 by radioimmunoassay (using a New England Nuclear Kit, Boston, MA). The recovery by this method was satisfactory (75%).

Measurement of AsA and cAMP. The other minced half-bladder samples were placed in 1.0 ml of ice-cold 6% trichloroacetic acid (TCA), homogenized, and centrifuged at 3000 r.p.m. for 10 min. Aliquots of the resultant supernatants were assayed for AsA by the 2,4-dinitro-phenylhydrazine colorimetric method and after removal of TCA by H_2O-saturated ether, used for measurement of cAMP by radioimmunoassay with dextran-coated charcoal (using a Yamasa RIA Kit, Japan).

Statistical analyses. The significances of intergroup differences in body weight, biochemistry values, and DNA synthesis levels were assessed using the two-sided Student's *t*-test. Insufficient homogeneity of variance was corrected with respect to the degrees of freedom according to Welch.

Results

Experiment 1

The results of urinalysis at week 4 are shown in Table 1. A significant increase in urine volume was observed in the $NaHCO_3$ and AsA + $NaHCO_3$ groups. Urine from rats given $NaHCO_3$, AsA + $NaHCO_3$, or AsA + K_2CO_3 showed significantly decreased osmolality. Urinary pH was significantly elevated in groups given $NaHCO_3$, or K_2CO_3, either alone or in combination with AsA, and AsA treatment itself caused a drop in pH. Large amounts of total ascorbic acid were detected by urine-testing strips in urine from AsA-treated groups. Increased levels of urinary electrolytes were associated with the individual dosing regimens. In addition, a decrease in urinary chloride was observed in groups given $NaHCO_3$, K_2CO_3, or $CaCO_3$ with or without AsA.

Table 1. Urine Characteristics in Rats Treated with Test Chemicals in Experiments 1 and 2.

Test chemical (% in diet)	No. of rats	Urine volume (g)	Urine osmolality (mosmol/kg H$_2$O)	Urine pH	Ascorbic acid in urine (mg/dl)[1]	Urinary level (mEq/litre) of:				Urinary level (mg/dl) of:	
						Na	K	Cl	Ca	P	Mg
Experiment 1											
None	5	1.6 ± 0.4	2086 ± 168	6.8 ± 0.4	0–10	177 ± 31	113 ± 66	124 ± 24	5 ± 3	11 ± 10	15 ± 4
NaHCO₃(3)	5	2.5 ± 0.6*	1361 ± 251**	8.2 ± 0.1**	0–10	502 ± 122**	113 ± 37	71 ± 28*	7 ± 2	28 ± 13	10 ± 4
K₂CO₃(3)	5	2.3 ± 0.5	1877 ± 391	8.1 ± 0.1**	0–10	149 ± 37	384 ± 76**	51 ± 16**	4 ± 2	26 ± 13	10 ± 4
MgCO₃(3)	5	1.2 ± 0.2	2138 ± 229	7.2 ± 0.6	25	134 ± 31	105 ± 10	104 ± 26	59 ± 19**	3 ± 1	258 ± 44**
CaCO₃(3)	5	1.2 ± 0.3	2012 ± 131	7.8 ± 0.6	0–10	135 ± 46	125 ± 45	123 ± 54	77 ± 13**	3 ± 1	76 ± 34**
AsA(5)	5	1.1 ± 0.4	2146 ± 210	6.1 ± 0.2*	150	144 ± 54	113 ± 37	140 ± 22	8 ± 2	24 ± 14	22 ± 8
AsA(5) + NaHCO₃(3)	5	2.7 ± 0.4**	1245 ± 385**	8.0 ± 0.3**	150	487 ± 105**	94 ± 24	45 ± 19**	10 ± 3	20 ± 17	20 ± 7
AsA(5) + K₂CO₃(3)	5	2.1 ± 0.7	1585 ± 178**	7.8 ± 0.4**	150	167 ± 29	288 ± 107*	50 ± 21**	5 ± 4	26 ± 11	14 ± 11
AsA(5) + MgCO₃(3)	5	1.8 ± 0.5	1801 ± 235	7.1 ± 0.3	75	103 ± 45	136 ± 31	113 ± 67	61 ± 21**	1 ± 1	219 ± 56**
AsA(5) + CaCO₃(3)	5	1.3 ± 0.4	2012 ± 131	7.4 ± 0.7	150	101 ± 63	90 ± 22	109 ± 45	77 ± 15**	3 ± 2	69 ± 77**
Experiment 2											
None	5	1.5 ± 0.3	1851 ± 253	6.9 ± 0.3	0–10	144 ± 53	274 ± 61	139 ± 50	7 ± 3	25 ± 22	51 ± 15
AsA-Na(5)	5	2.8 ± 0.7**	1246 ± 204**	8.1 ± 0.2**	150	316 ± 91*	113 ± 37**	88 ± 25	7 ± 3	24 ± 16	47 ± 31
NH₄Cl(1)	5	1.8 ± 0.4	1725 ± 192	5.9 ± 0.1**	0–10	100 ± 20	163 ± 60*	187 ± 60	4 ± 2	45 ± 26	30 ± 10
AsA-Na(5) + NH₄Cl(1)	5	2.9 ± 0.9*	1199 ± 137**	7.0 ± 0.4	150	264 ± 136	116 ± 34**	228 ± 113	7 ± 4	61 ± 34	29 ± 7

[1]Results are expressed as 0–10, 25, 50, or 150 mg/100 ml.

Values are means ± SD for results at week 4 (Experiment 1) or at week 8 (Experiment 2).

Values marked with asterisks differ significantly (Student's *t*-test) from those of the corresponding controls (*$P < 0.05$; **$P < 0.01$).

Macroscopically, no abnormalities were observed in the urinary bladder of any groups.

Estimates of urinary bladder DNA synthesis in treated and control rats, measured by incorporation of BrdU into DNA, are shown in Table 2. After 8 weeks, DNA synthesis was significantly elevated in rats treated with $NaHCO_3$, K_2CO_3, AsA + $NaHCO_3$, or AsA + K_2CO_3. In each case, a distinct increment in DNA synthesis was associated with the addition of AsA. No other treated groups demonstrated any significant changes in DNA synthesis.

Morphological findings are summarized in Table 3. Simple hyperplasia consisting of diffuse thickening of the epithelium with four to eight layers of epithelial cells affected, was observed in the $NaHCO_3$, K_2CO_3, AsA + $NaHCO_3$, and AsA + K_2CO_3 groups. Moreover, papillary hyperplasia with a delicate fibrovascular core demonstrated exophytic growth, as was noted in a single animal treated with AsA + K_2CO_3. Administration of $NaHCO_3$ or K_2CO_3 in combination with AsA produced more severe changes than did treatment with $NaHCO_3$ or K_2CO_3 alone.

Alterations of the luminal surface of the urinary bladder that were observed by scanning electron microscopy were classified as described previously (14,19). The normal epithelium appears flat and is composed of large polyclonal cells of relatively uniform size and shape; the luminal surfaces of the cells are covered with a complex network

Table 2. Estimation of DNA Synthesis in Bladder Epithelium of Rats Treated with Test Chemicals for 8 Weeks by Incorporation of BrdU (Experiments 1 and 2).

Test chemical (% in diet)	Flash labeling index (BrdU-incorporating cells, %)	Continuous labeling index (BrdU-incorporating cells, %)
Experiment 1		
None	0.06 ± 0.09	NE[1]
$NaHCO_3(3)$	$0.42 \pm 0.27^*$	NE
$K_2CO_3(3)$	$2.23 \pm 0.90^{**}$	NE
$MgCO_3(3)$	0.20 ± 0.20	NE
$CaCO_3(3)$	0.04 ± 0.05	NE
AsA(5)	0.02 ± 0.04	NE
AsA(5) + $NaHCO_3(3)$	$4.43 \pm 2.68^{*}$[2]	NE
AsA(5) + $K_2CO_3(3)$	$4.67 \pm 2.34^*$	NE
AsA(5) + $MgCO_3(3)$	0.32 ± 0.33	NE
AsA(5) + $CaCO_3(3)$	0.24 ± 0.16	NE
Experiment 2		
None	0.06 ± 0.08	0.30 ± 0.14
AsA-Na(5)	$0.93 \pm 0.51^*$	$1.30 \pm 0.14^{**}$
$NH_4Cl(1)$	0.04 ± 0.05	0.40 ± 0.28
AsA-Na(5) + $NH_4Cl(1)$	0.30 ± 0.17[3]	0.43 ± 0.06[4]

[1]NE, now examined.
Values are means ± SD for groups of five (flash labeling) or three (continuous labeling) rats after treatment for 8 weeks. Values marked with superscripts differ significantly (Student's t-test) from other groups as follows: significantly different from the corresponding control value, $^*P < 0.05$, $^{**}P < 0.01$; significantly different from corresponding $NaHCO_3$ group, [2]$P < 0.05$; significantly different from AsA-Na group, [3]$P < 0.05$, [4]$P < 0.01$.

of microridges. In contrast, the bladders of rats in groups demonstrating simple hyperplasia (the $NaHCO_3$, K_2CO_3, AsA + $NaHCO_3$, AsA + K_2CO_3 groups) presented a cobblestone appearance with the piling up of many small and round cells covered with ropy or leafy microridges, and/or short, uniform microvilli. Some cells had pleomorphic microvilli of various lengths and shapes on the luminal surface; these cells frequently also had uniform microvilli. Although the bladder epithelium of the majority of rats given AsA + $MgCO_3$ was normal, a single animal had leafy or ropy microridges on the luminal surface. No differences in bladder epithelium changes after treatment with or without AsA could be distinguished by scanning electron microscopy. No other chemicals produced any surface alterations of the bladder epithelium.

Experiment 2

As shown in Table 1, polyuria, hypotonic urine, crystalluria, and natriuresis were observed in rats treated with AsA-Na or AsA-Na + NH_4Cl. The urinary pH of rats given AsA-Na was significantly increased, whereas administration of NH_4Cl resulted in significant decrease in pH. The amount of potassium excreted was decreased in groups given AsA-Na, NH_4Cl, or AsA-Na + NH_4Cl. Large amounts of ascorbic acid were detected in AsA-Na–treated groups.

Regarding DNA synthesis, flash-labeling indices were significantly increased in the group given AsA-Na in comparison with control values (Table 2). Treatment with AsA-Na in combination with NH_4Cl resulted in a reduction in DNA synthesis in comparison with treatment with AsA-Na alone. As shown in Table 2, similar trends were observed for continuous labeling using miniosmotic pumps. Simple hyperplasia was observed in groups given AsA-Na or AsA-Na + NH_4Cl (Table 3). The severity of the hyperplasia was less in the group given AsA-Na + NH_4Cl than in that given AsA-Na alone. Under the scanning electron microscope, the bladder surfaces of rats given AsA-Na or AsA-Na + NH_4Cl showed alterations such as pleomorphic microvilli, short or uniform microvilli, and ropy or leafy microridges, but there were no differences between the treatment groups (AsA-Na vs. AsA-Na + NH_4Cl) in the severity of the alterations (Table 3). No morphological lesions were observed in the bladder epithelia of rats given NH_4Cl alone.

Experiment 3

Figure 1 shows labeling indices calculated as percent of bladder epithelium, as assessed by incorporation of BrdU into DNA in treated and control rats at different time points. Though AsA treatment did not elevate DNA synthesis at any time point, AsA-Na administration induced a significant increase at weeks 2–16, but not week 36. Rats receiving BHA demonstrated a significant increase at week 2, then a dramatic elevation from weeks 4–16; there were gradual decreases in DNA synthesis thereafter, although even at week 36 the level was significantly higher than the control values.

The results of measurement of prostaglandin E_2, cAMP, and AsA in bladder tissue, and of bladder weights for reference, are presented in Table 4. Each biochemical parameter is expressed as value per 1 mg bladder weight. A significant increase in bladder weight was noted in the AsA-Na group; we considered that this was caused by dilatation

Table 3. Morphological Findings in Bladder Epithelium Following Oral Administration of Test Chemicals to Rats (Experiment 1).

	LM finding		SEM finding					
	Simple hyperplasia		Pleomorphic microvilli		Short, uniform microvilli		Ropy or leafy microridges	
Test chemical (% in diet)	Incidence	Severity	Incidence	Severity	Incidence	Severity	Incidence	Severity
Experiment 1								
None	0/10[1]	− [2]	0/5	−	0/5	−	0/5	−
$NaHCO_3(3)$	6/10	+	2/5	+	4/5	+	3/5	++
$K_2CO_3(3)$	6/10	+	3/5	+	4/5	+	4/5	++
$MgCO_3(3)$	0/10	−	0/5	−	0/5	−	0/5	−
$CaCO_3(3)$	0/10	−	0/5	−	0/5	−	0/5	−
AsA(5)	0/10	−	0/5	−	0/5	−	0/5	−
AsA(5) + $NaHCO_3$	9/10	++	3/5	+	5/5	++	5/5	++
AsA(5) + $K_2CO_3(3)$	8/10	++	3/5	+	4/5	+	5/5	+++
AsA(5) + $MgCO_3(3)$	0/10	−	0/5	−	0/5	−	1/5	+
AsA(5) + $CaCO_3(3)$	0/10	−	0/5	−	0/5	−	0/5	−
Experiment 2								
None	0/11	−	0/3	−	0/3	−	0/3	−
AsA-Na(5)	9/11	++	2/3	+	3/3	+	3/3	++
$NH_4Cl(1)$	0/11	−	0/3	−	0/3	−	0/3	−
AsA-Na(5) + $NH_4Cl(1)$	6/11	+	2/3	+	3/3	+	3/3	++

LM = light microscopy; SEM = scanning electron microscopy.
[1]Number of rats affected/number examined.
[2]Graded (mean/group) as follows: − = no change; + = slight; ++ = moderate; +++ = severe.

of the bladder by polyuria. The bladders of rats given AsA-Na or BHA contained significantly greater amounts of prostaglandin E_2 and AsA; furthermore, AsA-Na induced an increase of cAMP. BHA treatment was also associated with a tendency for elevation of cAMP. No significant differences in any of the parameters were noted in rats treated with AsA.

Discussion

Increased DNA synthesis, simple hyperplasia, and proliferation-associated morphological alterations on the surfaces of bladder epithelial cells were typically seen in rats treated with $NaHCO_3$ or K_2CO_3 using scanning electron microscopy. Whereas administration of AsA in combination with $NaHCO_3$ or K_2CO_3 amplified the proliferative responses in the bladder epithelium, AsA itself did not induce any equivalent changes. In contrast, the degree of response in the bladder epithelium of rats given AsA-Na was reduced by simultaneous administration of NH_4Cl, which induced a drop in urinary pH. The present studies, moreover, showed that elevation of BrdU incorporation by AsA-Na was transient, an indication that no significant differences from normal epithelium levels had resulted after relatively long-term treatment. In addition, significant increases of prostaglandin E_2 and AsA in bladder tissue were noted for the AsA-Na or BHA, but

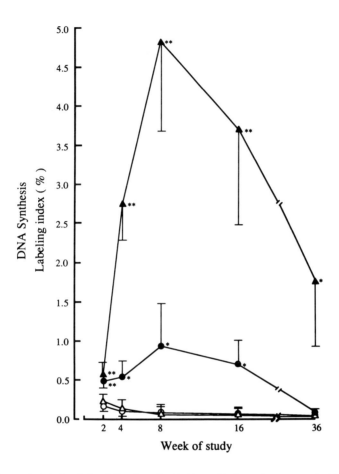

Figure 1. Labeling index (%) values for bladder epithelium of rats treated with test chemicals. 5% AsA (○); 5% AsA-Na (●); 2% BHA (△); control (▲). Data presented are mean ± SD values. Significantly different from control values at $P < 0.05$ (*) and $P < 0.01$ (**).

not AsA groups. Furthermore, cAMP levels in bladder tissue of rats exposed to AsA-Na or BHA were slightly higher than in the controls.

There have been many reports on the participation of Na^+, K^+, and alkalinity of the urine in mitogenesis or promotion of bladder carcinogenesis. Recent studies in vivo have indicated that while $NaHCO_3$ and K_2CO_3 both possess promoting potential, magnesium and calcium salts of carbonate do not exert any equivalent activity (3). Furthermore, Hasegawa and Cohen (20) have shown that of various salts of saccharin that were tested, the sodium and potassium salts are the most potent as bladder mitogens

Table 4. Bladder Weights, and Content of PGE_2, cAMP and AsA in Bladder Tissues of Rats Treated with Test Chemicals.[a]

Test chemical	No. of rats	Bladder weights (g)	PGE_2 (pmol/mg bladder)	cAMP (pmol/mg bladder)	AsA (μg/mg bladder)
AsA	5	0.063 ± 0.007	9.83 ± 9.75	0.80 ± 0.02	8.8 ± 1.5
AsA-Na	5	0.089 ± 0.012**	14.82 ± 7.41*	0.92 ± 0.05*	11.5 ± 1.7*
BHA	5	0.069 ± 0.006	14.52 ± 7.70	0.93 ± 0.27	11.2 ± 0.8*
Control	5	0.066 ± 0.004	2.46 ± 0.99	0.82 ± 0.03	8.5 ± 1.7

[a] Values are mean ± SD.
*Significantly different from control value at $P < 0.05$.
**Significantly different from control value at $P < 0.01$.

when assessed by [^{3}H]thymidine incorporation. A recent study further demonstrated that the promoting activity of AsA-Na is diminished by concurrent treatment with NH_4Cl used as a urine acidifier (2). In addition, it has been reported that NH_4Cl inhibits the induction of calculi and tumor formation by 4-ethylsulfonylnaphthalene-1-sulfonamide (39), and that NH_4Cl in combination with sodium o-phenylphenate (OPP-Na) reduces the tumorigenicity of OPP-Na for rat urinary bladder (40).

These results are therefore in agreement with the literature: The degrees of DNA synthesis and simple hyperplasia development in the bladder epithelium induced by AsA-Na ingestion were reduced by concurrent treatment with NH_4Cl. Previously it was reported that bladder epithelial cells exposed to sodium saccharin in vivo show an increase in membrane potential and related cellular Na/K ion pump activity (41). Further in vivo evidence indicated that sodium transport is increased in tumor cells and that sodium influx rises with intracellular pH due to activation of Na^+/H^+ exchange (42–47). The increased sodium influx activates Na-K ATPase (48,49), which in turn causes intracellular potassium to accumulate, resulting in DNA synthesis (50). In the current study, increased Na^+ or K^+ concentration and alkalinity in the urine might therefore be the direct mitogenic influence that caused cell proliferation in the bladder epithelium, as other researchers have suggested (51).

AsA acts as an antioxidant and reducing agent to protect cells from damage by free radicals (52); it has been suggested that high doses of AsA can therefore help prevent human cancer (53, 54). On the other hand, AsA has been reported to act as a co-promoter (an amplifier) in the N-butyl-N-(4-hydroxybutyl)nitrosamine–F344 rat model of two-stage bladder carcinogenesis, although AsA itself has no promoting activity (2,3, 55). Inhibition of gap-junction–mediated intercellular communication has been suggested to play an important role in the process of tumor promotion (56–58). However, we have shown that, contrary to expectation, AsA-Na has no effect on cell-to-cell communication in BALB/c3T3 cells in the normal pH range, although communication was inhibited with increasing pH of the medium (59). In our present study, we showed that increased DNA synthesis and simple hyperplasia in the bladder epithelium was induced by the administration of AsA under conditions of high urinary pH induced by $NaHCO_3$ or K_2CO_3 ingestion. These results suggest that in vivo, too, the effects of AsA occur only when this antioxidant is administered under conditions of increased urinary alkalinity and Na or K ion concentrations.

The results of the present investigation reveal a significant increase in prostaglandin E_2 levels within bladder tissue of rats treated with the promoters AsA-Na and BHA. A similar but less pronounced nonsignificant tendency for elevation was also found for the nonpromoter AsA. Since the latter has an enhancing effect in concert with $NaHCO_3$ and K_2CO_3 (2,3), the findings might suggest a role for prostaglandin synthesis in bladder tumor promotion. This is in line with earlier indications from in vivo studies (27–29). It was shown previously that bladder epithelial cells exposed to prostaglandin in vivo demonstrated an increase in cAMP levels (33). Since both prostaglandin E_2 and cAMP were elevated in bladder tissue of rats given AsA-Na or BHA, it is possible that the increased cAMP was a response to stimulation by prostaglandin E_2, as shown in our current study. Exactly how this might be related to bladder tumor promotion remains unclear, although numerous in vitro and in vivo investigations have demonstrated that cAMP plays a crucial role in differentiation processes (35).

The current study shows that AsA-Na increased intracellular levels of AsA, whereas no such result was evident with AsA itself. It is possible that Na^+ transport into the bladder cells of rats treated with AsA-Na is accompanied by movement of AsA or the chemical itself stimulates intracellular AsA synthesis. Accordingly, increased AsA levels in bladder tissue could alter normal cellular regulation of growth and differentiation in bladder epithelial cells. BHA treatment similarly increased the AsA content of bladder tissue, but since it is not associated with elevated urinary levels of this metabolite, the effect is presumably due to stimulation of synthesis in this case. In fact, BHA has also been found to cause a significant increase of AsA in the liver of rats (60). However, this point requires further investigation.

It is well documented that the promotion of bladder cancer effected by sodium salts may be mediated by increased Na^+ and pH (2,3,61), with sodium influx perhaps acting as the trigger for DNA synthesis (42,46). The present sequential investigation showed that whereas elevation of BrdU incorporation in the AsA-Na group was observed during the initial 16 weeks, this was transient; no significant difference from normal levels was observed at week 36. With BHA, however, DNA synthesis and surface alterations remained pronounced, suggesting a clear relation between the two parameters as indicated previously (7,17,61). However, the lack of obvious hyperplasia even after long-term BHA treatment, despite the high levels of BrdU incorporation observed, requires explanation. The reason is unclear at the present time although increased cell death, particularly in the superficial layers, is one possibility worthy of consideration. Apoptosis was, however, not apparent.

Conclusions

The results of the studies can be summarized as follows: 1) DNA synthesis and other proliferation-associated responses of bladder epithelium to treatment with various exogenously applied bases may be mediated via changes in urinary Na^+, K^+, and pH; 2) AsA amplifies proliferative responses in bladder epithelium induced by tumor promoters under conditions of increased urinary pH and Na^+ or K^+ concentration; 3) Biochemical parameters such as prostaglandin E_2 and total ascorbic acid may have significance for the promotion process in bladder carcinogenesis.

Acknowledgments

We are indebted to Professor N. Ito for helpful comments regarding this manuscript. The investigations were supported in part by Grants-in-Aid for Cancer Research from the Ministry of Education, Science, and Culture of Japan and from the Ministry of Welfare for the Comprehensive 10-Year Strategy for Cancer Control, Japan.

References

1. Ito N, Fukushima S. Promotion of urinary bladder carcinogenesis in experimental animals. Exp Pathol 36:1–15, 1989.
2. Fukushima S, Shibata M-A, Shirai T, Tamano S, Ito N. Roles of urinary sodium ion concentration and pH in promotion by ascorbic acid of urinary bladder carcinogenesis in rats. Cancer Res 46:1623–1626, 1987.
3. Fukushima S, Shibata M-A, Shirai T, Kurata Y, Tamano S, Imaida K. Promotion by L-ascorbic acid of urinary bladder carcinogenesis in rats under conditions of increased urinary K ion concentration and pH. Cancer Res 47:4821–4824, 1987.
4. Cohen SM, Arai M, Jacobs JB, Friedell GH. Promoting effect of saccharin and DL-tryptophan on urinary bladder carcinogenesis. Cancer Res 39:1207–1217, 1979.
5. Kurata Y, Asamoto M, Hagiwara A, Masui T, Fukushima S. Promoting effects of various agents in rat urinary bladder carcinogenesis initiated by N-butyl-N-(4-hydroxybutyl)nitrosamine. Cancer Lett 32:125–135, 1986.
6. Shirai T, Tagawa Y, Fukushima S, Imaida K, Ito N. Strong promoting activity of reversible uracil-induced urolithiasis on urinary bladder carcinogenesis in rats initiated with N-butyl-N-(4-hydroxybutyl)nitrosamine. Cancer Res 47:6726–6730, 1987.
7. Shibata M-A, Yamada M, Tanaka H, Kagawa M, Fukushima S. Changes in urine composition, bladder epithelial morphology and DNA synthesis in male F344 rats in response to ingestion of bladder tumor promoters. Toxicol Appl Pharmacol 99:37–49, 1989.
8. Imaida K, Fukushima S, Shirai T, Ohtani M, Nakanishi K, Ito N. Promoting activities of butylated hydroxyanisole and butylated hydroxytoluene on 2-stage urinary bladder carcinogenesis and inhibition of γ-glutamyl-transpeptidase-positive foci development in the liver of rats. Carcinogenesis 4:895–899, 1983.
9. Shibata M-A, Yamada M, Asakawa E, Hagiwara A, Fukushima S. Responses of rat urine and urothelium to bladder tumor promoters: possible roles of prostaglandin E_2 and ascorbic acid synthesis in bladder carcinogenesis. Carcinogenesis 10:1651–1656, 1989.
10. Fukushima S, Hagiwara A, Ogiso T, Shibata M, Ito N. Promoting effects of various chemicals in rat urinary bladder carcinogenesis initiated by N-nitroso-N-butyl-(4-hydroxybutyl)amine. Food Chem Toxicol 21:59–68, 1983.
11. Fukushima S, Thamavit W, Kurata Y, Ito N. Sodium citrate: A promoter of bladder carcinogenesis. Jpn J Cancer Res 77:1–4, 1986.
12. Fukushima S, Kurata Y, Shibata M-A, Ikawa E, Ito N. Promotion by ascorbic acid, sodium erythorbate and ethoxyquin of neoplastic lesions in rats initiated with N-butyl-N-(4-hydroxybutyl)nitrosamine. Cancer Lett 23:29–37, 1984.
13. Ito N. Early changes caused by N-butyl-N-(4-hydroxybutyl)nitrosamine in the bladder epithelium of different animal species. Cancer Res 36:2528–2531, 1976.
14. Jacobs JB, Arai M, Cohen SM, Friedell GH. Early lesions in experimental bladder cancer: Scanning electron microscopy of cell surface markers. Cancer Res 36:2512–2517, 1976.
15. Fukushima S, Arai M, Cohen SM, Jacobs JB, Friedell GH. Scanning electron microscopy of cyclophosphamide-induced hyperplasia of the rat urinary bladder. Lab Invest 44:89–96, 1981.
16. Fukushima S, Cohen SM., Arai M, Jacobs JB, Friedell GH. Scanning electron microscopic examination of reversible hyperplasia of the rat urinary bladder. Am J Pathol 102:373–380, 1981.
17. Fukushima S, Cohen SM. Saccharin-induced hyperplasia of the rat urinary bladder. Cancer Res 40:734–746, 1980.

18. Fukushima S, Shibata M-A, Kurata Y, Tamano S, Masui T. Changes in the urine and scanning electron microscopically observed appearance of the rat bladder following treatment with tumor promoters. Jpn J Cancer Res 77:1074–1082, 1986.
19. Cohen SM. Pathology of experimental bladder cancer in rodents. In: Bryan GT and Cohen SM (eds): The Pathology of Bladder Cancer. Vol. II., Boca Raton, FL: CRC Press, 1983, pp. 141–212.
20. Hasegawa R, Cohen SM. The effects of different salts of saccharin on the rat urinary bladder. Cancer Lett 30:261–268, 1986.
21. Knowles MA, Jani H, Hicks RM. Induction of morphological changes in the urothelium of cultured adult rat bladder by sodium saccharin and sodium cyclamate. Carcinogenesis 7:767–774, 1986.
22. Norman JT, Howlett AR, Spacey GD, Hodges GM. Effects of treatment with N-methyl-N-nitrosourea, artificial sweeteners, and cyclophosphamide on adult rat urinary bladder *in vitro*. Lab Invest 57:429–438, 1987.
23. Jaffe BM. Prostaglandins and cancer—an update. Prostaglandins 6:453–461, 1974.
24. Tutton PJM, Petry FM, Barkla DH. Prostaglandins and cell proliferation in intestinal tumors *in vivo*. In: Powles TJ, Bockaman RS, Honn KV, and Ramwell P (eds): Prostaglandins and Cancer, First International Conference, New York: Alan R. Liss, Inc., 1982, pp. 753–757.
25. Fürstenberger G, Gross M, Marks F. On the role of prostaglandins in the induction of epidermal proliferation, hyperplasia and tumor promotion in mouse skin. In: Powles TJ, Bockaman RS, Honn KV, and Ramwell P (eds): Prostaglandins and Cancer, First International Conference New York: Alan R. Liss, Inc., 1982, pp. 239–254.
26. Hubbard WC, Alley MC, McLemore TL, Boyd MR. Profiles of prostaglandin biosynthesis in sixteen established cell lines derived from human lung, colon, prostate, and ovarian tumors. Cancer Res 48:4770–4775, 1988.
27. Danon A, Zenser TV, Thomasson DL, Davis BB. Eicosanoid synthesis by cultured human urothelial cells: potential role in bladder cancer. Cancer Res 46:5676–5681, 1986.
28. Zenser TV, Thomasson DL, Davis BB. Characteristics of bradykinin and TPA increases in the PGE_2 levels of human urothelial cells. Carcinogenesis 9:1173–1177, 1988.
29. Cohen SM, Zenser TV, Murasaki G, Fukushima S, Mattammal MB, Rapp NS, Davis BB. Aspirin inhibition of N-[4-(5-nitro-2-furyl)-2-thiazolyl]formamide-induced lesions of the urinary bladder correlates with inhibition of metabolism by bladder prostaglandin endoperoxide synthetase. Cancer Res 41:3355–3359, 1981.
30. Brown WW, Zenser TV, Davis BB. Prostaglandin E_2 production by rabbit urinary bladder. Am J Physiol 239:1435–1440, 1980.
31. Hammarström S. Endogenous prostaglandin production and cell replication *in vitro*. In: Powles TJ, Bockman RS, Honn KV, and Ramwell P (eds): Prostaglandins and Cancer, First International Conference New York: Alan R. Liss, Inc., 1982, pp. 297–307.
32. Chlapowski FJ. The effects of hormones on cyclic 3′:5′-monophosphate accumulation in transitional epithelium of the urinary bladder. J Cyclic Nucleotide Res 1:193–205, 1975.
33. Hahn GL, Haynes L, Chlapowski FJ. Variations of adenosine 3′,5′-cyclic monophosphate levels in four chemically transformed rat transitional epithelial cell lines. J Natl Cancer Inst 65:657–662, 1980.
34. Chlapowski FJ, Nemecek GM. Aberrant cyclic adenosine 3′:5′-monophosphate metabolism in cultures of tumorigenic rat urothelium. Cancer Res 45:122–127, 1985.
35. Ekanger R, Ogreid D, Evjen O, Vintermyr O, Laerum OD, Doskeland SO. Characterization of cyclic adenosine 3′:5′-monophosphate-dependent protein kinase isozymes in normal and neoplastic fetal rat brain cells. Cancer Res 45:2578–2583, 1985.
36. Morstyn G, Hsu S-M, Kinsella H, Russo A, Mitchell JB. Bromodeoxyuridine in tumors and chromosomes detected with a monoclonal antibody. J Clin Invest 72:1844–1850, 1983.
37. Salmon JA. Analysis of arachidonic acid metabolites by radioimmunoassay and physicochemical methods. Mater Medic Pol 3:169–179, 1980.
38. Jaffe BM, Behrman HR, Parker CW. Radioimmunoassay measurement of prostaglandins E, A and F in human plasma. J Clin Invest 52:398–405, 1973.
39. Flaks A, Hamilton JM, Clayson DB. Effect of ammonium chloride on incidence of bladder tumors induced by 4-ethylsulfonylnaphthalene-1-sulfonamide. J Natl Cancer Inst 51:2007–2008, 1973.
40. Fujii T, Nakamura K, Hiraga K. Effects of pH on the carcinogenicity of O-phenylphenol and sodium ophenylphenate in the rat urinary bladder. Food Chem Toxicol 25:359–362, 1987.

41. Imaida K, Oshima M, Fukushima S, Ito N, Hotta K. Membrane potentials of urinary bladder epithelium in F344 rats treated with N-butyl- N-(4-hydroxybutyl)nitrosamine or sodium saccharin. Carcinogenesis 4:659–661, 1983.
42. Allemain GL, Paris S, Pouyssegur J. Growth factor action and intracellular pH regulation in fibroblasts. J Biol Chem 259:5809–5815, 1984.
43. Fehlman M, Canivet B, Freychet P. Epidermal growth factor stimulates monovalent cation transport in isolated rat hepatocytes. Biochem Biophys Res Commun 100:254–260, 1981.
44. Koch KS, Leffert HL. Increased sodium ion influx is necessary to initiate rat hepatocyte proliferation in cultured fibroblasts. Ann NY Acad Sci 339:175–190, 1980.
45. Moolenaar WH, Mummery CL, Van Der Saag PT, De Laat SW. Rapid ionic events and the initiation of growth in serum-stimulated neuroblastoma cells. Cell 23:789–798. 1981.
46. Moolenaar WH, Tsien RY, Van Der Saag PT, De Laat SW. Na$^+$/H$^+$ exchange and cytoplasmic pH in the action of growth factors in human fibroblasts. Nature 304:645–648, 1983.
47. Rothenberg P, Glaser L, Schlesinger P, Cassel D. Epidermal growth factor stimulates amiloride-sensitive ^{22}Na$^+$ uptake in A431 cells. Evidence for Na$^+$/H$^+$ exchange. J Biol Chem 258:4883–4889, 1983.
48. Rozengurt E, Gelerter TD, Legg A, Petticam P. Melittin stimulates Na entry, Na-K pump activity and DNA synthesis in quiescent cultures of mouse cells. Cell 23:781–788, 1981.
49. Rozengurt E, Heppel LA. Serum rapidly stimulates ouabain sensitive ^{86}Rb$^+$ influx in quiescent 3T3 cells. Proc Natl Acad Sci. USA 72:4492–4495, 1975.
50. Morgan K, Spurlock G, Brown RC, Mir MA. Release of sodium transport inhibitor (inhibitin) from cultured human cancer cells. Cancer Res 46:6095–6100, 1986.
51. Williamson DS, Nagel DL, Markin RS, Cohen SM. Effect of pH and ions on the electronic structure of saccharin. Food Chem Toxicol 25:211–218.
52. Woolley PV, Kumar S, Fitzgerald P, Simpson RT. Ascorbate potentiates DNA damage by 1-methyl-1-nitrosourea in vivo and generates DNA strand breaks in vitro. Carcinogenesis 8:1657–1662, 1987.
53. Cameron E, Pauling L. Cancer and Vitamin C. Menlo Park: Linus Pauling Institute, 1979, p. 108.
54. Cameron E, Pauling L, Leibovitz B. Ascorbic acid and cancer: A review. Cancer Res 39:663–681, 1979.
55. Fukushima S, Imaida K, Shibata M-A, Tamano S, Kurata Y, Ito N. L-ascorbic acid amplification of second-stage bladder carcinogenesis promotion by NaHCO3. Cancer Res 48:6317–6320, 1988.
56. Rivedal E, Sanner T, Yamasaki H. Inhibition of intercellular communication and enhancement of morphological transformation of Syrian hamster embryo cells by TPA. Use of TPA-sensitive and TPA-resistant cell lines. Carcinogenesis 6:899–902, 1985.
57. Trosko JE, Yotti LP, Warren ST, Tsushimoto G, Chang CC. Inhibition of cell-cell communication by tumor promoters. In: Hecker E, et al. (eds): Carcinogenesis—A Comprehensive Survey, vol. 7. New York: Raven Press, 1982, pp. 565–585.
58. Yamasaki H, Enomoto T, Martel N. Intercellular communication, cell differentiation and tumor promotion. In: Börzsönyi M, Day NE, Lapis K, and Yamasaki H (eds): IARC Scientific Publication no. 56 Lyon: International Agency for Research on Cancer, 1984, pp. 217.
59. Masui T, Fukushima S, Kato F, Yamasaki H, Ito N. Effects of sodium L-ascorbate, uracil, butylated hydroxyanisole and extracellular pH on junctional intercellular communication of BALB/c 3Tc cells. Carcinogenesis 7:1143–1146, 1988.
60. Horio F, Kimura M, Yoshida A. Effect of several xenobiotics on the activities of enzymes affecting acid synthesis in rats. J Nutr Sci Vitaminol 29:233–247, 1983.
61. Shibata M-A, Tamano S, Kurata Y, Hagiwara A, Fukushima S. Participation of urinary Na$^+$, K$^+$, pH, and L-ascorbic acid in the proliferative response of the bladder epithelium after the oral administration of various salts and/or ascorbic acid to rats. Food Chem Toxicol 27:403–413, 1989.

Chemically Induced Cell Proliferation:
Implications for Risk Assessment, pages 209-216
©1991 Wiley-Liss, Inc.

Liver Tumor Promoter Phenobarbital: A Biphasic Modulator of Hepatocyte Proliferation

Randy L. Jirtle, Sharon A. Meyer, and J. Scott Brockenbrough

A characteristic response of hepatocytes to liver tumor promoters is an increase in DNA synthesis. This proliferative response can be either compensatory or augmentative in nature. The promoting regimen of choline deficiency, for example, causes hepatocyte necrosis, which triggers a proliferative response to compensate for the loss of hepatic mass (1). The tumor promoter phenobarbital (PB), in contrast, induces both hepatocyte hyperplasia and hypertrophy without causing cell death (2–4). Thus, the total number of hepatocytes in the liver is augmented by PB treatment. These PB-induced hepatocyte responses do not, however, occur uniformly throughout the liver but are confined to the pericentral region of the lobules (Fig. 1) (5). The increased cell volume of the pericentral hepatocytes is maintained throughout the PB exposure period, but the DNA synthetic response is transient, maximizing by day 3 and returning to normal by 1 week (2–4).

The importance of this transient increase in DNA synthesis to tumor promotion is still unknown. Though transient hyperplasia may be a necessary component of the promotional process, alone it is clearly not sufficient to promote tumors. The reasons for this conclusion are that (a) the DNA synthetic response to PB is transient and complete by 1 week (2–4), whereas tumor promotion requires a continuous exposure to PB for at least 3 months (6); and (b) although only the pericentral hepatocytes proliferate in response to PB, the preneoplastic lesions, whose formation is promoted, occur more uniformly throughout the liver lobule. Because the ability of PB to promote tumor formation does not correlate either spatially or temporally with PB induction of DNA synthesis, we focused our attention on the modulation of hepatocyte proliferation that occurs with chronic exposure to PB.

Modulation of normal and preneoplastic hepatocyte proliferation

Although PB induces a temporary increase in DNA synthesis in the pericentral liver hepatocytes (Fig. 1) (5), continuous exposure to PB significantly reduces their proliferative response to mitogenic stimuli both in vivo (1,7) and in vitro (8). For example, the compensatory hyperplastic response to dietary choline deficiency has been shown to be inhibited by PB (1). In addition, Barbason and colleagues (7) demonstrated that, after chronic exposure to PB, the proliferative response to a partial hepatectomy was delayed and the magnitude of peak DNA synthesis was reduced. The hepatocytes' decreased ability to undergo DNA synthesis in PB-treated animals subsequent to a partial hepatectomy is shown clearly in Figs. 2A and B. Whether chronic PB exposure inhibits the proliferation of all but a small subpopulation of hepatocytes or whether the

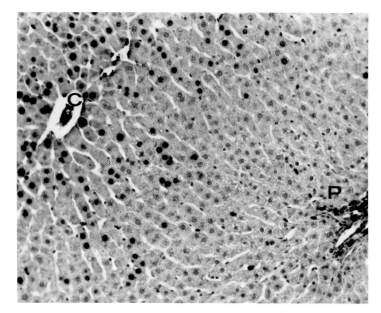

Figure 1. DNA synthesis in the liver of a F344 male rat exposed to PB for 2 weeks (0.1% in the drinking water). The anti-bromodeoxyuridine (BrdU) technique was used to detect hepatocytes that incorporated BrdU into their DNA during the 2-week period the animals were exposed to PB. BrdU was infused (6.9 µg/hr) with an Alzet osmotic pump (Alza Corp., Palo Alto, CA) placed intraperitoneally. The pericentral hepatocytes (C) but not the periportal hepatocytes (P) synthesized DNA in response to PB, ×125.

regenerative response is delayed relative to the DNA pulse-labeling period used in this study remains to be elucidated.

To investigate further the mechanism by which PB modifies the response of hepatocytes to mitogens, we used primary cultures of rat hepatocytes stimulated to proliferate with epidermal growth factor (EGF). Our results and those of others suggested that PB is not directly mitogenic but that it enhances the effectiveness of mitogenic substances such as EGF (9–11). Interestingly, PB facilitates EGF-induced hepatocyte proliferation only at low concentrations while it inhibits the growth of hepatocytes at higher concentrations. This biphasic response is of potential biologic importance in view of the mito-inhibitory effect observed after chronic PB exposure.

Using a 3-mM PB concentration, which is mito-inhibitory but not cytotoxic (12), we compared the ability of PB to inhibit EGF-dependent DNA synthesis in both normal and putative preneoplastic hepatocytes. Though 3-mM PB significantly reduced EGF stimulation of normal hepatocyte proliferation, preneoplastic cells were relatively refractory to inhibition of DNA synthesis (9). This suggested that chronic PB exposure may, in part, promote the formation of hepatocellular carcinomas by inhibiting the growth of normal and of preneoplastic cells differently. The importance of a difference in the reduction of normal hepatocyte growth in the promotional process is emphasized

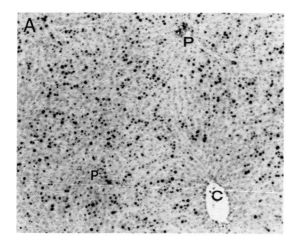

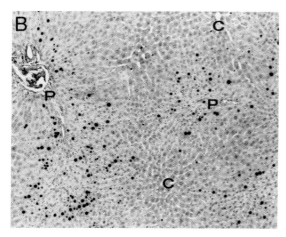

Figure 2. DNA synthesis in control (A) and PB-treated (B) male F344 rats after a two-thirds partial hepatectomy. The anti-BrdU technique was used to detect hepatocytes that incorporated BrdU into their DNA during a 6-hr interval starting 24 hr after the partial hepatectomy. The animals were injected intraperitoneally with BrdU (30 mg/kg). The pericentral (C) and periportai (P) areas of the liver lobule are marked, × 70.

further by the fact that other tumor-promoting regimens, including the Solt and Farber protocol (13) and that of feeding orotic acid (14), also reduced normal hepatocyte proliferation significantly. To elucidate the mechanism or mechanisms of PB's selectively inhibitory effect on EGF-induced DNA synthesis, we investigated the drug's ability to modulate elements of the signal transduction pathway known to mediate EGF-dependent mitogenesis.

Modulation of EGF-induced signal transduction

Normal hepatocytes. First step in the mitogenic signal-transduction pathway of EGF-induced proliferation is the binding of EGF to its receptor. We have demonstrated that PB does not compete with EGF for binding to the hepatocyte EGF receptor (15).

Furthermore, PB does not significantly alter either the relative magnitude or the kinetics of EGF-induced receptor down-regulation. Thus, PB does not influence these early steps in signal transduction.

Pretreatment of hepatocytes with PB was, however, found transiently to decrease the subsequent binding of EGF to its receptor in a dose-dependent manner (15,16). This PB-induced heterologous down-regulation of the EGF receptor is similar to that seen with the skin tumor promoter 12-O-tetradecanoylphorbol-13-acetate (TPA). When we tested for the additive nature of EGF receptor responses to TPA and PB to ascertain whether these two tumor promoters operate by a common mechanism, we observed that PB caused a dose-dependent reduction in hepatocyte EGF-binding both in the absence and presence of a saturating TPA concentration. Thus, PB and TPA elicited a transient reduction in EGF receptor-binding by independent mechanisms. The PB-induced mechanism seemed to be unique to normal hepatocytes; no similar effect was seen in A431 cells, HepG2 cells, or rat liver epithelial cells, whereas TPA caused a down-regulation of the EGF receptor in all four cell types (9). In addition, down-regulation of hepatocyte EGF receptors in response to barbiturates was specific to the tumor-promoting barbiturates phenobarbital and pentobarbital, while nonpromoting barbitur-ic acid and mono-substituted 5-ethyl-and 5-phenyl-barbituric acids were ineffective (17).

Activation of protein kinase C and subsequent phosphorylation of the EGF receptor resulted in the observed reduction of EGF-binding in response to TPA (18–20). Since the mechanisms responsible for the down-regulation of the EGF receptor are different for PB and TPA, we hypothesized that PB would not activate protein kinase C and confirmed this in studies measuring the translocation of protein kinase C activity from the cytosol to the membrane (15,16). Our results demonstrated, therefore, that PB is a non-TPA type of tumor promoter, and suggested that protein kinase C-independent mechanisms may contribute to liver tumor promotion.

Chronically PB-treated hepatocytes. The results described above were obtained with hepatocytes from untreated animals. However, to promote maximally hepatocellular tumor formation, PB must be delivered to animals continuously for at least 3 months (6). To advance our understanding of the PB-induced long-term effects required for tumor promotion, we examined whether chronic treatment of rats with PB affected (a) the responsiveness of hepatocytes to EGF receptor down-regulation by TPA, (b) the responsiveness of hepatocyte protein kinase C to activation by PB and TPA and (c) the subcellular hepatocyte distribution of protein kinase C.

We have shown that chronic treatment of animals with PB significantly sensitized hepatocytes to EGF receptor down-regulation by in vitro PB (21). These results are important because they demonstrated that the PB plasma concentration in chronically treated rats (i.e., 0.05–0.1 mM) is sufficient to cause a continuous down-regulation of the hepatocyte EGF receptor. This, combined with a PB-induced reduction in EGF receptor gene transcription (22), may account for the significant loss of hepatocyte EGF receptors observed in animals exposed chronically to PB (8,23).

In contrast to the EGF receptors' enhanced sensitivity to PB-induced down-regulation, hepatocytes chronically treated with PB were less responsive to TPA-induced EGF receptor down-regulation (21). Concomitantly, the ability of TPA to activate and tightly insert protein kinase C into the plasma membrane was also inhibited markedly by chronic PB exposure (24). However, neither total cellular protein kinase C activity nor its distribution between cytosol and membranes was found different for hepatocytes from PB-treated and control animals. Numerous nuclear proteins involved in mitogenesis, such as topoisomerase II, transcription factors, and proto-oncogenes are substrates of protein kinase C (25–28). Thus, the finding that chronic exposure of hepatocytes to PB severely compromises the ability of protein kinase C to be activated suggested that this may be an important target in the intracellular signal transduction pathway by which PB is inhibiting hepatocyte proliferation.

Modulation of transforming growth factor-β_1 (TGF-β_1) expression

TGF-β_1, a 25-kD homodimer, is a member of a family of five closely related polypeptides (29). It has a bifunctional role in modifying cellular proliferation—stimulating fibroblast growth while inhibiting that of epithelial cells including hepatocytes (29–32). Because chronic exposure of animals to PB also greatly reduced the ability of hepatocytes to respond to mitogenic stimuli (Fig. 2A and B), we investigated whether PB's growth-inhibitory effect was mediated in part through a change in hepatocyte sensitivity to TGF-β_1 or an increase in the intrahepatic concentration of TGF-β_1, or both.

The results of our studies showed that TGF-β_1 is 2 to 3 times more potent in inhibiting the growth of hepatocytes from animals chronically treated with PB than of those from control animals (9). To learn whether chronic exposure to PB increases the intrahepatic concentration of TGF-β_1, we stained liver sections immunohistochemically, using an antibody to the mature active portion of the TGF-β_1 molecule (anti-LC[1-30]) (33). In livers from control animals, hepatocytes stained moderately for TGF-β_1 (9). The relative absence of hepatocyte staining with an antibody to the amino-terminal region of the promolecule (anti-pre [266-278]) suggested, however, that the moderate staining observed with anti-LC[1-30] resulted mainly from hepatocyte uptake of TGF-β_1 rather than synthesis (9). In contrast, periductular cells and endothelial cells stained positive with both antibodies, implying that TGF-β_1 was synthesized constitutively by these nonparenchymal cells. These immunohistochemical staining patterns for TGF-β_1 in control liver were consistent with reported levels of TGF-β_1 gene transcription in parenchymal and nonparenchymal cells (34,35).

In contrast to the moderate staining observed in normal hepatocytes, periportal hepatocytes in PB-treated rats stained intensely for TGF-β_1 (Figs. 3A and B). Colocalization of staining with the anti-LC[1-30] and the anti-pre[266-278] suggested that PB induces either selective hepatocyte synthesis or uptake of the latent TGF-β_1 complex of TGF-β_1 (9). The mechanism by which PB regulates the intracellular concentration of TGF-β_1 in hepatocytes and to what degree the elevated periportal concentration of TGF-β_1 contributes to the hepatocytes' reduced ability to respond to mitogenic stimuli remains to be elucidated. However, the importance of TGF-β_1 in liver tumor promotion by PB was further strengthened by our finding that putative preneoplastic hepatocytes expresses significantly less TGF-β_1 than did the periportal hepatocytes (9).

In conclusion: PB is a potent promoter of hepatocellular tumor formation with a mechanism of action that is poorly understood. Although, initially, PB caused an increase in hepatocyte proliferation, this effect was transient and restricted to hepato-

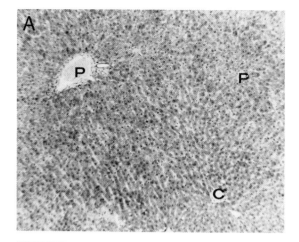

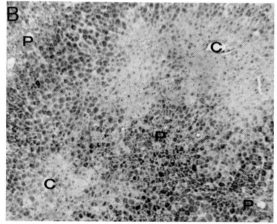

Figure 3. Immunohistochemical staining of TGF-β_1 in liver of a control animal (A) and one exposed to PB for 75 days (0.1% in the drinking water). TGF-β_1 was immunohistochemically localized with the anti-LC[1-30] antibody. Hepatocytes in the livers of control animals stained uniformly and moderately. In contrast, the periportal hepatocytes (P) in the PB-treated animals were intensely positive for TGF-β_1 while the pericentral cells (C) were relatively less stained, × 70.

cytes that reside in the liver's pericentral regions. In contrast, a chronic promotional PB regimen reduced the ability of normal hepatocytes to proliferate in response to mitogenic stimuli. This decreased proliferative capacity correlated with: 1) a significant reduction in EGF receptor number and the receptors' increased sensitivity to PB-induced down-regulation, 2) a loss in the ability of TPA to activate protein kinase C and 3) an elevation in the periportal hepatocyte concentration of TGF-β_1. Thus, chronic exposure to PB impaired two pathways involved in stimulating DNA synthesis and concordantly enhanced potential growth-inhibitory effects by elevating TGF-β_1. Putative preneoplastic hepatocytes appeared, however, to have acquired relative resistance to these PB-induced events. Although the importance of these alterations to hepatocellular tumor promotion remains to be clarified, they predict that clonal expansion of initiated cells results from a growth advantage because of their refractoriness to the net antiproliferative environment produced by PB.

Acknowledgment

We thank Dr. Michael Sporn, National Cancer Institute, for kindly providing the anti-LC[1-30] and anti-pre[266-278] antibodies, and we are grateful to Dr. Katherine Flanders for her assistance in using them in immunohistochemical studies. Our thanks also extend to Roxanne Scroggs for typing this manuscript. This work was supported by USPHS grants CA25951 and CA40172.

References

1. Abanobi SE, Lombardi B, Shinozuka H. Stimulation of DNA synthesis and cell proliferation in the liver of rats fed a choline-devoid diet and their suppression by phenobarbital. Cancer Res 42:412–415, 1982.
2. Peraino C, Fry RJM, Staffeldt E, Christopher JP. Comparative enhancing effects of phenobarbital, amobarbital, diphenylhydantoin, and dichlorodiphenyl-trichloroethane on 2-acetylaminofluorene-induced hepatic tumorigenesis in the rat. Cancer Res 35:2884–2890, 1975.
3. Argyris RS. Stimulators, enzyme induction and the control of liver growth. In: Clarkson B, Baserga R (eds): Control of Proliferation in Animal Cells. Cold Spring Harbor Conference on Cell Proliferation, 1974, pp 49–66.
4. Yager JD, Roebuck BD, Paluszcyk TL, Memoli VA. Effects of ethinyl estradiol and tamoxifen on liver DNA turnover and new synthesis and appearance of γ glutamyl transpeptidase-positive foci in female rats. Carcinogenesis 7:2007–2014, 1986.
5. Schulte-Hermann R, Timmermann-Trosiener I, Schuppler J. Facilitated expression of adaptive responses to phenobarbital in putative pre-stages of liver cancer. Carcinogenesis 7:1651–1655, 1986.
6. Preat V, Lans M, de Gerlache J, Taper H, Roberfroid M. Influence of the duration and the delay of administration of phenobarbital on its modulating effect on rat hepatocarcinogenesis. Carcinogenesis 8:333–335, 1987.
7. Barbason H, Rassenfosse C, Betz EH. Promotion mechanism of phenobarbital and partial hepatectomy in DENA hepatocarcinogenesis cell kinetics effect. Br J Cancer 47:517–525, 1983.
8. Eckl PM, Meyer SA, Whitcombe WR, Jirtle RL. Phenobarbital reduces EGF receptors and the ability of physiological concentrations of calcium to suppress hepatocyte proliferation. Carcinogenesis 9:479–483, 1988.
9. Jirtle RL, Meyer SA. Liver tumor promotion: Effect of phenobarbital on EGF and protein kinase C signal transduction and transforming growth factor-β_1 expression. Dig Dis Sciences, in press.
10. Edwards AM, Lucas CM. Phenobarbital and some other liver tumor promoters stimulate DNA synthesis in cultured rat hepatocytes. Biochem Biophys Res Commun 131:103–108, 1985.
11. Sawada N, Staecker JL, Pitot HC. Effects of tumor-promoting agents 12-O-tetradecanoylphorbol-13-acetate and phenobarbital on DNA synthesis of rat hepatocytes in primary cultures. Cancer Res 47:5665–5671, 1987.
12. Miyazaki M, Handa Y, Oda M, Yabe T, Miyano K, Sato J. Long-term survival of functional hepatocytes from adult rat in the presence of phenobarbital in primary culture. Exp Cell Res 159:176–190, 1985.
13. Solt D, Farber E. New principle for the analysis of chemical carcinogenesis. Nature 263:701–703, 1976.
14. Laconi E, Li F, Semple E, Rao Pm, Rajalakshini S, Sarma DSR. Inhibition of DNA synthesis in primary cultures of hepatocytes by orotic acid. Carcinogenesis 9:675–677, 1988.
15. Meyer SA, Gibbs TA, Jirtle, RL. Independent mechanisms for tumor promoters phenobarbital and 12-O-tetradecanoylphorbol-13-acetate in reduction of epidermal growth factor binding by rat hepatocytes. Cancer Res 49:5907–5912, 1989.
16. Meyer SA, Jirtle RL. Phenobarbital decreases hepatocyte EGF receptor expression independent of protein kinase C activation. Biochem Biophy Res Commun 158:652–659, 1989.
17. Meyer SA, Li C, Jirtle RL. Cytochrome P450-independent down-regulation of hepatocyte EGF receptors by liver tumor promoter phenobarbital. Proceedings of AACR 31:150, 1990.
18. Cochet C, Gill GN, Meisenhelder J, Cooper JA, Hunter T. C-kinase phosphorylates the epidermal

growth factor receptor and reduces its epidermal growth factor-stimulated tyrosine protein kinase activity. J Biol Chem 259:2553–2558, 1984.

19. Iwashita S, Fox CF. Epidermal growth factor and potent phorbol tumor promoters induce epidermal growth factor receptor phosphorylation in a similar but distinctly different manner in human epidermoid carcinoma A431 cells. J Biol Chem 259:2559–2567, 1984.

20. Davis RJ, Czech MP. Tumor-promoting phorbol diesters mediate phorphorylation of the epidermal growth factor receptor. J Biol Chem 259:8545–8549, 1984.

21. Meyer SA, Gibbs TA, Li C, Jirtle RL. In vivo phenobarbital alters hepatocyte EGF receptor down-regulation by in vitro phorbol ester (TPA) and phenobarbital. FASEB J 3:A1205, 1989.

22. Hsieh LL, Peraino C, Weinstein IB. Expression of endogenous retrovirus-like sequences and cellular oncogenes during phenobarbital treatment and regeneration in rat liver. Cancer Res 48:265–269, 1983.

23. Gupta C, Hattori A, Betschart JM, Virji MA, Shinozuka H. Modulation of epidermal growth factor receptors in rat hepatocytes by two liver tumor-promoting regimens, a choline-deficient and phenobarbital diet. Cancer Res 48:1162–1165, 1988.

24. Brockenbrough JS, Meyer SA, Jirtle RL. Specific and reversible inhibition of phorbol ester-induced protein kinase C translocation in hepatocytes from phenobabital treated rats. Proceedings AACR 31:151, 1990.

25. Sahyoun N, Wolf M, Bestermann J, Hsieh T, Sander M, Leviene H III, Chang KJ, Cuatracasas P. Protein kinase C phosphorylates topoisomerase II: Topoisomerase activation and its possible role in phorbol ester-induced differentiation of HL-60 cells. Proc Natl Acad Sci USA 83:1603–1607, 1986.

26. Imagawa M, Chiu R, Karin M. Transcription factor AP-2 mediates induction by two different signal-transduction pathways: Protein kinase C and cAMP. Cell 51:257–260, 1987.

27. McCaffrey P, Ran W, Campisi J, Rosner MR. Two independent growth factor-generated signals regulate c-*fos* and c-*myc* mRNA levels in Swiss 3T3 cells. J Biol Chem 262:1442–1445, 1987.

28. Fujiwara S, Fisher RJ, Bhat NK, Diaz SM, Papas TS. A short-lived nuclear phosphoprotein encoded by the human ets-2 proto-oncogene is stabilized by activation of protein kinase C. Mol Cell Biol 8:4700–4706, 1988.

29. Sporn MB, Roberts AB. Transforming growth factor-β. Multiple actions and potential clinical applications. JAMA 262:938–941, 1989.

30. Strain AJ, Frozen A, Hill DJ, Milner RDG. Transforming growth factor beta inhibits DNA synthesis in hepatocytes isolated from normal and regenerating rat liver. Biochem Biophys Res Commun 145:436–442, 1987.

31. Russell WE, Coffey RJ Jr, Ovellette AJ, Moses HL. Type β transforming growth factor reversibly inhibits the early proliferative response to partial hepatectomy in the rat. Proc Natl Acad Sci USA 85:5126–5130, 1988.

32. Houck KA, Michalopoulos GK. Altered responses of regenerating hepatocytes to norepinephrine and transforming growth factor type β. J Cell Physiol 141:503–509, 1989.

33. Flanders KC, Thompson NL, Cissel DS, van Obberghen-Schilling E, Baker CC, Kass ME, Ellingsworth LR, Roberts AB, Sporn MB. Transforming growth factor β1: Histochemical localization with antibodies to different epitopes. J Cell Biol 108:653–660, 1989.

34. Braun L, Mead Je, Panzica M, Mikumo R, Bell GI, Fausto N. Transforming growth factor b mRNA increases during liver regeneration: A possible paracrine mechanism of growth regulation. Proc Natl Acad Sci USA 85:1539–1543, 1988.

35. Nagy P, Evarts RP, McMahon JB, Thorgeirsson SS. Role of TGF-beta in normal differentiation and oncogenesis in rat liver. Molecular Carcinogenesis 2:345–354, 1989.

Chemically Induced Cell Proliferation:
Implications for Risk Assessment, pages 217-225
©1991 Wiley-Liss, Inc.

Chemically Induced Cell Proliferation and Carcinogenesis: Differential Effect of Compensatory Cell Proliferation and Mitogen-Induced Direct Hyperplasia on Hepatocarcinogenesis in the Rat

A. Columbano, G. M. Ledda-Columbano, P. Coni,
G. Pichiri-Coni, M. Curto, and P. Pani

Several lines of investigation have demonstrated that cell proliferation plays an important role in different phases of the carcinogenic process (Fig. 1). This discussion will be restricted to only those sequences of carcinogenic processes in which focal proliferations form precursor lesions such as nodules in the liver.

The role of cell proliferation in the initiation of liver carcinogenesis

The importance of cell proliferation in initiation has been documented by the observation that in the adult rat liver, which is essentially a quiescent organ, genotoxic carcinogens induced initiation only when their administration was coupled with a round of cell proliferation (1,2). Furthermore, cell proliferation has to occur prior to the repair of carcinogen-induced critical lesion(s) in DNA (3,4). The mechanism by which cell proliferation plays an important role in initiation is not yet clear. However, it is believed that either fixing a miscoding or a noncoding lesion—or enhancing the recombinational events or creating hypomethylated sequences in the newly made DNA strands—may be the mechanisms by which cell proliferation plays a crucial role in initiation (5–10). While each of these possibilities can account for the importance of cell proliferation during initiation, the latter seems most viable because agents such as 5-azacytidine, 5-azadeoxycitidine, and 2,3-adenosine dialdehyde that induce hypomethylation when administered during the time of carcinogen-induced repair, potentiated the initiation of liver carcinogenesis (11).

Role of cell proliferation during promotion phase of liver carcinogenesis

Tumor promotion may be defined operationally as the clonal expansion of initiated cells. Since promotion involves differential expansion of initiated hepatocytes, any hypothesis proposed needs to take into account this differential. The differential can be achieved by several ways; thus, a promoter may induce cell proliferation selectively in the initiated hepatocyte population (12). Alternatively, the promoter may differentially inhibit mitosis in the noninitiated surrounding hepatocytes while permitting the initiated hepatocytes to respond to growth stimuli and form hepatic foci/nodules (13). In the former mode, the promoter or the promoting regimen should be an inducer of cell proliferation, while in the latter mode it should be a mitosis inhibitor. Thus, tumor

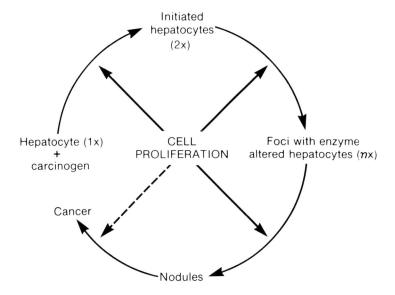

Figure 1. Schematic representation indicating the possible sites of action of cell proliferation in experimental liver carcinogenesis.

promoters do not always need to be mitogenic. Cell proliferation during promotion is not completely understood; for example, is its role only to achieve clonal expansion of the initiated hepatocytes or does it also modify the initiated cell? This modification, whether at the gene or the epigenetic level, may be achieved by the promoter or during multiple rounds of cell proliferation.

Role of cell proliferation during progression

Unfortunately, very little is known about the progression phase of liver carcinogenesis and the role that cell proliferation plays during this phase. However, it should be noted that the size of the proliferating compartment increased in hepatic nodules and not in the surrounding nonnodular tissue (14). This increase in the labeling index is accompanied with an increased incidence of cell death (14,15); the ratio, however, is skewed towards growth. Do nodular hepatocytes have to undergo a definitive number of cell cycles before they acquire neoplastic properties? Obviously, answers to these questions will help to understand the role of cell proliferation in the progression phase.

Cell proliferation induced by chemicals

Chemicals at necrogenic doses induce compensatory cell proliferation in such organs as the liver (Fig. 2). This regenerative growth is under the control of growth regulatory mechanisms and stops once the organ has reached the normal mass. Certain chemicals can also induce growth in organs such as liver and kidney without causing a prior cell loss. These agents, often called mitogens, obviously overcome the normally operating growth-controlling mechanisms and induce direct hyperplasia. Once the growth stimulus is removed, the organ returns to the original mass as a result of apoptosis, a particular mode of cell deletion (16–18). Thus, there are two groups of chemicals that induce liver cell proliferation; in one, cell loss precedes cell proliferation while in the other there is no cell loss prior to hyperplasia. Examples of the former group consist of a variety of necrogenic agents including carbon tetrachloride and chloroform. Several chemicals identified as capable of inducing direct hyperplasia in the liver include cyproterone acetate (CPA), lead nitrate, ethylene dibromide (EDB), nafenopin, phenobarbital, ethynyl estradiol, and α-hexachlorocyclohexane (α-HCH) (17,19–24). Depending on the strain and species of the animal and on the dose, some of these mitogens can induce liver cell necrosis. It is interesting to note that liver mitogens, for example, phenobarbital (25), induce only transient liver DNA synthesis; there is no sustained liver cell proliferation upon continuous exposure to these agents. In fact, prolonged exposure to phenobarbital inhibits mitosis in the rat liver (26).

Even though both types of stimuli induce liver cell proliferation, the mechanisms associated with these two types of stimuli must be different. For example, the mitogen-induced growth stimuli, unlike compensatory cell proliferative stimuli, should follow a signal transduction pathway that overcomes or bypasses normally operating growth

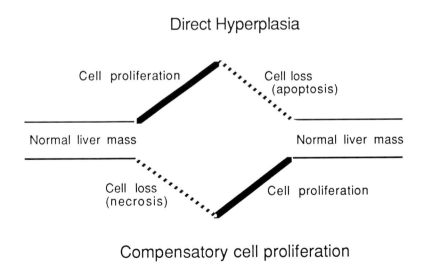

Figure 2. Schematic representation of two different types of liver cell proliferation.

regulatory mechanisms. We might speculate whether the signal for the apoptosis that occurs during the regression phase is induced by the hyperplastic state of the organ or by the mitogen itself.

Efficacy of chemically induced liver cell proliferation to support initiation

Since these two types of liver cell proliferation appear different, we were interested in assessing their ability to support carcinogen-induced initiation in the liver. The results obtained indicated that unlike compensatory liver cell proliferation induced by CCl_4 or partial hepatectomy, the direct hyperplasia induced by liver mitogens such as lead nitrate, EDB, CPA, and nafenopin was unable to support the initiation phase of liver carcinogenesis induced by non-necrogenic doses of carcinogens such as N-methyl-N-nitrosourea, benzo[a]pyrene, and diethylnitrosamine (27). A similar pattern of results was obtained whether the initiated hepatocytes were stimulated to grow using the resistant hepatocyte model, orotic acid, or phenobarbital, then monitored as foci of enzyme-altered hepatocytes, hepatic nodules, or hepatocellular carcinoma as the end point (28). These results are surprising because even though both types of proliferative stimuli induce liver cell proliferation, only the compensatory liver cell proliferative stimulus, not direct hyperplasia, supports carcinogen-induced initiation.

Efficacy of chemically induced liver cell proliferation to potentiate liver tumor promotion

In models of rat liver tumor promotion, the cell proliferative stimulus is often constitutive, as in the resistant hepatocyte model (13); in other cases, a proliferative stimulus given during promotion potentiates the efficacy of the tumor promoter, as is the case with phenobarbital (29,30) and orotic acid (31). One of the logical questions concerning chemically induced cell proliferation in the promotion phase is whether both the compensatory mode of liver cell proliferation and mitogen-induced direct hyperplasia potentiate the efficacy of the liver tumor promoter. Compensatory liver cell proliferation induced by partial hepatectomy or necrogenic doses of CCl_4 potentiates the promoting ability of phenobarbital (29,30), and orotic acid (31); it also is effective in the resistant hepatocyte model (31). On the contrary, direct hyperplasia induced by lead nitrate does not potentiate the tumor promotion in the above three models (32) (Fig. 3).

Currently, we are exploring two hypotheses to explain the differential effect of these two types of liver cell proliferative stimuli on the initiation and promotion phases of liver carcinogenesis. One hypothesis is that during mitogen-induced direct hyperplasia, the initiated hepatocytes are lost by apoptosis during the regression phase (27). This argument assumes that initiated hepatocytes are extremely sensitive to the apoptotic phenomenon. Alternatively, mitogen-induced direct hyperplasia is not conducive to the growth of carcinogen-induced initiated cells. This hypothesis argues that the signal transducing pathways for these two types of growth stimuli are different. While the normal hepatocytes respond to both types of signals, the initiated hepatocytes respond to those induced by compensatory liver cell proliferation but not to those induced by mitogen-induced direct hyperplasia. Attempts to explore the latter phenomenon indicated that mitogen-induced cell proliferative stimuli, like compensatory liver cell proliferative stimuli, induced serum growth factors. A partially purified fraction of platelet-

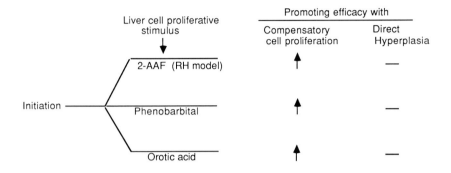

Figure 3. Schematic representation indicating the failure of lead nitrate induced hyperplasia to potentiate the promoting efficacy of three liver tumor-promoting regimens.

poor plasma from the rats treated with partial hepatectomy or with lead nitrate, CPA, or EDB added in vitro increased the labeling index of hepatocytes in culture (Table 1). It remains to be seen whether growth factor(s) purified from the plasma of rats treated with mitogens specifically promote the growth of normal hepatocytes but not that of hepatocytes from hepatic nodules.

In addition, the signal transducing pathways induced by these different growth stimuli appear different. For example, while a transient and sequential expression of c-*fos* and c-*myc* was observed in the rat liver following CCl_4 and partial hepatectomy, increased expression of c-*myc* but not c-*fos* was seen during liver hyperplasia induced by EDB. Interestingly, CPA-induced liver cell proliferation was not accompanied by an increased expression of either c-*fos* or c-*myc* (34). Lead nitrate–induced hyperplasia was accompanied by a poor expression of c-*fos* but by a persistent increase of c-*myc* (35). However, increased expression of c-Ha-*ras* and c-Ki-*ras* was seen in response to all the proliferative stimuli examined. These results indicate that unlike compensatory liver cell proliferative stimuli, the mitogen-induced direct hyperplasia was accompanied with little or essentially no increased expression of c-*fos*.

It will be interesting to determine whether these differences are a reflection of different pathways of signal transduction or if they exist because different growth factors were induced by different proliferative stimuli; we also wish to understand whether these differences affect the ability of a particular proliferative stimulus to support the growth

Table 1. Effect of 20% PPP Isolated 24 hr after Treatment with Various Proliferative Stimuli on DNA Synthesis of Primary Hepatocytes Cultures.

Treatment	Hepatocyte labelling Index (%)
Control	18.8 ± 1.56
CPA	37.9 ± 2.62
EDB	36.3 ± 4.65
Lead nitrate	38.0 ± 3.74
PH	37.5 ± 0.29

PPP was isolated as decribed by Semple et al. (33). CPA (60 mg/Kg, intragastrically), EDB (100 mg/kg, intragastrically) and lead nitrate (100 μmol/Kg, intravenously) were given 24 hr before sacrifice.

of initiated hepatocytes. It is equally important to ascertain whether initiated hepatocytes are more susceptible to apoptosis during the regression phase following mitogen-induced direct hyperplasia.

Even though the mechanisms are not fully understood, the results discussed here clearly suggest that chemicals can induce different types of cell proliferative stimuli, and that only some support the formation and growth of initiated hepatocytes. A technical point that merits consideration in this context concerns the use of the labeling index as a means to assess cell proliferation. This assay does not accurately differentiate compensatory cell proliferation from direct hyperplasia. Since this differentiation is mechanistically important, it may be useful to couple the labeling index assay with another approach, possibly one that is morphological, to monitor cell proliferation.

This discussion raises several important considerations concerning the role of chemically induced cell proliferation in liver carcinogenesis. If a chemical is genotoxic and necrogenic, it is very likely that the chemical is carcinogenic because not only does it induce DNA alterations in the initiation stage (if related to initiation), but it also induces compensatory cell proliferation; these are both prerequisites for initiation. However, if the chemical is genotoxic and nonnecrogenic, it is likely that the chemical is noncarcinogenic. If the chemical is genotoxic and nonnecrogenic but induces direct hyperplasia, then according to the data presented here it is unlikely that the chemical will be carcinogenic.

The next question is concerned with the chemical that is nongenotoxic but induces cell proliferation: Will it be a carcinogen? For this discussion, the term "nongenotoxic" is defined as an agent that does not induce DNA alterations related to initiation. We feel that the answer may be yes if one assumes the existence of initiated cells normally. The evidence for the existence of initiated cells is at best equivocal. In eukaryotes, spontaneous mutation rates have been estimated to be 10^{-10} to 10^{-12} errors per base pair per generation (36). In addition, because of the chemical environment in which we are living, it is likely that we may be susceptible to genetic damage. These genetic changes/mutations may accumulate with the age of the organism. It should be noted, however, that every mutation need not be a proinitiating lesion. Nonetheless, sustained cell proliferation has the potential to increase the risk of carcinogenesis by stimulating the growth of rare initiated cells when present. In this case, again, the differences in the cell proliferative stimuli need to be taken into account. If the nongenotoxic chemical is necrogenic and induces compensatory cell proliferation, it is likely that the existing initiated cells may not be amplified vigorously because they also may be lost during necrosis. On the other hand, if the nongenotoxic chemical is nonnecrogenic but induces hyperplasia, it is likely that the existing initiated cells may be amplified and accumulated. If these existing spontaneously initiated cells are like those induced by genotoxic agents, then they may not respond to mitogen-induced direct hyperplasia and grow to form tumors. If one assumes that they do respond to hyperplastic stimulus, then such a hyperplasia needs to be sustained; otherwise, when the stimulus is withdrawn, the excess number of cells may be eliminated, perhaps by a process involving apoptosis. Obviously, these arguments are valid only when the liver is used as the test organ; it is unproven whether similar arguments can be extended to other organs.

In conclusion, it may be said that only certain types of cell proliferative stimuli appear to increase the risk of carcinogenesis initiated by a carcinogen. We do not yet know whether cell proliferation alone in the absence of a carcinogen increases the risk of carcinogenesis.

Acknowledgments

We wish to thank Lori Cutler and Laura Giacomini for their excellent secretarial help. This work was supported in part by funds from Associazione Italiana Ricerca sul Cancro Italy, and from U.S. Public Health Service research grant CA 46261 from the National Cancer Institute and from the National Cancer Institute, Canada.

References

1. Cayama E, Tsuda H, Sarma DSR, Farber E. Initiation of liver carcinogenesis requires cell proliferation. Nature 275:60–61, 1978.
2. Columbano A, Rajalakshmi S, Sarma DSR. Requirement of cell proliferation for the initiation of liver carcinogenesis as assayed by three different procedures. Cancer Res 41:2079–2083, 1981.
3. Ishikawa T, Takayama S, Kitagawa T. Correlation between time of partial hepatectomy after a single treatment with diethylnitrosamine and induction of adenosine triphosphatase-deficient islands in rat liver. Cancer Res 40:4261–4264, 1980.
4. Columbano A, Ledda GM, Rao PM, Rajalakshmi S, Sarma DSR. Initiation of experimental liver carcinogenesis by chemicals: Are the carcinogen-altered hepatocytes stimulated to grow by different selection procedures identical? In Nicolini C (ed): Chemical Carcinogenesis. New York: Plenum Publishing Corporation, 1982, pp 167–178.
5. Loveless A. Possible relevance of O^6-alkylation of deoxyguanosine to the mutagenicity and carcinogenicity of nitrosamines and nitrosamides. Nature 223:206–207, 1969.
6. Swendberg JA, Dryoff MC, Bedell MA, Popp JA, Huh N, Kirstein U, Rajewsky MF. O^4-ethyldeoxythimidine but not O^6-ethyldeoxyguanosine accumulates in hepatocyte DNA of rats exposed continuously to diethylnitrosamine. Proc Natl Acad Sci USA 81:1692–1695, 1984.
7. Rajalakshmi S, Sarma DSR. Replication of hepatic DNA in rats treated with diethylnitrosamine. Chem Biol Interact 11:245–252, 1975.
8. Columbano A, Ledda-Columbano GM, Rao PM, Rajalakshmi S, Sarma DSR. In vivo replication of carcinogen-modified DNA: Presence of dimethylnitrosamine-induced N-7-methylguanine and O^6-methylguanine in the parental and daughter strands of the in vivo replicated hybrid DNA. Biochemical Archives 1:121–130, 1985.
9. Boehm TL, Drahovsky D. Alteration of enzymatic-methylation of DNA cytosines by chemical carcinogens: a mechanism involved in the initiation of carcinogenesis. J Natl Cancer Inst 71:429–433, 1983.

10. Kastan MB, Gowans BJ, Lieberman MW. Methylation of deoxycytidine incorporated by excision-repair synthesis of DNA. Cell 30:509–516, 1982.
11. Denda A, Rao PM, Rajalakshmi S, Sarma DSR. 5-azacytidine potentiates initiation induced by carcinogens in rat liver. Carcinogenesis 6:145–146, 1985.
12. Schulte-Hermann R, Ohde G, Schuppler J, Timmermann-Trosiener I. Enhanced proliferation of putative preneoplastic cells in rat liver following treatment with the tumor promoters phenobarbital, hexachlorocyclohexane, steroid compounds and nafenopin. Cancer Res 41:2556–2562, 1981.
13. Solt DB, Farber E. New principle for the analysis of chemical carcinogenesis. Nature 263:702–703, 1976.
14. Rotstein J, Sarma DSR, Farber E. Sequential alterations in growth control and cell dynamics of rat hepatocytes in early precancerous steps in hepatocarcinogenesis. Cancer Res 46:2377–2385, 1986.
15. Columbano A, Ledda-Columbano GM, Rao PM, Rajalakshmi S, Sarma DSR. Occurrence of cell death (apoptosis) in preneoplastic and neoplastic liver cells: A sequential study. Am J Pathol 116:441–446, 1984.
16. Columbano A, Ledda-Columbano GM, Coni P, Faa G, Liguori C, Santacruz G, Pani P. Occurrence of cell death (apoptosis) during the involution of liver hyperplasia. Lab Invest 52:670–675, 1985.
17. Bursch W, Laurer B, Timmermann-Trosiener I, Barthel G, Schuppler J, Schulte-Hermann R. Controlled death (apoptosis) of normal and putative preneoplastic cells in rat liver following withdrawal of tumor promoters. Carcinogenesis 6:453–458, 1984.
18. Wyllie AH, Kerr JFR, Currie AR. Cell death: the significance of apoptosis. Int Rev Cytol 68:251–306, 1980.
19. Columbano A, Ledda G, Sirigu P, Perra T, Pani P. Liver cell proliferation induced by a single dose of lead nitrate. Am J Pathol 110:83–88, 1983.
20. Nachtomi E, Farber E. Ethylene dibromide as a mitogen for liver. Lab Invest 38:279–283, 1978.
21. Levine WG, Ord MG, Stocken A. Some biochemical changes associated with nafenopin-induced liver growth in the rat. Biochem Pharmacol 26:939–942, 1977.
22. Peraino C, Fry RJM, Staffeldt E, Cristopher JP. Comparative enhancing effects of phenobarbital, amobarbital, diphenylhydantoin and dichlorodiphenyltrichloroethane on 2-acetylaminofluorene-induced hepatic tumorigenesis in the rat. Cancer Res 35:2884–2890, 1975.
23. Ochs H, Dusterberg B, Gunzel P, Schulte-Hermann R. Effect of tumor promoting contraceptive steroids on growth and drug metabolizing enzymes in rat liver. Cancer Res 46:1224–1232, 1986.
24. Schulte-Hermann R. Reactions of the liver to injury: adaptation. In Farber E, Fisher MM (eds): Toxic injury of the Liver. New York: Marcel Dekker, 1979, pp 385–444.
25. Schulte-Hermann R, Schuppler J, Timmermann-Trosiener I, Ohde G, Bursch W, Berger H. The role of growth of normal and preneoplastic cell populations for tumor promotion in rat liver. Environ Health Perspect 50:185–194, 1984.
26. Barbason H, Rassenfosse C, Betz EH. Promotion mechanism of phenobarbital and partial hepatectomy in DENA hepatocarcinogenesis, cell kinetics effect. Br J Cancer 47:517–525, 1983.
27. Columbano A, Ledda-Columbano GM, Lee G, Rajalakshmi S, Sarma DSR. Inability of mitogen-induced liver hyperplasia to support the induction of enzyme-altered islands induced by liver carcinogens. Cancer Res 47:5557–5559, 1987.
28. Ledda-Columbano GM, Columbano A, Curto M, Ennas GM, Coni P, Sarma DSR, Pani P. Further evidence that mitogen-induced cell proliferation does not support the formation of enzyme-altered islands in rat liver by carcinogens. Carcinogenesis 10:847–850, 1989.
29. Ford JO, Pereira MA. Short-term in vivo initiation/promotion bioassay for hepatocarcinogens. J Environ Pathol Toxicol Oncol 4:39–46, 1980.
30. Tatematsu M, Nakanishi K, Murasaki G, Miyata Y, Hirose M, Ito N. Enhancing effect of inducers of liver microsomal enzymes on induction of hyperplastic liver nodules by N-2-fluorenylacetamide in rats. J Natl Cancer Inst 63:1411–1416, 1979.
31. Columbano A, Ledda GM, Rao PM, Rajalakshmi S, Sarma DSR. Dietary orotic acid, a new selective growth stimulus for carcinogen altered hepatocytes in rat. Cancer Lett 16:191–196, 1982.
32. Columbano A, Ledda-Columbano GM, Coni P, Pichiri G, Curto M, Ennas MG, Pani P, Sarma DSR. Failure of mitogen-induced hyperplasia to substitute for partial hepatectomy during promotion in the phenobarbital and resistant hepatocyte model. Proceedings of the American Association for Cancer Research 30:845, 1989.

33. Semple E, Hayes MA, Rushmore TH, Harris L, Farber E. Mitogenic activity in platelet-poor plasma from rats with persistant liver nodules or liver cancer. Biochim Biophys Res Commun 148:449–455, 1987.
34. Coni P, Pichiri G, Ledda-Columbano GM, Rao PM, Rajalakshmi S, Sarma DSR, Columbano A. Expression of cell cycle dependent proto-oncogene during mitogen-induced liver cell proliferation. Proceedings of the American Association for Cancer Research 30:746, 1989.
35. Coni P, Bignone FA, Pichiri G, Ledda-Columbano GM, Columbano A, Rao PM, Rajalakshmi S, Sarma DSR. Studies on the kinetics of expression of cell cycle dependent proto-oncogenes during mitogen-induced liver cell proliferation. Cancer Lett 47:115–119, 1989.
36. Wabl M, Burrows PD, von Gabain A, Steinberg C. Hypermutation at the immunoglobulin heavy chain locus in a pre-B-cell line. Proc Natl Acad Sci USA 82:479–482, 1985.

Chemically Induced Cell Proliferation:
Implications for Risk Assessment, pages 227-236
©1991 Wiley-Liss, Inc.

Control of Hepatocyte Proliferation in Regeneration, Augmentative Hepatomegaly, and Neoplasia

G. Michalopoulos

The role of cell proliferation in chemical carcinogenesis has been illustrated in several tissues and with a variety of chemicals. Of these tissues, the liver is perhaps the one in which the issue first became apparent. In this organ, the specific factors involved are better defined and the potential misconceptions more deeply entrenched. In this paper I will review the evidence for the role of hepatocyte proliferation as a component of the mode of action of initiating and promoting carcinogenic chemicals. I will also examine the mechanisms that regulate hepatocyte proliferation in the more controlled environment of chemically or surgically induced liver regeneration and in the completely controlled environment of hepatocyte cultures in chemically defined media.

Physiologic regulators of hepatocyte proliferation

Much knowledge gained recently about the mechanisms that control hepatocyte proliferation has come from two models. The first is the model of hepatocyte cultures in chemically defined media. When hepatocytes are kept in serum-free conditions, the rate of DNA synthesis is very low. As specific substances are added, their effect on hepatocyte replication may be assessed without the influence of other interfering factors. A second source of information has been the study of gene expression during liver regeneration stimulated by two-thirds partial hepatectomy. Specific growth factors, growth amplifiers, and growth inhibitors have been identified by both of these approaches (for a complete review see ref. 1). Based on these agents' mode of action in chemically defined media in culture, they can be categorized as (A) complete hepatocyte mitogens, (B) growth inhibitors, and (C) growth triggers (comitogenic substances or incomplete mitogens).

Complete hepatocyte mitogens

Complete mitogens are substances that are capable—by themselves in chemically defined media and in the absence of serum—to stimulate hepatocyte DNA synthesis and mitosis in otherwise quiescent hepatocyte populations. They are described below.

Epidermal growth factor (EGF): EGF stimulates proliferation of most epithelial cells, and it stimulates DNA synthesis in hepatocytes (2). EGF was, in fact, the first substance shown to have this effect, and it still is the polypeptide hormone most frequently used to induce hepatocyte DNA synthesis in cultures. In addition to its mitogenic effect, EGF affects several other functions of hepatocytes, including amino acid transport and protein synthesis. Transforming growth factor-beta (TGF-β) suppresses EGF-stimulated mitogenesis but not the EGF-stimulated increase in protein synthesis (3). Although questions have been raised whether EGF is the "natural" mitogen that induces the complex changes associated with liver regeneration, injection of EGF results in increased DNA synthesis in liver (4). EGF is, in fact, the only complete hepatocyte mitogen that fulfills this function.

Transforming growth factor-alpha (TGF-α): EGF and TGF-α share the same receptor, and they are both mitogenic for the same cell types, including hepatocytes. Mitogenic effects of TGF-α in hepatocytes are also inhibited by TGF-β as in the case of EGF.

In the whole animal, the role of TGF-α in liver regeneration recently became a focus of attention after regenerating hepatocytes were shown to produce TGF-α actively (5). Since TGF-α is a complete hepatocyte mitogen, the hypothesis is that TGF-α might stimulate proliferation of hepatocytes as part of an autocrine loop.

Hepatopoietin A/Hepatocyte growth factor (HPTA/HGF): This protein of 100,000 kDa was isolated from rat, rabbit, and human serum and plasma. It is more abundant in serum but exists in plasma in measurable levels. We originally identified it as HPTA, a fraction seen by chromatography of serum from hepatectomized rats (6). Purification methods and the structure of HPTA were recently described (7). HPTA is a heterodimer composed of one chain of 70,000 kDa and another of 35,000 kDa, held together by disulfide bonds. In terms of the molar concentration required to reach maximum nuclear labeling index (70–80%), this substance is about 10 times more powerful than EGF. A substance similar in properties to HPTA was isolated from rat serum by Nakamura et al. in 1984 (8) and described as "hepatotropin." These researchers (9) also purified a substance with a heterodimer structure similar to that of HPTA from rat platelets and named it *Hepatic growth factor* (HGF) in 1987. A similar substance, one that increases in the plasma of patients in fulminating hepatic failure, was named human hepatic growth factor (hHGF) by Gohda et al. in 1986 (10). The work on the structure of these substances showed that all three are heterodimers of a heavy and a light chain with molecular weights in the range of 70,000 and 35,000, respectively. Recent publications on the amino acid structure of rabbit HPTA (11) and the structure of the cloned and sequenced gene of human HGF (12,13) strongly suggest that HPTA and HGF are the same molecule. An 87% homology (3 of 24 amino acids) in the sequence of the first 24 amino acids from the amino terminus of the light chain was seen between rabbit HPTA and human HGF. This extensive homology suggests that HPTA and HGF are identical, and that the differences seen reflect differences of species origin. I shall use the term HPTA/HGF for this growth factor, to reflect its origin of discovery.

The amino acid sequence of the heavy chain of HPTA/HGF reveals extensive homology with plasminogen and other coagulation-related proteases containing structures known as "kringles." The light chain of this molecule is in the superfamily of serine protease homologues. These are molecules similar to proteases but lack the amino acids histamine, aspartate, and serine in characteristic locations; when present in true proteases, these amino acids form the catalytic site.

HPTA/HGF has receptors that differ from those of EGF or acidic fibroblast growth factor (FGF). Its mitogenic effect is also inhibited by TGF-β, and its increased bioactivity was also noted in humans with fulminating hepatic failure. In human and rabbit serum, direct measurement of HPTA/HGF by ELISA gave a concentration of 0.5 ng/ml. In plasma, its concentration is considerably lower, but it increases prior to hepatic DNA synthesis in regeneration stimulated by either two-thirds hepatectomy or gavage of CCl_4 (P. Linolroos and G.K. Michalopoulos, unpublished observations). Recent studies (14) showed that the major tissue sources of HPTA are the pancreas (exocrine portion), the brain (large neurons of the occipital lobe), and interfollicular cells of the thyroid.

Heparin-binding growth factor-1 (HBGF-1 [acidic FGF]): This growth factor of 16,000 kDa also stimulates DNA synthesis in hepatocytes, acting only on hepatocyte subpopulations, however, because only half of the cells respond to HBGF-1 (15). It requires heparin for its activity and is totally inactive without it (16). Recent evidence gathered by Kan et al. (16) showed that this HBGF is also secreted by regenerating hepatocytes, with the highest secretion rate occurring at the peak of DNA synthesis. The factor is produced by parenchymal hepatocytes and nonparenchymal cells and its secretion persists for 7 days after two-thirds partial hepatectomy.

Hepatopoietin B (HPTB): This is the activity found in serum of hepatectomized rats in addition to that of HPTA/HGF (17). HPTB is smaller than 500 kDa and does not contain amino acids in its molecule. Its properties are those of a glycolipid. It is a complete hepatocyte mitogen but less active than EGF and HPTA, and it interacts with them in a synergistic manner. Its origin is still unknown.

Growth inhibitors

TGF-β: This is the main growth inhibitor shown to inhibit the DNA synthesis of hepatocytes stimulated by either EGF or HPTA/HGF. Most studies of hepatocytes have been done with TGF-β_1, and three or more other members of the TGF-β family of polypeptides have been identified. Their molecular weight is about 26,000 kDa.

Strong in vivo evidence exists for TGF-β's role as an inhibitor of DNA synthesis in liver regeneration. TGF-β mRNA production by nonparenchymal hepatocytes first becomes detectable at 4 hr, remains at low levels until 18–20 hr, then rises sharply, peaking at 72 hr and remaining at high levels for more than 96 hr (18,19). Injection of TGF-β at different times before and soon after two-thirds partial hepatectomy inhibited the peak of DNA synthesis seen at 24 hr of regeneration. Repeated and stronger doses of TGF-β failed, however, to inhibit DNA synthesis completely, a delayed peak appearing at 72 hr (20).

Comitogenic growth factors (growth triggers)

This group consists of substances that affect hepatocyte growth in a positive direction but in an indirect manner. Best characterized as growth triggers, these substances have the following properties: They enhance the mitogenic effect of growth stimulators (EGF, HPTA, etc.); they decrease the inhibitory effect of growth inhibitors; and they have no direct mitogenic effects of their own in serum-free cultures.

Based on the first two properties, these substances have the potential of tilting a balance between the stimulative and inhibitory growth factors described above, so that the effect of growth stimulators becomes predominant and the growth process is triggered. The three properties listed above have not been demonstrated for all of these substances, and more often the studies are limited to demonstrating the first and third characteristics. Substances that fit in this category are the following.

Norepinephrine: This, the well-characterized neurotransmitter of the sympathetic nervous system, is the stronger and best characterized comitogen for hepatocytes. Mediated through the α-1 adrenergic receptor, its effects in culture cover all three of the listed criteria. A role for the sympathetic nervous system and its neurotransmitter in liver regeneration was shown by several studies in the past. More recently, blockade of the α-1 adrenergic receptor by prazosin was shown to abolish the 24-hr peak of DNA synthesis seen during liver regeneration (21). This demonstrated clearly that the α-1 adrenergic receptor has an essential function during the early stages of liver regeneration. When hepatocytes isolated from regenerating liver are kept in balanced concentrations in the presence of EGF and TGF-β, so that no DNA synthesis takes place, the addition of norepinephrine alone increases the labeling index from less than 4% to more than 70%. Norepinephrine, a nonmitogen per se, clearly can tilt the balance between growth stimulators and inhibitors and act as a trigger for hepatocyte mitogenesis. The ability of a nonmitogenic substance to act as a mitogen in the presence of other complete mitogens may be a model for the mode of action of xenobiotics that induce DNA synthesis during augmentative hepatomegaly. Most xenobiotics are not mitogenic in culture, and they induce DNA synthesis in an indirect manner, possibly by tilting the balance between mitotic stimulators, analogous to norepinephrine's action.

Vasopressin, angiotensin II, and angiotensin III: These hormones act through receptors with the same intracellular second messengers as the α-1 receptor. Overall, norepinephrine is much more potent than vasopressin or angiotensin II and III, both in terms of stimulating EGF mitogenesis and of decreasing or inhibiting the effect of TGF-β (3).

Estrogens: Substantial evidence supports a role for estrogens in liver regeneration (22–24). Estrogen levels rise after two-thirds partial hepatectomy, reaching a peak at 24–48 hr. Conversely, testosterone levels decrease. Tamoxifen given soon after this operation blocks hepatic DNA synthesis. Finally, estrogens added to primary cultures with serum or EGF enhance mitogenesis (24). Estrogen receptors and their retention time in the nucleus increase after two-thirds partial hepatectomy, while nuclear androgen receptors decrease. Hepatocytes from male rats, however, are more responsive to EGF than those from female rats. Ethinyl estradiol, which potentiates the effect of EGF in culture, promotes hepatic tumorigenesis in the whole animal.

Insulin and glucagon: Insulin does not stimulate hepatocyte proliferation in culture, despite strong tropic effects on hepatocyte physiology and viability; in chemically defined media, hepatocytes degenerate and die in the absence of insulin. Pancreatectomy results in diminished hepatic weight, but administration of insulin and glucagon partially reverses this atrophy. Pancreatectomy is also associated with decreased DNA synthesis during liver regeneration, an effect that is reversed by insulin and glucagon administration. Despite strong evidence that insulin and glucagon are required as permissive factors for optimal DNA synthesis and liver regeneration, there is no evidence that these substances have any mitogenic effects on the liver. Studies of intact rats (4) have shown that injection of insulin and glucagon do not cause DNA synthesis, whereas injection of EGF does.

Types of hepatocyte proliferation induced by chemicals

Many chemicals induce proliferation of hepatocytes when administered to the whole animal, the degree of cell replication ranging from barely detectable to very high levels of DNA synthesis, comparable to those induced in liver regeneration after partial hepatectomy. The chemicals that function in this fashion can be divided into two categories, based on the mechanism by which hepatocyte proliferation is induced. Cell proliferation is the main means by which hepatic mass is regulated. The two conditions in which hepatocyte proliferation is induced by chemicals are the following.

Regenerative hyperplasia: This condition is triggered by chemicals that are toxic to hepatocytes, which of course includes carcinogenic substances that induce liver tumors. The site of toxicity is usually centrilobular, but other sites, such as the midzonal and periportal, may also be targets, site varying with specific chemicals. Acute administration of hepatotoxic chemical dosages sufficient to induce loss of more than 5% of hepatic parenchyma is followed by a proportionate and measurable DNA synthesis in the surviving hepatocytes, so that the total mass of hepatic parenchyma is restored. Continuous administration of hepatotoxic chemicals is associated with continuous loss of hepatic parenchyma, with resultant continual hepatocyte proliferation proportionate to the amount of hepatocytes lost. Following multiple rounds of toxic reaction and hepatocyte proliferation, many of these chemicals will induce cirrhosis of the liver. When stable cirrhosis is established, continually higher rates of hepatocyte proliferation may become permanent. Cirrhosis is associated with continuously high rates of parenchymal proliferation caused by anoxic changes in hepatocytes due to decreased blood flow through the cirrhotic nodules.

There is a clear-cut association of carcinogenicity in liver with chemicals capable of generating DNA adducts and causing regenerative DNA synthesis in the liver (25). Such genotoxic chemicals as polycyclic aromatic hydrocarbons, which are not toxic to the liver and thus do not stimulate regenerative DNA synthesis, are inefficient carcinogens in the liver, but their carcinogenicity is enhanced by concomitant procedures that stimulate DNA synthesis (e.g., partial hepatectomy and hepatic growth in neonatal animals) (26).

The mechanisms by which these chemicals stimulate DNA synthesis are probably similar to the mechanisms associated with hepatic DNA synthesis after two-thirds partial hepatectomy. Although the mechanisms brought on by chemically induced hepatectomy have not been compared with those of surgical hepatectomy, it is assumed that the operating mechanisms are the same because the driving force of regeneration, loss of hepatic parenchyma, is the same in both instances. Differences in cell proliferation kinetics between regeneration induced by surgery and that induced by chemicals have been described (27); following administration of carbon tetrachloride, DNA synthesis proceeded slower by 24 hr compared to that induced by partial hepatectomy (27). These differences are assumed to result from the removal of dying hepatocytes and other cells before DNA synthesis begins in the surviving cells. Other potential differences include the site of DNA synthesis. The liver's periportal region is the site of the earliest identifiable DNA synthesis in hepatocytes. In chemically induced hepatic toxicity, the damage is zonally selective—where DNA synthesis begins might vary with the site of damage.

Since the hepatotoxic chemicals induce DNA synthesis indirectly by decreasing the number of hepatocytes, these chemicals cannot be considered hepatic mitogens. As Novicki et al. (28) showed, these chemicals inhibit DNA synthesis in hepatocytes when added to cultures in which hepatocytes are stimulated by growth factors to proliferate. Hepatocytes derived from early neoplastic foci, identified as staining positively with γ-glutamyl transpeptidase, are more resistant to these chemicals' mito-inhibitory effect than normal hepatocytes. For the initiated neoplastic hepatocytes, this should create a selective proliferative advantage leading to clonal expansion. Since the total mass of the liver needs to be maintained, initiated neoplastic hepatocytes resistant to the chemical carcinogens' inhibitory effect would then bear a proportionately heavier burden in the effort to maintain homeostasis of the hepatic mass. This advantage is probably the reason chemical carcinogens are efficient liver carcinogens only if they are toxic to the liver.

Augmentative hepatomegaly: In this condition, induced by many xenobiotic chemicals, hepatic mass increases from normal to an additional 60–100%, depending on the chemical and the duration of exposure. Chemicals inducing this phenomenon do not usually cause hepatic toxicity. Administration of the chemicals is followed by a transient period of DNA synthesis that lasts from 2 to 7 days, after which the final liver weight is reached. Because most of these chemicals also cause hepatocyte enlargement, the increase in final liver weight results from this as well as an increase in hepatocyte numbers (29).

Although chemicals that induce augmentative hepatomegaly fall into several categories of structure and function, most induce an increase in specific hepatocyte organelles. A large group of these chemicals induces a broad spectrum of cytochrome P450 isozymes and an increase in membranes of the smooth endoplasmic reticulum. Phenobarbital exemplifies these compounds. Others of different structure but similar effects include the antiepileptic drug phenytoin, the muscle relaxant diazepam, and several other well or less known medications and chemicals. Another group is composed of compounds that induce peroxisome proliferation as well as selective forms of cytochrome P450 (for review see ref. 30). All these compounds strongly promote carcinogenesis in the liver. Their initiating potential is either low or absent (e.g., in the case of phenobarbital) or strong enough to allow them to be classified as complete liver carcinogens (this includes many of the peroxisome proliferators).

Although these chemicals induce profound changes in liver mass and an increase in DNA synthesis, they exert these effects only when given to the whole animal. When the same compounds are administered to cultures of hepatocytes in the absence of other mitogens, they are not usually mitogenic for hepatocytes, which strongly suggests that these compounds require other growth factors for their effects. The only exception to this finding is cyproterone acetate (see chapter by Schulte-Hermann et al. in this volume and ref. 31). These chemicals' precise mode of interaction with defined growth factors is not entirely clear. Phenobarbital may be the best studied example. Given to the whole animal, phenobarbital leads to a wave of DNA synthesis that peaks at 3–5 days (32). Blockade of the α-1 adrenergic receptor abolishes the peak but not the increase in liver weight.

When DNA synthesis is induced, hepatocytes acquire increased sensitivity to EGF (33). Following this early period, this sensitivity decreases progressively to a point at which hepatocytes isolated from rats kept for 60 days on a phenobarbital protocol lose sensitivity to insulin EGF and do not respond to EGF when exposed to this growth factor in culture (34,35). The numbers of EGF receptors decrease in parallel with the hepatocytes' loss of responsiveness to EGF. The mechanism by which phenobarbital induces this biphasic change of sensitivity to EGF is not clear. Added to hepatocytes in culture, phenobarbital slightly increases the effectiveness of EGF (36), while at higher doses it abolishes the EGF response. The biphasic change seen in the whole animal as a function of time seems to be reproduced in culture as a function of concentration, a parallelism that suggests phenobarbital might have to accumulate at critical sites (perhaps at plasma membranes) before it diminishes responsiveness to EGF. It might do so, therefore, when animals have undergone prolonged exposure to this drug.

There may, however, be other reasons for these observations. The tumor-promoting effects of phenobarbital require prolonged exposure too, and prolonged exposure of phenobarbital is associated with diminished responses to EGF. These findings imply that the tumor-promoting effect of phenobarbital is caused by its mitogen inhibition. Although this association is paradoxical, it is less so when examined carefully. After prolonged exposure to phenobarbital, the mitogenesis inhibition of normal hepatocytes might give neoplastic hepatocytes a proliferative advantage. This is the same situation as in the case of the toxic carcinogenic chemicals: because the liver mass must be maintained, initiated neoplastic hepatocytes resistant to the inhibitory effect of phenobarbital will bear a heavier burden in maintaining homeostasis of the hepatic mass. This should lead to clonal expansion of the initiated cells over that of normal cells. Therefore, although toxic chemicals and tumor promoters differ in the mechanisms by which they induce DNA synthesis in hepatocytes, the reasons they lead to greater clonal expansion of initiated cells might be the same. A difference in sensitivity to phenobarbital between normal and neoplastic hepatocytes has indeed been shown recently by Jirtle et al. (37). Similar biphasic changes in sensitivity to EGF may be induced by α-hexachlorocyclohexane (W.H. Tsai and G.K. Michalpoulos, unpublished observations).

How these chemicals induce the early wave of DNA synthesis is also not clear. In hepatocyte cultures maintained in the presence of EGF and TGF-β so that no cell replication takes place, addition of norepinephrine, which is nonmitogenic by itself, leads to hepatocyte DNA synthesis because norepinephrine amplifies the effect of EGF and diminishes that of TGF-β (3). This may be a mechanism by which the xenobiotics induce DNA synthesis in hepatocytes, although other possibilities exist. The processes leading to DNA synthesis in regeneration and those induced by the xenobiotics have basic similarities: both depend on α-1 receptor function (32) and both produce an increased sensitivity to EGF (33; Tsai and Michalopoulos, unpublished observations). But the early induction of DNA synthesis is probably not critically related to these chemicals' tumor-promoting effects. Indeed, as Marsman et al. found (38), the same magnitude of early DNA synthesis is induced by the peroxisome proliferators di(2-ethylhexyl)phthalate (DEHP) and [4-chloro-6-(2,3-xylidino)-2-pyrimidinylthio]acetic acid (Wy-14,643), despite the fact that the first compound is a weaker carcinogen than the second. In fact, after early DNA synthesis, prolonged DNA synthesis is induced by Wy-14,643 and not by DEHP.

Categorizing chemicals that induce hepatic DNA synthesis according to regen-erative hyperplasia or augmentative hepatomegaly might not always be correct; quite possibly some chemicals operate both ways. Such compounds such as lead nitrate (39) and Wy-14,643 cause a prolonged stimulation of DNA synthesis after the early wave associated with augmentative hepatomegaly. These compounds might induce augmentative hepatomegaly as well as prove toxic to the enlarged liver on prolonged administration, thus leading to the high cellular turnover of prolonged exposure, like that seen with use of toxic chemicals.

The association of DNA synthesis with hepatic carcinogenesis is strong, although a basic question, whether DNA synthesis alone is capable of inducing liver cancer, remains to be answered. Such an association needs to be verified for all chemicals for which this thesis is proposed. DNA synthesis is easy to demonstrate and to study, but quantitating genetic damage of hepatocytes induced by chemicals is more difficult to do. Our available methods focus on DNA damage, as measured by unscheduled DNA synthesis (40) and assessment of DNA fragmentation (41). Few studies have dealt with the possibility that some of the carcinogenic agents for which DNA damage cannot be demonstrated might be clastogenic. Compared to all other available methods, sister chromatid exchange in hepatocytes was recently shown by far the most sensitive system (by two to three orders of magnitude of chemical concentration) for the detection of genotoxic potential in hepatocytes (42). The effect of apparently nonmutagenic (nongenotoxic) carcinogens on hepatocyte chromosome fragmentation needs to be assessed before recruitment of endogenously initiated cells by continuously induced DNA synthesis becomes the accepted mode of studying these chemicals' actions.

Conclusions

Chemicals associated with increased DNA synthesis in hepatocytes often tend to be associated with increased incidence of liver cancer. These chemicals should not be treated as hepatic mitogens. In fact, their carcinogenic—promoting or initiating— potential is more apt to be associated with inhibition of DNA synthesis than with stimulation. Differences in resistance by initiated and normal hepatocytes to the chemicals' effects might be the operative mechanisms by which these chemicals induce hepatic neoplasia, as Farber (26) originally proposed. As the growth factors associated with hepatocyte proliferation become better identified, their involvement and triggering of hepatic DNA synthesis is bound to be better understood.

References

1. Michalopoulos GK. Liver regeneration: Molecular mechanisms of growth control. F.A.S.E.B. in press, 1990.
2. McGowan JA, Strain AJ, Bucher NLR. DNA synthesis in primary cultures of adult rat hepatocytes in a defined medium: Effects of epidermal growth factor, insulin, glucagon, and cyclic-AMP. J Cell Physiol 180:353–363, 1981.
3. Houck KA, Michalopoulos GK. Altered responses of regenerating hepatocytes to TGF-β. J Cell Physiol 141:503–509, 1989.
4. Bucher NLR. Thirty years of liver regeneration: A distillate. In: Cold Spring Harbor Conferences on Cell Proliferation, vol. 9, Growth of Cell in Chemically Defined Media, pp. 15–26, 1982.
5. Mead JE, Fausto N. Transforming growth factor TGF-α may be a physiological regulator of liver regeneration by means of an autocrine mechanism. Proc Natl Acad Sci USA 86:1558–1562, 1989.

6. Michalopoulos G, Houck K, Dolan M, Novicki DL. Control of proliferation of hepatocytes by two serum hepatopoietins. Fed Proc 42:1023, 1983.

7. Zarnegar R, Michalopoulos G. Purification and biological characterization of human hepatopoietin A, a polypeptide growth factor for hepatocytes. Cancer Res 49:3314–3320, 1989.

8. Nakamura T, Nawa K, Ichihara A. Partial purification and characterization of hepatocyte growth factor from serum of hepatectomized rats. Biochem Biophys Res Commun 122:1450–1459, 1984.

9. Nakamura T, Nawa K, Ichihara A, Kaise N, Nishino T. Purification and subunit structure of hepatocyte growth factor from rat platelets. FEBS Lett 224:311–316, 1987.

10. Gohda E, Tsubouchi H, Nakayama H, Horono S, Sakiyama O, Takahashi K, Miyazaki H, Hashimoto S, Daikuhara Y. Purification and partial characterization of hepatocyte growth factor from plasma of a patient with hepatic failure. J Clin Invest 81:414–419, 1988.

11. Zarnegar R, Muga S, Enghild J, Michalopoulos GK. NH2-terminal amino acid sequence of rabbit hepatopoietin A, a heparin-binding polypeptide growth factor for hepatocytes. Biochem Biophys Res Commun 163:1370–1376, 1989.

12. Miyazawa K, Tsubouchi H, Naka D, Takahashi K, Okigaki M, Arakaki N, Nakayama H, Hirono S, Sakiyama O, Takahashi K, Gohoda E, Daikuhara Y, Kitamura N. Molecular cloning and sequence analysis of cDNA for human hepatocyte growth factor, Biochem Biophys Res Commun 163:967–973, 1989.

13. Nakamura T, Nishizawa T, Hagiya M, Seki T, Shimonishi M, Sugimura A, Tashiro K, Shimizu S. Molecular cloning and expression of human hepatocyte growth factor. Nature 342:440:443, 1989.

14. Zarnegar R, Muga S, Rahija R, Michalopoulos GK. Tissue distribution of HPTA, a heparin-binding polypeptide growth factor for hepatocytes. Proc Natl Acad Sci USA, in Press.

15. Houck K, Zarnegar R, Muga S, Michalopoulos GK. Acidic fibroblast growth factor (HBGF-1) stimulates DNA synthesis in primary rat hepatocyte cultures. J Cell Physiol, in press.

16. Kan M, Huan J, Mansson P, Yasumitsu H, Carr B, McKeehan W. Heparin-binding growth factor type 1 (acidic fibroblast growth factor): A potential biphasic autocrine and paracrine regulator of hepatocyte regeneration. Proc Natl Acad Sci USA 86:7432–7436, 1989.

17. Michalopoulos G, Houck KA, Dolan ML, Luetteke NC. Control of hepatocyte replication by two serum factors. Cancer Res 44:4414–4419, 1984.

18. Braun L, Mead JE, Panzica M, Mikumo R, Bell GI, Fausto N. Transforming growth factor ß mRNA increases during liver regeneration: A possible paracrine mechanism of growth regulation. Proc Natl Acad Sci USA 85:1539–1543, 1988.

19. Carr BI, Huang TH, Itakura K, Noel M, Marceau N. TGF-β gene transcription in normal and neoplastic liver growth. J Cell Biochem 39:477–487, 1989.

20. Russell WE, Coffey RJ, Ouellette AJ, Moses HL. Type beta transforming growth factor reversibly inhibits the early proliferative response to partial hepatectomy in the rat. Proc Natl Acad Sci USA 85:5126–5130, 1988.

21. Cruise JL, Knechtle SJ, Bollinger RR, Kuhn C, Michalopoulos GK. Alpha 1-adrenergic effects and liver regeneration. Hepatology 7:1189–1194, 1987.

22. Francavilla A, Gavaler JS, Makowka L, Barone M, Mazzaferro V, Ambrosino G, Iwatsuki S, Guglielmi FW, DiLeo A, Balestrazzi A. et al. Estradiol and testosterone levels in patients undergoing partial hepatectomy. A possible signal for hepatic regeneration? Dig Dis Sci 34:818–822, 1989.

23. Francavilla A, Eagon PK, DiLeo A, Polimeno L, Panella C, Aquilino AM, Ingrosso M, Van Thiel DH, Starzl TE. Sex hormone-related functions in regenerating male rat liver. Gastroenterology 91:1263–1270, 1986.

24. Shi YE, Yager JD. Effects of the liver tumor promoter ethinyl estradiol on epidermal growth factor-induced DNA synthesis and epidermal growth factor receptor levels in cultured rat hepatocytes. Cancer Res 49:3574–3580, 1989.

25. Lewis JG, Swenberg JA. The kinetics of DNA alkylation, repair and replication in hepatocytes, Kupffer cells, and sinusoidal endothelial cells in rat liver during continuous exposure to 1,2-dimethylhydrazine. Carcinogenesis 4:529–536, 1983.

26. Farber E. Chemical carcinogenesis. N Engl J Med 305:1379–1389, 1981.

27. Clawson GA. Mechanisms of carbon tetrachloride hepatotoxicity. Pathol Immunopathol Res 8:104–112, 1989.

28. Novicki DL, Rosenberg MR, Michalopoulos G. Inhibition of DNA synthesis by chemical carcinogens in cultures of initiated and normal proliferating hepatocytes. Cancer Res 45:337–344, 1985.

29. Michalopoulos G, Eckl PM, Cruise JL, Novicki L, Jirtle RL. Models of rodent liver carcinogenesis. Toxicol Ind Health 3:119–127, 1987.
30. Reddy JK, Rao MS. Xenobiotic-induced peroxisome proliferation: Role of tissue specificity and species differences in response in the evaluation of the implications for human health. Arch Toxicol Suppl 10:43–53, 1987.
31. Parzefall W, Monschau P, Schulte-Hermann R. Induction by cyproterone acetate of DNA synthesis and mitosis in primary cultures of adult rat hepatocytes in serum free medium. Arch Toxicol, in press.
32. Tsai WH, Cruise JL, Michalopoulos GK. Blockade of alpha-1 adrenergic receptor inhibits hepatic DNA synthesis stimulated by tumor promoters. Carcinogenesis 10:73–78, 1989.
33. Francavilla A, Ove P, Polimeno L, Sciascia C, Coetzee ML, Starzl TE. Epidermal growth factor and proliferation in rat hepatocytes in primary culture isolated at different times after partial hepatectomy. Cancer Res 46:1318–1323, 1986.
34. Eckl PM, Meyer SA, Whitcombe WR, Jirtle RL. Phenobarbital reduces EGF receptors and the ability of physiological concentrations of calcium to suppress hepatocyte proliferation. Carcinogenesis 9:479–483, 1988.
35. Gupta C, Hattori A, Betschart JM, Virji MA, Shinozuka H. Modulation of epidermal growth factor receptors in rat hepatocytes by two liver tumor-promoting regimens, a choline-deficient and a phenobarbital diet. Cancer Res 48:1162–1165, 1988.
36. Sawada N, Staecker JL, Pitot HC. Effects of tumor-promoting agents 12-O-tetradecanoyl-phorbol-13-acetate and phenobarbital on DNA synthesis of rat hepatocytes in primary culture. Cancer Res 47:5665–5671, 1987.
37. Jirtle RL. Dig Dis Sci, in press.
38. Marsman DS Cattley RC, Conway JG, Popp JA. Relationship of hepatic peroxisome proliferation and replicative DNA synthesis to the hepatocarcinogenicity of the peroxisome proliferators di(2-ethylhexyl)phthalate and [4-chloro-6-(2,3-xylidino)-2-pyrimidinylthio]acetic acid (Wy-14,643) in rats. Cancer Res 48:6739–6744, 1988.
39. Columbano A, Ledda-Columbano GM, Coni PP, Vargiu M, Faa G, Pani P. Liver hyperplasia and regression after lead nitrate administration. Toxicol Pathol 12:89–95, 1984.
40. Butterworth BE, Ashby J, Bermudez E, Casciano D, Mirsalis J, Probst G, Williams G. A protocol and guide for the in vitro rat hepatocyte DNA-repair assay. Mutat Res 189:113–121, 1987.
41. Sina JF, Bean CL, Dysart GR, Taylor VI, Bradley MO. Evaluation of the alkaline elution/rat hepatocyte assay as a predictor of carcinogenic/mutagenic potential. Mutat Res 113:357–391, 1983.
42. Eckl PM, Strom SC, Michalopoulos G, Jirtle RL. Induction of sister chromatid exchanges in cultured adult rat hepatocytes by directly and indirectly acting mutagens/carcinogens. Carcinogenesis 8:1077–1083, 1987.

Chemically Induced Cell Proliferation:
Implications for Risk Assessment, pages 237-244
©1991 Wiley-Liss, Inc.

Mitogenesis and Programmed Cell Death as Determinants of Carcinogenicity of Nongenotoxic Compounds

R. Schulte-Hermann, W. Bursch, and W. Parzefall

Stimulation of growth in their target organs is a common property of most nongenotoxic carcinogens. That chemicals can induce "additive" or "adaptive" liver growth has been known for more than 40 years, and the role of cell proliferation, cell hypertrophy, and functional changes was investigated in some detail three and four decades ago (1–9). After the discovery that many hepatomitogens can cause tumor formation in rodent liver upon long-term treatment, many additional studies on a variety of chemicals were initiated, and compilations of compounds active on the liver were published (9,10).

Three points relevant to carcinogenesis by nongenotoxic mitogens must be stressed:

a) *Mitogenesis and carcinogenesis.* Most or all of the nongenotoxic carcinogens do not simply induce liver growth but stimulate, at the same time, profound functional changes in the organ. In other words, activation of gene programs, or pleiotropic responses, and not simply enhanced cell proliferation, seem to be responsible for these agents' carcinogenic activity (10–12).

b) *Roles of cell proliferation in carcinogenesis.* Cell proliferation in cells may have a critical role at several steps of the multiple-stage cancer development process, namely during initiation ("co-initiation"—by errors during replication, by "fixation" of genotoxic insults of non-compound–related origin, or other means) or during promotion (11). The "co-initiating" activity of most chemical mitogens is probably of little relevance because usually they induce only a short-lived, early increase in cell replication, which returns to normal even if the treatment continues. Obviously, an effective feedback mechanism prevents excessive cell multiplication in the liver even if growth stimulatory signals by continuous mitogen treatment are steadily present (10,13,14). Therefore, the cell number of the whole organ increases only during initial phases of treatment and then remains constant at an enhanced level (14). This means that the hyperplasia resulting from the early burst of replication is sustained, rather than the stimulation of cell proliferation. It is this condition of sustained hyperplasia that seems to favor tumor development during long-term exposure to a mitogen, and the most likely explanation is that, in this condition, promotion of tumor development occurs through preferential stimulation of the multiplication of initiated or preneoplastic cells (9–11,14). Such initiated cells may be induced experimentally by treatment with genotoxic carcinogens, or they may arise for unknown reasons ("spontaneously") (15,16). The relation between mitogenesis and tumor promotion has long been uncertain for the group of peroxisome proliferators. In some earlier studies, these agents did not appear to have promoting activity in the liver, despite strong hepatomitogenic potential and carcinogenic activity. It now seems that they promote growth of a specific, hitherto neglected subtype of foci characterized by weak diffuse basophilia and with properties different from those of previously studied foci (17–20).

These observations emphasize the need to take into account the whole gene program, which is expressed by the chemical, rather than merely its mitogenic activity.

c) *Cell proliferation and cell death.* Organ growth is usually believed to result from cell multiplication and cell enlargement. Increasing evidence suggests, however, that cell death may also be an important growth determinant in normal liver as well as in preneoplastic foci or malignant tumors. The type of cell death involved is not the "classical" necrosis as it occurs after massive injury to cells, but rather the so-called "apoptosis" or "programmed cell death". The term apoptosis was coined by Wyllie, Kerr, and Currie (21) and describes the type of cell death that occurs during certain developmental stages to remove excessive tissues, such as the Mullerian duct in the male embryo. Apoptosis is also involved in cell turnover in normal tissues and in involution of such hormone-dependent organs as the adrenal after hypophysectomy (21,22). Some findings on apoptosis as related to carcinogenesis will be considered here.

Apoptosis in normal liver

As mentioned above, prolonged treatment with a hepatomitogen results in enlargement and hyperplasia of the liver. The liver seems to "know" that it is too big, however, and upon withdrawal of the mitogen its size returns to normal, and much of the hyperplasia disappears as well. The rate of involution depends on the half-life of the chemical. With compounds like cyproterone acetate (CPA), which has a biological half-life of about 8 hr, as much as 25% of the total liver DNA may disappear within a few days. With compounds like α-hexachlorocyclohexane (biological half-life several days), the decline of organ mass and cell number are much slower (23,24). The disappearance of DNA as seen after CPA treatment is far too rapid to be explained by normal cell turnover; rather, an enhanced rate of cell death must be assumed. In fact, a steep increase of apoptosis, coinciding with the maximum of DNA elimination, has been found in the liver after cessation of CPA treatment. Most important, retreatment with CPA or other hepatomitogens readily interrupted the process of DNA elimination and inhibited apoptosis. This showed that DNA elimination is not caused by a delayed type of damage-induced cell death (23–25). How many cells are eliminated in the liver per unit of time after CPA treatment ceases? To answer this question one needs to know, in addition to the number of dead cells present in histologic sections, the duration of the histologically visible parts of apoptosis. To measure the duration of apoptosis, we studied the kinetics of disappearance of cell residues after inhibition of apoptosis by CPA and found a half-life of about 2 hr and a total duration of about 3 hr (25). Based on this, calculating the rate of cell loss per hour through apoptosis, we found that in the hyperplastic liver during regression 0.5% of hepatocytes undergo apoptosis per hour (25). Although the apoptosis incidence per day cannot be calculated directly because of its possible circadian rhythmicity, we assume the loss of 5–10% of hepatocytes per day, which agrees quite well with the 25% loss of DNA as determined biochemically (see above). It seems pertinent to emphasize that caution should be exerted in the use of the term apoptosis. It is becoming popular to call various signs of cell death apoptosis. However, morphology is not necessarily specific for this type of cell death (26). Therefore, we urgently need biochemical and molecular markers. A useful biochemical marker appears to be the activation of an endonuclease. This enzyme cleaves chromatin into nucleosomes, and may be responsible for the chromatin condensation seen histologically (28) (Table 1).

However, endonuclease activation is certainly not specific for apoptosis; the enzyme has been shown to be activated also by calcium ionophores and may be activated under a variety of other conditions associated with increased cellular calcium. Another possible marker is the appearance of the enzyme transglutaminase in apoptotic cells (29). The most reliable marker at this time is a functional one, namely the ability of mitogens to inhibit apoptosis (10,23,27). Further markers of apoptosis will become available when the molecular characteristics of the process are better established. Recently we found that a gene called TRPM 2 (testosterone repressed prostate message 2) is strongly expressed in rat liver during the peak of apoptotic activity (Table 1). This gene was originally found in regressing prostate tissue after orchiectomy (30,31). It may be involved in organ involution; its exact function is not yet known.

Apoptosis in preneoplastic foci in the liver

Foci of phenotypically altered cells can be identified in rat liver by a variety of markers and are believed to represent preneoplastic lesions. Numerous nongenotoxic carcinogens have been shown to promote preferential growth of these foci. To understand the mechanism of this preferential growth, we determined cell replication rates. As we and others found, even "early" foci show enhanced proliferative activity (10,32), and these results, despite some dispute (33) have been confirmed. Long-term studies at multiple time points from early foci up to carcinoma formation revealed that, without promoter, foci grew much less than expected from cell replication rates; obviously, cell loss occurred. In contrast, during phenobarbital (PB) treatment, the observed growth rates of foci fit quite well with those calculated from cell replication rates (34,35).

Studies of apoptosis in this model revealed the following: A) The incidence of histologic signs of apoptosis was always much higher in foci than in normal liver (23),

Table 1. Characteristics and Indicators of Apoptosis.

Functional markers
  • Occurrence during tissue involution
  • Inhibition by growth stimuli
Morphologic markers
  • Separation of cell from neighboring cells
  • Condensation of chromatin
  • Cell fragmentation into "apoptotic bodies"
  • Phagocytosis of apoptotic bodies by neighboring epithelial cells and phagocytes
Biochemical and genetic markers
  • Initiation of apoptosis prevented by inhibitors of RNA and protein synthesis
  • Appearance of specific sugar residues on outer cell membrane
  • DNA fragmentation into nucleosomes
  • Expression of transglutaminase (?)
  • Expression of TRPM-2 gene (?)

and recently we showed that the duration of apoptotic stages in foci is similar to that of normal liver (26). We can now conclude, therefore, that the rate of apoptosis in foci is much higher than in normal liver and that it counterbalances to some extent the increased replicative activity found in foci (35). B) Administration of PB tended to lower the incidence and rate of apoptosis in foci, and, after withdrawal of the tumor promoter, the incidence of cell death was greatly increased. Retreatment with PB prevented apoptosis, which indicated that apoptosis and not a necrotic type of cell death was occurring, and led to the conclusion that the promoter prolongs the life span of preneoplastic hepatocytes. In other words, the promoter seems to protect preneoplastic cells from elimination (23,26,35). C) Our quantitative data provided rough estimates of the number of focal cells dying by apoptosis.

At the highest rate, up to 1–3% of putative preneoplastic cells may be eliminated by apoptosis per hour. Such estimates may be helpful for mathematical modeling of carcinogenesis. We hope, in addition, that these findings will help to answer the question of whether tumor promotion is reversible, and, if so, in what time period this will occur after the tumor promoter is withdrawn.

Apoptosis in tumors

Cells dying by apoptosis are frequently seen in neoplastic nodules and hepatocellular carcinomas in the liver. We also studied apoptosis in another tumor model, the transplantable tumor H301, which was originally derived from a hamster kidney tumor. This tumor's growth depends strictly on the presence of estrogens, which in our model were provided by implanted pellets of diethylstilbestrol (DES). Removal of the DES pellets induced rapid loss of tumor mass; readministration reinduced tumor growth. Signs of cell death were quite frequent in this tumor, and we reported elsewhere (36) the incidence of cell death increased after DES was removed and decreased dramatically when DES treatment was resumed. This proved, in this tumor model also, that apoptosis rather than (or in addition to) necrosis is involved in tumor growth and regression. Furthermore, it showed that, in a frankly malignant tumor, a nongenotoxic carcinogen can shift the balance of cell multiplication and cell death toward multiplication and can protect tumor cells from being eliminated. These findings on the roles of cell proliferation and cell death in the growth of normal and neoplastic tissues are schematically depicted in Figure 1. The important point is that mitogens can have two effects: stimulation of cell replication and inhibition of apoptosis. Withdrawal of the mitogen produces the opposite: decrease of cell generation and increase of cell death.

DNA synthesis in isolated hepatocytes

The ability to stimulate tissue growth (by cell proliferation or by inhibition of cell death) is probably a necessary, but not sufficient, property of tumor promoters. This suggests that induction of DNA synthesis can be used as an indicator of the possible tumor-promoting activity of chemical compounds. We were interested, therefore, in developing a culture system with isolated hepatocytes from rat or human sources to test for tumor-promoting activity. As shown in Figure 2, CPA is a potent inducer of DNA synthesis in isolated hepatocytes from rats in a completely defined medium, in

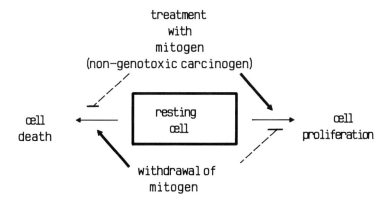

Figure 1. Redefinition of growth stimulus (or mitogen) as a signal inducing either cell generation or inhibition of cell death (apoptosis). (->) stimulation, (- - l) inhibition.

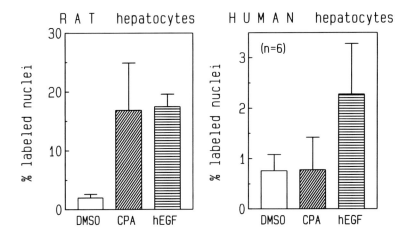

Figure 2. Mitogen effects on DNA synthesis in rat and human hepatocytes. Rat hepatocytes were cultured on collagen gel under serum-free conditions as described (37). Cells were treated with 10 μM CPA or dimethylsulfoxide (DMSO) (0.2%) at 20 to 68 hr or with 20 ng of EGF/ml at 20 to 44 hr. At between 44 and 68 hr, cells were labeled with [^{3}H]thymidine. Liver cells from 6 persons were cultured under the same conditions. At 18 hr after plating, continuous treatment with EGF (20 ng/ml), DMSO (0.2%), or CPA (10 μM) began. Between 44 and 68 hr, cells were labeled with [^{3}H]thymidine. DNA synthesis was evaluated in autoradiographs counterstained with hematoxylin.

accordance with its tumor promoting activity in this rodent species (37). In human hepatocytes, in contrast, CPA seemed to be inactive as an inducer of DNA synthesis even though the epidermal growth factor (EGF) was effective. This result, although still preliminary, would not support the hypothesis that the risk of humans treated with CPA is similar to that of rats for developing hepatic tumors.

Conclusion

We studied the regulation of cell death by apoptosis in three different models— normal liver, altered hepatic foci, and a hormone-dependent malignant kidney tumor. In all of them, the evidence was that the incidence of apoptosis is reduced by mitogens. Inhibition of apoptosis, in addition to enhanced cell replication, therefore seems to be involved in formation and maintenance of tissue hyperplasia and (pre-)tumor growth. The term "growth stimulus" should be redefined as meaning stimulation of cell replication or inhibition of apoptosis, or both. The two effects are schematically shown in Figure 1. Quantitative data on cell generation and apoptosis are becoming available and may help to understand growth kinetics of (pre)neoplastic lesions in quantitative terms; they may provide the data needed for mathematical modeling of carcinogenesis (38,39). Finally, growth-stimulatory potential as defined above may be an indicator of the compound's possible tumor-promoting activity. Measuring the stimulation of DNA synthesis by a promoter in such cultured cells as human hepatocytes may help to improve risk assessment for humans.

References

1. Wilson JW, Leduc EH. The effect of coramine on mitotic activity and growth in the liver of the mouse. Growth 14:31–48, 1950.
2. Rachmilewitz M, Rosin A, Doljanski L. Observations on the mitotic reaction induced in the livers of rats by thiourea. Am J Pathol 26:937–945, 1950.
3. Doljanski F. The growth of the liver with special reference to mammals. Int Rev Cytol 10:217–241, 1960.
4. Golberg L. Liver enlargement produced by drugs: its significance. Proc Eur Soc for Study of Drug Toxicity, vol 7. Amsterdam: Excerpta Medica Foundation, 1966, p 171–184.
5. Kunz W, Schaude G, Schmid W, Siess M. Lebervergrösserung durch Fremdstoffe. Naunyn-Schmiedebergs Arch Pharmacol Exp Pathol 254:470–488, 1966.
6. Argyris TS. Stimulators, enzyme induction and the control of liver growth. In: Clarkson B, Baserga R (eds): Control of Proliferation in Animal Cells. Cold Spring Harbor: Cold Spring Harbor Laboratory, 1974.
7. Schlicht I, Koransky W, Magour S, Schulte-Hermann R. Grösse und DNS-Synthese der Leber unter dem Einfluss körperfremder Stoffe. Naunyn-Schmiedebergs Arch Pharmakol Exp Pathol 261:26–41, 1968.
8. Schulte-Hermann R, Thom R, Schlicht I, Koransky W. Zahl und Ploidiegrad der Zellkerne der Leber unter dem Einfluss körperfremder Stoffe. Naunyn-Schmiedebergs Arch Pharmakol Exp Pathol 261:42–58, 1968.
9. Schulte-Hermann R. Induction of liver growth by xenobiotic compounds and other stimuli. Crit Rev Toxicol 3:97–158, 1974.
10. Schulte-Hermann R. Tumor promotion in the liver. Arch Toxicol 57:147–158, 1985.
11. Schulte-Hermann R. Reactions of the liver to injury: Adaptation. In: Farber E, Fisher MM (eds): Liver: Normal function and Disease, vol 2, Toxic Injury of the Liver. New York: Marcel Dekker, 1979, pp 385–444.

12. Schulte-Hermann R, Timmermann-Trosiener I, Schuppler J. Facilitated expression of adaptive responses to phenobarbital in putative pre-stages of liver cancer. Carcinogenesis 7:1651–1655, 1986.
13. Schulte-Hermann R, Schmitz E. Feedback inhibition of hepatic DNA synthesis. Cell Tissue Kinet 13:371–380, 1980.
14. Schulte-Hermann R, Parzefall W. Failure to discriminate initiation from promotion of liver tumors in a long-term study with the phenobarbital-type inducer α-hexachlorocyclohexane and the role of sustained stimulation of hepatic growth and monooxygenases. Cancer Res 41:4140–4146, 1981.
15. Schulte-Hermann R, Timmermann-Trosiener I, Schuppler J. Promotion of spontaneous preneoplastic cells in rat liver as a possible explanation of tumor production by nonmutagenic compounds. Cancer Res 443:839–844, 1983.
16. Ward JM. Increased susceptibility of livers of aged F344/NCr rats to the effects of phenobarbital on the incidence, morphology, and histochemistry of hepatocellular foci and neoplasms. J Natl Cancer Inst 71:815–822, 1983.
17. Schulte-Hermann R, Bursch W, Gerbracht U, Kraupp-Grasl B, Timmermann-Trosiener I. Effects of nongenotoxic hepatocarcinogens on phenotype and growth of different populations of altered foci in rat liver. Toxicol Pathol 17, part 1, 1989.
18. Kraupp-Grasl B, Huber W, Putz B, Gerbracht U, Schulte-Hermann R. Tumor promotion by the peroxisome inducer nafenopin in rat liver may involve a new subtype of phenotypically altered foci. Cancer Res 50:3701–3708, 1990.
19. Marsman DS, Popp JA. Importance of basophilic hepatocellular foci in the development of hepatic tumors induced by the peroxisome proliferator Wy-14,643. Proc Am Assoc Cancer Res 30:193, 1989.
20. Gerbracht U, Bursch W, Kraus P, Putz B, Reinacher M, Timmermann-Trosiener I, Schulte-Hermann R. Effects of hypolipidemic drugs on phenotypic expression and cell death (apoptosis) in altered foci of rat liver. Carcinogenesis 11:617-624, 1990.
21. Wyllie AH, Kerr JFR, Currie AR. Cell death: The significance of apoptosis. Int Rev Cytol 68:251–306, 1980.
22. Bursch W. Cell death by apoptosis: Significance for the regulation of homeostasis of cell number and its disturbance during cancer development. In: Paukovits W (ed): Growth Regulation and Carcinogenesis. Boca Raton: CRC Press, in press.
23. Bursch W, Lauer B, Timmermann-Trosiener I, Barthel G, Schuppler J, Schulte-Hermann R. Controlled death (apoptosis) of normal and putative preneoplastic cells in rat liver following withdrawal of tumor promoters. Carcinogenesis 5:453–458, 1984.
24. Bursch W, Düsterberg B, Schulte-Hermann R. Growth, regression and cell death in rat liver as related to tissue levels of the hepatomitogen cyproterone acetate. Arch Toxicol 59:221–227, 1986.
25. Bursch W, Taper HS, Lauer B, Schulte-Hermann R. Quantitative histological and histochemical studies on the occurrence and stages of controlled cell death (apoptosis) during regression of rat liver hyperplasia. Virchows Arch [B] 50:153–166, 1985.
26. Bursch W, Paffe S, Putz B, Barthel G, Schulte-Hermann R. Determination of the length of the histological stages of apoptosis in normal liver and in altered hepatic foci of rats. Carcinogenesis, 11:847-853,1990.
27. Schulte-Hermann R, Bursch W. Cell death through apoptosis and its relationship to carcinogenesis. In: Volans GN, Simms J, Sullivan FM, Turner P (eds): Basic Science in Toxicology. London, New York, Philadelphia: Taylor and Francis, 1990.
28. Wyllie AH, Morris RG, Smith AO, Dunlop D. Chromatin cleavage in apoptosis: Association with condensed chromatin morphology and dependence on macromolecular synthesis. J Pathol 142:67–77, 1984.
29. Fesus L, Thomazy W, Autuori F, Ceru MP, Tarsca E, Piancetini M. Apoptotic hepatocytes become insoluble in detergents and chaotropic agents as a result of transglutaminase action. FEBS Lett 245:150–154, 1989.
30. Leger J, Le Guellec R, Tenniswood PR. Treatment with antiandrogens induces an androgen-repressed gene in the rat ventral prostate. The Prostate 13:131–142, 1988.
31. Tenniswood M, Montpetit M, Leger J, Wong P, Pineault J, Rouleau M. Epithelial-stromal interactions and cell death in the prostate. In: Farnsworth W and Ablin R (eds): Prostate as an Endocrine Gland. Baca Raton: CRC Press, 1990.
32. Schulte-Hermann R, Ohde G, Schuppler J, Timmermann-Trosiener I. Enhanced proliferation of putative preneoplastic cells in rat liver following treatment with the tumor promoters phenobarbital, hexachlorocyclohexane, steroid compounds and nafenopin. Cancer Res 41:2556–2562, 1981.

33. Bannasch P, Moore MA, Klimek F, Zerban H. Biological markers of preneoplastic foci and neoplastic nodules in rodent liver. Toxicol Pathol 10:19–36, 1982.
34. Schulte-Hermann R, Timmermann-Trosiener I, Schuppler J. Response of liver foci in rats to hepatic tumor promoters. Toxicol Pathol 10:63–70, 1982.
35. Schulte-Hermann R, Timmermann-Trosiener I, Barthel G, Bursch W. DNA synthesis, apoptosis and phenotypic expression as determinants of growth of altered foci in rat liver during phenobarbital promotion. Cancer Res 50:5127–5135, 1990.
36. Bursch W, Liehr J, Sirbasku D, Schulte-Hermann R. Role of cell death for growth and regression of hormone-dependent H-301 hamster kidney tumors. In: Feo F (ed): Chemical Carcinogenesis: Models and Mechanisms. New York: Plenum Press, New York, 1988, pp 275–280.
37. Parzefall W, Monschau P, Schulte-Hermann R. Induction by cyproterone acetate of DNA synthesis and mitosis in primary cultures of adult rat hepatocytes in serum free medium. Arch Toxicol 63:456–461, 1989.
38. Moolgavkar SH. Multistage models for cancer risk assessment. In: Travis CC (ed): Biologically Based Methods for Cancer Risk Assessment. New York: Plenum Press 159:9–20, 1989.
39. Moolgavkar SH. The role of somatic mutations and cell replication kinetics in quantitative cancer risk assessment. In: Slaga T and Butterworth B (eds): Chemically Induced Cell Proliferation. New York: Alan R. Liss, 1991.

Chemically Induced Cell Proliferation:
Implications for Risk Assessment, pages 245-251
©1991 Wiley-Liss, Inc.

Chemically Induced Cell Proliferation as a Criterion in Selecting Doses for Long-Term Bioassays

James A. Swenberg and Robert R. Maronpot

The major focus of this volume is on the role of cell proliferation in cancer risk assessment. That cell proliferation is required for both initiation of the carcinogenic process and clonal expansion of initiated cells is well established. As such, cell proliferation is intimately involved in modulating the shape of the dose response curve for carcinogenicity. It seems mandatory, then, to know a chemical agent's dose-response curve for cell proliferation in order to better interpret the dose response for carcinogenesis and, ultimately, to extrapolate from these data the chemical's potential cancer risk to human beings.

When one examines results of the past decade's cancer bioassays conducted by the National Toxicology Program (NTP), one cannot help but be amazed that potent genotoxic agents such as butadiene, which induce cancer over exposure concentrations covering several orders of magnitude, are given the same classification as chemicals such as *d*-limonene which are not genotoxic and only cause increases in tumors at doses that cause target organ toxicity. What does this tell us about these chemicals regarding the mechanisms involved in tumor induction and the potential risk for carcinogenesis to humans?

Obviously, these questions will not have simple answers. However, reducing human cancer through risk management requires being able to rank risks and to evaluate where the greatest gains will be made per dollar expended. To achieve the highest possible risk reduction in the presence of financial limits, different degrees of risk management will be required for different chemicals. We may progress faster by first reducing exposures that result in the greatest and most efficient risk reduction. Efficient risk management systems will, however, require a better understanding than we have of the mechanisms involved in positive carcinogen bioassays.

Spontaneous mutations leading to cancer are well documented in rodents (1–7) and human beings (7–10). Persistent increases in cell proliferation that result from high-dose chemical toxicity can markedly alter both initiation of carcinogenesis and clonal expansion of spontaneously initiated cells. If the carcinogenic response is caused by increases in cell proliferation that are not relevant to human exposure, these chemicals do not pose human health concerns. Spending public or private funds for risk management of these chemicals would therefore dilute efforts aimed at cancer control. The best way to deal with such issues is to have a cancer control policy that utilizes scientific data on mechanisms. When agents are carcinogenic in animals due to secondary factors that do not occur in humans, they would not be regulated in the same manner as agents likely to have carcinogenic potential in humans. Cell proliferation data may be of great importance for determining whether or not an agent falls into this category. In addition, knowing dose-response relationships for cell proliferation adds tremendous insight to downward extrapolation of high-dose risks for carcinogens posing potential risk to humans.

Role of cell proliferation in mutagenesis and carcinogenesis

DNA synthesis is required for causing mutations, that is, converting DNA damage to heritable events passed on to the daughter cell (11). Most data that support this conclusion were developed using genotoxic agents that covalently bind to DNA, forming adducts. It is now recognized that DNA-damaging events also occur frequently in normal cells. Estimates of these events' occurrence range from 50,000 (12) to nearly 250,000 (13) per cell per day (Table 1). Cells have several DNA repair pathways that correct this spontaneous DNA damage efficiently, so that the many spontaneous DNA-damaging events cause few mutations (12). DNA repair is a time-dependent process. Synchronized cells exposed to mutagens at the G_1/S interface develop much higher mutation frequencies than cells exposed in early G_1 interface (14,15). Likewise, cells deficient in DNA repair capability have higher mutation frequencies than normal cells (16–18). Anything, therefore, that reduces the time a cell has available for DNA repair will raise the probability of mutation. If cell proliferation is increased by chemical intoxification, clearly the time available to such cells for DNA repair will be reduced. Thus, more DNA adducts will remain as the cell enters S-phase, increasing the probability of mutational events. When such mutations occur at critical sites in the genome, the carcinogenic process is initiated. Critical mutations may confer a selective

Table 1. Approximate Rates of DNA Damage and Repair in Human Cells.

Type of damage	Estimated occurrences of damage per hour per cell[a]	Estimated maximal repair rate, base pairs per hour per cell[b]
Endogenous		
Depurination	1,000	b
Depyrimidination	55	b
Cytosine deamination	15	b
Single-strand breaks	5,000	2×10^5
N^7-methylguanine	3,500	Not reported
O^6-methylguanine	130	10^4
Oxidation products	120	10^5
Exogenous		
Background ionizing radiation		
Single-strand breaks	10^{-4}	2×10^5
Oxidation damage	10^{-4}–10^{-3}	10^5
Ultraviolet damage of skin (noon Texas sunlight)		
Primidine dimers	5×10^4	5×10^4

Source: Modified from *Drinking Water and Health: Selected Issues in Risk Assessment* (13).
[a] Might be higher or lower by a factor of 2.
[b] Not reported, but rates are at least 10^4, to judge from concentration of repair activities in cell extracts.

growth advantage, loss of homeostatic controls, genetic instability, and other predisposing characteristics on these cells.

Stimulation of cell proliferation may also result in clonal expansion of the initiated cells, which then increases the probability of additional genetic events occurring in these cells, a factor that appears to be involved in the progression from initiation to benign, malignant, and metastatic neoplasms (Fig. 1) (19).

Use of cell proliferation in setting doses for chronic studies

Many chemicals cause toxicity in target organs that result in individual cell necrosis. The tissue responds to the cell loss by increasing the rate of cell proliferation. Routine pathologic examination is a rather insensitive tool for assaying these changes—at best it is qualitative. Recent advances in the methods of quantitating cell proliferation permit the generation of valuable data with minimal impact on the time, cost, and personnel required for subchronic and chronic toxicity testing. Therefore, given the importance of cell proliferation to the temporal development of tumors, it is important that we incorporate the collection of cell proliferation data in protocols for evaluating carcinogenic potential.

The preferred protocols for evaluating cell proliferation are discussed in other chapters of this book. Suffice it to say here that the use of osmotic minipumps that deliver [^{3}H]thymidine ([^{3}H]Tdr) or bromodeoxyuridine (BrdU) offer the greatest sensitivity in that they label all cells passing through S-phase for a period of days. This alleviates problems with circadian rhythms, increases the number of labeled over unlabeled cells,

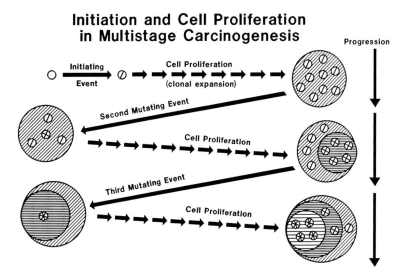

Figure 1. Initiation and cell proliferation in multistage carcinogenesis.

and reduces the margins of error. In general, 7–10 animals should be added to each dose group of a subchronic study. These animals should be treated like other members of the dose group, except for pump implantation during the last week of exposure. BrdU has several advantages over [^{3}H]Tdr: First, it is without radioactive hazard; second, commercially available antibodies and well-established immunohistochemical methods permit any laboratory to set up the technique; and, finally, while both methods can be applied to all tissues, immunohistochemistry is much less time consuming. The pathologist can get a qualitative impression by scanning the slides and then quantitating target tissues and any other tissues which appear to show increased labeling.

Interpretation and use of quantitative data on cell proliferation will undoubtedly evolve during the next few years as more information becomes available. This data will be helpful in better defining the MTD, which is a complex process with multiple endpoints requiring consideration. Meanwhile, however, we must begin to collect and use quantitative cell proliferation data in setting doses for carcinogenicity studies in rodents. It is unreasonable to expect a tissue subjected to 10- to 20-fold increases in cell proliferation for months to years to accurately reflect human health risks resulting from very much lower exposure to the same chemical. The exact point at which an MTD based on cell proliferation should be set can only be approximated at this time, but a sustained three- to four-fold increase is likely to be both statistically and biologically significant. Increases in cell proliferation of this magnitude change the tumor response slope of genotoxic carcinogens (20–22). Based on the few examples of nongenotoxic carcinogens that result from secondary mechanisms that increase cell proliferation, i.e., saccharin, d-limonene, and unleaded gasoline, it seems that the carcinogenic effect requires five- to 20-fold increases in cell proliferation (23–28). In addition to dose-response relationships in toxicity, a recent study by Bogdanffy et al. (29) demonstrated that cell proliferation data also provides information on saturation of metabolic activation.

Cell proliferation data should be used also when setting the middle and low doses. Because neither of these doses increases cell proliferation, secondary mechanisms involving cell proliferation should not be invoked to explain positive results at middle- and low-exposure doses. In addition, if human exposure to the chemical under investigation occurs only at comparably low doses, quantitative risk assessment can be based on data from the two lower doses, with confidence that the results will not be confounded by cell proliferation.

Perspectives

Advances in methods and understanding of multistage carcinogenesis provide a strong rationale for redesigning subchronic toxicity protocols so that they evaluate sustained effects on cell proliferation. Many chemicals induce only transient increases in cell proliferation. It is unlikely that these increases cause enough spontaneous genetic events to result in increased initiation, promotion and progression of carcinogenesis. For this reason, use of acute-administration data is less desirable and may confound the approach proposed above.

Not all chemicals that increase cell proliferation are expected to be carcinogenic. If initiated cells are more sensitive to intoxication, they will be killed selectively and not progress to malignancy. In addition, some mitogenic responses are followed by programmed cell death when the mitogen is removed (which is discussed in other chapters), and these cells do not appear to form neoplasms.

Among new methods for quantitating cell proliferation that are evolving is the use of antibodies to proliferating cell nuclear antigen (PCNA) to identify cycling cells (30–32). The advantage of this antigen is that it is present naturally, and no exogenous substance needs to be administered to the test animals. Use of PCNA would make retrospective studies of previously tested chemicals possible. An auxiliary protein of DNA polymerase *delta*, PCNA is present in high concentration in nuclei of cells in late G_1/S-, S-, G_2-phase, and mitosis (33). Thus, immunohistochemically, PCNA identifies a larger segment of the cell cycle of proliferating cells than methods using [^{3}H]Tdr or BrdU. The PCNA technique does not permit an accumulation of labeled cells as is done with minipumps, and, currently, PCNA immunohistochemical analysis still suffers from problems of reproducibility from tissue to tissue, of fixation, and other difficulties (34–36). Reproducible results are likely when the original methods are modified (Foley, Maronpot, Swenberg, Dietrich, paper in preparation).

In summary, incorporation of cell proliferation data into dose-setting for and interpretation of chronic carcinogenicity studies represents an exciting opportunity to improve the scientific basis of cancer risk assessment in human beings. More accurate predictions of human risk will permit prioritizing chemicals and the extent of risk management necessary to maximize risk reduction in humans.

References

1. Balmain A, Ramsden M, Bowden G, Smith J. Activation of the mouse cellular Harvey-*ras* gene in chemically induced benign skin papillomas. Nature 307:658–660, 1984.
2. Sukumar S, Notario V, Martin-Zanca D, Barbacid M. Induction of mammary carcinomas in rats by nitroso-methyurea involves malignant activation of H-*ras*-1 locus by single point mutation. Nature 306:658–661, 1983.
3. Wiseman R, Stowers S, Miller E, Anderson M, Miller J. Activating mutations of the c-Ha-*ras* proto-oncogene in chemically induced hepatomas of the male B6C3F1 mouse. Proc Natl Acad Sci 83:5285–5289, 1986.
4. Stowers SJ, Glover PL, Reynolds SH, Boone LR, Maronpot RR, Anderson MW. Activation of the K-*ras* proto-oncogene in lung tumors from rats and mice chronically exposed to tetranitromethane. Cancer Res 47:3212–3219, 1987.
5. Reynolds SH, Stowers SJ, Patterson RM, Maronpot RR, Aaronson SA, Anderson MW. Activated oncogenes in B6C3F1 mouse liver tumors: Implications for risk assessment. Science 11:1309–1316, 1987.
6. You M, Candrian U, Maronpot RR, Stoner GD, Anderson MW. Activation of the Ki-*ras* proto-oncogene in spontaneously occurring and chemically induced lung tumors of the strain *A* mouse. Proc Natl Acad Sci 86:3070–3074, 1989.
7. Anderson MW, Maronpot RR, Reynolds SH. Role of oncogenes in chemical carcinogenesis: Extrapolation from rodents to humans. In: Bartsch H, Hemminiki K, O'Neill IK (eds): Methods for Detecting DNA Damaging Agents in Humans: Applications in Cancer Epidemiology and Prevention. Lyon: IARC Scientific Publications, 1988, pp. 477–485.
8. Vogelstein B, Fearon ER, Hamilton SR, Kern SE, Preisinger AC, Leppert M, Nakamura Y, White R, Smits AMM, Bos JL. Genetic alterations during colorectal-tumor development. N Engl J Med 319:525–532, 1988.
9. Rodenhuis S, Slebos RJ, Boot AJ, Evers SG, Mooi WJ, Wagenaar SS, Van Bodegom PC, Bos JL. Incidence and possible clinical significance of K-*ras* oncogene activation in adenocarcinoma of the human lung. Cancer Res 48:5738–5741, 1988.

10. Forrester K, Almoguera C, Han K, Grizzle W, Perucho M. Detection of high incidence of K-*ras* oncogenes during human colon tumorigenesis. Nature 327:298–303, 1987.
11. Swenberg JA, Fedtke N, Fennell TR, Walker VE. Relationships between carcinogen exposure, DNA adducts and carcinogenesis. In: Clayson DB, Munro IC, Shubik P, Swenberg JA (eds): Progress in Predictive Toxicology. Amsterdam: Elsevier Science Publishers, 1990, pp. 161–184.
12. Loeb L. Endogenous carcinogenesis: Molecular oncology into the twenty-first century: Presidential address. Cancer Res 49:5489–5496, 1989.
13. Drinking Water and Health: Selected Issues in Risk Assessment, vol. 9, Washington, D.C.: National Academy Press, 1989.
14. Maher VM, McCormick J. Role of DNA lesions and excision repair in carcinogen-induced mutagenesis and transformation in human cells. In: Grein H, Jung R, Kramer M, Marquardt H, Oesch F (eds): Biochemical Basis of Chemical Carcinogenesis. New York: Raven Press, 1984, pp. 143–158.
15. Yang LL, Maher VM, McCormick JJ. Relationship between excision repair and the cytotoxic and mutagenic effect of the anti-7,8-diol-9,10-epoxide of benzo[*a*]pyrene in human cells. Mutat Res 94:435–447, 1982.
16. Simon L, Hazard RM, Maher VM, McCormick JJ. Enhanced cell killing and mutagenesis by ethylnitrosourea in xeroderma pigmentosum cells. Carcinogenesis 2:567–570, 1981.
17. Domoradzki J, Pegg AE, Dolan ME, Maher VM, McCormick JJ. Depletion of O^6-methylguanine-DNA-methyltransferase in human fibroblasts increases the mutagenic response to N-methyl-N'-nitro-N-nitrosoguanidine. Carcinogenesis 6:1823–1826, 1985.
18. Maher VM, Domoradzki J, Corner RC, McCormick JJ. Correlation between O^6-alkylguanine-DNA alkytransferase activity and resistance of human cells to the cytotoxic and mutagenic effects of methylating and ethylating agents. In: Harris CC (ed): Biochemical and Molecular Epidemiology of Cancer. Philadelphia: Alan R. Liss, 1986, pp.411–418.
19. Swenberg JA, Richardson FC, Boucheron JA, Deal FH, Belinsky SA, Charbonneau, Short BG. High-to low-dose extrapolation: Critical determinants involved in the dose-response to carcinogenic substances. Environ Health Perspect 76:57–63, 1987.
20. Deal FH, Richardson FC, Swenberg JA. Dose response of hepatocyte replication following continuous exposure to diethylnitrosamine. Cancer Res 49:6985–6988, 1989.
21. Monticello TM, Morgan KT, Everitt JI, Popp JA. Effects of formaldehyde gas on the respiratory tract of rhesus monkeys. Am J Pathol 134:515–527, 1989.
22. Cohen SM, Ellwein LB. Proliferative and genotoxic cellular effects in 2-acetylaminofluorene bladder and liver carcinogenesis: Biological modeling of the ED01 study. Toxicol Appl Pharmacol 104:79–93, 1990.
23. Cohen SM, Ellwein LB. Cell growth dynamics in long-term bladder carcinogenesis. Toxicol Lett 43:151–173, 1988.
24. Ellwein LB, Cohen SM. A cellular dynamics model of experimental bladder cancer: Analysis of the effect of sodium saccharin in the rat. Risk Anal 8:215–221, 1988.
25. Ellwein LB, Cohen SM. Comparative analyses of the timing and magnitude of genotoxic and nongenotoxic cellular effects in urinary bladder carcinogenesis. In: Travis CC (ed): Biologically-Based Methods for Cancer Risk Assessment. New York: Plenum, 1989, pp. 181–192.
26. Short BG, Burnett VL, Cox MG, Bus JS, Swenberg JA. Site-specific renal cytotoxicity and cell proliferation in male rats exposed to petroleum hydrocarbons. Lab Invest 57:564–577, 1987.
27. Short BG, Burnett VL, Swenberg JA. Elevated proliferation of proximal tubule cells and localization of accumulated $\alpha_{2\mu}$-globulin in F344 rats during chronic exposure to unleaded gasoline or 2,2,4-trimethylpentane. Toxicol Appl Pharmacol 101:414–431, 1989.
28. Dietrich DR, Swenberg JA. Alpha$_{2\mu}$-globulin is necessary for d-dimonene promotion of male rat kidney tumors. Toxicologist, in press.
29. Bogdanffy MS, Kee CR, Kelly DP, Carakostas MC, Sykes GP. Subchronic inhalation study with vinyl fluoride: Effects on hepatic cell proliferation and urinary fluoride excretion. Fundam Appl Toxicol 15:394–406, 1990.
30. Ogato K, Kurki P, Celis JE, Nakamura RM, Tan EM. Monoclonal antibodies to a nuclear protein (PCNA/cyclin) associated with DNA replication. Exp Cell Res 168:475–486, 1987.
31. Robbins BA, de la Vega D, Ogata Kenji, Tan EM, Nakamura RM. Immunohistochemical detection of proliferating cell nuclear antigen in solid human malignancies. Arch Pathol Lab Med 111:841–845, 1987.
32. So AG, Downey KM. Mammalian DNA polymerases alpha and delta: Current status in DNA replication. Biochemistry 27:4591–4595, 1988.

33. Celis JE, Madsen P, Celis A, Nielsen HV, Gesser B. Cyclin (PCNA, auxiliary protein of DNA polymerase delta) is a central component of the pathway(s) leading to DNA replication and cell division. Federation European Biochemical Society 220:1–7, 1987.

34. Galand P, Degraef C. Cyclin/PCNA immunostaining as an alternative to tritiated thymidine pulse labelling for marking S-phase cells in paraffin sections from animal and human tissues. Cell Tissue Kinet 22:383–392, 1989.

35. Garcia RL, Coltrera MD, Gown AM. Analysis of proliferative grade using anti-PCNA cyclin monoclonal antibodies in fixed, embedded tissues: Comparison with flow cytometric analysis. Am J Pathol 134:733–739, 1989.

36. Thaete LG, Ahmen DJ, Malkinson AM. Proliferating cell nuclear antigen (PCNA/cyclin) immunocytochemistry as a labeling in mouse lung tissues. Cell Tissue Res 256:167–173, 1989.

Chemically Induced Cell Proliferation:
Implications for Risk Assessment, pages 253-284
©1991 Wiley-Liss, Inc.

Guidelines for Measuring Chemically Induced Cell Proliferation in Specific Rodent Target Organs

Thomas L. Goldsworthy, Kevin T. Morgan, James A. Popp, and Byron E. Butterworth

The importance of induced cell proliferation in toxicology and carcinogenesis

Carcinogenesis is a complex process involving sequential mutations in normal cellular growth control genes with subsequent clonal growth of the preneoplastic or neoplastic cells. Chemical carcinogens may act both by inducing mutations and altering cellular growth control genes. Increasing attention has been focused on chemicals that induce cancer in rodent bioassays yet do not exhibit the traditional characteristics of genotoxicity. Cell proliferation induced by such nongenotoxic carcinogens is a common denominator in the pathogenesis of many rodent tumors. The induction of cell proliferation is also being implicated in the formation of many human tumors (see the chapter by Preston-Martin et al. in this volume). Since carcinogens seem to act through various mechanisms and at different stages in the process of carcinogenesis, the ability to distinguish the carcinogens' mechanism of action and to establish whether these events are likely to occur in human beings becomes critical.

A glossary of terms describing events related to chemically induced cell proliferation is presented in Table 1. Induced cell replication has been conceptually hypothesized or experimentally demonstrated to play a role in every step of chemical carcinogenesis (1–5). Such chemicals might induce a proliferative response by interacting with cellular receptors and growth factors, causing cell death and subsequent regenerative growth, interrupting tissue growth control mechanisms such as cell-to-cell communication, and inhibiting programmed cell death (apoptosis).

A chemical that does not exhibit genotoxic activity may produce tumors nevertheless when it is subjected to a long-term bioassay. Although the mechanisms of such nongenotoxic carcinogens remain largely unknown, tumors observed in bioassays often seem to be related to the organ-specific toxicity resulting from administration of high doses of a chemical. This raises concern about the relevance of some of these observations to predicting carcinogenesis in people exposed to low levels of the chemical. Gathering data on chemically induced cell proliferation in studies that precede a cancer bioassay could provide valuable information for the rational selection of both high and low doses for long-term studies. All biologically relevant information on the test chemical must be used when choosing appropriate test dosages. Further, information on a chemical's ability to induce proliferation in the target organ may be critical for interpreting the final outcome of a rodent bioassay.

Table 1. Glossary of Terms.

Additive hyperplasia: Cell growth induced by a mitogenic stimulus.

Apoptosis: Physiological process of programmed single-cell death.

Cell proliferation: Enhanced growth of a selected population of cells as observed in a growing or regenerating tissue through increased cell replication.

Cell replication: Production of two daughter cells by the process of replicative DNA synthesis and subsequent cell division.

Cell turnover: The steady-state rates of cell replication and cell death in a tissue.

Cytotoxicants: Chemicals that cause cell toxicity or cell death or both.

Hyperplasia: Increase in the size of a tissue through an increase in cell number.

Hypertrophy: Increase in the size of a tissue through an increase in cell size.

Labeling index (LI): Percentage of labeled cells.

Mitogens: Chemicals that induce cell proliferation with little or no cytotoxicity.

Mitotic index (MI): Percentage of cells undergoing mitosis.

Regenerative proliferation: Cell division required to replace dead cells.

S phase: Synthesis phase portion of the cell cycle in which nuclear DNA is replicated. During S phase, DNA precursors [^{3}H]thymidine and analogues such as bromodeoxyuridine (BRdU) are incorporated into the DNA.

Unit length-labeling index (ULLI): Number of labeled cells per unit length of basement membrane.

Although the cell replication rate is intricately involved in the carcinogenic process, the body contains rapidly proliferating tissues in which cancer is rare. In the small intestine, for example, where cells proliferate at a very high rate, spontaneous tumor frequency is low. Cell populations that normally proliferate at a high rate must have inherent mechanisms to repair genetic damage or eliminate altered cells before cancer progression can occur. Thus, the magnitude or altered induction of proliferation, or both, over that of normal cellular processes may be critical in the development of cancer.

To date, short-term tests for carcinogens rely almost entirely on genotoxic end points. It is becoming increasingly clear that assays of mutagenicity are inappropriate for detecting carcinogens whose primary biologic activity is not genotoxicity. Short-term tests based on chemically induced cell proliferation might have predictive value for certain classes of nongenotoxic carcinogens (see the chapter by Butterworth in this volume). At the present time, however, it is not possible to use induced cell proliferation as a short-term test for carcinogenic potential because of the lack of a quantitative data base that relates the extent and duration of chemically induced cell proliferation under bioassay conditions to carcinogenic activity. For example, chemicals may induce only brief alteration in cell proliferation or induce proliferation in nonsusceptible cells in the target tissue—neither event may be adequate to lead to an increased tumor incidence. Furthermore, growth alterations exhibited early in nonlesion tissue may not reflect activity exhibited later in preneoplastic lesions. The predictive value of in vitro and in vivo genotoxicity assays is often judged by simplistic plus/minus versus carcinogen/noncarcinogen comparisons. In the case of chemically induced cell proliferation, experimental conditions, target organ specificity, and quantitative dose response relationships must be evaluated.

Chemically induced cell proliferation

In general, two broad classes of chemicals induce cell proliferation. In the first class are directly mitogenic agents; in the liver, this includes such agents as α-hexachlorocyclohexane and polybrominated biphenyls. Mitogens induce additive hyperplasia (increased organ-to-body weight ratios) with little or no cytotoxicity; in the liver this is indicated by a lack of detectable liver-specific enzymes in the serum (6,7). As the liver reaches its new larger size, the rate of hepatocyte cell turnover may return to background levels or remain elevated. In preneoplastic foci of altered cells, however, cell turnover rates may remain substantially elevated as long as the chemical continues to be administered. A peak of S-phase DNA synthesis usually occurs in hepatocytes at about 24–36 hr following a single administration of one of these agents. As a class, these compounds range from very weak carcinogenic agents such as di(2-ethylhexyl)phthalate to potent carcinogens such as ciprofibrate (8–10).

In the second class of chemicals that induce cell proliferation are agents that produce cytotoxicity or cytolethality, or both, and result in regenerative cell growth. Administration of hepatotoxic chemicals results in histopathologic lesions and the release of enzymes into the serum, which indicates toxicity (11). Regenerative hyperplasia occurs to replace the damaged tissue. In hepatocytes, a peak of cell proliferation is usually seen at about 48 hr after a single administration of one of these agents. Examples of such chemicals are carbon tetrachloride and furan (12,13).

Among the many procedures for studying chemically induced cell proliferation are two commonly used methods for assessing the extent of cell replication: the labeling index (LI), which measures the percentage of cells that have incorporated a specific DNA precursor label over a period of time, and the mitotic index (MI), which measures the percentage of cells undergoing mitosis at a given time (14,15). The MI is a more precise measure of cell replication, but the LI is more sensitive to increases in cell replication because mitosis is a more transient event in the cell cycle and results in the observation of a low number of mitotic figures. Cells labeled in the DNA-synthesis phase of the cell cycle (S phase) are more readily recognized than those in mitosis and thus provide a clearer identification of the labeled cell (Fig. 1).

Currently, our information is insufficient to define quantitatively the relationship between extent and duration of chemically induced cell proliferation and carcinogenic potential in different species and target organs. Measurement of the extent and duration of chemically induced proliferation in conjunction with such other parameters as histopathology, oncogene and growth-factor expression, and enzyme induction is likely to be important in understanding the relationship of cell replication to carcinogenesis. That chemicals may influence the likelihood of cancer by affecting either or both genotoxic and proliferative activity should be emphasized. The available data on chemically induced cell proliferation have been obtained by use of widely divergent protocols, making comparisons among the different data sets difficult, if not impossible (16–19). We present suggested protocols and guidelines that focus on methods to measure cell proliferation related to nasal, renal, and hepatic carcinogenesis, with the goal of readily comparing information generated by different laboratories in the future. Many laboratories already measure cell proliferation or could easily incorporate this end point into acute or 90-day studies.

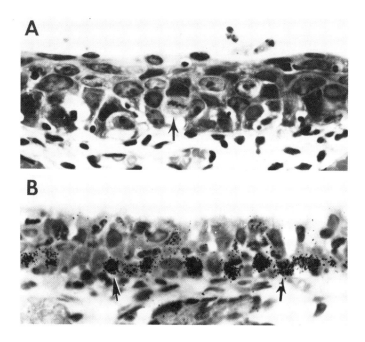

Figure 1. Photomicrographs of rat nasal septum, following exposure to 10 ppm of formaldehyde, demonstrating relative frequency and detection of (A) mitotic figure, and (B) labeled replicating cells (arrows).

Measuring cell proliferation

Animals

If a cancer bioassay has been performed or the laboratory has a historic data base for a particular strain of rodent, it is rational to continue using that strain. But if the laboratory has no such data or experience, the use of F344 rats and B6C3F1 mice is reasonable because the National Toxicology Program (NTP) provides an extensive historic data base. When examining a known carcinogen, the gender and strain employed in the bioassay should be used. If tumors were produced in one gender or species but not the other, the corresponding comparison for induction of cell replication would be valuable for correlating cell proliferation and carcinogenicity. Whenever possible, animal husbandry factors used during the conduct of the cell replication experiments should be like those used in the chronic bioassay. Rodents known to be pathogen-free should be used because murine diseases may markedly affect cell turnover in important target organs.

The animals' age is critically important. During the first 8 weeks of the post-weaning growth period the LI in liver and other organs is high, and it may remain somewhat elevated for up to 10 weeks. Mature adult rodents 10–12 weeks of age should be used to avoid variations in control baseline LI values. Since some bioassays begin with animals as young as 6 weeks, young animals should be used to match bioassay conditions. Irrespective of the age of the animals used, appropriate controls should be included at each time point. Experiments should be designed so that at least five animals per group are available for analysis of cell proliferation.

Dose selection

In correlating S-phase response with carcinogenesis, the same doses and dosing regimen employed in the bioassay should be chosen. If one can produce cell proliferation at massive doses that were not or would not be used in a bioassay, the results will have limited value in mechanistic considerations or in developing a predictive risk model. Multiple dose groups are recommended. It is particularly instructive to compare cell proliferation results obtained from a high dose of chemical that produced tumors to those of a low dose that did not. If no cancer data or preliminary studies are available for the chemical of interest, the high dose should be one that is expected to be chosen as the maximum tolerated dose. If it is possible to test additional doses, a lower dose should be selected that probably would not be toxic to nor cause cell proliferation in the target organ in question. The basis for this decision may require a preliminary study of the cell proliferation or histopathology, or both, of tissue from a pilot experiment. An agent's route of administration and pharmacokinetic factors also may greatly affect the animal's response to the chemical. Whenever possible, the route of administration used in the bioassay should be employed. If no cancer data or other relevant information is available, the human exposure route for that particular agent should be used.

Treatment

Everyday chemical administration. In the case of daily oral administration, the chemical is continually available by incorporation in the animal's food or water. Because rodents usually feed at night, chemical ingestion takes place at that time. The baseline LI in the livers of control rats shifts throughout the day (Fig. 2). Many environmental factors including diet, light exposure, and hormonal status can modify the observed chemically induced cell proliferation response, and such factors may be responsible in part for the large variation in LI often seen among animals seemingly treated alike. When attempting to reduce variation, lighting cycles and the timing of food consumption should be kept consistent. Animals must be adequately adapted to lighting and feeding schedules before chemical treatment begins.

Schulte-Hermann (20) demonstrated that hepatic cell proliferation induced by α-hexachlorocyclohexene in female Wistar rats was influenced by food intake, which in turn was influenced by the lighting cycle. As a study (11) of the influences of feeding and light cycles in the liver of male F344 rats exposed to trimethylpentane (TMP) showed, rat hepatic replicative DNA synthesis activity induced by TMP peaked at 13 hr following the change from light to dark on the previous night, irrespective of controlled feeding times. The response pattern indicated that, in this case, the light-dark rhythm and not the time of food administration was the dominant influence on timing the TMP-induced replicative response. Controlled feeding schedules are useful for understanding diurnal rhythms and other factors involved in the proliferative response (21,22), but the

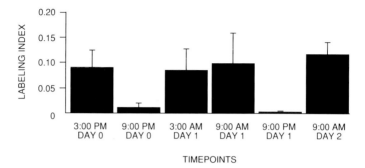

Figure 2. Time course of cell replication in hepatocytes after administration of a single dose of corn oil to male F344 rats. Animals ($N = 5$) were given 1 ml of corn oil by gavage at 9 A.M. (day 0). [3H]Thymidine (1 mCi/kg of body weight[BW]) was administered by intraperitoneal injection 2 hr before each scheduled sacrifice. Labeling index (mean ± SEM) was calculated from scoring at least 2,000 hepatocyte nuclei from computer-generated, randomly selected fields in the left hepatic lobe of each rat.

disadvantage of this procedure is that it no longer conforms to chronic chemical administration under bioassay conditions.

The DNA precursor label must be administered during the same time of day before each animal's sacrifice because various chemical treatments may shift the labeling pattern. This problem can be minimized by using the pump-labeling method rather than the pulse technique. Our recommendation is that animals be sacrificed in the morning and that each study adhere to a consistent time frame.

Five days/week chemical administration. Many inhalation and gavage studies are conducted based on only Monday-through-Friday exposures. For the Five Days/Week Chemical Administration—Six-Day Pump Label protocol (see appendix), Sunday implant times were chosen to avoid surgical procedures on the day of an inhalation exposure or gavage treatment. The Saturday sacrifice time results in [3H]thymidine or 5-bromodeoxyuridine (BRdU) delivery throughout the 5-day chemical treatment period with necropsy the morning after the last day of treatment. If working on the weekend is an insurmountable problem, the labeling period could be shifted to implantation on Wednesday, with sacrifice the following Tuesday, or a similar weekday schedule. Such a 6-day labeling period will, however, include the 2 weekend days during which there was no treatment, and it may result in a lower LI response. Note that for the 5-day/week dosing schedule, a Monday sacrifice would mean no chemical administration during the preceding 2 days. Stopping chemical administration may result in a very rapid return of LI to baseline. A Monday sacrifice should therefore be avoided, particularly with pulse labeling, because it will probably result in substantial reductions either in the percentage of cells in S phase or in such ancillary parameters as serum enzymes, number of hepatocyte peroxisomes, or gene expression. The Five Days/Week Chemical Administration—Three-Day Pump Label procedure (see appendix) that can be conducted during a single exposure week may be the preferred protocol if the above-mentioned situations are to be avoided.

Single dose of chemical. A small data base for cell proliferation following a single chemical treatment has been generated using the in vivo–in vitro hepatocyte DNA repair assay (18), and others have examined the stimulation of DNA synthesis at 24 hr after a single chemical treatment (23). Although the latter protocol provides insight as to whether a chemical's single dose is capable of inducing proliferation, it provides little information on chemically induced proliferation after chronic exposure or under bioassay conditions.

Mitogenically induced liver hyperplasia generally has a maximal S-phase response at about 24 hr following a single dose of chemical, with no hepatocyte necrosis or liver-specific enzymes in the serum (11). 4-Acetylaminofluorene (4-AAF) produces a mitogenic response (Fig. 3) with no observed toxicity as indicated histopathologically and by a lack of liver-specific enzymes in the serum (Fig. 4) (24). Regenerative liver hyperplasia generally does not show a maximal S-phase response until 48 hr following a single dose of chemical. Hepatocyte necrosis and liver-specific enzymes in the serum may be seen before S-phase synthesis peaks after administration of a cytotoxic agent. Furan produces hepatic cell regeneration (Fig. 3) following significant hepatocytotoxicity (Fig. 4) (13). The occurrence of a significant proliferative response induced by a chemical without histopathologic lesions or serum enzyme elevations demonstrates how sensitive the assessment of proliferative changes may be.

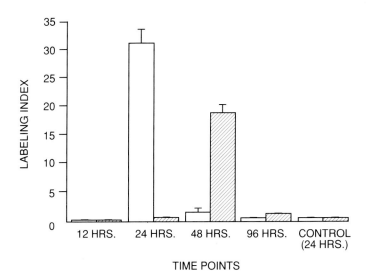

Figure 3. Mitogenic versus regenerative chemically induced cell proliferation response in rat liver. Male F344 rats ($N = 5$) were administered a single dose of 4-AAF (500 mg/kg BW) (open bar) or furan (300 mg/kg BW) (hatched bar) in corn oil by gavage at 10 A.M. ($t = 0$) and sacrificed 12, 24, 48, and 96 hr later. [^{3}H]thymidine (1 mCi/kg BW) was administered intraperitoneally 2 hr before each scheduled sacrifice. LI (mean ± SEM) was calculated from scoring at least 2,000 hepatocyte nuclei from computer-generated, randomly selected fields in the left lobe of each rat. Note the sharp LI peak that occurs at different times after 4-AAF and furan administration.

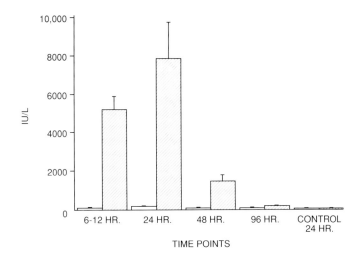

Figure 4. Effects of 4-acetylaminofluorene (4-AAF, open bar) and furan (hatched bar) on serum enzyme levels in male F344 rats. Animals (*N* = 5) were administered a single dose (500 mg/kg BW) of 4-AAF or furan (30 mg/kg BW) in corn oil by gavage at 10 A.M.(t = 0) and sacrificed 6 (4-AAF), 2 (furan), 24, 48, and 96 hr later. Blood collected by cardiac puncture was allowed to coagulate at room temperature for at least 30 min. Samples were spun at 2,000 × *g* to separate red blood cells from serum, and serum was stored at 4°C. Alanine aminotransferase (ALT) values (IU/liter) were determined on an Abbott VP Biochromatic Analyzer using an activated reagent in a modification of the methods described by Bergmeyer et al. (65). Note the large increase in ALT levels seen only after furan treatment despite the relatively similar magnitude of LI (Fig. 3). Similar results (data not shown) are observed with AST serum levels.

Nasal epithelium, after multiple exposures to cytotoxic agents, may undergo an initial reparative phase that may last from days to weeks. This repair process is associated with a burst of cell proliferation that declines rapidly (25,26). Induction and decline of the cell proliferation response depends, in part, on the severity of the insult. Thus, optimization of postexposure time for S-phase determination is a difficult process that is chemical and organ dependent.

Choice of protocol. Suggested protocols for Everyday Chemical Administration and Five Days/Week Chemical Administration are presented in the appendix. Observations thus far indicate that, for these dosing regimens, the pump labeling method is the most sensitive and reliable technique for detecting the LI response after chronic chemical administration (16).

Several sacrifice times are suggested for the 90-day treatment schedules. Sacrifices at all time points may not be feasible because of the large number of animals needed. If only a limited number of sacrifice times can be scheduled, we suggest that cell proliferation responses at the start, middle, and end of a study (i.e., weeks 1, 6, and 13) provide the most useful information.

Control and treatment groups should be run at every time point. Erroneous conclusions may be drawn when data obtained in control animals at only one time point are compared to data obtained from treated animals at multiple times (27). Deleting selected treatment groups is preferable to reducing the numbers of animals per group to fewer than five.

The animals' health must be monitored throughout chemical administration. In the case of continuous oral chemical treatment, body weights should be recorded biweekly and consumption of feed or water containing the chemical monitored. Body and organ weights at sacrifice provide useful information. If other parameters such as serum enzymes or enzyme induction are measured, they should correspond to one or more of the sacrifice times given in the appendix.

Although the Single Dose of Chemical protocol (see appendix) is easier to follow than the other proliferation studies described, this assay has disadvantages when one interprets the significance of the data. Following a single administration, the LI response depends closely on the dose of chemical used, which precludes the use of such data in understanding the role of cell replication in neoplasia under bioassay conditions. Single administration of a chemical hardly reflects the tissue- and site-specific alterations or the complex S-phase patterns that often occur with chronic administration of a chemical. Marsman et al. (16) demonstrated the importance of measuring the extent and duration of chemically induced hepatic cell proliferation with the peroxisome-proliferating agents di(2-ethylhexyl)phalate (DEHP) and Wy-14,643 (WY). Both the weak carcinogen DEHP and the potent carcinogen WY induced a short burst of hepatic DNA synthesis, but only WY maintained enhanced hepatocyte replication upon its further administration. For these two agents, persistent elevation of cell proliferation exhibited the best correlation with carcinogenic potential; measurement of LI response after single doses would not provide the information needed to contrast the activity of these two chemicals adequately. Monticello and Morgan (28; see also the chapter by Monticello et al. in this volume) also demonstrated the importance of sustained increases in cell proliferation in the induction of formaldehyde-induced nasal carcinogenesis.

As laboratory teams design protocols that fit their needs best, the suggested protocols presented in the appendix may serve as guidelines. If, for example, additional time points are included, labeling and sacrifice times could be consistent with the given protocols. The more similar the protocols, the easier will it be to compare and contrast data generated by their use.

Labeling methods

Pulse labeling. This refers to a single administration of the DNA precursor label before an animal's sacrifice. In the case of [³H]thymidine, the label remains as thymidine in the body for only up to 30 min, resulting in a relatively brief labeling period (14). Since the pulse-labeling method gives an indication of the level of cell replication taking place at a specific time, pulse labeling would be the method of choice to define the shape of the LI curve after a single dose of chemical or during continuous chemical treatment. Advantages of the pulse-labeling technique compared to pump labeling include lower costs, lower amounts of label required, and fewer containment safety problems. When using [³H]thymidine, autoradiographic exposure periods tend to be shorter for pulse-labeled than for pump-labeled studies.

A critical issue in using the pulse-label technique to measure LI is knowing when to sacrifice animals in relation to chemical treatment. For example, if the period of elevated S-phase synthesis is short, such as at 24 hr following a single dose of a mitogen (Fig. 3) or only during morning hours following chronic chemical treatment (11), pulse labeling at slightly different times will give different results. One concern is the possibility that some chemicals will shift the period of peak DNA synthesis in an unknown manner.

According to the protocols suggested in the appendix, animals are administered label 2 hr before sacrifice. Although a pulse-administration time before sacrifice may be shortened to 30 min, a 2-hr pulse usually allows investigators time to inject and sacrifice a relatively large number of animals without an overlap of the two procedures. In general, sacrifices should be performed at a consistent time, for example, between 9 A.M. and noon. Animals should be sacrificed in the order in which they were pulsed to maintain a constant time between injection of the label and sacrifice. The pulse-dosing schedule may be staggered according to the time required for necropsy. Some investigators have employed multiple pulse-label doses to increase LI measurement sensitivity (15,29,30). The pulse-labeling technique has been used successfully in many organs including the liver, kidney, and nose.

Continuous labeling. As used in this chapter, this term refers to the continuous administration, for several days, of DNA-precursor by an osmotic pump placed under the animal's skin. Continuous labeling may also be achieved by repeated pulse injections or administration of DNA precursor by an implanted pellet. One advantage of continuous labeling is that all cells going into S phase during the period the pump is in place will be labeled and accumulated. Accordingly, diurnal variations in cell proliferation will affect the labeling index data minimally because the cells in S phase are summed over a substantial time period. The longer labeling period is most suitable for detecting slight changes in chemically induced S-phase rates.

Osmotic pumps, which deliver a solution continuously for a period of days or weeks, may be implanted subcutaneously or intraperitoneally. Pump specifications and rapid implant procedures are described in the suppliers' literature. Briefly, the animal is anesthetized and prepared for an aseptic surgical procedure. For subcutaneous implantation, the mid-dorsal lumbar area is shaved and prepared for surgery. An incision is made through the skin and a pocket is formed in the subcutaneous tissue. The pump is inserted into the incision with the pump opening forward. The incision is stapled or sutured closed. Subcutaneously implanted pumps have been used successfully to label cells in a variety of organs including the liver, kidney, and nose (16,31-34). The type of anesthetic drug used for the surgical implantation procedure should not interfere with the biologic endpoints being examined. For example, a gaseous respiratory tract irritant such as ether should not be used for anesthesia when respiratory cell proliferation is evaluated. Parenteral anesthetics (i.e., xyalzine/ketamine) may be used to avoid upper respiratory tract irritation induced by gas anesthetics. We have found isoflurane to be an excellent gas anesthetic for most proliferation studies because the depth of anesthesia can be accurately controlled by use of a precision vaporizer, and the animals recover quickly.

The Five Days/Week Chemical Administration—Six-Day Pump Label protocol in the appendix is designed for pump implant surgery to be performed on the night before the chemical treatment regimen begins, to avoid the interplay and overlap of anesthesia with chemical administration. In the Five Days/Week Chemical Administration—Three-Day Pump Label protocol for gavage studies, pumps should be implanted at least an hour before or after treatment. In the Five Days/Week Chemical Administration—Three-Day Pump Label protocol for inhalation studies, pumps might be implanted either on the night before or several hours before inhalation exposure and the animals allowed to recover from surgery before inhalation exposure. When using pump-labeling methods, one must be certain that the pump will not run out of label before the animal's sacrifice.

Choice of labeling method. Enhanced sensitivity of the continuous label compared to the pulse label was recently reported in a study by Marsman et al. (16), who measured hepatocyte LI after pulse- and pump-label [^{3}H]thymidine administration after 8, 18, or 39 days in control and WY-treated animals (Fig. 5). Only the WY-treated, pump-labeled animals (Fig. 5B) showed consistent LI elevations at all time points measured. The pulse-labeled, treated animals showed a slight increase in LI over controls only at day 18 (Fig. 5A). These results demonstrate the utility and enhanced sensitivity of the longer labeling period through use of an osmotic pump and raise some concerns about studies that depend only on the pulse-labeling method.

Because the pulse technique provides only a brief period of label availability, this method may result in a higher percentage of cells that are lightly labeled (i.e., a higher proportion of labeled cells just entering or leaving the S-phase period of the cell cycle). Consequently, pump-label studies may tend to score more accurately because of the fewer number of minimally labeled cells.

In the design of experimental protocols, a critical issue in measuring LI is determining when and how to investigate the induced proliferative response in relation to the chemical treatment regimen (Fig. 6). Thus, the decision to use pulse- or pump-label administration in a cell proliferation study depends on the experimental objective in question. Pulse studies are required when determining a relatively short time course in induction of cell proliferation and are most useful for defining the shape of an induced proliferation peak. Pump-label methods are capable of detecting initial peak LI responses as well as slight, sustained LI increases but will not give the shape of an initial peak. For evaluating the magnitude and extent of proliferation in longer-term studies, the pump-labeling procedure seems to be the method of choice.

Specific nuclear proteins are present in actively dividing but not resting cells. Recently, several monoclonal antibodies to cell cycle-related nuclear proteins have been developed that label proliferating cells preferentially. The proliferating cell nuclear antigen (PCNA), with peak concentrations seen in late G1/S phase, may prove to be one of the most versatile antibodies because it may be used to detect proliferating cells in both fixed, embedded tissues and frozen tissue samples (35-37). Similar to the immunohistochemical detection of nuclear protein antibodies in identifying proliferating cells is the use of in situ hybridization techniques to determine cellular mRNA level of proliferation-dependent genes (38). Both methods are microscopic slide-based analyses that allow joint evaluation of cell kinetics and histologic parameters. In addition, both methods may potentially be used for retrospective cell proliferation analyses of previously studied material. The two techniques, which do not require administration of a DNA precursor label, should result in an LI response similar to that of a pulse label for identifying chemically induced cell proliferation.

A

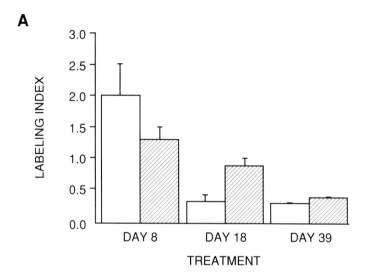

B

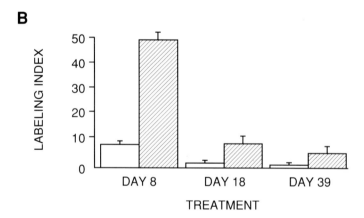

Figure 5. Comparison of LI determined by pulse- and pump-labeling methods (data taken from Marsman et al. [16]). Male F344 rats were fed NIH-07 chow (control, open bar) or NIH-07 chow blended with 0.2% WY-14,643 (WY, hatched bar). Animals were sacrificed on days 8, 18, and 39 of treatment. (A) LI determined in rats administered a pulse injection of [^{3}H]thymidine 2 hr before sacrifice. (B) LI determined in rats administered [^{3}H]thymidine via implanted osmotic pump 7 days before sacrifice. Note that scale on y-axis is much larger in graph (B). WY induced a statistically significant LI over controls in pump-labeled (B) but not pulse-labeled rats (A) at all time points measured.

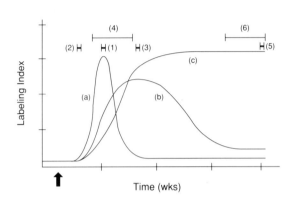

Figure 6 Selected hypothetical chemically induced cell proliferation scenarios. This graph demonstrates the complexity of experimental design with respect to time and type of label administration, and its relation to the interpretation of chemically-induced cell proliferation responses. ↑, start of chemical treatment; ⊢———⊣, single pulse-label administration; ⊢—⊣, continuous label administration (3–7 days) via implanted osmotic pump. Rapid peak of cell proliferation (curve a) would be detected by pulse label (1) but would be missed by pulse labels (2) and (3). Continuous pump label (4) would detect the cell proliferation response of curves (a), (b), or (c) but would not readily distinguish among them. At later time points, a clear response (curve c) would be detected by a pulse label (5), whereas a more subtle but still potentially important cell proliferation response (curve b) might be unobservable by pulse (5) and detected by pump label (6).

Label

[³H]*Thymidine.* This is the most commonly used radiolabeled DNA precursor. Its widespread use in cell proliferation studies is due to its availability in highly specific activity, the fact that its incorporation is restricted to DNA, and that its incorporation can be measured by a variety of techniques. Although perturbations of cell-cycle dynamics have been reported, it is generally assumed that low doses of [³H]thymidine do not affect normal cell function (39). The most common form of [³H]thymidine used is labeled on the methyl group. Ring-labeled thymidine is also available and may result in lower grain background problems because demethylation does not yield a labeled one-carbon product. In rodent cell-proliferation studies, the typical products for methyl-[³H]thymidine would have specific activities in the range of 25-90 Ci/mM and a concentration of 1 mCi/ml. Radioactive agents undergo chemical as well as radioactive decomposition that depends in part on temperature, sterility, and length of storage (15) so that, in general, [³H]thymidine should be refrigerated and stored no longer than one month.

An intraperitoneal (i.p.) injection of [³H]thymidine (1- or 2-mCi/kg body weight [BW]) can be used in pulse-label rodent experiments. For pump-label experiments with rats, an osmotic pump of 2-ml capacity with a pump rate of 10 μl/hr may be used. For pump-label experiments with mice, an osmotic pump of 200-μl capacity with a pump rate of 1 μl/hr for 6 days or an osmotic pump of 100-μl capacity with a pump rate of 1 μl/hr for 3 days may be used. The [³H]thymidine concentration used to fill pumps is 1 mCi/ml, and it may be used as received from the supplier without dilution.

Bromodeoxyuridine. BRdU is a thymidine analogue that has been used instead of [³H]thymidine to label a variety of tissues in vivo (19,31,40,41). BRdU-labeled DNA is visualized with immunohistochemical techniques (31). BRdU's hepatic proliferative activity (LI) in control and treated rodents was shown to be similar when compared to [³H]thymidine-labeling techniques (41,42). The relatively recent use of BRdU-labeling methods indicates, however, that caution should be used in selecting this technique and interpreting the results. Researchers should examine the dosages and methods described here and be aware of potential BRdU dose-related chemical interactions and toxicity on LI data. In our laboratory to date, BRdU methods have proved to be effective and reproducible.

BRdU is light-sensitive and should be handled only under incandescent lighting in a dark container wrapped in foil. BRdU (20 mg/ml) is dissolved in phosphate-buffered saline (PBS) while stirring and must be dissolved completely. Raising the pH slightly with 0.1N NaOH will help solubilize it. For pulse-labeled animals, 100 mg/kg BRdU is given by i.p. injection. Osmotic pumps filled with a 20 mg/ml BRdU solution may be used to deliver 10 μl/hr to rats or 1 μl/hr to mice over a period of days.

Detection and quantitation of label

Autoradiography. This topic, described extensively in the literature, will be discussed here only briefly. Tissue sections (2–8μ) are deparaffinized for autoradiography, dipped in nuclear track emulsion, and exposed in a dark, desiccated container at −15°C to −20°C for periods that are tissue- and treatment-dependent and range widely. For slides pump-labeled with [³H]thymidine as described here, the exposure period is about 4–10 weeks. In the case of pump [³H]thymidine-labeled rat livers, increasing the length of autoradiographic exposure from 1–7 weeks increases the LI dramatically, presumably because faintly labeled cells eventually release sufficient radiation to produce more silver grains (D.S. Marsman, personal communication). In general, shorter exposure periods are required for tissue sections from pulse-treated animals than for those from pump-treated animals. Two slides should be prepared per block of animal tissue so that the second set may serve as a backup. To choose the correct exposure time, additional test slides should be cut from a few of the tissue blocks and developed periodically; slides should be exposed to the point at which cells with labeled nuclei have a density of at least 10 silver grains. If the slides are underexposed, many cells will have few observable silver grains, which makes the decision whether to score a cell as undergoing DNA synthesis difficult and labor-intensive. If slides are overexposed, the silver grains may obscure visualization of the size and shape of the nucleus in the target cell type. Identification of the cell type is important because nontarget cells, including interstitial and inflammatory cells, may also be labeled. Of overriding importance in the process of autoradiography is the need for all control and treatment groups in an experiment to be processed identically. Specific factors, proper internal controls and potential problems in the use of [³H]thymidine and autoradiography have been reviewed by others (15,39).

Dark-field microscopy, in which the silver grains in labeled cells illuminate brightly against a dark background, may be used to scan an autoradiogram for areas to be scored. This allows the investigator to visualize cell-specific labeling sites and localized labeling patterns with ease.

Scintillation counting. These techniques of measuring [³H]thymidine incorporation are relatively easy to perform and have been used in many studies. One major disadvantage of the method is that it prevents simultaneous histopathologic evaluation of the same tissue area. A toxic insult to the liver may result in incorporation of DNA precursor into bile-duct cells, interstitial cells, and inflammatory cells in addition to hepatocytes. Furthermore, the cells' architecture may be changed dramatically by chemical treatment, and site-specific changes will not be detected. For example, when rats or mice are administered furan under treatment conditions similar to those that yielded tumors in a bioassay, areas of hepatic necrosis are infiltrated by inflammatory cells (43). Multiple cell types in addition to the hepatocyte are labeled, thereby artificially increasing the measure of thymidine incorporation by scintillation counting. When scintillation counting is done, a rigorous DNA extraction procedure should be used and time points should correspond to those presented in the appendix.

Bromodeoxyuridine immunohistochemistry. Immunohistochemical procedures are used to visualize BRdU-labeled DNA in a variety of tissues (31,41,44,45). The immunohistochemical methods to detect BRdU-labeled rat liver DNA at the Chemical Industry Institute of Toxicology (CIIT) are presented below (R. Randall and O. Lyght, personal communication). Tissue sections are fixed in 10% neutral buffered formalin and paraffin-embedded. Five- to seven-micron sections are cut and mounted on slides coated with 3-aminopropyltriethyloxysilane (APTS), to which the tissue adheres. Tissue sections are deparaffinized and rehydrated in graded alcohols. Slides are allowed to air-dry, and each section is circled with wax pen. Since the anti-BRdU antibody binds only to single-stranded DNA, tissue sections are treated with 1 N HCl for 1 hr at 40°C. After DNA denaturation, slides are rinsed in PBS. Tissue sections are treated with 0.05% protease for 20 min at 37°C to remove formalin-induced protein crosslinks (BRdU staining following enzyme digestion of formalin-fixed tissues has been shown to be as sensitive as with ethanol-fixed tissue [45]). Then the slides are washed in PBS, endogenous peroxidase is inhibited with 3% hydrogen peroxide in distilled water, and this is followed by another washing in PBS. Potential nonspecific binding sites are blocked with normal horse serum. Tissue sections are then flooded with the primary antibody, monoclonal mouse anti-BRdU diluted from 1:25–1:100 in PBS containing 0.5% Tween 20 and 1% bovine serum albumin (pH 7.6) at room temperature for 1 hr. Optimal antibody concentrations will vary among species and organs. Following a wash in PBS, tissue sections are flooded with a horse antimouse-avidin-biotinylated peroxidase complex for 30 min at room temperature. This secondary antibody may be diluted 1:100 or 1:200. The blocking serum and secondary antibody are available from various manufacturers as a kit. BRdU incorporation is visualized after a final incubation for 5–10 minutes in the peroxidase substrate, 3,3′-diaminobenzidine tetrahydrochloride (DAB) plus nickel chloride, or for 10 min in 3-amino-9-ethylcarbazole (AEC), followed by a rinse in distilled water. Tissue sections may be counterstained by various agents including hematoxylin or contrast green. Tissue sections are then dehydrated in graded ethanol, cleared in xylene, and coverslipped. If AEC is used, tissue should not be dehydrated, and coverslipped with an aqueous mounting medium. Cells that have incorporated BRdU are identified as having dark brown to black (DAB) or red (AEC) pigment over their nuclei.

Defining a cell nucleus as being labeled depends on the fixation and immunohistochemical procedures used, and these must be optimized for each tissue. Staining intensity depends greatly on enzyme treatment to remove protein crosslinks and the concentration of primary and secondary antibodies. Choice of counter-stain is important, and care should be taken not to mask the labeled cells.

Choice of label. The use of [³H]thymidine has an advantage over BRdU because the [³H]thymidine technique has been the method of choice for many years and has accumulated a substantial historic data base and experience. One disadvantage is that the amount of [³H]thymidine label needed for a chronic pump-label experiment presents serious, and sometimes prohibitive, problems in safety, cost, containment, and decontamination. Another disadvantage is that autoradiographic exposure periods may range from weeks to months.

The BRdU technique has the advantage of not presenting the radiation hazard, containment, or decontamination problems inherent in [³H]thymidine. Further, results from BRdU use are more rapidly obtained because tissue sections can be processed immediately for BRdU-immunohistochemical staining. A disadvantage of the BRdU technique is that there is no definitive or quantitative lower-end cut-off for determining whether a cell is to be scored as labeled.

Tissue preparation

Among the known or expected target tissues for cancer induction that are the focus of research, the liver ranks high, and much of the current proliferation data have been collected for this organ. Since the epithelium of the gut exhibits rapid cell turnover, it provides a good control that should be taken and processed with the tissue of interest to confirm that the DNA precursor was actually delivered to the animal. Sectioning, fixation, and preparation for microscopic evaluation are specific for each tissue and target-cell population. Consistent collection and sectioning techniques should be followed. Certain tissues, like those from the kidney, may require perfusion fixation to preserve morphologic integrity. In general, formalin-fixed, paraffin-embedded tissue sections cut at 5–7μ are adequate for cell proliferation evaluation. Certain tissues may need to be examined in finer detail, and they can be embedded in glycol methracrylate or paraffin and sectioned at 2-μ thickness. Other procedures may be followed to prepare sections for electron-microscopic or histopathologic examination. Frozen sections should be taken if additional histopathologic parameters or end points such as enzyme or oncogene expression are of interest. Listed below are tissue preparation procedures used at our institution for liver-, kidney- and nasal-cell replication studies in the rat.

Liver. Animals are sacrificed and whole livers immediately removed, weighed, and examined. Midlobe radial sections (1–2 mm of the left, right median, and right anterior liver lobes) are cut and placed overnight in 10% buffered formalin or Omnifix® along with a 2-mm cross-section of gut taken just below the stomach. Remaining liver may be frozen in liquid nitrogen and stored at –70°C for further analysis. The three liver-lobe sections and gut are embedded in paraffin and sectioned at a thickness of 5–7μ. Sections of each lobe are mounted on a single slide. One set is deparaffinized and stained with hematoxylin and eosin (H/E).

When using autoradiography, the tissue is deparaffinized before being dipped in the photographic emulsion. In a dark, light-tight box containing dessicant, slides are exposed for 4–8 weeks for pulse-labeled cells and 6–10 weeks for pump-labeled cells. The slides are developed, and emulsion is scraped from the back of the wet slides. Then the slides are thoroughly dried, stained with H/E, and cover-slipped with mounting medium. Since lobe differences in LI and carcinogenic effects have been observed (46–50), finding out whether a lobular difference existed before the LI was determined has been useful. Normally, only the left lobe is scored, but it is useful to save the extra lobes, especially of mouse liver; one may need the extra tissue to count the desired number of cells. Labeled hepatocyte nuclei are recorded as a fraction of all hepatocyte nuclei counted in random fields of nonlesion tissue until a minimum of 1000–2000 hepatocyte nuclei are counted per animal. One must be aware that other cell types such as interstitial cells, inflammatory cells, and bile-duct cells are also present in the liver. Nonhepatic cell labeling may be scored independently in the same field if the data appear relevant.

Kidney. A growing number of chemicals has been shown specifically to increase cell proliferation in the P2 segment of the proximal tubule (32,33,51). Cell proliferative effects of three chemicals known to induce tumors in male rat kidneys were measured following 7-day osmotic pump infusion of [^{3}H]thymidine (Fig. 7) (33). Labeling indices were reported for individual segments (P1, P2, P3) of the proximal tubule, for proximal tubule data grouped together (P1 + P2 + P3), and for all kidney cell types

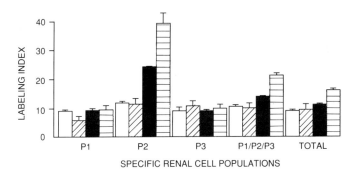

Figure 7. Effect of trichloroethylene, perchloroethylene, and pentachloroethane on cell proliferation in specific cell populations of kidneys of male F344 rats (33). Three animals per group were gavaged daily for 10 days. Seven-day osmotic pumps filled with tritiated thymidine were implanted on day 3 in control and treated animals. Perchloroethylene and pentachloroethane specifically increased LI in the P2 segment of the rat kidney. Pooling of the renal cell types significantly diluted the LI response when LI was scored without regard to cell type or tubular segment. Open bar, control; diagonally hatched bar, trichloroethylene, 1000 mg/kg BW; solid bar, perchloroethylene, 1000 mg/kg BW; horizontally hatched bar, pentachloroethane, 150 mg/kg BW.

measured collectively. Perchloroethylene and pentachloroethane, but not trichloroethylene, specifically increased the LI in the P2 segment of the rat kidney; this large increase was seen only when the individual P2 segment data were analyzed. Pooling of the cell types significantly diluted the effect when the LI was scored without regard to cell type or tubular segment. These data demonstrate the need to identify specific tubule cell populations in the rat kidney to determine certain chemically induced cell proliferative effects.

Procedures for measuring cell proliferation in the kidney have been described previously (32,51). Kidney evaluation may be performed on nonperfused formalin-fixed median-transverse kidney sections to determine cell replication indices within the cortex and medulla. In most experimental situations, care in sectioning and immediate fixation procedures will allow the gathering of adequate LI data and the distinction of proximal versus distal tubular populations in control and chemically treated rats. However, because the quality of such tissue preparation does not usually permit identification of specific tubule cell populations and subtle toxic manifestations, the kidney perfusion method is described below. Note that this technique is labor-intensive and should be used only when identification of specific tubular cell populations is required.

For perfused kidney sections, rats are anesthetized, and the kidneys are flushed in situ by retrograde perfusion of the caudal abdominal aorta (32,33,51). Osmium sodium phosphate buffer (200 mM, pH 7.4) is perfused via a rotary infusion pump for 5–10 sec, followed immediately by 50 ml of a fixative solution containing 2% paraformaldehyde–1% glutaraldehyde in the same buffer at a perfusion pressure of 80 mm Hg. Animals are exsanguinated, kidneys removed, and 1–2 mm median transverse sections of perfused kidneys are immersed in fresh fixative at 4°C for 24 hr. Kidney slices are embedded in glycol methacrylate, sectioned at 2μ, and stained with either H/E or with Lee's methylene blue-basic fuchsin for detection of protein droplets in the proximal tubules.

Each animal's most completely perfused left or right kidney section is used to quantify labeled and unlabeled cells. Cell labeling and cell type are scored at 400× on randomly generated fields extending from the cortex to the inner medulla. Cells from the proximal tubule are classified into 3 segments termed P1, P2, and P3, and they are identified by cytoplasmic vacuoles, length of microvilli, and the topographic location of the tubular segment within the cortex and the outer medulla. P1 tubular segments are located in the cortical labyrinth (occasionally surrounding glomeruli) and characterized by intermediate length of microvilli, multiple apical vacuoles of various sizes, and a small number of small, round protein droplets. P2 segments are located randomly in the cortical labyrinth and in tips of medullary rays. P2 cells have shorter microvilli, fewer small apical vacuoles than P1 cells, and varying amounts of protein droplets. The P3 segments are located at the base of the medullary rays and the outer stripe of the medulla (OSOM). P3 cells are characterized by a homogeneous dark cytoplasm with a tall, dense brush border and rare lysosomes or apical vacuoles. Cell proliferation is quantitated by counting about 2,000 labeled and unlabeled nuclei of the proximal tubule segments. About 1,000 interstitial cells (IC) and 2,000 cells from distal tubules and collecting ducts (DT/CD) from cortex to inner medullary zone may also be scored if that information is desired. LI is calculated as the percentage of labeled cells per total number of cells counted for each respective cell type.

Nasal epithelium. The interesting challenges associated with assessment of epithelial cell proliferation in the nasal passages arise from the complexity and nature of this tissue and from the technical aspects of histopathologic study and autoradiography of dense materials like the nasal bones. Before undertaking cell proliferation studies of the nose, it is essential to become familiar with normal nasal histology and potential toxic responses. This knowledge will permit appropriate selection of section levels and regions to be used for S-phase determinations. The nasal passages contain several different epithelial cell types that cover a tortuous airway surface. Nasal air flow patterns and regional metabolism often result in highly localized toxic responses in the respiratory tract. Inappropriate sectioning may miss major lesions or make their interpretation difficult. A number of articles addressing these issues are included in the reference list (52–55), and the chapter by Monticello et al. in this volume, which contains a more detailed discussion of this topic. Identification of respiratory tract cells in S-phase by labeling with [3H]thymidine and analysis by histoautoradiography (26,34,56,57) or labeling with BRdU and analysis by immunohistochemistry have been described (58). Nasal toxicology was also the subject of several recently published symposium proceedings (59–61).

Consultation with other workers in this field is recommended if knowledge of the rodent nose is limited. Principal difficulties encountered during studies of nasal cell proliferation concern (1) the selection of section levels for tissue trimming; (2) generation of high-quality histologic sections, with a minimum of folds; and (3) selection or development of a counting procedure.

The histologic methods described by Young et al. (52) are a useful guide for sectioning the nose. The procedure does not cover all regions, however, and additional section levels should be considered. Some investigators use up to six section levels for the rat nose, including the nasal vestibule. In contrast, the National Toxicology Program uses three levels. Section levels should include representative samples of squamous, respiratory (ciliated and nonciliated), and olfactory mucosa. If wet material is stored appropriately, additional sections may be taken at a later date. Consistency of section level and section angle are important in tissue trimming, a process that also provides a good opportunity for gross observations of nasal lesions.

Immersion fixation is generally recommended for light microscopy, since vascular perfusion fixation may induce artifacts in the olfactory epithelium (62). The nasal cavity is flushed gently with 10–20 ml of an appropriate fixative such as 10% neutral buffered formalin. The head is then trimmed to remove the jaw and excess soft tissue and is placed in fresh fixative. If the brain is to be removed, great care should be taken to avoid damaging the nose, especially when collecting the olfactory bulb. After fixation, the skull is decalcified in 5% formic acid, with ion-exchange resin. Adequate decalcification is essential and will take one to several weeks depending on the animal's age.

Cell proliferation data from the nasal mucosa may be difficult to obtain because nasal lesions are often highly site-specific. Different chemicals or exposure conditions may induce unique lesions or lesion distribution, so that sites for S-phase determinations must be selected carefully (63). Lesion distribution should be assessed first and the information used for site selection of S-phase counts (examples of different approaches are presented in references 26 and 57).

S-phase determinations may use the LI, which is based on the total study cell population as the denominator. This approach may involve counting large numbers of unlabeled nuclei and is therefore time-consuming. Another method involves using the unit length labeling index (ULLI), defined as the number of labeled cells per millimeter of basement membrane (57). When the basement-membrane length is used as the ULLI denominator, it is not influenced by changes in the total cell population. Furthermore, this method eliminates the labor-intensive total cell-counting procedure. The induction of olfactory epithelial cell proliferation in response to inhalation exposure to methyl bromide (26) illustrates the advantage of the ULLI approach, as does the influence of changes in total cell population as discussed by Monticello et al. (57) and illustrated in Fig. 8. After 3 days of exposure to methyl bromide, the number of labeled olfactory cells increased and the total cell population decreased markedly (Fig. 8). While the LI increased more than 20-fold over controls, the ULLI was increased only eight fold. The LI, in this particular situation, indicated an artificially elevated cell-proliferation response during the early stages of olfactory epithelial recovery from methyl-bromide exposure. Much of this effect was attributed to changes in the total cell population, which had decreased by about 50% as a result of acute cell death, resulting in an increase in the calculated LI.

Procedures for determining the ULLI have been described in detail by Monticello et al. (57). Specific sites of the nasal mucosa are selected on the basis of nasal lesion distribution and cell type of interest. The basement membrane for each site is measured in millimeters, using an image analysis system by tracing the magnified projected image onto a digitizing tablet. Labeled cells are quantitated in these specific sites and the ULLI is expressed as the number of labeled cells divided by the length of basement membrane (for each site). Monticello et al. (34) applied a similar approach to study the respiratory epithelium.

Positive controls

Positive controls are valuable and may be used also to compare the responses obtained by different laboratory teams. For the male rat liver, partial hepatectomy and pulse label at 24 hr would be an ideal control. Other positive controls might be: (1) Nafenopin, 100 mg/kg gavage by corn oil, pulse label at 24 hr; 75 mg/kg/day gavage by corn oil, pump label during the first week; (2) WY-14,643, 100 mg/kg orally, pulse label at 24 hr; 0.1% in the diet, pump label during the first week; (3) 4-acetylaminofluorene, 500 mg/kg in corn oil by gavage, pulse label at 24 hr; 0.5% in the diet, pump label during the first week; (4) carbon tetrachloride, 2,000 mg/kg in corn oil by gavage, pulse label at 48 hr.

For the male rat kidney, positive controls might be: (a) 1.5 mg/kg mercuric chloride by subcutaneous injection or 10 mg/kg mercuric chloride by gavage 4 days before the pulse label; (b) 2,2,4-trimethylpentane, 500 mg/kg/day by gavage, pump label after day 3; (c) pentachloroethane, 150 mg/kg/day by gavage, pulse or pump label after day 3.

For the male rat nasal epithelium positive controls might be instillation of 40 μl of 40 mM glutaraldehyde into the nose; pulse label 3 days later.

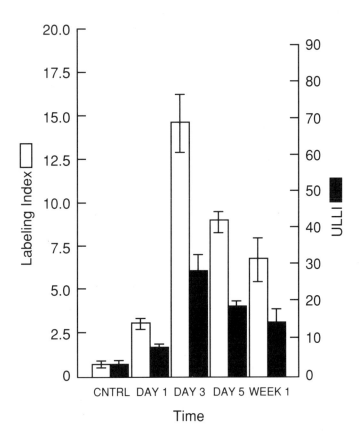

Figure 8. Bar graph comparing mean cell proliferation rates obtained by the LI (open bar) or ULLI (solid bar) method, for olfactory epithelium of F344 rats exposed during days 1, 3, and 5 and week 1 after inhalation exposure to 200 ppm methyl bromide (taken in part from reference 57). Measurement of cell proliferation by the LI method overdramatized the effect of methyl bromide on the olfactory cell proliferation because such treatment decreases the total cell population, resulting in a relatively high LI (20-fold higher than control).

Reporting the data

Labeling indices are generally reported as the percentage of cells in S phase. The LI value for a tissue from a single treatment group is represented by the mean of the animals in that group plus or minus the standard deviation (animal-to-animal). At this point no statistical test has been agreed on as a standard for determining the significance of cell proliferation data. The unpaired t test of the equality of two means (control vs.

treated groups) is one test of statistical significance. Transformation of the data to the square root of $(Y + 0.5)$ may be required to satisfy conditions of normal distribution and equal variance (64). An analysis of variance (ANOVA) and the Dunnett's multiple-comparison procedure of the transformed data provide a more rigorous test of statistical significance. A similar approach involves the arc sine square root transformation of the data, followed by ANOVA and either the Dunnett's or Newman-Keuls multicomparison tests.

The phrase *fold increase in LI over control* is often used in cell proliferation studies. The presentation of cell proliferation data in this manner is useful in comparing LI responses across strains and species and for assessing results obtained in various laboratories. But this approach may also contribute to misleading impressions of the results. Since control LI values are often near zero, small changes in these values will yield large changes in the calculated fold increase over control that may have no biologic relevance. In scoring a control slide, for example, it is common to see only one or two labeled cells per 1,000 counted, so that counting similar fields on the same slide may yield a control LI of 0.1 or 0.2. Yet, using a control of 0.1 instead of 0.2 would yield a 100% higher value in the calculated fold increase over control LI for the treated liver. The absolute value of the LI provides an indicator of the biologic activity and magnitude of response occurring in the target organ. Cell replication responses are best assessed when the cell proliferation data include the absolute value of the LI and not just the fold increase in LI over control.

Summary

A larger data base will be required to relate the extent, duration, and nature of chemically induced cell proliferation to carcinogenic potential and to establish the importance of this end point in chemical carcinogenesis. As that relationship becomes clearer, the information gained will become valuable in investigations of mechanisms of carcinogenesis, development of short-term tests for nongenotoxic carcinogens, selection of appropriate doses for cancer bioassays, and in the formulation of improved risk-assessment models. Because the quality of chemically induced cell replication data depends on the procedures and protocols followed for these labor-intensive studies, efforts among laboratories must be coordinated so that the work and the expenditure of substantial resources will yield a cohesive data base.

Acknowledgments

For providing expertise, examples, and editorial suggestions in the preparation of this paper we thank Sandy Eldridge, Jeffery Everitt, Betsy Gross, Otis Lyght, Daniel Marsman, Thomas Monticello, Holly Randall, Mary Beth St. Clair, Lorraine Tilbury, and Daniel Wilson. We are grateful to Linda Smith and Sadie Leak for typing the manuscript.

Disclaimer

Any stated or implied reference to a particular product, supplier, or manufacturer is meant only as an example, not an endorsement.

References

1. Columbano A, Rajalakshmi S, Sarma DSR. Requirement of cell proliferation for the initiation of liver carcinogenesis as assayed by three different procedures. Cancer Res 41:2079–2083, 1981.
2. Pitot HC, Goldsworthy T, Moran S. The natural history of carcinogenesis: Implications of experimental carcinogenesis in the genes of human cancer. Journal of Supramolecular and Structural Cell Biochemistry 17:133–146, 1981.
3. Slaga TJ (series ed): Mechanisms of Tumor Promotion, vols. 1–4. Boca Raton: CRC Press, 1983–1984.
4. Argyris TS. Regeneration and the mechanism of epidermal tumor promotion. CRC Crit Rev Toxicol 4:211–248, 1985.
5. Farber E, Sarma DSR. Biology of disease. Lab Invest 56:4–22, 1987.
6. Schulte-Hermann R. Induction of liver growth by xenobiotic compounds and other stimuli. CRC Crit Rev Toxicol 3:97–158, 1974.
7. Schulte-Hermann R, Parzefall W, Bursch W. Role of stimulation of liver growth by chemicals in hepatocarcinogenesis. In: Butterworth BE, Slaga TJ (eds): Nongenotoxic Mechanisms in Carcinogenesis. Banbury Report 25. Cold Spring Harbor, New York: Cold Spring Harbor Laboratory, 1987.
8. Reddy JK, Lalwani ND. Carcinogenesis by hepatic peroxisome proliferators: Evaluation of the risk of hypolipidemic drugs and industrial plasticizers to humans. CRC Crit Rev Toxicol 12:1–58, 1983.
9. Butterworth BE. The genetic toxicology of di(2-ethylhexyl)phthalate (DEHP). In: Butterworth BE, Slaga TJ (eds): Nongenotoxic Mechanisms in Carcinogenesis. Banbury Report 25. Cold Spring Harbor, New York: Cold Spring Harbor Laboratory, 1987, pp. 257–276.
10. Conway JG, Cattley RC, Popp JA, Butterworth BE. Possible mechanisms in hepatocarcinogenesis by the peroxisome proliferator di(2-ethylhexyl)phthalate. Drug Metab Rev 21:65–102, 1989.
11. Loury DJ, Goldsworthy TL, Butterworth BE. The value of measuring cell replication as a predictive index of tissue-specific tumorigenic potential. In: Butterworth BE, Slaga TJ (eds): Nongenotoxic Mechanisms in Carcinogenesis. Banbury Report 25. Cold Spring Harbor, New York: Cold Spring Harbor Laboratory, 1987.
12. Doolittle DJ, Muller G, Scribner HE. The relationship between hepatotoxicity and induction of replicative DNA synthesis following single or multiple doses of carbon tetrachloride. J Toxicol Environ Health 22:63–78, 1987.
13. Wilson DM, Butterworth BE. Evaluation of genotoxicity and induced cell proliferation in hepatocytes from rats and mice treated with furan. Environ Mol Mutagen 14:219, 1989.
14. Baserga R, Wiebel F. The cell cycle of mammalian cells. Int Rev Exp Pathol 7:1–25, 1969.
15. Bisconte JC. Kinetic analysis of cellular populations by means of quantitative radioautography. Int Rev Cytol 57:75–126, 1979.
16. Marsman DS, Cattley RC, Conway JG, Popp JA. Relationship of hepatic peroxisome proliferation and replicative DNA synthesis to the hepatocarcinogenicity of the peroxisome proliferators di(2-ethylhexyl)phthalate and [4-chloro-6-(2,3-xylidino)-2-pyrimidinylthio]acetic acid (Wy-14,643) in rats. Cancer Res 48:6739–6744, 1988.
17. Lutz WK, Büsser MT, Sagelsdorff B. Potency of carcinogens derived from covalent DNA binding and stimulation of DNA synthesis in rat liver. Toxicol Pathol 12:106–111, 1986.
18. Mirsalis JC. In vivo measurement of unscheduled DNA synthesis and S-phase synthesis as an indicator of hepatocarcinogenesis in rodents. Cell Biol Toxicol 3:165–173, 1987.
19. Ward JM, Hagiwara A, Anderson LM, Lindsey K, Diwan BA. The chronic hepatic or renal toxicity of di(2-ethylhexyl)phthalate, acetaminophen, sodium barbital, and phenobarbital in male B6C3F1 mice: Autoradiographic, immunohistochemical, and biochemical evidence for levels of DNA synthesis not associated with carcinogenesis or tumor promotion. Toxicol Appl Pharmacol 96:494–506, 1988.
20. Schulte-Hermann R. Two-stage control of cell proliferation in rat liver by α-hexachlorocyclohexane. Cancer Res 37:166–171, 1977.
21. Hopkins HA, Campbell HA, Barbiroli B, Potter VR. Thymidine kinase and deoxyribonucleic acid metabolism in growing and regenerating livers from rats on controlled feeding schedules. Biochem J 136:955–966, 1973.
22. Bursch W, Schulte-Hermann R. Synchronization of hepatic DNA synthesis by scheduled feeding and lighting in mice treated with the chemical inducer of liver growth α-hexachlorocyclohexane. Cell Tissue Kinet 16:125–134, 1983.
23. Busser M, Lutz WK. Stimulation of DNA synthesis in rat and mouse liver by various tumor promoters. Carcinogenesis 8:1433–1437, 1987.

24. Goldsworthy TL, Butterworth BE. Mitogenic activity induced by 4-acetylaminofluorene (4-AAF) in rat liver. Proceedings of the American Association of Cancer Research 30:210, 1989.
25. Swenberg JA, Gross EA, Randall HW. Localization and quantitation of cell proliferation following exposure to nasal irritants. In: Barrow CS (ed): Toxicology of the Nasal Passages. New York: Hemisphere Publishing Co., 1986, p. 291.
26. Hurtt ME, Thomas DA, Working PK, Monticello TM, Morgan KT. Degeneration and regeneration of the olfactory epithelium following inhalation exposure to methyl bromide: Pathology, cell kinetics and olfactory function. Toxicol Appl Pharmacol 94:311–328, 1988.
27. Burns ER. A critique of the practice of comparing control data obtained at a single time point to experimental data obtained at multiple time points. Cell Tissue Kinet 14:219–224, 1981.
28. Monticello TM, Morgan KT. Correlation of cell proliferation and inflammation with nasal tumors in F344 rats following chronic formaldehyde exposure. Proceedings of the American Association of Cancer Research 31:139, 1990.
29. Goldfarb S, Pugh TD, Koen H, He YZ. Preneoplastic and neoplastic progression during hepatocarcinogenesis in mice injected with diethylnitrosamine in infancy. Environ Health Perspect 50:149–161, 1983.
30. Hanigan MH, Kemp CJ, Ginsler JJ, Drinkwater, NR. Rapid growth of preneoplastic lesions in hepatocarcinogen-sensitive C3H/HeJ male mice relative to C57BL/6J male mice. Carcinogenesis 9:885–890, 1988.
31. DeFazio A, Leary JA, Hedley DW, Tattersall MHN. Immunohistochemical detection of proliferating cells in vivo. J Histochem Cytochem 35:571–577, 1987.
32. Short BG, Burnett VL, Cox MG, Bus JS, Swenberg JA. Site-specific renal cytotoxicity and cell proliferation in male rats exposed to petroleum hydrocarbons. Lab Invest 57:564–577, 1987.
33. Goldsworthy TL, Lyght O, Burnett VL, Popp JA. Potential role of α-2μ-globulin, protein droplet accumulation, and cell replication in the renal carcinogenicity of rats exposed to trichloroethylene, perchloroethylene, and pentachlorethane. Toxicol Appl Pharmacol 96:367–379, 1988.
34. Monticello TM, Morgan KT, Everitt JE, Popp JA. Effects of formaldehyde gas on the respiratory tract of rhesus monkeys: Pathology and cell proliferation. Am J Pathol 134:515–527, 1989.
35. Celis JE, Celis A. Cell cycle dependent variations in the distribution of the nuclear protein cyclin proliferating cell nuclear antigen in cultured cells: Subdivision of S phase. Proc Natl Acad Sci USA 82:3262–3266, 1985.
36. Garcia VJ, Caltrera MD, Gown AM. Analysis of proliferative grade using anti-PCNA/cyclin monoclonal antibodies in fixed, embedded tissues. Am J Pathol 134:733–739, 1989.
37. Takasaki Y, Deng JS, Tan EM. A nuclear antigen associated with cell proliferation and blast transformation: Its distribution in synchronized cells. J Exp Med 154:1899–1909, 1981.
38. Chou MY, Chang AL, McBride J, Donoff B, Gallagher GT, Wong DTW. A rapid method to determine proliferation patterns of normal and malignant tissues by H3 mRNA in situ hybridization. Am J Pathol 136:729–733, 1990.
39. Maurer HR. Potential pitfalls of [^{3}H]thymidine techniques to measure cell proliferation. Cell Tissue Kinet 14:111–120, 1981.
40. Wynford-Thomas D, Williams ED. Use of bromodeoxyuridine for cell kinetic studies in intact animals. Cell Tissue Kinet 19:179–182, 1986.
41. Lanier TL, Berger EK, Eacho PI. Comparison of 5-bromodeoxyuridine and [^{3}H]thymidine in rodent hepatocellular proliferation studies. Carcinogenesis 10:1341–1343, 1989.
42. Eldridge SR, Tilbury LF, Goldsworthy TL, Butterworth BE. Measurement of chemically induced cell proliferation in rodent liver and kidney: A comparison of 5-bromo-2'-deoxyuridine and [^{3}H]thymidine administered by injection or osmotic pump. Carcinogenesis 11:2245–2251, 1990.
43. Wilson DM, Goldsworthy TL, Popp JA, Butterworth BE. Evaluation of genotoxicity, cytotoxicity, and cell proliferation in hepatocytes from rats and mice treated with furan. Proceedings of the American Association of Cancer Research 31:103, 1990.
44. Gratzner HG. Monoclonal antibody to 5-bromo- and 5-iododeoxyuridine: New reagent for detection of DNA replication. Science 218:474–475, 1982.
45. Sugihara H, Hattori T, Fukuda M. Immunohistochemical detection of bromodeoxyuridine in formalin-fixed tissues. Histochemistry 85:193–195, 1986.
46. Deal FH, Richardson FC, Swenberg JA. Dose-response of hepatocyte replication following continuous exposure to diethylnitrosamine. Cancer Res 49:6985–6988, 1989.
47. Garvey LK, Lyght O, Popp JA. Evaluation of deoxycholic acid (DCA) promotion in rat liver.

Toxicologist 8:195, 1988.

48. Richardson FC, Boucheron JA, Dyroff MC, Popp JA, Swenberg JA. Biochemical and morphologic studies of heterogeneous lobe responses in hepatocarcinogenesis. Carcinogenesis (London) 7:247–251, 1986.

49. Richardson FC, Morgan PH, Boucheron JA, Deal FH, Swenberg JA. Hepatocyte initiation during continuous administration of diethylnitrosamine and 1,2-sym-dimethylhydrazine. Cancer Res 48:988–992, 1988.

50. Watanabe K, Williams GM. Enhancement of rat hepatocellular-altered foci by the liver tumor promoter phenobarbital: Evidence that foci are precursors of neoplasms and that the promoter acts on carcinogen-induced lesions. J Natl Cancer Inst 61:1311–1314, 1978.

51. Short B, Burnett VL, Swenberg JA. Histopathology and cell proliferation induced by 2,2,4-trimethylpentane in the male rat kidney. Toxicol Pathol 14:194–203, 1986.

52. Young JT. Histopathologic examination of the rat nasal cavity. Fundam Appl Toxicol 1:309–312, 1981.

53. Jiang XA, Morgan KT, Beauchamp RO Jr. Histopathology of acute and subacute nasal toxicity. In: Barrow CS (ed): Toxicology of the Nasal Passages. New York: Hemisphere Publishing Co., 1986, pp. 51–89.

54. Randall HW, Bogdanffy MS, Morgan KT. Enzyme histochemistry of the rat nasal mucosa embedded in cold glycol methacrylate. Am J Anat 179:10–17, 1987.

55. Reznik G, Stinson SF (eds). Nasal tumors in animals and man. Boca Raton: CRC Press, 1983.

56. Chang JCF, Gross EA, Swenberg JA, Barrow CS. Nasal cavity deposition, histopathology, and cell proliferation after single or repeated formaldehyde exposures in B6C3F1 mice and F344 rats. Toxicol Appl Pharmacol 68:161–176, 1983.

57. Monticello TM, Morgan KT, Hurtt ME. Unit length as the denominator for quantitation of cell proliferation rates in nasal epithelium. Toxicol Pathol 18:24–31, 1990.

58. St Clair MB, Gross EA, Morgan KT. Interactions of glutaraldehyde with nasal epithelium. Toxicologist 9:37, 1989.

59. Barrow CS. Toxicology of the nasal passages. New York: Hemisphere Publishing Co., 1986.

60. Feron VJ, Bosland MC. Nasal carcinogenesis in rodents: Relevance to human health risk. Proceedings of the TNO-CIVO/NYU Symposium. Veldhoven, The Netherlands: Pudoc, Wageningen, 1988.

61. Uriah L, Morgan KT, Maronpot R. Toxicologic pathology of the upper respiratory system. Proceedings of the National Toxicology Program Symposium. Environ Health Perspect, in press.

62. Hurtt ME, Morgan KT, Working PK. Histopathology of acute toxic responses in selected tissues from rats exposed by inhalation to methyl bromide. Fundam Appl Toxicol 9:352–365, 1987.

63. Buckley LA, Jiang XZ, James RA, Morgan KT, Barrow CS. Respiratory tract lesions induced by sensory irritants at the RD50 concentration. Toxicol Appl Pharmacol 74:417–429, 1984.

64. Steel RGD, Torrie JH. Principles and Procedures of Statistics, a Biometrical Approach. New York: McGraw-Hill Book Company, 1980, p. 235.

65. Bergmeyer HJ, Scheibe P, Waklefeld AW. Optimization of methods for aspartate aminotransferase and alanine aminotransferase. Clin Chem 24:58–73, 1978.

Appendix: Suggested protocols

Protocol designs are based on observations of labeling kinetics for a variety of chemicals studied at CIIT, with an emphasis on hepatocyte proliferation. As much as possible, schedules minimize working on weekends. To provide flexibility, a variety of time points have been included for each protocol, so that the investigator may do as little or as much as he or she desires while still adhering to the common time frame. The optional stop-studies are designed to see whether cell turnover rates return to baseline after chemical treatment is stopped. If additional parameters are measured, such as enzyme induction, oncogene expression, peroxisomal proliferation, or serum enzymology, they should be measured at one or more of the sacrifice times of the cell proliferation studies. In every case, the S-phase data should be interpreted along with a corresponding histopathologic evaluation of the target tissue.

Everyday chemical administration—pulse label

Monday	Tuesday		Repeat injection and sacrifice as on day 1 on the following days:
t = 0, morning start treatment	t = 1 day, morning inject label		
		Wednesday	- day 2
		Friday	- day 4
	2 hr later sacrifice	Tuesday	- day 8
		Friday	- day 18
		Friday	- day 39
		Friday	- day 88

Test chemical is in the diet or drinking water.

Stop experiment. Stop experiments can be done at any point in the study, but they must be done in parallel with both treated and untreated controls. Chemical administration is stopped one week preceding one of the standard pulse label time points. The example given is to stop chemical administration at the beginning of the working day on Friday, day 32, and to pulse-label in the morning on Friday, day 39, resulting in 7 night feeding periods without chemical.

Sun	Mon	Tue	Wed	Thu	Fri	Sat	Sun	Mon	Tue	Wed	Thu	Fri	Sat
	0	1	2	3	4	5	6	7	8	9	10	11	12
	c	c	c	c	c	c	c	c	c	c	c	c	c
		pls	pls		pls				pls				

Sun	Mon	Tue	Wed	Thu	Fri	Sat	Sun	Mon	Tue	Wed	Thu	Fri	Sat
13	14	15	16	17	18	19	20	21	22	23	24	25	26
c	c	c	c	c	c	c	c	c	c	c	c	c	c
					pls								

Sun	Mon	Tue	Wed	Thu	Fri	Sat	Sun	Mon	Tue	Wed	Thu	Fri
27	28	29	30	31	32	33	34	35	36	37	38	39
c	c	c	c	c	c	c	c	c	c	c	c	c
												pls

Stop												
		...	Thu	Fri	Sat	Sun	Mon	Tue	Wed	Thu	Fri	
		...	31	32	33	34	35	36	37	38	39	
		...	c								pls	

90-Day timepoint												
					...	Sun	Mon	Tue	Wed	Thu	Fri	
					...	83	84	85	86	87	88	
					...	c	c	c	c	c	pls	

c = chemical administered on that day, pls = injection of label with sacrifice 2 hr later.

Everyday chemical administration—three-day pump label

Pump week 1 (days 1–4)			Pump week 3 (days 15–18)
Monday	Tuesday	Friday	Implant Tuesday, day 15
			Sacrifice Friday, day 18
t = 0, morning	t = 1 day, morning	t = 4 days,	**Pump week 6 (days 36–39)**
start treatment	implant pump	morning	
		sacrifice	Implant Tuesday, day 36
			Sacrifice Friday, day 39
			Pump week 13 (days 85–88)
			Implant Tuesday, day 85
			Sacrifice Friday, day 88

Test chemical is in the diet or drinking water.

Stop experiment. Stop experiments may be done at any point in the study, but they must be done in parallel with both treated and untreated controls. Chemical administration is stopped one week preceding the end of one of the standard pump label time periods. The example given is to stop chemical administration at the beginning of the working day on Friday, day 32, implant the pump on Tuesday morning, day 36, and sacrifice on Friday morning, day 39.

Sun	Mon	Tue	Wed	Thu	Fri	Sat	Sun	Mon	Tue	Wed	Thu	Fri	Sat		
0	1	2	3	4	5	6	7	8	9	10	11	12			
c	c	c	c	c	c	c	c	c	c	c	c	c			
		imp	—	—	sac										

Sun	Mon	Tue	Wed	Thu	Fri	Sat	Sun	Mon	Tue	Wed	Thu	Fri	Sat		
13	14	15	16	17	18	19	20	21	22	23	24	25	26		
c	c	c	c	c	c	c	c	c	c	c	c	c	c		
		imp	—	—	sac										

Sun	Mon	Tue	Wed	Thu	Fri	Sat	Sun	Mon	Tue	Wed	Thu	Fri	Sat	Sun	Mon
27	28	29	30	31	32	33	34	35	36	37	38	39	40	41	42
c	c	c	c	c	c	c	c	c	c	c	c	c	c	c	c
									imp	—	—	sac			

Stop

				Thu	Fri	Sat	Sun	Mon	Tue	Wed	Thu	Fri	Sat	Sun	Mon
...				31	32	33	34	35	36	37	38	39	40	41	42
...				c					imp	—	—	sac			

90 -day timepoint

							Sun	Mon	Tue	Wed	Thu	Fri	Sat	Sun	Mon
...							83	84	85	86	87	88	89	90	91
...							c	c	c	c	c	c	c	c	c
									imp	—	—	sac			

c = chemical administered on that day, imp = implant pump, sac = sacrifice animal.

Everyday chemical administration—six-day pump label

Pump week 1 (days 1–7)			Pump week 3 (days 15–21)
Monday	Tuesday	Monday	Implant Tuesday, day 15
			Sacrifice Monday, day 21
t = 0, morning	t = 1 day, morning	t = 7 days,	
start treatment	implant pump	morning	Pump week 6 (days 36–42)
		sacrifice	
			Implant Tuesday, day 36
			Sacrifice Monday, day 42
			Pump week 13 (days 85–91)
			Implant Tuesday, day 85
			Sacrifice Monday, day 91

Test chemical is in the diet or drinking water.

Stop experiment. Stop experiments can be done at any point in the study, but they must be done in parallel with both treated and untreated controls. Chemical administration is stopped one week preceding the midpoint of one of the standard pump label time periods. The example given is to stop chemical administration at the beginning of the working day on Friday, day 32, implant the pump on Tuesday morning, day 36, and sacrifice on Monday morning, day 42.

	Sun	Mon	Tue	Wed	Thu	Fri	Sat	Sun	Mon	Tue	Wed	Thu	Fri	Sat	Sun	Mon
		0	1	2	3	4	5	6	7	8	9	10	11	12		
		c	c	c	c	c	c	c	c	c	c	c	c	c		
			imp	—	—	—	—	—	sac							
	Sun	Mon	Tue	Wed	Thu	Fri	Sat	Sun	Mon	Tue	Wed	Thu	Fri	Sat		
	13	14	15	16	17	18	19	20	21	22	23	24	25	26		
	c	c	c	c	c	c	c	c	c	c	c	c	c	c		
			imp	—	—	—	—	—	sac							
	Sun	Mon	Tue	Wed	Thu	Fri	Sat	Sun	Mon	Tue	Wed	Thu	Fri	Sat	Sun	Mon
	27	28	29	30	31	32	33	34	35	36	37	38	39	40	41	42
	c	c	c	c	c	c	c	c	c	c	c	c	c	c	c	c
										imp	—	—	—	—	—	sac
Stop				...	Thu	Fri	Sat	Sun	Mon	Tue	Wed	Thu	Fri	Sat	Sun	Mon
				...	31	32	33	34	35	36	37	38	39	40	41	42
				...	c					imp	—	—	—	—	—	sac
90-day timepoint				...				Sun	Mon	Tue	Wed	Thu	Fri	Sat	Sun	Mon
				...				83	84	85	86	87	88	89	90	91
				...				c	c	c	c	c	c	c	c	c
										imp	—	—	—	—	—	sac

c = chemical administered on that day, imp = implant pump, sac = sacrifice animal.

Five-day/week chemical administration—pulse label

Monday	Tuesday	Repeat injection and sacrifice as on day 1 on the following days:
t = 0, morning start treatment	t = 1 day, morning inject label	Wednesday - day 2
		Friday - day 4
	2 hr later sacrifice	Tuesday - day 8
		Friday - day 18
		Friday - day 39
		Friday - day 88

Chemical is not administered to animals on the day of their sacrifice.

Stop experiment. Stop experiments can be done at any point in the study, but they must be done in parallel with both treated and untreated controls. Chemical administration is stopped one week before one of the standard pulse label time points. The example given is to stop chemical administration at the end of the working day on Thursday, day 31, and to pulse label on Friday morning, day 39, resulting in 7 days without chemical.

Sun	Mon	Tue	Wed	Thu	Fri	Sat	Sun	Mon	Tue	Wed	Thu	Fri	Sat
	0	1	2	3	4	5	6	7	8	9	10	11	12
	c	c	c	c	c			c	c	c	c	c	
		pls	pls	pls				pls					

Sun	Mon	Tue	Wed	Thu	Fri	Sat	Sun	Mon	Tue	Wed	Thu	Fri	Sat
13	14	15	16	17	18	19	20	21	22	23	24	25	26
	c	c	c	c	c			c	c	c	c	c	
				pls									

Sun	Mon	Tue	Wed	Thu	Fri	Sat	Sun	Mon	Tue	Wed	Thu	Fri
27	28	29	30	31	32	33	34	35	36	37	38	39
	c	c	c	c				c	c	c	c	c
												pls

Stop				Thu	Fri	Sat	Sun	Mon	Tue	Wed	Thu	Fri
		...		31	32	33	34	35	36	37	38	39
		...		c								pls

90-day timepoint							Sun	Mon	Tue	Wed	Thu	Fri
						...	83	84	85	86	87	88
						...	c	c	c	c	c	pls

c = chemical administered on that day, pls = injection of label with sacrifice 2 hr later.

Five days/week chemical administration—three-day pump label

	Pump week 1 (days 1–4)		Pump week 3 (days 15–18)
Monday	Tuesday	Friday	Implant Tuesday, day 15
			Sacrifice Friday, day 18
$t = 0$, morning	$t = 1$ day, morning	$t = 4$ days,	
start treatment	implant pump	morning	Pump week 6 (days 36–39)
		sacrifice	
			Implant Tuesday, day 36
			Sacrifice Friday, day 39
			Pump week 13 (days 85–88)
			Implant Tuesday, day 85
			Sacrifice Friday, day 88

Chemical is not administered to animals on the day of their sacrifice.

Stop experiment. Stop experiments can be done at any point in the study, but they must be done in parallel with both treated and untreated controls. Chemical administration is stopped 4 days before the beginning of one of the standard pump label time periods. The example given is to stop chemical administration at the end of the work day on Thursday, day 31, implant the pump on Tuesday morning, day 36, and sacrifice on Friday morning, day 39.

Sun	Mon	Tue	Wed	Thu	Fri	Sat	Sun	Mon	Tue	Wed	Thu	Fri	Sat
	0	1	2	3	4	5	6	7	8	9	10	11	12
	c	c	c	c	c			c	c	c	c		
		imp	—	—	sac								

Sun	Mon	Tue	Wed	Thu	Fri	Sat	Sun	Mon	Tue	Wed	Thu	Fri	Sat
13	14	15	16	17	18	19	20	21	22	23	24	25	26
	c	c	c	c	c			c	c	c	c	c	
		imp	—	—	sac								

Sun	Mon	Tue	Wed	Thu	Fri	Sat	Sun	Mon	Tue	Wed	Thu	Fri	Sat
27	28	29	30	31	32	33	34	35	36	37	38	39	40
	c	c	c	c	c			c	c	c	c	c	
									imp	—	—	sac	

Stop		Tue	Wed	Thu	Fri	Sat	Sun	Mon	Tue	Wed	Thu	Fri	Sat
		29	30	31	32	33	34	35	36	37	38	39	40
		c	c	c					imp	—	—	sac	

90-day timepoint					...		Sun	Mon	Tue	Wed	Thu	Fri	Sat
					...		83	84	85	86	87	88	89
					...			c	c	c	c	c	
									imp	—	—	sac	

c = chemical administered on that day, imp = implant pump, sac = sacrifice animal.

Five day/week chemical administration—six-day pump label

	Pump week 1 (days 1–5)		Pump week 3 (days 13–19)
Monday	Sunday	Saturday	Implant Sunday, day 13
			Sacrifice Saturday, day 19
t = 0, morning	t = 1 day, morning	t = 5 days,	**Pump week 6 (days 34–40)**
start treatment	implant pump	morning	
		sacrifice	Implant Sunday, day 34
			Sacrifice Saturday, day 40
			Pump week 13 (days 83–89)
			Implant Sunday, day 83
			Sacrifice Saturday, day 89

Chemical is not administered to animals on the day of their sacrifice.

Stop experiment. Stop experiments can be done at any point in the study, but they must be done in parallel with both treated and untreated controls. Chemical administration is stopped one week before the midpoint of one of the standard pump label time periods. The example given is to stop chemical administration at the end of the work day on Tuesday, day 29, implant the pump on Sunday morning, day 34, and sacrifice on Saturday morning, day 40.

Sun	Mon	Tue	Wed	Thu	Fri	Sat	Sun	Mon	Tue	Wed	Thu	Fri	Sat
	0	1	2	3	4	5	6	7	8	9	10	11	12
	c	c	c	c	c			c	c	c	c	c	
imp	—	—	—	—	—	sac							
Sun	Mon	Tue	Wed	Thu	Fri	Sat	Sun	Mon	Tue	Wed	Thu	Fri	Sat
13	14	15	16	17	18	19	20	21	22	23	24	25	26
	c	c	c	c	c			c	c	c	c	c	
imp	—	—	—	—	—	sac							
Sun	Mon	Tue	Wed	Thu	Fri	Sat	Sun	Mon	Tue	Wed	Thu	Fri	Sat
27	28	29	30	31	32	33	34	35	36	37	38	39	40
	c	c	c	c	c			c	c	c	c	c	
							imp	—	—	—	—	—	sac
Stop		Tue	Wed	Thu	Fri	Sat	Sun	Mon	Tue	Wed	Thu	Fri	Sat
		29	30	31	32	33	34	35	36	37	38	39	40
		c					imp	—	—	—	—	—	sac
90-day timepoint						...	Sun	Mon	Tue	Wed	Thu	Fri	Sat
						...	83	84	85	86	87	88	89
						...		c	c	c	c	c	
							imp	—	—	—	—	—	sac

c = chemical administered on that day, imp = implant pump, sac = sacrifice animal.

Single dose of chemical—pulse label

Monday	Tuesday	Repeat injection and sacrifice as on day 1 on the following days:
t = 0, morning treat	t = 1 day, morning inject label	Wednesday - day 2 Friday - day 4 Tuesday - day 8
	2 hr later sacrifice	

Sun	Mon	Tue	Wed	Thu	Fri	Sat	Sun	Mon	Tue
	0 c	1	2	3	4	5	6	7	8
		pls	pls		pls				pls

c = chemical administered on that day, pls = injection of label with sacrifice 2 hr later.

Chemically Induced Cell Proliferation:
Implications for Risk Assessment, pages 285-289
©1991 Wiley-Liss, Inc.

Evaluation of Bromodeoxyuridine Labeling in Hepatomegaly Produced by Peroxisomal Proliferation or P-450 Induction in Rodents

P. F. Smith, K. A. O'Brien, and K. P. Keenan

A growing number of nongenotoxic compounds are being identified as carcinogens in certain rodent strains. This finding has major implications for drug development, although the relevance of nongenotoxic carcinogenicity in rodents to human beings is difficult to establish. An often-encountered response to nongenotoxic compounds is organomegaly with multiple pleiotropic responses (e.g., microsomal enzyme induction and peroxisome proliferation), which may or may not be related to the ultimate carcinogenicity of these agents in the test species. Moreover, and perhaps most importantly, there are currently no well-validated, short-term methods for screening drug development candidates in terms of their potential to produce carcinogenicity by nongenotoxic mechanisms. Some examples of nongenotoxic rodent hepatocarcinogens are found in a number of drug classes including the barbiturates (phenobarbital), benzodiazepines (ripazepam), fibrates (nafenopin, clofibrate), certain antibiotics (rifampiocin), and synthetic hormones (cyproterone acetate, ethinyl estradiol). The nongenotoxic carcinogenicity of these agents is often species-, strain-, and even gender-specific in rodents.

Not all compounds that induce acute cell proliferation and hyperplasia have the same ability to induce tumor formation in target tissues. Simple repeated wounding of the skin or trachea to induce sustained cell turnover, rather than hyperplasia per se, yields the highest tumor-promoting potency in several rodent systems (1,2). In studies of two peroxisome proliferators with very different abilities to induce hepatic cancer in F344 rats but equivalent abilities to induce acute cell proliferation, sustained hepatomegaly, persistent peroxisome proliferation, and long-term increases in fatty acyl-CoA oxidase activity, the only strong correlation between the two compounds' hepatocarcinogenicity was the ability of the potent carcinogen, WY-14,643 ([4-chloro-6-(2,3-xylidino)-2-pyrimidinylthio]acetic adic), to induce persistent, long-term, replicative DNA synthesis in hepatocytes. This difference in cell proliferation was not detected by single pulse-labeling with [3H]thymidine, but only by the continuous administration of [3H]thymidine by osmotic minipumps (3). Many short-term tests tend to be viewed in simple terms of plus/minus, carcinogen/noncarcinogen results. However, the analysis of chemically induced persistent cell proliferation in rodent carcinogenesis will require a quantitative analysis of the location, extent, duration, and specific cell types involved in that proliferation. This analysis will be necessary if a predictive assay for some classes of potentially nongenotoxic carcinogens is to be developed into a meaningful data base that will correlate with the results of long-term carcinogenic bioassays.

To test alternative methods of evaluating sustained hyperplasia and cell proliferation and their potential relationship to nongenotoxic carcinogenesis in rodents, we conducted a pilot study in 10-week-old Sprague-Dawley (SD) rats and CD-1 mice. Persistent DNA synthesis was determined following osmotic mini-pump (Alza, Palo Alto, California) administration of the thymidine analogue, bromodeoxyuridine (BrdUrd), and immunohistochemical staining of target tissues from rats and mice fed either the potent peroxisome proliferator, WY-14,643 (WY), or the microsomal enzyme inducer, phenobarbital (PB), at 0.1% in the diet.

Materials and methods

Animals included SD rats and CD-1 mice obtained from Charles River Laboratories (Raleigh, North Carolina) and fed either control meal (Purina 5002) or meal mixed with the test articles (WY from Chemsyn, Lenexa, Kansas, or PB from Sigma) at 0.1%. 5-Bromo-2-deoxyuridine (BrdUrd, Sigma) was administered continuously for 1 week by osmotic minipumps (pumps contained BrdUrd dissolved in 0.5 N sodium bicarbonate at a final concentration of 50 mg/ml), and animals were necropsied after 1 or 5 weeks of treatment. At necropsy, the liver was collected for immunohistochemical staining of paraffin-embedded sections cut at 5 microns, mounted on 3-aminopropyl-triethyloxysilane (Sigma)-coated slides.

BrdUrd immunohistochemical staining was performed following 0.04% pepsin digestion and DNA hydrolysis in 4 M hydrochloric acid. Mouse anti-BrdUrd γ-globulin (Becton Dickinson Cat. #7580) was used as a primary antibody, and a standard procedure was followed using the Vector Vectastain ABC kit and 3,3-diaminobenzidine as the chromogen (4). One thousand hepatocyte nuclei were scored for BrdUrd staining to obtain a percentage labeling index (LI).

Results

Feeding WY or PB produced marked sustained hepatomegaly in SD rats and CD-1 mice after 1 and 5 weeks of treatment (Fig. 1). Male and female SD rats fed WY had high hepatocyte LI at week 1 that remained elevated above controls at week 5 in males only. Rats of both genders fed PB had high hepatocyte LI at week 1 that declined at 5 weeks (Fig. 2).

CD-1 mice of both gender fed WY, in contrast to rats, had high sustained hepatocyte LI at both 1 and 5 weeks. Mice fed PB had high hepatocyte LI at week 1, which declined to control values by week 5 (Fig. 2). The distribution of BrdUrd hepatocyte nuclear labeling was similar in rats and mice. WY-fed animals had panlobular labeling with periportal labeling seen in rats by week 5. PB-fed animals had labeling in centrilobular hepatocytes that showed typical centrilobular hypertrophy. In both rats and mice, considerable nonhepatocyte labeling was noted in both control and treated animals. In female control mice, a very high LI was noted compared to that of male mice. This difference was seen at both time points and has been observed by others, but it remains unexplained.

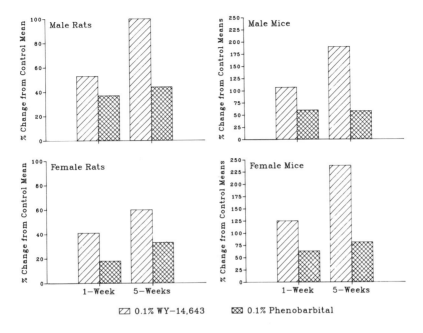

Figure 1. Liver weights (percentage change from control) obtained from SD rats and CD-1 mice after 1 or 5 weeks of treatment with WY or PB (0.1% of diet). Values indicate percentage change from control means with n = 5 animals per group.

Discussion

Continuous BrdUrd delivery by osmotic minipumps coupled with immunohistochemical staining and determination of LI of target tissues and cell types seems to provide a useful method for determining chemically induced persistent DNA synthesis in the rodent strains examined. Sustained proliferative changes with WY but not PB in rats are consistent with the greater hepatocarcinogenicity shown for WY in other rat strains (e.g., F344, 3). However, determination of later time points will be necessary to establish the relationship of sustained DNA synthesis and carcinogenic potential of the test compound for the specific strains of the two species studied.

These differences in LI could not be detected with the more traditional pulse-labeling of animals with thymidine analogs. The use of osmotic minipumps allows the measurement of low but real differences in DNA synthesis in the liver. Cell proliferation is considered important in the initiation, promotion, and progression of cancer. It has long been known that numerous chemicals and treatments induce transient bursts of cell proliferation, as measured by single pulse methods, which return to control levels

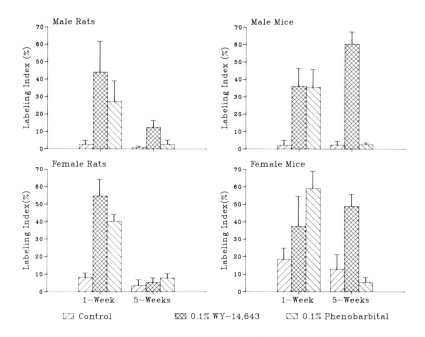

Figure 2. Hepatocyte labeling indices (percentage of labeled cells) determined by counting 1000 hepatocyte nuclei from SD rats or CD-1 mice after 1 or 5 weeks of treatment with control diet (control) or either WY or PB (0.1% of diet). Values indicate the mean ± standard deviation from n = 5 animals per group.

following continued treatment. Only some of these treatments have been associated with carcinogenicity (5). Using continuous labeling with BrdUrd or tritiated thymidine in osmotic minipumps should make it possible to determine whether a compound induces elevated, persistent levels of cell proliferation, and whether this event is associated with the compounds' known or potential carcinogenicity.

Conclusion

Application of these methods should be considered for several areas including: 1) determination of dose-response relationships, e.g., maximum tolerated dose levels and no-effect levels; 2) differentiation of the relative contribution of hypertrophy versus hyperplasia in specific types of organomegaly; and 3) distinction of different compounds of a specific chemical class based on their ability to induce sustained proliferation in target organs of a test species and, thus, determination of their carcinogenic potential at earlier time points than the two-year bioassay.

References

1.   Argyris TS. Regeneration and the mechanism of epidermal tumor promotion. CRC Crit Rev Toxicol 14:211–258, 1985.
2.   Keenan KP, Saffiotti U, Stinson SF, Riggs CW, McDowell EM. Multifactorial hamster respiratory carcinogenesis with interdependent effects of cannula-induced mucosal wounding, saline, ferric oxide, benzo[*a*]pyrene and N-methy-N-nitrosourea. Cancer Res 49:1528–1540, 1989.
3.   Marsman DS, Cattley RC, Conway JG, Popp JA. Relationship of hepatic peroxisome proliferation and replicative DNA synthesis to the hepatocarcinogenicity of the peroxisome proliferators di(2-ethylhexyl) phthalate and 4-chloro-6-(2,3-xylidino)-2-pyrimidinylthio acetic acid (WY-14,643) in rats. Cancer Res 48:6739–6744, 1988.
4.   Schutte B, Reynders MMJ, Bosman FT, Blijham GH. Effect of tissue fixation on anti-bromodeoxyuridine immunohistochemistry. J Histochem Cytochem 35:1343–1345, 1987.

Chemically Induced Cell Proliferation:
Implications for Risk Assessment, pages 291-301
©1991 Wiley-Liss, Inc.

Evaluation of the Form of the Cell Growth Rate Function of the Two-Stage Model for Carcinogenesis

Gail Charnley and James D. Wilson

The two-stage model for carcinogenesis described by Moolgavkar and Knudson (1) and adapted for cancer risk assessment (2) has advantages over standard empirical modeling techniques in that it can incorporate information on the biologic mechanisms of action of an agent into dose-response equations. For example, suspected nongenotoxic tumor promoters can be modeled according to their effects on cell proliferation and the mutagenic effects of genotoxic carcinogens by transition rates between cell types (normal, initiated, transformed). For nongenotoxic carcinogens, assumptions must be made about the shape of the dose-response relationship when the number of susceptible cells goes beyond the observable range. One such assumption has been that the dose-response relationship is a bounded log-logisticlike function; at low carcinogen doses, it is bounded by the background number of stem cells, while at high doses, proliferation, and therefore the number of susceptible cells, probably plateaus. This logic has yet to be validated. In fact, although the effects of exposure to a number of chemicals on both cell proliferation and cell number have been evaluated, few dose-response data are available. We conclude that the available data are insufficient to allow evaluation of the nature of the cell growth rate function.

Background

A number of nongenotoxic carcinogens, including 2,3,7,8-tetrachlorodibenzo-*p*-dioxin (TCDD), polychlorinated biphenyls (PCB), and saccharin, can elicit cellular alterations that affect the number of proliferating cells in their target organs (3,4). These agents may increase tumor incidence partly by virtue of their abilities to increase the number of mitotic divisions within the target organ, which would increase the likelihood of expression of cells with a neoplastic phenotype (5). Under these assumptions, the probability of tumor development would be proportional to the number of susceptible cells (stem cells) multiplied by the cell proliferation rate (which can be determined via flow cytometry or autoradiography). If the number of stem cells is not known, as often is the case, it can be estimated from the organ weight as a first approximation. If we assume that the number of susceptible cells has reached equilibrium at each exposure level, the effects of exposure to an agent at level "x" on the total number of mitotic divisions of a susceptible cell population in an organ may be expressed as

$$C_0(x) = vW_0(x)r(x),$$

where $W_0(x)$ and $r(x)$ are the organ weight and the autoradiographically determined labeling index, respectively, and "v" is proportional to the number of susceptible cells per unit of weight.

In their discussion of dose-response functions for nongenotoxic agents, Thorslund et al. (2) used a log-logisticlike function for the relationship between organ weight and exposure to 2-(diethylhexyl)phthalate (DEHP), and assumed the labeling index did not vary with exposure. The resulting alpha-form for the dose-response function for tumor formation allowed a good fit to the data. No comparison of fits with other functional forms was made.

In their application of the two-stage model to TCDD-induced rat liver tumor rates, Thorslund and Charnley (6) obtained equally good fits for the imputed cell growth rate from tumor data using log-logistic or one-hit models. The log-logistic form provided an adequate fit for chlordane-induced mouse liver tumors, although the estimation procedure used was not 100% efficient.

The validity of the assumption that a log-logisticlike (alpha-form) function is the most appropriate for the cell growth rate function has not been addressed adequately. The two-stage model has been applied to only a limited number of nongenotoxic carcinogens, with results that are promising but inadequate to properly validate the assumption. Since standard cancer dose-response models are empirical, they make no assumptions about an agent's effects on any biologic parameters. The two-stage model has the potential to introduce more biologic information into the low-dose extrapolation procedure. However, only if such information comes from independent experiments on cell proliferation will the results provide any improvement over empirical fitting of models directly to tumor data.

Results

Nasal mucosa

Phenacetin, which is not a genotoxin, can induce nasal and renal tumors in rats when administered as 1.25% or 2.5% of the diet for 2 years (7). Its early cell proliferative effects on rat olfactory epithelium were demonstrated when 2-week daily gavage with 100-, 625-, or 1250-mg/kg/day phenacetin increased cell replication in that tissue by 62.4%, 174%, and 763%, respectively (8) (Fig. 1). The dose-response relationships for cell proliferation and tumor formation were similar. These data could be used to determine a cell growth rate function if the total number of cells in the olfactory mucosa with and without treatment could be estimated. However, this study was too short to determine a steady-state growth rate.

Formaldehyde also induces epithelial tumors, DNA-protein cross-links, and increased cell turnover (9–11). Figure 2 shows the effects on the rat nasal mucosa of exposure to 0-, 0.5-, 2-, or 6-ppm formaldehyde 6 hr/day for 9 days by inhalation (12). The maximal proliferation rates could be used to calculate a cell growth rate function if some assumptions are made on the number of cells in the nasal mucosa. At 9 days, the data indicated a steady state had been reached. In addition, no effect on proliferation was seen at the lowest dose, indicating that the effect may have been a logistically-bounded high-dose phenomenon.

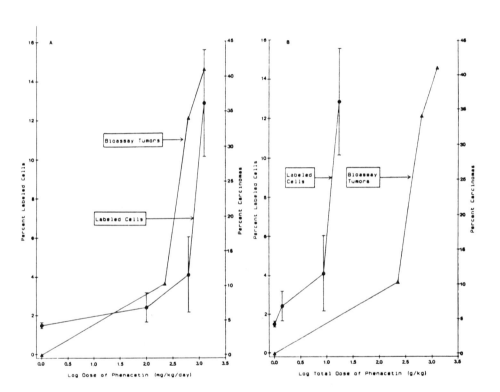

Figure 1. Effects of phenacetin on the rat nasal mucosa. (A) Labeling index of olfactory mucosa in rats treated with phenacetin for 2 weeks and percentage carcinoma incidence from bioassay data (Isaka et al., 1979) versus phenacetin dose. The dose-response curves for the two endpoints are similar and demonstrate that increases in both are high-dose effects. (B) Labeling index and bioassay tumor data plotted against cumulative dose. This figure demonstrates that cell replication is occurring in the nasal olfactory mucosa at cumulative doses far lower than those that result in tumors. Source: Bogdanffy et al., 1989.

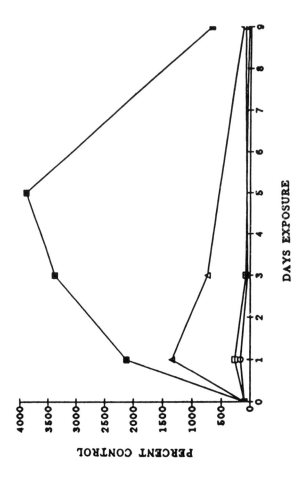

Figure 2. Effects of formaldehyde on the rat nasal mucosal epithelium. Compilation of all rat cell turnover data using the 18-hr [³H]thymidine pulse. Exposures were 0.5 (□), 2 (○), and 6 (△) ppm formaldehyde 6 hr/day and the combined data from 12 ppm 3 hr/day and 15 ppm 6 hr/day (■). Source: Swenberg et al., 1987.

Kidney

Subacute inhalation exposure to trimethylpentane, the component of unleaded gasoline that induces nephrotoxicity and renal tumors in male rats (13), has been associated with crystalloid body accumulation, degeneration, necrosis, and increased cell proliferation in the proximal convoluted tubular epithelium (13). Table 1 shows the relationship between trimethylpentane exposure for 21 days by gavage and the labeling indices in male rat kidneys. The total number of cells likely could be calculated, given assumptions about the number of cells in the unexposed proximal convoluted tubular epithelium. However, without time-course data, it is impossible to tell whether the steady state has been reached.

Table 1. Effects of Trimethylpentane on the Male Rat Kidney.

Kidney location	Zone 1			Zone 2			Zone 3			Zone 4		
TMP dose (mg/kg)	0	50	500	0	50	500	0	50	500	0	50	500
Glomerulus	0.14	0.31	0.25									
Proximal convoluted tubule (P$_1$)	0.16	0.32	0.45[ab]									
Proximal convoluted tubule (P$_2$)	0.30	1.73	1.61[a]									
Proximal straight tubule (P$_3$)				0.29	0.52	0.76[ab]						
Thin limb of Henle							0.33	0.59	0.46	0.07	0.33	0.16
Distal tubule	0.29	0.73	0.33	0.12	0.17	0.20	0.23	0.84	0.56[a]	0.04	0.11	0.00
Interstitium	0.28	0.30	0.93[ab]	0.13	0.91	0.77[a]	0.42	0.73	0.62	0.18	0.50	0.26
Mean	0.25	0.82	0.85[a]	0.21	0.54	0.75[ab]	0.31	0.76	0.57[a]	0.11	0.34	0.16

[a] Significant trend test ($P < 0.05$).
[b] Significant dose relationship ($P < 0.05$).
Source: Short et al., 1986.

Liver

TCDD is a nongenotoxic agent that can increase liver tumor incidence in rats and mice (14, 15). Increases in relative liver weight have also been observed among exposed rats (16), presumably reflecting increases in cell proliferation rates. Increases in the relative liver weight can be assumed to be proportional to increases in the total number of hepatocytes. Table 2 shows the effects of exposure to 0.05-, 0.5-, or 5-µg TCDD/ kg once weekly by gavage for 2 weeks on relative liver weight in rats. These values could be used to calculate a growth rate function, but without time-course data, it is unclear whether a steady state has been reached. In addition, liver weights are expressed relative to body weight, not to control liver weights. Since the data indicate treatment affected body weight gain, these values would have to be adjusted to reflect only changes in liver weight.

DEHP has been demonstrated in chronic bioassays using F344 rats and B6C3F1 mice to be tumorigenic when given in the diet (17,18). DEHP has been shown to induce a burst of mitosis in the liver immediately after the start of treatment; the extent of this burst is dose dependent and transient (19). The relative liver weight of DEHP-treated animals, however, increases and remains increased, indicating that the overall number of hepatocytes is greater in DEHP-treated than in control animals (20). The potency of DEHP as a mitotic agent has been correlated with its potency as a hepatocarcinogen (21). The species most sensitive to DEHP-induced hepatocarcinogenesis is the mouse. However, relative liver weight data exist only for the rat and hamster (Tables 3 and 4) (22, and Butterworth, personal communication). Thus, although growth rate functions can be calculated with these data, they are not useful for cancer risk assessment. The data in Table 3 are too sparse to reliably establish the shape of a dose-response relationship. In Table 4, the data do not indicate whether a steady state has been reached and are expressed relative to body weight rather than control liver weight. Thus, no treatment-related differences in body weight could be assumed.

Table 2. Effects of TCDD on Rat Relative Liver Weight.

Exposure	No. of rats	Weight gain (g)	Relative liver weight	Nonprotein SH groups (nmol/g wet wt)
DMSO, control	4	17.5 ± 1.4	3.01 ± 0.10	5.18 ± 0.04
MCPA, 100 mg/kg	4	6.3 ±13.4	3.03 ± 0.08	5.17 ± 0.15
2,4-D, 100 mg/kg	3	5.0 ± 5.0*	3.22 ± 0.19	5.74 ± 0.35
Ky-5, 100 mg/kg	5	10.0 ± 4.2	3.53 ± 0.06**	5.87 ± 0.05*
2,3,7,8-TCDD, 5μg/kg	4	17.5 ± 4.3	3.47 ± 0.09*	6.21 ± 0.20*
2,3,7,8-TCDD, 0.5 μg/kg	4	32.5 ± 4.3*	3.30 ± 0.07*	5.92 ± 0.24
2,3,7,8-TCDD, 0.05 μg/kg	4	33.8 ±10.5	3.03 ± 0.10	5.85 ± 0.14

DMSO, dimethyl sulfoxide
Difference from controls (two-tailed Student's t-test): *$P < 0.05$, ** $P < 0.01$.
Source: Mustonen et al., 1989.

Table 3. Effects of DEHP on Relative Liver Weight.

Dose (ppm)	Relative liver weight
0	1
6,000	1.73

Source: B. Butterworth, personal communication.

Diethylnitrosamine (DEN) is a genotoxic hepatocarcinogen in rodents that induces hepatocellular proliferation (12). Increasing the DEN dose increases the extent of hepatocyte labeling; labeling returns to control levels except when high doses are used (although the experiment may have been too short to show a similar pattern) (Fig. 3). Evaluation of this effect on the total number of hepatocytes, perhaps by determining changes in liver weight, would be necessary in order to calculate a growth rate function.

The genotoxic hepatocarcinogen ridelline (a pyrrolizidine alkaloid) increases the number of hepatocytes in S phase after short-term administration (Fig. 4) (23). Similar results have been obtained with a number of other hepatocarcinogens, both genotoxic and nongenotoxic (Tables 5 and 6) (24,25). Studies of the effect of these increases on the total number of hepatocytes that exist after chronic administration are needed before growth rate functions can be calculated.

Urinary bladder

The ability of dietary administration of sodium saccharin to induce rat urinary bladder epithelial tumors has been attributed to the compound's cell proliferative effects in this tissue (4,26). The bladder epithelial labeling index increases approximately linearly with dose and remains elevated after 18 weeks' dosing (Table 7) (4,27). The effect on the total number of bladder epithelial cells could be estimated, although at the doses used the effect is essentially linear. Data on effects of lower doses are needed to evaluate possible nonlinearity.

Table 4. Effects of DEHP on Relative Liver Weight in the Rat and Hamster.

				Treatment[ab]			
Species	Parameter	Control (corn oil)	DEHP 25 mg/kg	DEHP 100 mg/kg	DEHP 250 mg/kg	DEHP 1000 mg/kg	
Rat	Relative liver weight (g/100 g body wt)	3.3 ± 0.1	3.5 ± 0.1 (107)	3.9 ± 0.1[c] (118)	4.8 ± 0.1[c] (146)	5.8 ± 0.2[c] (176)	
	Cytochrome P-450 (nmol/mg microsomal protein)	1.39 ± 0.06	1.36 ± 0.08 (98)	1.65 ± 0.06 (119)	1.78 ± 0.11[c] (129)	1.86 ± 0.07[c] (134)	
	7-Ethoxycoumarin O-deethylase (nmol/hr/mg microsomal protein)	177 ± 6	176 ± 17 (100)	212 ± 15 (120)	210 ± 22 (119)	312 ± 68[d] (177)	
Hamster	Relative liver weight (g/100 g body wt)	3.9 ± 0.2	4.1 ± 0.1 (105)	3.9 ± 0.1 (101)	4.3 ± 0.2 (112)	4.7 ± 0.1[c] (122)	
	Cytochrome P 450 (nmol/mg microsomal protein)	1.69 ± 0.07	1.69 ± 0.10 (100)	2.09 ± 0.20 (123)	2.06 ± 0.08 (122)	2.54 ± 0.08[c] (150)	
	7-Ethoxycoumarin O-deethylase (nmol/hr/mg microsomal protein)	410 ± 24	456 ± 59 (111)	611 ± 29[c] (149)	403 ± 21 (98)	484 ± 22 (118)	

[a] DEHP was administered by daily gastric intubation for 14 days at the dose levels indicated. Control animals received corresponding quantities (5 ml/kg) of the corn oil vehicle.
[b] Results are expressed as mean ± SEM for groups of five animals, with percentage of control values being shown by the figures in parentheses.
[c] Significantly different (Dunnett's test) from control: $P < 0.01$.
[d] Significantly different (Dunnett's test) from control: $P < 0.05$.
Source: Lake et al., 1984.

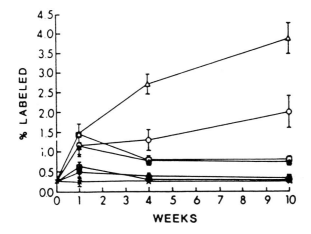

Figure 3. Effect of diethylnitrosamine on rat hepatocyte labeling index. The percent of hepatocytes labeled with [³H]thymidine during exposure to 0(X), 0.4 (■), 1 (●), 4 (▲), 10 (□), 40 (○), or 100 (△) ppm DEN. *Source:* Swenberg et al., 1987.

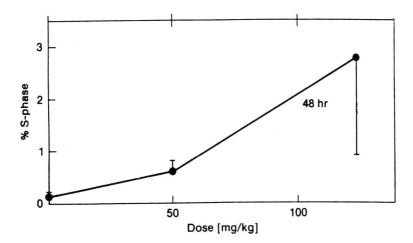

Figure 4. Effect of riddeline on the percent of rat hepatocytes in S-phase. Source: Mirsalis, 1987.

Conclusion

In conclusion, available data are too limited to calculate a cell growth rate function for any particular chemical without making a number of assumptions and are completely inadequate for evaluating the nature of the log-logistic assumption.

Table 5. Effect of Methapyrilene on Rat and Mouse Hepatocyte S-phase Induction.

Treatment	Rat dose (mg/kg)	Mouse time (hr)	%S ± SE	%S ± SE
Control	0	48	0.10 ± 0.08	0.27 ± 0.08
Methapyrilene	50	24	0.50 ± 0.20	–
		48	0.67 ± 0.32	–
	75	48	–	0.32 ± 0.10
	225	24	1.24 ± 0.34	–
		48	6.28 ± 0.71	1.37 ± 0.51
		72	4.11 ± 0.45	–

Male F344 rats and female B6C3F1 mice were administered MP in water at the times indicated prior to sacrifice. Each point represents the mean of three animals; %S = percent of cells in S-phase synthesis, standard errors (SE) represent the variation among animals. Source: Steinmetz et al., 1988.

Table 6. Effect of Several Hepatocarcinogens on Hepatic Cell Proliferation.

Treatment	Dose (mg/kg)	Time (hr)	Male mice %S ± SE (n)	Female mice %S ± SE (n)	Male rats %S ± SE (n)
Control corn oil	0	48	0.16 ± 0.04 (11)	0.21 ± 0.08 (5)	0.05 ± 0.02 (5)
CCl	20	48	0.11 ± 0.07 (3)	0.33 ± 0.21 (2)	–
	100	48	9.42 ± 0.95 (17)	11.04 ± 1.86 (8)	0.46 ± 0.19 (3)
	400	48	–	–	4.90 ± 2.37 (4)
DMN	10	24	0.74 ± 0.18 (3)	–	0.72 ± 0.19 (3)
	10	48	1.09 ± 0.31 (3)	–	2.37 ± 0.56 (3)
2,6-DCPD	200	24	0.02 ± 0.01 (3)	–	–
	200	48	0.43 ± 0.33 (4)	0.22 ± 0.17 (3)	–
	400	24	0.04 ± 0.02 (3)	–	–
	400	48	0.92 ± 0.73 (3)	–	–
	500	48	TOXIC	3.76 ± 1.11 (3)	–
PBB	200	48	2.57 ± 0.82 (3)	6.31 ± 1.49 (3)	–
	1000	48	1.98 ± 0.42 (3)	13.51 ± 1.99 (4)	–
TCE	200	24	0.40 ± 0.16 (3)	–	–
	200	48	0.30 ± 0.04 (3)	0.45 ± 0.36 (3)	–
	1000	24	0.63 ± 0.50 (3)	–	–
	1000	48	2.23 ± 1.19 (3)	0.69 ± 0.18 (4)	–

Animals were treated by gavage at 24 or 48 hr prior to sacrifice. DMN was administered in water; all other compounds were administered in corn oil. %S is the percentage of cells in S phase; (n) is the number of treated animals in each group. At least 6000 cells were scored for each animal. SE represents variation between animals. Source: Mirsalis et al., 1985.

The role of cell proliferation in carcinogenesis is well known, and the effect of cell proliferation on tumor incidence at the high doses used for carcinogenesis bioassays in rodents is critical. Dose-response evaluations for genotoxic carcinogens will greatly overestimate risk of low-dose exposure if the contribution of cell proliferation at high doses is not adequately characterized. Failing to account for the effects of nongenotoxic carcinogens on cell proliferation fails to consider the mechanisms of action of such

Table 7. Effect of Sodium Saccharin on the Rat Urinary Bladder Epithelial Labeling Index.

Level of sodium saccharin in the diet (%)	No. of rats	No. of rats with simple hyperplasia	Labeling index[b]
5.0	5	4 (80)[a]	0.36 ± 0.13[c]
2.5	5	3 (60)	0.19 ± 0.07[d]
1.0	5	1 (20)	0.12 ± 0.05[e]
0.5	5	0	0.12 ± 0.03[d]
0.1	4	0	0.06 ± 0.03[f]
0	4	0	0.04 ± 0.03

[a] Numbers in parentheses, percentage.
[b] Mean ± 0.005.
[c] $P < 0.005$
[d] $P < 0.01$
[e] $P < 0.05$
[f] $P < 0.4$

Labeling Index of Urinary Bladder Epithelium in Rats Fed 5% Sodium Saccharin.

Duration (wk)	Saccharin	Control
1	0.36 ± 0.18[ab]	0.05 ± 0.02
5	0.28 ± 0.12[b]	0.06 ± 0.04
9	0.42 ± 0.20[b]	0.05 ± 0.03
18	0.41 ± 0.24[c]	0.04 ± 0.03

[a] Mean ± SD of labeled cells/100 cells.
[b] $P < 0.05$, saccharin versus control.
[c] $P < 0.06$, saccharin versus control.
Sources: Murasaki and Cohen, 1981; Fukushima and Cohen, 1980.

chemicals, as they are now understood. Generating adequate data for the characterization of dose-response relationships for cell proliferation should be a priority if cancer risk assessment is to reflect the underlying biologic mechanisms of carcinogenesis.

References

1. Moolgavkar SH, Knudson AG. Mutation and cancer: A model for human carcinogenesis. JNCI 66:1037–1052, 1981.
2. Thorslund TW, Brown CC, Charnley G. Biologically motivated cancer risk models. Risk Anal 7:109–119, 1987.
3. Poland A, Knutson JC. 2,3,7,8-Tetracholorodibenzo-*p*-dioxin and related halogenated aromatic hydrocarbons: Examination of the mechanism of toxicity. Annu Rev Pharmacol Toxicol 22: 517–554, 1982.
4. Fukushima S, Cohen SM. Saccharin-induced hyperplasia of the rat urinary bladder. Cancer Res 40:734–736, 1980.
5. Peraino C, Richards WL, Stevens FJ. Multistage hepatocarcinogenesis. In: Slaga TJ (ed): Mechanisms of Tumor Promotion, Vol. 1. Tumor Promotion in Internal Organs. Boca Raton, FL: CRC Press, 1983.

6. Thorslund TW, Charnley G. Quantitative dose-response models for tumor promoting agents. In: Banbury Report 31. Carcinogen Risk Assessment: New Directions in the Qualitative and Quantitative Aspects. Cold Spring Harbor, NY: Cold Spring Harbor Laboratory, 1988.

7. Isaka H, Yoshii H, Otsuji A, Koike M, Nagai Y, Koura M, Sugiyasu K, Kanabayashi T. Tumors of Sprague-Dawley rats induced by long-term feeding of phenacetin. Gann 70:29–36, 1979.

8. Bogdanffy MS, Mazaika TJ, Fasano WJ. Early cell proliferative and cytotoxic effects of phenacetin on rat nasal mucosa. Toxicol Appl Pharmacol 98:100–112, 1989.

9. Swenberg JA, Gross EA, Randall HW. Localization and quantitation of cell proliferation following exposure to nasal irritants. In: Barrow CS (ed): Toxicology of the Nasal Passages. Washington, DC: Hemisphere Publishing, 1966.

10. Swenberg JA, Kerns WD, Mitchell RI, Gralla EJ, Pavkov KL. Induction of squamous cell carcinomas of the rat nasal cavity by inhalation exposure to formaldehyde vapor. Cancer Res 40:3398–3402, 1980.

11. Feldman MY. Reactions of nucleic acids and nucleoproteins with formaldehyde. Prog Nucleic Acids Res Mol Biol 13:1–49, 1973.

12. Swenberg JA, Richardson FC, Boucheron JA, Deal FH, Belinsky SA, Charbonneau M, Short BG. High-to low-dose extrapolation: Critical determinants involved in the dose response of carcinogenic substances. Environ Health Perspect 76:57–63, 1987.

13. Short BG, Burnett VL, Swenberg JA. Histopathology and cell proliferation induced by 2,2,4-trimethylpentane in the male rat kidney. Toxicol Pathol 14:194–203, 1986.

14. Kociba RJ, Keyes DG, Beyer JE, Carreon RM, Wade CE, Dittenber DA, Kalnins RP, Frauson LE, Park CN, Barnard SD, Hummel RA, Humiston CG. Results of a two-year chronic toxicity and oncogenicity study of 2,3,7,8-tetrachlorodibenzo-p-dioxin in rats. Toxicol Appl Pharmacol 46:279–303, 1978.

15. National Cancer Institute (NCI). Bioassay of 2,3,7,8-Tetrachlorodibenzo-p-dioxin for Possible Carcinogenicity. Washington, DC: CHHS Publ. No. 80-1765, 1980.

16. Mustonen R, Elovaara E, Zitting A, Linnainmaa K, Vainio H. Effects of commercial chlorophenolate, 2,3,7,8-TCDD, and pure phenoxyacetic acids on hepatic peroxisome proliferation, xenobiotic metabolism and sister chromatid exchange in the rat. Arch Toxicol 63:203–208, 1989.

17. National Toxicology Program (NTP). Carcinogenesis bioassay of DEHP (CAS No. 117-81-7) in F344 rats and B6C3F1 mice (feed study). NTP 80-37. Research Triangle Park, NC: NIH Publication 82-1772, 1982.

18. Kluwe KM, Haseman JK, Douglas JF, Huff JE. The carcinogenicity of dietary di(2-ethylhexyl) phthalate (DEHP) in Fischer 344 rats and B6C3F1 mice. J Toxicol Environ Health 10:797–815, 1982.

19. Mitchell FE, Price SC, Hinton RH, Grasso P, Bridges JW. Time and dose-response study of the effects on rats of the plasticizer di(2-ethylhexyl) phthalate. Toxicol Appl Pharmacol 81:371–392, 1985.

20. Smith-Oliver T, Loury D, Butterworth BE. Measurement of DNA repair and cell proliferation in hepatocytes from mice treated with di(2-ethylhexyl) phthalate (DEHP). Environ Mutagen 7(Suppl):71, 1985.

21. Marsman DS, Cattley RC, Conway JG, Popp JA. Relationship of hepatic peroxisome proliferation and replicative DNA synthesis to the hepatocarcinogenicity of the peroxisome proliferators di(2-ethylhexyl) phthalate and [4-chloro-6-(2,3-xylidino)-2-pyrimidinylthio]acetic acid (Wy-14,643) in rats. Cancer Res 48:6739–6744, 1988.

22. Lake BG, Gray TJB, Foster JR, Stubberfield CR, Gangolli SD. Comparative studies on di(2-ethylhexyl) phthalate-induced hepatic peroxisome proliferation in the rat and hamster. Toxicol Appl Pharmacol 72:46–60, 1984.

23. Mirsalis JC. In vivo measurement of unscheduled DNA synthesis and S-phase synthesis as an indicator of hepatocarcinogenesis in rodents. Cell Biol Toxicol 3:165–173, 1987.

24. Steinmetz KL, Tyson CK, Meierhenry EF, Spalding JW, Mirsalis JC. Examination of genotoxicity, toxicity and morphologic alteration in hepatocytes following in vivo or in vitro exposure to methapyrilene. Carcinogenesis 9:959–963, 1988.

25. Mirsalis JC, Tyson CK, Loh EN, Steinmetz KL, Bakke JP, Hamilton CM, Spak DK, Spalding JW. Induction of hepatic cell proliferation and unscheduled DNA synthesis in mouse hepatocytes following in vivo treatment. Carcinogenesis 6:1521–1524, 1985.

26. Greenfield RE, Ellwein LB, Cohen SM. A general probabilistic model of carcinogenesis: Analysis of experimental urinary bladder cancer. Carcinogenesis 5:437–445, 1984.

27. Murasaki G, Cohen SM. Effect of dose of sodium saccharin on the induction of rat urinary bladder proliferation. Cancer Res 41:942–944, 1981.

Chemically Induced Cell Proliferation:
Implications for Risk Assessment, pages 303-322
©1991 Wiley-Liss, Inc.

New methods for studying the proliferation and differentiation of epidermal keratinocytes from adult mice

Rebecca J. Morris, Susan M. Fischer, and Thomas J. Slaga

Introduction and background

A single subtumorigenic exposure to a carcinogen and subsequent chronic regenerative epidermal hyperplasia of sufficient magnitude can induce on the backs of mice benign and malignant cutaneous neoplasms. Tumor initiation is thought to convert some of the epidermal keratinocytes into latent neoplastic cells whereas promotion elicits expression of the neoplastic change (1-3). Effective initiators of skin carcinogenesis such as benzo[a]pyrene (B[a]P) and 7,12-dimethylbenz[a]anthracene (DMBA) can, as activated electrophiles, bind covalently to cellular DNA and thereby irreversibly alter the genome of epidermal keratinocytes (4-8). Any expressions of the consequences of this carcinogen–induced genomic alteration in the absence of promotion have not yet been identified. Moreover, the tumor responses evoked whether promotion is begun one week or one year after the exposure to the carcinogen are surprisingly similar (9-18). Considering that the normal epidermis is characterized by continual turnover and cyclic growth and regression of the hair follicles, why and how the latent neoplastic cells remain in the epidermis for so long presents something of an enigma (19-21). The identification of cellular targets maintaining the lifelong potential to form tumors following an exposure to carcinogen is consequently an objective with considerable significance for future molecular and biological studies on the regulation of epidermal growth. It appeared from the carcinogenesis experiments that a potential target cell was almost surely one having a high potential for proliferation relative to most of the proliferative population. It also seemed reasonable to conjecture that the target cell was a cell that normally remained in the epidermis for long periods of time despite the continual turnover.

Two new sets of methods have been developed towards meeting this objective: i) *in vivo* methods that use radioactive labeling of specific epidermal cells followed by light microscopic autoradiography so that their persistence and their responses under various conditions might be studied and ii) *in vitro* techniques to characterize the primary *in vitro* clonogenic keratinocytes, epidermal cells with high proliferative potential. These methods were developed in the context of the two-stage carcinogenesis experiments described below.

Two-stage carcinogenesis experiments

To provide a comprehensive background for present and future experiments, to confirm in our laboratory the work of other investigators, and to relate eventually the results of in *vivo* and in *vitro* experiments, two-stage carcinogenesis experiments were performed to determine in CD–1 and SENCAR mice the effects upon the tumor responses of an interval delay between initiation and tumor promotion (9-18). Briefly, CD–1 mice were treated topically with 200 nmol of DMBA in 200 μl of acetone. SENCAR mice were treated with 10 nmol of DMBA. Control mice of both stocks were treated with 200 μl of acetone. After intervals of 1, 3, 20, and 51 weeks for the CD-1 mice and intervals of 1 and 51 weeks for the SENCAR mice, groups were treated twice weekly with either 200 μl of acetone or TPA in 200 μl of acetone (17 nmol for the CD–1 mice; 3 nmol for the SENCAR) for twenty weeks. Several observations from the results of this study are specifically relevant and are described below.

Firstly, regardless of the time between exposure to the carcinogen and tumor promotion, the first "pinpoint" (≤1 mm diameter) lesions were observed at five weeks of promotion and the first "countable" (≥1 mm diameter) papillomas appeared at six weeks in both the CD–1 and the SENCAR mice (Figure 2). The first cutaneous malignancies were also identified after similar intervals in all groups (Table 1). There were no obvious differences observed in the size or the morphology of the lesions among any experimental groups.

Secondly, there was no statistically significant difference in the final tumor responses at forty weeks regardless of the delay interval (Figure 2a, b, Table 1). Similarly, there was little difference in the incidence of carcinoma and other cutaneous malignancies except among the older animals, which, having a shorter period of observation, were usually terminated because of weight loss, ruffled fur, or signs of stress at an earlier stage in the experiment.

Thirdly, despite the similar final tumor responses in the CD–1 mice, there was a reduction in the maximal number of tumors of approximately 50% between the 1- and 3- week interval groups and the 20- and 51- week interval groups. The maximal number of tumors was counted at 15, 13, 18, and 16 weeks for the 1-, 3-, 20-, and 51- week interval groups, respectively. The reduction in the maximal number of papillomas was not observed in the SENCAR mice (Figure 2c, d).

Figure 1. A) The percentage of mice with papillomas as a function of an increasing delay interval between initiation and promotion. These data demonstrate that virtually all of the mice in all four groups had developed papillomas by 20 weeks. B) Effects on the tumor responses of CD-1 female mice of an increasing delay interval between initiation at eight weeks of age with 200 nmol of DMBA and promotion with 17 nmol of TPA twice weekly for 20 weeks after intervals of 1, 3, 20, and 51 weeks. These data demonstrate: i) a similar latency until the appearance of the first 2-mm papillomas in all four groups (the first pinpoint lesions appeared at 5 weeks); ii) a similar papilloma response at 39 to 40 weeks of promotion (P = 0.5964 by Student's *t* test); iii) a significantly (P = 0.0205) decreased maximal number of papillomas when the delay interval between initiation and promotion was increased from 3 to 20 weeks. C) The percentage of SENCAR female mice with papillomas as a function of an increasing delay interval between initiation and promotion. These data confirm those of the CD-1 mice. All SENCAR mice in the 51 week group had been terminated by 34 weeks of promotion. D. The deffects of the papilloma responses of SENCAR mice of an increasing interval delay between initiation at 8 weeks of age with 10 nmol of DMBA and promotion with 3 nmol of TPA twice weekly for 20 weeks. These data confirm those shown for the CD-1 mice except that the maximal responses of both groups of SENCAR were virtually identical. E) The percentage of CD-1 mice with papillomas as a function of age at initiation with 200 nmol of DMBA at eight or 61 weeks of age and subsequent promotionone week later with 17 nmol of TPA twice weekly for 20 weeks. These data demonstrate: i) that virtually all of the mice in both groups had developed papillomas by 20 weeks of promotion; ii) that the mice developed papillomas at virtually the same rate regardless of the age at initiation. All of the mice in the 60-week group were terminated by 38 weeks of promotion. →

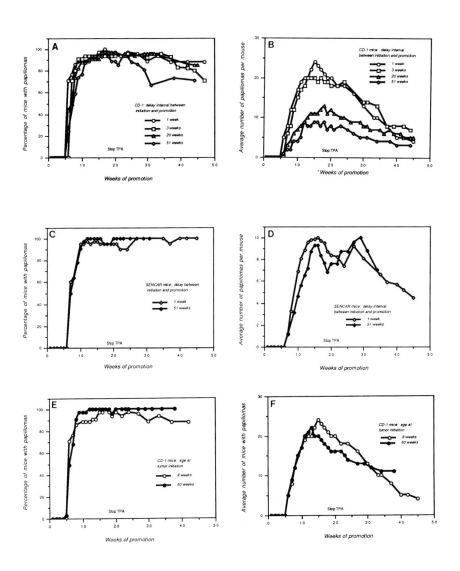

Table 1. Effects of increasing the interval between initiation and promotion or of the age at initiation upon the formation of cutaneous malignancies in CD-1 or in SENCAR female mice.

	CD-1 delay interval (weeks) [b]				SENCAR delay interval (weeks) [c]		CD-1 age at initiation (weeks) [d]		
	1	3	20	51	1	51	8	28	60
Week of promotion when 10% of mice were observed to have cutaneous malignancy [a]	22	24	23	23	31	35	22	22	25
Number of mice terminated with cutaneous malignancy	18	23	17	5	18	3	18	15	7

[a] Squamous cell carcinomas and other cutaneous malignancies were identified grossly by their broad base, elevated margin, and intracutaneous infiltration. They were verified at autopsy and were confirmed histopathologically.

[b] Groups of CD-1 female mice were treated with a topical application of 200 nmol of DMBA and were promoted twice weekly for 20 weeks with 17 nmol of TPA after intervals of 1, 3, 20, and 51 weeks.

[c] Groups of SENCAR female mice were treated with 10 nmol of DMBA and were promoted twice weekly for 20 weeks with 3 nmol of TPA after 1 and 51 weeks. The SENCAR mice initiated at 51 weeks of age were all terminated at 35 weeks of promotion.

[d] Groups of CD-1 female mice were initiated with 200 nmol of DMBA when 8, 28, and 60 weeks of age. They were treated twice weekly for 20 weeks with 17 nmol of TPA beginning 1 week later.

Finally, virtually all of the mice developed papillomas regardless of the interval between initiation and promotion (Figure 2). The overall incidence of papillomas among control mice initiated with acetone and promoted twice weekly with TPA for twenty weeks was five to eight mice per group and 0.1 to 0.5 papillomas per mouse regardless of the stock of mouse or the length of the interval delay. The average number of papillomas among control mice initiated with 200 nmol of DMBA and promoted twice weekly with acetone for twenty weeks was 0.02. No papillomas developed in mice treated with acetone for both the initiation and promotion steps.

To ascertain whether the decreased maximal tumor responses of the CD–1 mice as a function of increasing the delay interval between initiation and tumor promotion could possibly reflect a diminishing responsiveness to TPA in the older animals, we determined the effects on the tumor responses of age at initiation (Figure 2e, f). The results of this experiment demonstrated the similar latency as well as the similar incidence of papillomas whether the mice were initiated at eight or sixty weeks of age.

Thus, we have confirmed that the consequences of a topical exposure to a carcinogen are essentially irreversible, are not expressed in the absence of tumor promotion, and are very similar whether tumor promotion is begun quite soon following initiation or one year later. To determine how the latent neoplastic lesions are maintained requires first understanding cellular turnover in the epidermis. Are there any basal keratinocytes present in the normal, untreated epidermis that would have characteristics such as a long cell cycle time, persistence on the basal layer, or would have a greater potential for proliferation than most other epidermal keratinocytes? If there are, then these keratinocytes could maintain the latent neoplastic lesion following an exposure to a carcinogen.

Cellular kinetics of adult murine epidermis

The epidermis is a continually renewing tissue, normally balancing cellular proliferation in the basal layer with cellular loss from the suprabasal layer through a program of terminal differentiation (20-22). The basal layer of adult murine epidermis consists primarily of keratinocytes, although Langerhans cells (about 10%), melanocytes (about 3%), and Merkel cells (rare) are also present (20). The hair follicles are highly specialized epidermal appendages contiguous with both the interfollicular epidermis and the sebaceous glands. Each basal cell was formerly believed to contribute equally to the balanced epidermal proliferation; displacement from the basal layer was believed to be random; and mitosis was considered to provide the "force" necessary for displacement (23, 24). More recently, several laboratories including ours (25-30) have presented evidence of proliferative heterogeneity within the basal layer compatible with the hierarchical stem cell pattern of cellular replacement originally described by Gilbert and Lajtha for the bone marrow (31, 32) in which a small population of self-renewing stem cells also produces proliferative cells that undergo a series of amplification divisions prior to terminal maturation.

Investigation by light microscopy of whole mounts of epidermal sheets and vertical cross sections through the skin has disclosed that the dorsal epidermis of adult mice is organized into morphologically defined proliferative units (30, 33). Thus, well prepared vertical cross sections reveal a single layer of basal cells covered over by a suprabasal layer with regularly spaced columns of three flattened nucleated cells and occasional cells between the columns. Epidermal proliferative units are most easily visualized in silver stained epidermal whole mounts (33, 34) as groups of ten to twelve basal cells positioned within usually hexagonal margins of the flattened suprabasal cells (Figure 2). Two or three of the basal cells in each group are close to the central column of suprabasal nuclei. The remaining basal cells in each proliferative unit are usually more than one nuclear diameter from the center; these nuclei are designated "peripheral". Approximately 5% of the peripheral nuclei are readily labeled in light microscopic autoradiographs with a single injection of [³H]thymidine in the morning hours. Mitotic figures are also easy to find among the peripheral nuclei. We have shown that most pulse-labeled nuclei remain on the basal layer for four to five days before they are displaced to the suprabasal layers and are found in the columns (35), but nuclei labeled with [3H]thymidine in the morning hours rarely remain in the basal layer for as long as one month. Therefore, these cells behave as though they were more mature or more differentiated than the central cells.

In contrast, continuous administration of [³H]thymidine for at least one week is required to label the central nuclei of the proliferative units, and they are rarely found in mitosis in the normal epidermis (30). This latter observation suggested that these central cells might be more slowly cycling than the peripheral cells (34). This suggestion was born out by the work of Bickenbach and Mackenzie (27) and shortly thereafter by Potten (29, 30, and this laboratory. We used different labeling methods and different

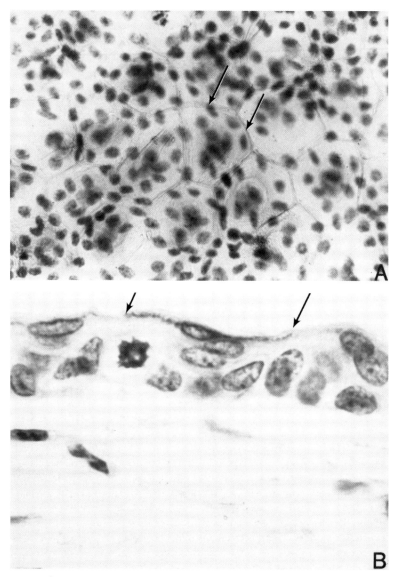

Figure 2. A) A surface view of the dorsal epidermis of an untreated CD-1 mouse demonstrating the hexagonal arrangement of the platelike cells in the stratum corneum (arrows) following silver impregnation of an epidermal whole mount. Note the nuclei of the underlying basal cells here stained with hematoxylin. B) A routine paraffin cross section through the skin of an untreated CD-1 mouse. Note the columnar arrangement of the differentiating suprabasal cells. The edges of the outermost cell would correspond to the silver stained edges above. Note the mitotic basal cell beneath the edge of the flattened suprabasal cell.

ages of mice, but we all observed that if the entire basal layer were labeled by continuous administration of [³H]thymidine, then the central cells retained the [³H]thymdine label for one to six months longer than the peripheral cells (36). Bickenbach, McCutecheon, and Mackenzie demonstrated that the reduction in grain count over these label-retaining cells was consistent with a slow cell cycle for this population (36).

The forgoing observations of the "maturing" and the slowly cycling label-retaining basal cells suggested that the methods of cellular kinetics could be used to focus on epidermal populations that might be significant in the initiation and promotion of skin carcinogenesis.

Evidence that heterogeneity among epidermal basal cells is germane to research in chemical carcinogenesis

There are at least two different subpopulations of proliferating epidermal cells with different responses to TPA

Despite substantial evidence suggesting that basal keratinocytes within the murine epidermal proliferative units comprise a maturation sequence of epidermal stem cells, transit (amplifying) cells, and postmitotic maturing keratinocytes very little was known about possible relationships between the maturity of keratinocytes within the proliferative units and their responsiveness to treatments effective in skin tumor promotion. We, therefore, used well recognized differences in the kinetics of [³H]thymidine labeling within the proliferative units to identify in the normal, dorsal epidermis of adult SENCAR mice two classes of basal cells: (i) those with characteristics expected of a slowly cycling population, and (ii) those with cellular kinetic features of maturing keratinocytes prior to displacement from the basal layer (29).

The purpose of the study was to determine what happened to the [³H]thymidine label-retaining basal cells and the "maturing" classes of basal cells from the dorsal epidermis of adult SENCAR mice and to compare their early cellular kinetic responses to topical application of the tumor promoter, TPA. Autoradiography of epidermal whole mounts and cross sections demonstrated that injection of [³H]thymidine every six hours of one week labeled 95% of the basal nuclei, including those in the central region of the epidermal proliferative units. One month later, the labeling index was reduced to 2%; 90% of the label-retaining cells were within one nuclear diameter of the central suprabasal column of the proliferative units. When mice were treated with 2 µg of TPA one month after labeling, seventy-five percent of the label–retaining cells remained on the basal layer through the twenty-eight hour experimental period (Figure 3a). Label-retaining cells were found in mitosis by 23 hours after treatment with TPA (Figure 3b). In contrast, the basal labeling index following a one hour pulse of [³H]thymidine was 5%. Eighty-five percent of the labeled cells were found in the periphery of the proliferative units. By four days after pulse labeling, most of the originally labeled epidermal cells ("maturing" basal cells) had divided, although vertical cross sections indicated that 92% remained on the basal layer. Following a single application of TPA, 60% of the labeled cells were displaced to the suprabasal layers (Figure 3a). When mice were treated with TPA on day four, labeled cells were rarely found in mitosis throughout the 28 hour experimental period. (Figure 3b). These

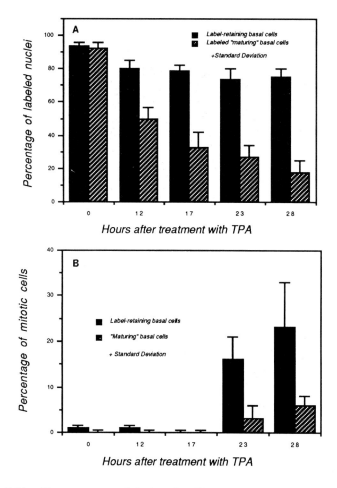

Figure 3. A) The different responses of slowly cycling [3H]thymidine label-retaining basal cells and [3H]thymidine pulse-labeled "maturing" basal cells from SENCAR female mice following treatment with 2 mg of TPA. Note that approximately 80% of the label-retaining basal cells remain on the basal layer through 28 hours after treatment with TPA. Each bar represents the average + S.D. from four to six mice. In contrast, the "maturing" basal cells are rapidly displaced from the basal layer and undergo terminal differentiation.(29). Each bar represents the average + S.D. from three to six mice. B) The different mitotic responses of [3H]thymidine label-retaining basal cells and [3H]thymidine pulse labeled "maturing" basal cells following treatment with TPA. Whereas approximately 20% of the label-retaining basal cells were found in mitosis following treatment with TPA, few of the "maturing" basal cells divide: they have undergone terminal differentiation. Each bar represents the average of three to six determinations + S.D. Colchicine was injected intraperitoneally five hours before the animals were killed. Experimental details are presented in reference 29.

observations suggested that two classes of epidermal basal cells differed not only with respect to their positions in the tissue architecture and relative time spent on the basal layer, they had different early responses to TPA treatment: the label-retaining cells proliferated, and most of the "maturing" cells continue to differentiate.

Evidence that slowly cycling epidermal basal cells retain carcinogen

We next confirmed and extended these studies with regard to the distribution and persistence of radioactively labeled B[a]P in the skin of adult SENCAR female mice (37). This was investigated by autoradiography of epidermal whole mounts and cross sections at intervals following a single initiating application of 200 nmol of either [^{3}H]B[a]P (2 mCi) or [^{14}C]B[a]P (23 μCi). One day after treatment, the entire thickness of the skin was labeled, although the grain density was greatest over the hair follicles, sebaceous glands, and interfollicular epidermis. At one and two weeks, decreases in the nuclear grain density were consistent with the overall pattern of epidermal renewal. One month after treatment, carcinogen label-retaining cells comprised approximately 2% of the interfollicular basal cells; they were also present in the hair follicles (Figure 4). Carcinogen label-retaining cells were compared with the slowly cycling [^{3}H]thymidine label-retaining cells and the "maturing" basal cells, two distinct proliferative subsets of adult murine epidermis. Carcinogen label-retaining cells were found to have characteristics of the slowly cycling cells: i) most of the carcinogen labeled nuclei were found in the central regions of the epidermal proliferative units; ii) treatment of the carcinogen label-retaining cells with 2 μg of TPA elicited labeled mitoses within one day as well as a general decrease in grain density over basal nuclei. In contrast, "maturing" basal cells four days after a single injection of [^{3}H]thymidine were found at the periphery of the epidermal proliferative units. Within one day after treatment with 2 μg of TPA, "maturing" basal cells were displaced to the suprabasal layers. Double isotope - double emulsion autoradiographs demonstrated doubly labeled cells one month after continuous labeling with [^{3}H]thymidine and treatment with [^{14}C]B[a]P and provide evidence that the radioactively labeled carcinogen is retained by the slowly cycling [^{3}H]thymidine label-retaining cells. These observations suggested that a slowly cycling population of epidermal cells may be relevant to the initiation phase of two-stage carcinogenesis, not necessarily because they retain the carcinogen adducts, but because they are immature and farther from terminal differentiation than other cell populations.

Evidence that slowly cycling epidermal basal cells from adult mice may be clonogenic in vitro

Differences between the two distinct subpopulations of epidermal basal cells from adult mice are thus germane not only to the functional biology of normal epidermis, but also to the initiation and promotion of skin carcinogenesis. Whereas slowly cycling basal cells retain [^{3}H]B[a]P adducts, remain on the basal layer at least five weeks longer than other basal cells, and are mitotically activated following exposure to TPA; most pulse labeled (maturing) basal cells remain on the basal layer less than one week and are displaced suprabasally within one day after treatment with TPA. In collaboration with Dr. Christopher Potten at the Paterson Institute for Cancer Research, Manchester England, we compared the fates *in vitro* of these two labeled populations. Slowly cycling

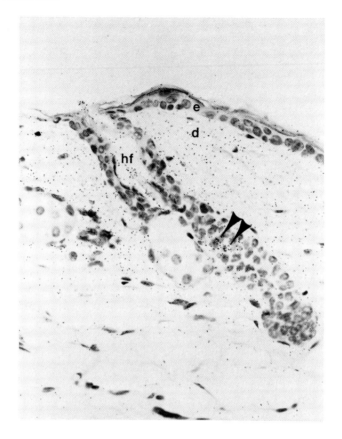

Figure 4. Carcinogen label-retaining cells in the hair follicle. Mice were treated with a single topical application of 200 nmols of [³H]B[a]P (2 mCi) in 200 ml of acetone. Four weeks later, samples of the dorsal skin were fixed in aqueous 10% formalin and paraffin cross sections were prepared. The slides were prepared for light microscopic autoradiography following extraction with ethyl acetate. Note the label-retaining cells (arrows) in the hair follicle (hf); e, epidermis; d, dermis.

(label-retaining) epidermal cells were identified by light microscopic autoradiography six weeks after twice daily injection with [3H]thymidine on days three through five after birth (27, 30). Pulse labeled maturing epidermal cells were identified in seven to eight week old mice forty minutes after a single injection of [³H]TdR. Epidermal cells including those from the hair follicles were isolated by trypsinization and cultured at low density on feeder layers of irradiated 3T3 in Dulbecco's minimal essential medium according to the method of Rheinwald and Green (38). At daily intervals, some of the cultures were fixed, processed for light microscopic autoradiography, and the distribution of labeled nuclei quantitated. After four days, cultures from mice with label-retaining cells had labeled nuclei in pairs and clusters with grain counts consistent with their division (Table 2). In contrast, cultures from mice with pulse-labeled epidermal cells showed that the labeled nuclei remained primarily as single cells (Table 3). Labeling the mice with [14C]TdR gave similar results, indicating that our observations were not a consequence of radiation damage induced by the tritium. These results demonstrate that two distinct subpopulations of basal keratinocytes, pulse-labeled and label-retaining, maintain one of their important *in vivo* characteristics when cultivated *in vitro*.

Table 2. Are SCLRC (*in vivo*)[a] clonogenic (*in vitro*)?[b]

	Distribution of labeled nuclei (percentage)[c]		
Days *in vitro*	Singles	Pairs	Clusters
1	95	3	2
2	47	23	30
4	26 ± 6.7	38 ± 7.0	36 ± 7.2
5	not done	not done	not done
7	_d	_d	_d

a To identify SCLRC, BDF$_1$ mice were injected subcutaneously with 10 μCi of [3H]thymidine twice daily for three days beginning the third day after birth. Six weeks later, the female mice were used for isolation of epidermal cells. The use of [14C]thymidine gave similar results.
b Isolation and cultivation of the epidermal cells was performed as in the accompanying legend for pulse-labeled epidermal cells.
c Quantitative light microscopic autoradiography was performed as for pulse labeled cells. The values represent the averages ± S.D. of one to eight flasks.
d Nuclei labeled with > 3 silver grains were rarely observed at seven days.

Table 3. Are pulse labeled epidermal keratinocytes (*in vivo*)[a] clonogenic (*in vitro*)?[b]

	Distribution of labeled nuclei (percentage)[c]		
Days in vitro	Singles	Pairs	Clusters
1	94 ± 6.0	6 ± 6	0 ± 0
2	89 ± 4.2	11 ± 4.2	0 ± 0
4	80 ± 5.3	11 ± 6.5	9 ± 6
5	68 ± 8.5	20 ± 14	12 ± 4.5
7	70 ± 4.8[d]	16 ± 5.6[d]	14 ± 4.6[d]

a To identify pulse-labeled keratinocytes, BDF$_1$ female mice eight weeks of age (The Paterson Institute for Cancer Research, Manchester, ENGLAND) were injected with 25 μCi of [3H]thymidine between 9:00 am and 10:00 am, 40 min before killing.
b Epidermal cells were isolated as we have described (62), plated at 5x10^5 per T75 flask, and cultivated on 5x10^5 irradiated Swiss 3T3 in DMEM with 10% fetal bovine serum , cholera toxin, and hydrocortisone (64). At intervals thereafter, the 3T3 were remover, the flasks were fixed in formalin, and were processed for light microscopic autoradiography.
c Microscopy was performed with a Zeiss Standard microscope equipped with 40x and 100x planapochromatic objectives and 10x eyepieces. Silver grains on or within the nuclear margin were counted over 300 to 700 consecutive single or clustered keratinocytes (containing ≤ 20 cells).. Limits on the grain counts in this experiment were ≥ 10 grains per cluster and ≥ 3 grains per labeled nucleus. The values are the average of three to five flasks. Other choices of limits on the grain counts gave similar results, as did the use of [14C] thymidine.
d Many labeled nuclei appeared to be "suprabasal" (nonproliferating) by seven days.

Pulse labeled keratinocytes maintain for the most part a very limited capacity for proliferation whereas label-retaining (slowly cycling) keratinocytes have relatively greater potential for proliferation. These results have considerable significance for present and future studies in carcinogenesis and in skin biology, especially as related to the identification of cells able to maintain lifelong the "latent neoplastic lesion". The slowly cycling, label-retaining cells are particularly interesting in this regard. The pulse labeled cells are also interesting because of their apparently limited proliferative capacity *in* vivo and *in vitro* and because they respond so quickly to TPA (*in vivo*) by terminal differentiation.

Development of new in vitro methods for adult murine epidermal cells

The development of new culture media

With rare exceptions (39-42), long–term primary cultures of epidermal cells from normal, untreated adult mice have been notoriously difficult to establish and to maintain except under conditions in which the concentration of calcium in the medium has been reduced such that the keratinocytes neither stratify nor make desmosomes (43, 44), two distinctive characteristics of their terminal differentiation *in vivo*. The addition of calcium to such cultures has been found to induce rapid terminal differentiation and sloughing of nearly all proliferative keratinocytes except those from mice treated with chemical carcinogens (45-47). Although these culture conditions have provided the basis for excellent assays of carcinogen-treated epidermal cells, as well as studies of calcium dependent factors involved in the induction of terminal differentiation of epidermal cells from newborn mice (43-44), they are inappropriate for comparison of proliferative subpopulations of epidermal keratinocytes from untreated adult murine epidermis, studies designed for coculture of dermal and epidermal cells, or for biochemical, toxicological, or metabolic studies requiring calcium (48, 49).

A culture medium has been formulated to support the long-term proliferation and differentiation of epidermal cells in primary cultures from normal and treated adult mice. This formulation is based upon MCDB-151 modified by the addition of 1.2 mM $CaCl_2$, 0.1% purified bovine serum albumin (BSA), trace elements, and growth supplements. For four to twelve weeks, cultures demonstrate desmosomes, keratin fibers, basal proliferation, and stratification characteristic of keratinocytes. The addition of 0.1 µg/ml of TPA resulted in approximately 70% cellular detachment, but with continued treatment, the remaining cells proliferated to confluence and stratified. This culture medium has application to a number of studies related to skin carcinogenesis in the murine model system that have not previously been possible.

Epidermal colonies may be grown from freshly isolated epidermal cells from normal as well as treated adult mice in SPRD-105 medium with feeder layers of irradiated Swiss 3T3 fibroblasts (38). Three types of colony morphology are observed (Figure 5). Those appearing within the first week tend to be small and consist of flattened cells having a "mature" appearance. Type II colonies usually appear in the second week, consist of highly proliferative "immature" epidermal cells, are candidate stem cells colonies. Type III colonies have characteristics of Types I and II. The reproducibility of this technique suggested its use as an assay for comparing clonogenic cells among treatment groups *in vivo*. Normalizing the cell yields upon harvesting, the number of colonies, and histological determination of basal nuclear counts per centimeter squared of epidermis will permit further biologically meaningful comparison of the different treatment groups.

Characterization of adult murine epidermal cells by density gradient sedimentation

Lineage or maturation markers are not yet characterized for murine epidermal keratinocytes and the use of radioactive labels for long periods of time is not without potential problems. We have therefore explored the use of density and size as a means of separating basal cells that might have different properties of growth and differentiation. There is good biological precedence for this approach. Sun and Green (50) first described the relationship between decreasing buoyant density and increasing size and maturity of cultured human keratinocytes. As reviewed by Klein-Szanto et al. (51), all of the subsequent investigations were focused primarily on the suprabasal rather than the proliferative population (52-56). Barrandon and Green (57) have reported that the smallest of cultured human foreskin keratinocytes have the highest clonogenic potential on fibroblast feeder layers. They also presented evidence that a relationship between size of basal cells and clonogenicity exists *in vivo*.

Epidermal cells from adult mice were isolated by trypsinization and sedimented through a Percoll density gradient designed to elicit maximal separation among basal cells. The gradients were characterized with regard to i) morphology of the sedimented cells, ii) enrichment for label-retaining cells, iii) for cells that could proliferate in the presence of TPA, iv) for clonogenic cells from normal and initiated mice, and v) for cells with particular antigenic determinants.

Quantitative and qualitative characterization. Table 4 summarizes some of the characteristics of untreated adult murine epidermal cells isolate by trypsinization and then separated on 61.5% Percoll gradients. The recovery of nucleated cells was approximately 76% with the greatest loss of nucleated spinous and granular cells. Three fractions containing >93% viable basal cells were recovered. All three fractions demonstrated some heterogeneity with regard to size (fraction 5, 3-5 μm; fraction 4, 3-6 μm; fraction 3, 4-7 μm) and morphology as determined by light microscopy. Electron microscopy demonstrated the cells of the lower three fractions consisted of basal keratinocytes, but otherwise showed few outstanding morphological characteristics; in general, the more dense cells appeared to have higher ratio of nucleus to cytoplasm and somewhat more ribosomes. Interactive sedimentation of fraction 4 cells demonstrated that most of them return to that density range.

Enrichment for slowly cycling and carcinogen label-retaining cells. Autoradiographic analysis of sedimented epidermal cells from mice that had been labeled with [^{3}H]thymidine demonstrated that pulse-labeled epidermal cells are distributed fairly uniformly throughout the lower four fractions of the gradients. Those labeled cells in fraction 1 are large, round cells with a basal rather than a differentiated morphology. The labeled "maturing" basal cells four days following a single pulse of [^{3}H]thymidine are also fairly evenly distributed throughout the gradient, with an increase in the number of labeled basaloid cells in fraction 1. In contrast, we observed a density-dependent enrichment in fraction 5 for the slowly cycling [^{3}H]thymidine label-retaining cells. Carcinogen label-

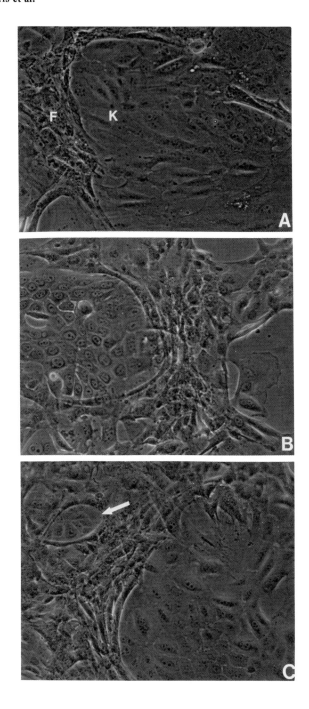

Table 4. Density gradient sedimentation of epidermal basal cells from adult mice. [a]

			% basal cells[e]			[3H]BaP label-retaining cells[f]			
Gradient fraction[b] and density (g/ml)	Distribution of cells[c] (%)	Viability[d] (%)	Griffonia simplici-folia	Bullous pemphi-goid	K14	Exp1	Exp2	Exp3	%[g] clonogenic
1 (1.017-1.062)	41 ± 9.4	15 ± 4.6	20	14	39	-	-	-	24 ± 8.1
2 (1.062-1.076)	11 ± 4.4	78 ± 6.6	67	35	63	1	15	10	36 ± 9.4
3. (1.076-1.088)	8 ± 2	93 ± 2.9	95	88	94	6	4	3	42 ± 14
4 (1.088-1.097)	13 ± 2.6	94 ± 1.1	91	90	89	8	3	4	72 ± 22
5 (10.97-1.143)	3 ± 1	95 ± 1.8	90	89	81	10	8	12	88 ± 17

[a] Thirty million freshly harvested epidermal cells from CD-1 female mice were sedimented through continuous, preformed density gradients having a starting density of 1.086 g/ml of Percoll.

[b] Density marker beads supplied for use with Percoll were used to define the fractions.

[c] Average percentage recovery of the total number of cells loaded onto the gradients (viable plus nonviable) ± S.D. of seven separate determinations. The cells were counted in a hemacytometer.

[d] The viability was assessed by ability to exclude trypan blue dye. The values represent the the average percentage of viable cells in each fraction ± S.D. of seven separate determinations.

[e] The cells were fixed with 1% paraformaldehyde and then incubated with the FITC conjugate of the lectin or with the appropriate antiserum followed by the FITC conjugated secondary antibody, and then were counterstained with propidium iodide. Cells to be incubated with K14 were first permeabilized with acetone. Seventy-five to five humdred consecutive single cells in each fraction were scored as available with a Zeiss standard microscope with epifluorescence and 25x and 40x immersion objectives. Cells with bright relative fluorescence were scored as positive. Values are the average of two or three separate experiments whose variation was within 20% for fractions 1 and 2 and was within 10% for fractions three through five.

[f] Epidermal cells were harvested and sedimented four weeks after a single topical application of 200 nmol of [3H]BaP. Values are the counts of at least 1000 cells in each fraction labeled with ≥5 grains in 28-day autoradiographs.

[g] Epidermal cells from untreated CD-1 female mice were sedimented through Percoll density gradients, were seeded at a density of 8000 viable cells per 60-mm dish onto 2-5x106 irradiated 3T3 cells, were cultured for two weeks in SPRD-105 medium, were fixed, and were stained. Keratinocyte colonies between 0.5 and 2.0 mm in diameter were counted and were verified by microscopy. The values represent the average number of colonies ± S.D. from sixteen to nineteen dishes in three separate experiments. The mice in these experiments were seven to nine weeks of age.

Figure 5. Micrographs of keratinocyte colonies from normal untreated epidermis of CD-1 female mice. A) Colonies of Type I morphology appear after five to seven days in vitro and exhibit cellular features of morphological maturation: large, flat, frequently binucleated keratinocytes (K) that often grow beneath the irradiated 3T3 fibroblasts (F). Colonies of Types II (B) and III (C) may be found after seven to eleven days. Type II colonies consist almost entirely of very small basal cells. Type III colonies have features of both types I and II (arrow).
←

retaining cells also demonstrated a density-dependent enrichment (Table 4).

Enrichment for epidermal cells that proliferate in the presence of TPA in vitro. We were intrigued by the observation that following treatment with TPA *in vitro* (40), some small basal cells from normal epidermis did not slough from the dish, but instead remained attached and apparently unscathed by the TPA, and capable of long-term proliferation upon continued treatment. Such a characteristic might be expected of a fairly immature population of epidermal basal cells. We therefore performed density gradient sedimentation of normal epidermal basal cells from adult mice and seeded the same number of trypan blue excluding cells from fractions 2-5 and from the unseparated mixture in SPRD-109 medium onto collagen coated dishes. Twenty-four hours later, similar numbers of attached cells were observed microscopically in fractions 3-5, as observed on previous occasions (fraction 3-5 contain basal cells). The dishes from the various fractions were divided into two experimental groups and treated with either acetone or TPA. Twenty-four hours after treatment, fractions 3-5 in the acetone treated group retained similar numbers of attached cells (judged microscopically), as previously observed for normal, untreated fractions. In the TPA-treated group, however, fraction 5 retained many more attached cells than fraction 3. The cultures were maintained with continued treatment at each change of the medium for two weeks. These results suggest that the Percoll density gradients also enrich for basal cells that are either inherently resistant to TPA, or that respond to it primarily by proliferation. Somehow, these cells and their progeny must be able to "adapt" to the TPA because the TPA-treated cultures eventually stratify and are practically indistinguishable (morphologically) from the control cultures. Whether these "resistant" cells are also resistant to other treatments such as a calcium selection medium, or whether they are label-retaining cells is not known at this time. We hope to continue these experiments; we would expect these cells might be generally less responsive to other treatments.

Enrichment for clonogenic epidermal cells. As demonstrated in Table 4 there was a slight density-dependent enrichment in Fraction 5 for keratinocytes that can form colonies *in vitro* on irradiated 3T3 fibroblasts.

Primary in vitro clonogenic keratinocytes during two-stage carcinogenesis

The formation of colonies *in vitro* by freshly harvested epidermal cells was studied because this is a well-recognized, quantifiable indicator of both the number of cells with high growth potential relative to other proliferative cells and also the relative growth potential of single cells. These *in vitro* experiments were performed with the carcinogenesis studies described above. From normal, untreated CD-1 female mice nine to fifty-nine weeks of age, single cell suspensions of freshly harvested epidermal cells were seeded at clonal density onto Swiss 3T3 feeder layers, cultivated for two weeks in SPRD-105 medium, fixed, and stained with rhodamine B. As shown by Figure 6a, the number of primary epidermal clonogens from untreated mice determined in this culture system remains essentially unchanged during adult life with an average cloning efficiency of 0.45%. As an internal technical control, some of the determinations were made in parallel with epidermal cells harvested from age-matched mice treated with 200 µl of acetone one month earlier. Any difference in the cloning efficiency from ten of eleven such experiments was not statistically significant.

To determine whether a single initiating application of 200 nmol of DMBA might bring about a change in the number of primary epidermal clonogens, CD-1 female mice were exposed to eight weeks of age to either 200 µl of acetone or to 200 nmol of DMBA when eight weeks of age. At intervals of seven to sixty-one weeks thereafter, the number of primary clonogens was determined, and as shown in Figure 6b , remained essentially within the control values for the duration of the experiment. In contrast, twelve treatments of the mice with 17 nmol of TPA resulted in an increase at least two-fold in the number of colonies detected one month after the last treatment.

Conclusions

Two new experimental approaches have been designed to address problems of the proliferation of epidermal cells from the normal and the treated adult mouse within the context of the two-stage model for skin carcinogenesis. The first approach uses the techniques of cellular kinetics, labeling cells in *vivo* with radioactive isotopes followed over time by light microscopic autoradiography, to focus on a subpopulation of epidermal cells from normal epidermis that remains in the proliferative population far longer than most basal cells. This slowly cycling population also retains carcinogen adducts covalently bound to the DNA. Although these cells probably retain the carcinogen because they are slowly cycling, they are nevertheless of interest as regards persistence of the "latent neoplastic lesion". The second approach uses culture media formulated to support concomitant proliferation and terminal differentiation of primary epidermal cells from normal as well as treated adult mice and density gradient sedimentation to separate primary epidermal basal cells with high proliferative poten-tial.. One of the culture media is useful for quantitating the primary keratinocytes from different *in vivo* treatment groups that can make a colony from a single cell. These primary *in vitro* clonogenic keratinocytes are important because they are epidermal cells with far greater proliferative capacity than most epidermal basal cells. We are using these developments in the context of the two-stage model for skin carcinogenesis in the mouse. Our results demonstrate that these methods should greatly extend the range of experiments that can now be performed with primary epidermal cells from the adult mouse.

Figure 6. A) The number of primary *in vitro* clonogenic epidermal cells from normal untreated CD-1 female mice nine to fifty-nine weeks of age. Single cell suspensions of freshly isloated epidermal cells from three to five mice were seeded at clonal density onto Swiss 3T3 fibroblasts, were cultivated for two weeks in SPRD-105 medium, were fixed, and were stained with rhodamine. Each bar represents the average number of keratinocyte colonies 0.5 to 2.0 mm in diameter per 10^4 viable cells in five to ten dishes plus the standard deviation. These data demonstrate that the number of primary *in vitro* clonogenic keratinocytes from normal mice remains essentially unchanged for the duration of the experiment. This number of colonies was not different statistically (p.0.1074) in ten of eleven experiments performed simultaneously with matched acetone-treated controls. B. The number of primary *in vitro* clonogenic keratinocytes from CD-1 female mice exposed at eight weeks of age to a topical application of either 200 µl of acetone or to 200 nmol of DMBA and harvested seven to sixty-one weeks later. These data demonstrate that initiation of the mice with 200 nmol of DMBA did not detectably affect the number of primary epidermal clonogens for sixty-one weeks. Qualitative differences in the growth of the colonies were observed and are under investigation. In nine of thirteen parallel experiments there was not significant difference (p>0.05 in the number of colonies from mice exposed to either acetone or to DMBA.

$\rightarrow$

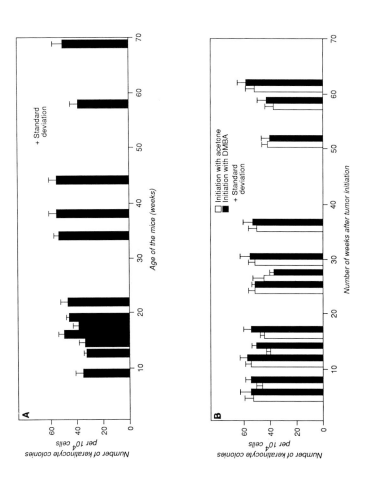

Figure 6.

References

1. Boutwell, R.K. CRC Crit. Rev. Toxicol. 2: 419-443, 1974.
2. Scribner, J.D., and Suss, R. Int. Rev. Exp. Pathol. 18: 137-198.
3. Slaga, T.J. In: T.J. Slaga (ed.), Mechanisms of Tumor Promotion, Vol. 2, pp. 1-16. CRC Press, Inc., Boca Raton, FL, 1984.
4. Dipple, A., Mosch, R.C., and Bigger, C.A.H. In: C.E. Searle (ed.), Chemical Carcinogens, Ed. 2, Vol. 1, ACS Monograph 182, pp. 41-163. Washington, D.C.: American Chemical Society, 1984.
5. Miller, E.C. and Miller, J.A. Cancer (Phila.), 47: 2327-2345, 1981.
6. Osborn, M.R. In: C.E. Searle (ed.), Chemical Carcinogens, Ed. 2, Vol. 1, ACS Monograph 182, pp. 485-524. Washington D.C.: American Chemical Society, 1984.
7. Ashurst, S.W., Cohen, G.M., Nesnow, S., DiGiovanni, J., and Slaga, T.J. Cancer Res., 43: 1024-1029, 1982.
8. Nakayama, J., Yuspa, S.H., and Poirier, M.C. Benzo(a)pyrene-DNA adduct formation in mouse epidermis. Cancer Res., 43:1024-1029, 1982.
9. Boutwell, R.K. Some biological aspects of skin carcinogenesis. Prog.Exp. Tumor Res., 4: 207-250, 1964.
10. Roe, F.J.C., Carter, R.N., Mitchley, B.V.C., Peto, R., and Hecker, E. Int. J. Cancer, 9:624-673, 1972.
11. Stenback, F., Peto, R., and Shubik, P. Br. J. Cancer, 44: 1-14, 1981.
12. Van Duuren, B.L., Sivak, A., Katz, C., Deidman, I., and Melchionne, S. Cancer Res., 35:502-505, 1975.
13. Loehrke, H., Schweizer, J., Dederer, E., Hesse, B., Rosenkranz, G., and Goerttler, K. Carcinogenesis (Lond.), 4:771-775, 1983.
14. Hennings, H. and Boutwell, R.K. Cancer Res., 30:312-320, 1985.
15. Argyris, T.S. Amer. J. Indust. Med., 8: 329-337, 1985.
16. Hennings, H. and Yuspa, S.H. JNCI, 74: 735-740, 1985.
17. Stenback, F. and Arranto, A. IARC Sci. Publ. 58:151-166, 1985.
18. Morris, R.J., Tacker, K.C., Fischer, S.M., and Slaga, T.J. Cancer Res. 48: 6285-6290, 1988.
19. Argyris, T.S. Natl. Cancer Inst. Monogr., 10: 23-43, 1963.
20. Potten, C.S. In: C.S.Potten (ed.), Stem Cells: Their Identification and Characterization, pp. 200-232. New York: Churchill-Livingstone, 1983.
21. Iversen, O.H., Bjerknes, R., and Devik, J. Cell Tissue Kinet., 1: 352-367, 1968.
22. Leblond, C.P. Natl. Cancer Inst. Monogr., 14: 119-150, 1964.
23. Leblond, C.P., Greulich, R.C., and Pereira, J.P. In: W. Montagna and R.E. Billingham, (editors) Advances in Biology of the Skin Vol. 5. "Wound Healing" pp. 39-67, Pergamon Press, 1964.
24. Mitrani, E. Br. J. Dermatol. 109: 635-642, 1983.
25. Christophers, E. J. Invest. Dermatol. , 56: 165-170, 1971.
26. Mackenzie, I.C. Nature (London), 226: 653-655, 1970.
27. Bickenbach, J.R. J. Dental Res., 60: 1611-1620, 1981.
28. Mackenzie, I.C. and Bickenbach, J.R. Cell Tissue Res., 242: 551-556, 1985.
29. Morris, R.J., Fischer, S.M., and Slaga, T.J. J. Invest. Dermatol., 34: 277-281, 1985.
30. Potten, C.S. Cell cycles in cell hierarchies. Int. J. Radiat. Biol. Relat. Stud. Phys. Chem. & Med., 49: 257-278, 1986.
31. Gilbert, C.W. and Lajtha, L.G. Cellular Radiation Biology, pp. 118-154, Williams and Wilkins, Baltimore, 1965.
32. Lajtha, L.G. Differentiation 4: 23-24, 1979.
33. Allen, T.D. and Potten, C.S. J. Cell Sci. 15: 291-319, 1974.
34. Potten, C.S. Cell Tissue Kinet. 7: 77-80, 1974.
35. Morris, R.J. and Argyris, T.S. Cancer Res. 43: 4935-4942, 1983.
36. Bickenbach, J.R., McCutecheon, J., and Mackenzie, I.C. Cell Tissue Kinet. 19: 325-333, 1986.
37. Morris, R.J., Fischer, S.M., and Slaga, T.J. Cancer Res. 46: 3061-3066, 1986.
38. Rheinwald, J.G., and Green, H. Cell 6: 331-344, 1975.
39. Fischer, S.M. In: Webber, M.M. (editor) In Vitro Models for Cancer Research Vol. 3. CRC Press, Inc., Boca Raton, FL, pp. 275-300, 1985.
40. Morris, R.J., Tacker, K.C., Baldwin, J.K., Fischer, S.M., and Slaga, T.J. Cancer Lett. 34: 297-304, 1987.
41. Pera, M.F. and Gorman, P.A. Carcinogenesis 5: 671-682, 1984.

42. Hennings, H. Holbrook, K., and Yuspa, S.H. J. Cell Physiol. 116: 265-281, 1983.
43. Hennings, H. and Holbrook, K. Exp. Cell Res. 143: 127-142, 1983.
44. Hennings, H., Michael, D., Cheng, C., Steinert, P., Holbrook, K., and Yuspa, S.H. Cell 19: 245-254, 1980.
45. Kawamura, H., Strickland, J.E., Yuspa, S.H. Cancer Res. 45: 2748-2757, 1985.
46. Miller, D.R., Viaje, A., Rotstein, J., Aldaz, C.M., Conti, C.J., and Slaga, T.J. Cancer Res. 49: 410-414, 1989.
47. Yuspa, S.H. and Morgan D.L. Nature, 293: 72-74, 1981.
48. Yuspa, S.H., Lichti, U., Hennings, H. In: I.A. Bernstein and M. Seij (editors) Biochemistry of normal and abnormal epidermal differentiation, S.Karger, Basel, pp. 171-191, 1980.
49. DiGiovanni, J., Gill, R.D., Nettikumara, A.N., Colby, A.B., and Reiners, J.J., Jr. Cancer Res. 49: 5567-5574, 1989.
50. Sun, T.-T. and Green, H. Cell, 9: 511-521, 1976.
51. Clausen, O.P.F., Lindmo, T., Sandnes, K., and Thorud, E. Virchows Arch. B. Cell Pathol., 20: 261-275, 1976.
52. Clausen, O.P.F., Kirkhus, B., Thorud, E., Schjolberg, A., Moen, E., and Cromarty, A. J. Invest. Dermatol., 86:266-270, 1986.
53. Watt, F.M. and Green H. J. Cell Biol., 90: 738-742, 1981.
54. Brysk, M.M., Snider, J.M., and Smith, E.B. J. Invest. Dermatol., 77: 205-209, 1981.
55. Goldenhersh, M.A., Good, R.A., Sarkar, N.H., and Safai, B. Anal. Biochem., 119:246-252, 1982.
56. Schweizer, J., Kinjo, M., Furstenburger, G., and Winter, H. Cell, 37: 159-170, 1984.
57. Furstenberger, G., Gross, M., Schweizer, J., Vogt, I., and Marks, F. Carcinogenesis, 7:1745-1753, 1986.
58. Fischer, S.M., Nelson, K.D.G., Reiners, J.J., Viaje, A., Pelling, J.C., and Slaga, T.J. J. Cutaneous. Pathol., 9: 43-49, 1982.
59. Reiners, J.J. and Slaga, T.J. Cell, 32:247-255, 1983.

Chemically Induced Cell Proliferation:
Implications for Risk Assessment, pages 323-335
©1991 Wiley-Liss, Inc.

Chemically Induced Cell Proliferation in Upper Respiratory Tract Carcinogenesis

Thomas M. Monticello, Roger Renne, and Kevin T. Morgan

Epithelial injury followed by cell proliferation is a prominent feature of many toxicant-induced regenerative and adaptive responses in the respiratory system. This proliferative response is needed to replace damaged epithelium and to protect the airway mucosa from further insult by repairing and adapting the epithelial barrier. Cell proliferation, an essential component of the multistage process of carcinogenesis, is required for both initiation and promotion of neoplasia in certain organs (1,2), and it plays an essential role in the later stages of carcinogenesis, including the progression of benign lesions to malignancy and metastasis (3). Cell proliferation may also be a significant component of and contributor to the enhancement of respiratory carcinogenesis, as indicated, for example, by the role of promoterlike factors in cigarette smoke (4).

A number of chemicals induce neoplasms in the nasal cavity of the rat (Table 1), but quantitative information characterizing proliferative responses of the respiratory epithelium to nasal carcinogens in rodents is minimal (5-17). There is also a lack of information regarding cell proliferation during tumor development in the upper respiratory tract. This chapter will focus on toxicant-induced alterations in cell proliferation in the upper respiratory tract and the potential role it may play in carcinogenesis, with special reference to formaldehyde-induced nasal cancer in rodents.

The mucosal epithelium of the upper respiratory tract, including that of the nasal passages, is normally in a steady state of cell renewal, in which cell production balances cell loss (18). Under normal conditions, the cell turnover time of the upper respiratory tract epithelium is very long (19). Increases in cell proliferation rate are seen, however, in chronically irritated respiratory airway epithelium, which is also a common site for malignant transformation (2). Malignancies are most common in tissues composed of cell populations that either have a high endogenous rate of proliferation, or, like the mucosa of the respiratory tract, can be induced to proliferate at increased rates following exposure to irritating air pollutants (2). Moreover, there is substantial evidence that neoplasia often develops in chronically injured tissue. In humans, both maxillary sinusitis (20) and chronic bronchitis (21) have been associated with neoplasia in their respective locations.

Methods of evaluation

Nasal passages

The nasal passages of laboratory animals and human beings are complex and consist of a variety of epithelial types, including squamous, respiratory and olfactory.

Table 1. Rodent Nasal Carcinogens in Rodents.

Chemical	Cell proliferation study[a]	Reference
Benzo[a]pyrene	no	5
p-Cresidine	no	6
1,2-Dibromo-3-chloropropane	no	7
1,2-Dibromoethane	no	8
1,4-Dioxane	acute	9
Dimethylcarbamyl chloride	no	7
Epichlorohydrin	no	10
Formaldehyde	acute	11
	acute, subchronic, chronic	12,13
Hexamethylphosphoramide	no	14
Nitrosamines	no	15
Phenacetin	acute	16
Procarbazine	no	6
Propylene oxide	no	7
Tetrachlorodibenzodioxin	no	17

[a]In vivo cell proliferation study of the upper respiratory tract epithelium using a DNA precursor label.

Stratified squamous epithelium, which is fairly resistant to inhaled irritant gases, lines the most anterior portion of the rat nasal cavity. In the rodent's nasal respiratory epithelium, which is a common target tissue following exposure to irritant gases (22,23), morphologic characteristics differ from area to area (24–26). In a region just posterior to the nasal vestibule and extending to the anterior one-third of the maxilloturbinate, for example, the lateral aspects of the nasoturbinate and the lateral wall are covered by a pseudostratified cuboidal epithelium with rare secretory and ciliated cells. The remaining lined portions of the respiratory system are more characteristic of upper airway epithelium and consist of a pseudostratified columnar epithelium with cilia and varying numbers of secretory cells. Evaluation of the different types of epithelium in the nasal passages requires, therefore, that at least four or five standard nasal sections be examined (27,28).

Both neoplastic and nonneoplastic chemically induced lesions in the rat nasal mucosa vary considerably in location and nature. The distribution of these lesions is believed to be a consequence of regional deposition of the inhaled material, local tissue susceptibility, or a combination (23). In the case of highly water-soluble or reactive gases, such as formaldehyde, nasal airflow patterns probably play a major role in determining the distribution of lesions (23). In other cases, regional metabolism may play the major role. Because of the site-specificity of toxicant-induced lesions, and site-specific morphologic variation in rodent respiratory epithelium, a working knowledge of rodent nasal anatomy and histology is important, as is systematic examination of rodent nasal tissue for histopathologic and cell proliferation studies.

Larynx

The microscopic anatomy of the rodent larynx has received much attention because of the frequent use of rodents in inhalation toxicology studies. The types of epithelium lining the laryngeal lumen of the rat (29–32), the mouse (33), and the Syrian golden hamster (34) have been described in detail. Although the anatomy of the larynx is less complex than that of the nose, one must be aware of certain anatomic features when examining this organ for evidence of cell proliferation or other cellular changes induced by inhaled xenobiotics. As in the nose, the epithelium lining the laryngeal lumen changes caudally from stratified squamous to pseudostratified ciliated, columnar respiratory epithelium. In rodents, several intermediate types of epithelium have been described in the areas of transition from stratified squamous to respiratory epithelium; the type of intermediate epithelium present depends on anatomic location and rodent species. In the rat, mouse, and hamster, the epithelium covering the surface of the epiglottis caudal to the area of stratified squamous epithelium is composed mostly of cuboidal cells, with some ciliated columnar cells and flattened squamoid cells. This area is among the most sensitive to cellular changes such as degeneration, squamous metaplasia, or hyperplasia of epithelium in response to inhaled xenobiotics (35). As in the rodent nose, the predilection of this site for lesions is probably caused by airflow characteristics and regional epithelial sensitivity (32,35,36). Failure to examine this area carefully microscopically may result in an underestimation of the effects of inhaled xenobiotics on upper respiratory tract epithelium. Histologic preparation and microscopic evaluation of this area of the larynx require extreme care because the "normal" border between stratified squamous and intermediate types of epithelium at the base of the epiglottis lacks clear, consistent landmarks. Therefore, to differentiate exposure-induced squamous metaplasia from normal stratified squamous epiglottal epithelium, sections must be prepared and examined meticulously and strictly compared to similar sections from unexposed control rats.

Cell proliferation quantitation

Tissue growth and maintenance can be described quantitatively when three parameters are known: the length of the cell cycle in the proliferative compartment, the growth fraction (obtained from the labeling index), and the rate of cell loss (37). For hyperplastic responses leading to potential tumor formation, one important disturbance may involve the recruiting of resting cells (Go) into the proliferative pool, which reflects a disturbance of control in the growth fraction (37). Since, at best, cell loss is difficult to measure in the upper respiratory tract epithelium, cell-kinetic measurements are based largely on cell proliferation using such DNA precursor labels as tritiated thymidine or bromodeoxyuridine, combined, respectively, with histoautoradiographic or immunohistochemical examination.

Cell proliferation in the upper respiratory tract mucosa may be assessed in several ways: by the mitotic index (MI), the percentage of cells in mitosis at a given time; the labeling index (LI), the percentage of labeled cells in the study population that have incorporated a DNA precursor; and the unit length labeling index (ULLI), expressed as the number of labeled cell profiles per millimeter of basement membrane (38). For studies of cell proliferation in tissues with relatively long generation times, such as the upper respiratory tract mucosa (39), the LI and ULLI may provide a more sensitive indicator of cell proliferation than the MI because of the small number of mitotic figures observed in this tissue. Other advantages of an LI or ULLI measure over an MI include the indices' higher numerical value, and a greater ease of recognizing and identifying the proliferating cell type more definitively (40). Suggested protocols for measuring cell proliferation have been described (41).

Obtaining cell proliferation data from the epithelial lining of the upper respiratory tract may be labor-intensive because of the region's extensive surface area and the large number of cells that need to be examined and counted. This work may be reduced somewhat by careful selection of specific areas, which will also strengthen the meaning of the collected data. When obtaining labeling indices from the respiratory mucosa, an important concern is that the total cell population may be altered in response to treatment, either through cell loss (by cytotoxicity and exfoliation) or increase in cell number (e.g., hyperplasia). Alterations in the total cell count may influence the LI. If such changes occur in a nondividing component of the epithelium (i.e., ciliated respiratory epithelial cells) in the absence of a true proliferative response in the progenitor cell population, an apparent increase in cell proliferation may occur simply because the denominator for the LI calculation has changed (38). Furthermore, when selecting an approach to S-phase determination, it is important to consider potential effects on cellular hypertrophy on the labeling indices.

Unit-length labeling index

The LI method requires quantitation of the total number of cells in the population under study and is time-consuming; we therefore recently assessed an alternative method of studying cell proliferation using the ULLI (38). Rats were exposed by inhalation to formaldehyde or methyl bromide, and alterations in cell proliferation were determined in the respiratory and olfactory epithelia, respectively. Results based on basement membrane length as the denominator appeared not to be influenced by changes in total cell population either through cell loss or hyperplasia after treatment with the test chemicals, and they had a high degree of correlation with results obtained by the LI method. The ULLI method also had the advantage of eliminating the need for a laborious total cell count. Since LI data are required for calculating other cell kinetic parameters such as cell cycle time (37), a combination of the LI and ULLI may be considered useful for some cell proliferation studies of the upper respiratory tract, with the ULLI method employed for rapid total cell assessment, followed by the LI method for selected areas.

Proliferation of the laryngeal epithelium

Proliferative lesions of the epithelium lining the laryngeal lumen have been reported in many rodent inhalation studies, often as accompanying similar lesions in the nasal epithelium. The epithelial lesions most frequently observed to be induced by inhalation exposure are squamous metaplasia and hyperplasia with superficial keratinization. In rats and hamsters, proliferative lesions of laryngeal epithelium following repeated inhalation exposure to tobacco smoke have been described in detail (32,42–46). In rats exposed to this type of smoke, squamous metaplasia apparently occurs as a sequel to degeneration of the epithelium covering the base of the epiglottis (47–49), and is often accompanied by acanthosis and hyperkeratosis of the metaplastic epithelium and the adjacent normal squamous epithelium.

The fate of laryngeal epithelium induced to undergo proliferation or metaplasia, or both, by exposure to a xenobiotic agent seems to depend, at least partly, on the agent, the concentration and duration of exposure, and the test animal species. For example, although laryngeal metaplasia has been reported in the rat following chronic tobacco inhalation, even prolonged exposure has not been reported to cause laryngeal neoplasia in this species (43,45,46,50). In hamsters, in contrast, lifetime exposure to tobacco smoke inhalation induces squamous cell neoplasms of laryngeal epithelium in association with squamous metaplasia and hyperplasia (42,44).

Although the morphology of the epithelium lining the rodents' laryngeal lumen has been described in detail, little information is available regarding laryngeal epithelial cell kinetics. Lewis (31) reported mitotic indices for the various types of epithelium lining the larynx of young, specific pathogen-free Sprague-Dawley rats using colchicine to induce mitotic arrest in metaphase. The mean MI (percentage of total nucleated epithelial cells in mitosis) was 5.6% for the stratified squamous epithelium covering the cranial epiglottis and arytenoid projections, 2.4% in the squamoid epithelium covering the vocal folds, 2.2% in the cuboid epithelium covering the ventrolateral region at the base of the epiglottis, 1.5% in the cuboid epithelium of the ventral pouch, and 0.6% in the ciliated respiratory epithelium. For isolated islands of respiratory epithelium at the base of the epiglottis, the MI was 2.6%, an increased mitotic rate that was believed to represent the high cell production necessary to maintain epithelial continuity in an area subjected to increased insult from inhaled material (31). The MI of respiratory epithelium in the caudal larynx correlated well with the MI cited for cranial trachea (51).

Formaldehyde-induced increases in cell proliferation

Altered cell proliferation is a sensitive indicator of respiratory epithelial cell toxicity. Formaldehyde has been shown to increase cell proliferation in the rat (11,12), monkey (52), and xenotransplanted human respiratory epithelium (53). Little is known, however, about the mechanisms of these responses, which may involve autocrine and paracrine growth factors, mutations in growth regulatory genes, and/or regenerative stimuli brought about by death of adjacent cells and tissues (54,55). It is also possible that the increases in cell proliferation seen after exposure to high concentrations of this gas are related to effects of other promoters or enhancers of respiratory carcinogenesis (56,57).

Formaldehyde gas is cytotoxic and carcinogenic to the nasal respiratory epithelium of rats chronically exposed to extremely high (>10 ppm) concentrations (58,59), whereas human beings cannot tolerate atmospheric formaldehyde concentrations of more than about 1–5 ppm. An important feature of formaldehyde-induced toxicity and carcinogenicity (58,60) is the steep, nonlinear concentration-response relationship. Animals exposed to 2 ppm in a chronic formaldehyde toxicity study had no tumors, but as exposure concentrations increased from 6–14.3 ppm formaldehyde, the tumor incidence increased 50-fold (58). After acute exposure (e.g., for 9 days) to formaldehyde, a nonlinear concentration response was also observed for cell proliferation in the nasal respiratory epithelium of rodents (11), which correlated with formaldehyde-induced lesions of the respiratory epithelium. These nonlinear responses may be attributed to formaldehyde-induced cytotoxicity and the overloading of protective mechanisms at higher formaldehyde concentrations (61). Following the deposition of inhaled formaldehyde on the nasal mucosa, saturation of detoxification pathways probably plays an important role in the subsequent toxic and carcinogenic responses of the rat nasal respiratory epithelium (61). Glutathione-mediated detoxification of formaldehyde, for example, becomes saturated at exposures above 4 ppm (62), which results in disproportionately more DNA-protein crosslinks per part per million of formaldehyde at exposures of 6 ppm or above than occur at 4 ppm or less (63). Crosslinks may be regarded as a measure of the internal dose of formaldehyde received by the target tissue, as opposed to inhaled or delivered dose.

The occurrence of formaldehyde-induced rat nasal cancer is nonlinear between 6 and 15 ppm (58), the difference between these concentrations being the extent of cell proliferation in the nasal respiratory epithelium (11,12). Formaldehyde is weakly mutagenic (64), binds covalently in vitro to DNA and associated proteins, and reacts preferentially with single-stranded DNA (65,66). Formaldehyde-induced elevations in nasal cell proliferation may therefore have special relevance to formaldehyde-induced nasal carcinogenesis. Increases in cell proliferation may enhance the likelihood of formaldehyde's interaction with DNA and the conversion of promutagenic damage to mutations before DNA repair can occur (61). More significant, perhaps, is that sustained elevations in cell proliferation may promote carcinogenesis by increasing the clonal expansion of initiated cells to a large enough population to allow multiple critical mutational events to occur (3). To determine the potential role of cell proliferation in formaldehyde-induced nasal carcinogenesis, our chronic inhalation study was designed, in part, to investigate the association between formaldehyde-induced lesions, including nasal cancer, and alterations in the cell proliferation rate of nasal respiratory epithelium of F344 rats.

Acute to subchronic formaldehyde exposure

Formaldehyde-induced lesions and increases in cell proliferation following acute to subchronic exposure occur in specific regions of the anterior nasal passages, primarily the wall of the lateral meatus and nasal septum in the region of the middle meatus. Increases in cell proliferation were associated with respiratory epithelial lesions, which included cellular degeneration and necrosis, hyperplasia, and early squamous metaplasia. After either 4 days or 6 weeks of exposure, significant elevations in cell proliferation were observed in the 6, 10, and 15 ppm concentration groups (12). However, after 3 months' exposure, elevations in cell proliferation were present only in the groups exposed to 10 and 15 ppm (12). These results demonstrated that low levels of formaldehyde (0.7 and 2 ppm) did not increase cell proliferation in the rat nasal respiratory epithelium, and that 6 ppm formaldehyde induced a transient increase in cell proliferation that returned to control levels at 3 months. The transient increases seen at 6 ppm highlighted the importance of evaluating multiple time points in cell proliferation studies. Other workers studying the effects of respiratory toxicants on cell kinetics in airway epithelium (67,68) have also demonstrated a dose-related response, suggesting that the magnitude of proliferation is related to the amount of injury in these tissues. Finally, another potentially important result from the subchronic formaldehyde exposures was that only the clearly carcinogenic concentrations of formaldehyde, 10 and 15 ppm (58,59), induced sustained elevations in nasal respiratory epithelial cell proliferation.

Putative preneoplastic lesions

That the respiratory epithelium of both laboratory animals and humans responds to exposure to carcinogens with various metaplastic-dysplastic or preneoplastic lesions is well documented (56,69–71). Preneoplastic lesions are generally believed to be precursor lesions that have a high probability of developing into neoplasms. As recent in vivo studies at the Chemical Industry Institute of Toxicology (CIIT) demonstrated, potentially preneoplastic lesions may be induced in F344 rat nasal respiratory epithelium by exposing the animal to carcinogenic (15 ppm) concentrations of formaldehyde for several months (72). This work led us to investigate the cellular kinetics of these lesions (72).

Morphologically, the preneoplastic nasal lesions resembled those of extranasal respiratory epithelium, and they were characterized by epithelial hyperplasia-metaplasia with atypia (often termed dysplasia). Many of the putative preneoplastic lesions were highly keratinized, a potentially relevant finding because formaldehyde induces highly keratinized squamous cell carcinomas (58). Cell proliferation rates in the preneoplastic lesions were significantly higher than those of control nasal respiratory epithelium, and the labeled cells of the various lesions showed different autoradiographic patterns (72). Labeled cells in the hyperplastic-metaplastic lesions with atypia were primarily basal in location, while the markedly keratinized lesions were labeled throughout, including in the superficial layers.

Cell proliferation results from the formaldehyde-induced preneoplastic lesions, in addition to results reported by other workers for rat tracheal epithelium exposed to chemical carcinogens (70), suggested that preneoplastic lesions in respiratory epithelium exhibit two key characteristics: disturbed cell maturation and an increased rate of cell proliferation (56,70,72). The disturbance of maturation accompanied by increased cell proliferation indicated some type of alteration in growth control. This hypothesis is supported by in vitro studies of the effects of rat tracheal epithelial cells to peptide growth factors such as transforming growth factor beta (TGF-β) (73,74). The role of TGF-β or other molecular events regulating formaldehyde-induced nasal respiratory cell proliferation is as yet not known.

Promotional effects of formaldehyde during chronic exposure

Chemical carcinogenesis is generally believed to be a multistep process that can be separated operationally into three stages described as initiation, promotion, and progression (75). Initiation concerns mutational events that lead to altered expression or function of growth-control genes. The experimentally defined process of promotion is the clonal expansion of inititated preneoplastic or neoplastic cells. In normal tissue, injury from xenobiotics like formaldehyde may result in mild or severe metaplasia and minor disturbance of growth control (76). If the tissue was initiated previously, however, clonal expansion of carcinogen-altered cells may occur, with benign lesions or preneoplastic cell foci as the the end-products (77). All promoters in the mouse skin two-stage model result in the production of a chronic regenerative hyperplasia following damage by the repeated application of the promoter (78). Cell proliferation, then, and in particular selective proliferation of carcinogen-altered cells, seems to be an essential feature of the promotion process (2).

By definition, formaldehyde is classified as a complete carcinogen. But because it is only a weak initiator (64), induction of nasal cancer in rats may primarily result from its role as a promoting agent secondary to induced cell proliferation (64,79). In our laboratory's ongoing chronic inhalation study, 6- or 12-month exposure to formaldehyde has resulted in statistically significant elevations in cell proliferation in the two highest concentration groups only, those exposed to 10 and 15 ppm (13). The incidence of nasal tumors (reported up to and including 16-month exposure) were also present only in the 10 and 15 ppm groups. These data are consistent with the proposal that sustained increases in cell proliferation may be the driving force or promoter of formaldehyde-induced cancer. The exact mechanism of the promoting activity is not known, but it may involve the induction of restorative growth caused by the cytotoxicity (80) seen at higher formaldehyde concentrations.

Tissue damage and cancer

Sustained elevations in cell proliferation in association with chronic wounding may play important roles in respiratory carcinogenesis. If injury to the respiratory epithelium is mild and acute, an orderly progression occurs of localized death and inflammation, followed by epithelial cell migration, proliferation, and transient hyperplasia, with a subsequent return to normal structure and function (81–83). If the injury is severe or chronic, however, the normal temporal sequence of events of regeneration and repair is disrupted. The morphology and cytokinetics of regeneration in respiratory tract epithelium of hamsters following mechanical injury, have been studied extensively (81–85), as has the role of cell proliferation in respiratory tract carcinogenesis induced by exposure to chemical carcinogens (86,87). Keenan and coworkers (86,87) demonstrated that laryngeal or tracheal epithelial cell proliferation, induced by damage to the mucosa by intralaryngeal or intratracheal cannulation, is a major determinant of the carcinogenic response in the hamster respiratory tract after repeated instillation of benzo[a]pyrene, methylnitrosourea, or both. Most respiratory tract tumors occurred at or near sites of wounding (and subsequent focal cell proliferation) in the larynx or trachea, even though the entire respiratory tract was exposed to the carcinogen. The authors speculated that, in this model, the critical mechanisms probably were related to local release of paracrine peptide growth factors in the wound areas (87).

Malignant tumors induced in the nasal epithelium by irritating carcinogens such as formaldehyde (58) and acetaldehyde (88) have been found to arise from surface epithelium that is severely damaged. These findings, in addition to other examples that showed cancer to develop in chronically injured tissue (2,89), led Feron, Wouterson, and coworkers (59,90) to investigate the role of tissue damage in formaldehyde-induced nasal carcinogenesis. In a long-term inhalation study, male rats with severely damaged or undamaged nasal mucosa were exposed to 10 ppm formaldehyde (59). The damage was induced by bilateral intranasal electrocoagulation of the anterior third of the nasal passages. Rats with damaged nasal mucosa exhibited increases in formaldehyde-induced rhinitis, hyperplasia, and metaplasia of the respiratory epithelium. More important, exposure to 10 ppm formaldehyde for 28 months produced approximately an 8-fold higher increase in nasal squamous cell carcinomas in rats with damaged noses than in those with intact noses (e.g., not pretreated with nasal electrocautery but similarly exposed) (59). The conclusion from these studies was that both severe damage to the nasal mucosa and hyperproliferation are important in the development of nasal tumors in rats exposed to formaldehyde (59).

Conclusions

Cell death and renewal are predominant features of most toxicologic injuries to the respiratory epithelium (91). Toxicant-induced cell necrosis, followed by regeneration, could therefore be a major determinant in chemical carcinogenesis in the respiratory epithelium. Our studies of cell proliferation in nasal respiratory epithelium in formalde- hyde-exposed rats demonstrated a good correlation of cellular injury and cell proliferation, and a response dependent on formaldehyde concentration. Since cell proliferation is clearly involved in chemical carcinogenesis, these dose-responsive changes represent potentially important data that should be included in the risk-assessment process (63). Furthermore, quantitative information obtained through cell proliferation studies may be used in mathematical models of carcinogenesis (92), providing a key biologic variable to improve low-dose and interspecies extrapolation of risk.

References

1. Rajewsky MF. Tumorigenesis by exogenous carcinogens: Role of target cell proliferation and state of differentiation. In Likhachev A (ed): Age-Related Factors in Carcinogenesis. Lyon: IARC Scientific Publication 58, 1985, pp. 215–223.
2. Grisham JW, Kaufmann WK, Kaufman DG. The cell cycle and chemical carcinogenesis. Survey and Synthesis of Pathology Research 1:49–66, 1983.
3. Farber E, Sarma DRS. Hepatocarcinogenesis: A dynamic cellular perspective. Lab Invest 56:4–22, 1987.
4. Trump BF, McDowell EM, Harris CC. Chemical carcinogenesis in the tracheobronchial epithelium. Environ Health Perspect 55:77–84, 1984.
5. Thyssen J, Althoff J, Kimmerle G, Mohr U. Inhalation studies with benzo[a]pyrene in Syrian golden hamsters. J Natl Cancer Inst 66:575–577, 1981.
6. Soderman JV. Handbook of Identified Carcinogens and Noncarcinogens: Carcinogenicity-Mutagenic- ity Database. Boca Raton: CRC Press, 1982.
7. Brown HR. Neoplastic and hyperplastic changes in the upper respiratory tract-NTP archives. Environ Health Perspect, in press, 1990.
8. Stinson SF. Nasal cavity cancer in laboratory animal bioassays of environmental compounds. In: Reznik G, Stinson SF (eds): Nasal Tumors in Animals and Man, vol. 3, Chapter 7. Boca Raton: CRC Press, 1983.
9. Goldsworthy TL, Monticello TM, Jackh R, Smith-Oliver T, Bermudez E, Morgan KT, Butterworth BE. Assessment of 1,4-dioxane-induced carcinogenicity, genotoxicity and cell replication in rat nose and liver (abstract). Proc Amer Cancer Res 29:85, 1988.
10. Laskin S, Sellakumar R, Kuschner M, Nelson N, La Mendola S, Rusch GM, Katz GV, Dulak NC, Albert RE. Inhalation carcinogenicity of epichlorohydrin in noninbred Sprague-Dawley rats. J Natl Cancer Inst 65:751–757, 1980.
11. Swenberg JA, Gross EA, Randall HW. Localization and quantitation of cell proliferation following exposure to nasal irritants. In Barrow CS (ed): Toxicology of the Nasal Passages. Washington, DC: Hemisphere Publishing, 1986, pp. 291–300.
12. Monticello TM, Morgan KT. Cell proliferation in rat nasal respiratory epithelium following three

months exposure to formaldehyde gas. Toxicologist 10:181, 1990.

13. Monticello TM, Morgan KT. Correlation of cell proliferation and inflammation with nasal tumors in F-344 rats following chronic formaldehyde exposure (abstract). Proceedings of the American Association of Cancer Research 31:139, 1990.

14. Lee KP, Trochimowicz HJ. Induction of nasal tumors in rats exposed to hexamethylphosphoramide by inhalation. J Natl Cancer Inst 68:157–164, 1983.

15. Magee PN, Montesano R, Preussman R. N-Nitroso compounds and related carcinogens. In Searle CE (ed): Chemical Carcinogens—ACS Monograph 173. Washington, DC: American Chemical Society, 1976.

16. Bogdanffy MS, Mazaika TJ, Fasano WJ. Early cell proliferative and cytotoxic effects of phenacetin on rat nasal mucosa. Toxicol Appl Pharmacol 98:100–112, 1989.

17. Kociba RJ, Keyes DG, Beyer JE, Carreon RM, Wade CE, Ditlenber DA, Kalnins RP, Frauson LE, Park CN, Barnard SD, Hummel RA, and Humiston CG. Results of a two-year chronic toxicity and oncogenicity study of 2,3,7,8-tetrachlorodibenzo-p-dioxin in rats. Toxicol Appl Pharmacol 46:279–303, 1978.

18. Fabrikant JI, Cherry J. The kinetics of cellular proliferation in normal and malignant tissues: X Cell proliferation in the nose and adjoining cavities. Ann Otol Rhinol Laryngol 79:572–578, 1970.

19. Shorter G, Titus JL, Divertie MB. Cytodynamics in the respiratory tract of the rat. Thorax 21:32, 1966.

20. Sato T. High-risk factors in the development of head and neck cancers. Gan To Kagaku Ryoho 14:2626–2631, 1987.

21. Campbell H, Lee EJ. The relationship between lung cancer and chronic bronchitis. British Journal of Diseases of the Chest 57:113–119, 1963.

22. Buckley LA, Jiang XZ, James RA, Morgan KT, Barrow CS. Respiratory tract lesions induced by sensory irritants at the RD50 concentration. Toxicol Appl Pharmacol 74:417–429, 1984.

23. Morgan KT, Monticello TM. Airflow, gas deposition, and lesion distribution in the nasal passages. Environ Health Perspect 85:209–218, 1990.

24. Monteiro-Riviere NA, Popp JA. Ultrastructural characterization of the nasal respiratory epithelium in the rat. Am J Anat 169:31–43, 1984.

25. Morgan KT, Jiang XZ, Patterson DL, Gross EA. The nasal mucociliary apparatus. Correlation of structure and function in the rat. Am Rev Respir Dis 130:275–281, 1984.

26. Morgan KT, Monticello TM. Formaldehyde toxicity: Respiratory epithelial injury and repair. In Thomassen DG (ed): Biology, Toxicology and Carcinogenesis of Respiratory Epithelium. Washington, DC: Hemisphere Publishing, 1990, pp. 155–171.

27. Young JT. Histopathologic examination of the rat nasal cavity. Fundam Appl Toxicol 1:309–312, 1981.

28. Young JT. Light microscopic examination of the rat nasal passages. In Barrow CS (ed): Toxicology of the Nasal Passages. Washington, DC: Hemisphere Publishing, 1986, pp. 27–36.

29. Smith G. Structure of the normal rat larynx. Lab Anim 11:223–228, 1977.

30. Lewis DJ, Prentice DE. The ultrastructure of rat laryngeal epithelia. J Anat 130:617–632, 1980.

31. Lewis DJ. Mitotic indices of rat laryngeal epithelia. J Anat 132:419–428, 1981.

32. Lewis DJ. Factors affecting the distribution of tobacco smoke-induced lesions in the rodent larynx. Toxicol Lett 9:189–194, 1981.

33. Nakano T, Muto H. The transitional zone in the epithelium lining the mouse epiglottis. Acta Anat 130:285–290, 1987.

34. Brockmeyer C, Thiedmann KV, Heinrich U, Mohr U. Light and scanning electron microscopic investigation of the laryngeal mucosa of Syrian golden hamsters. Exp Pathol 36:237–245, 1989.

35. Gopinath C, Prentice DE, Lewis DJ. The respiratory system. In Gresham GA (ed): Current Histopathology, vol. 13, Atlas of Experimental Toxicologic Pathology. Norwell: MTP Press, 1987, chapter 3.

36. Chevalier HJ, Dontenwill W. Experimental studies on the accumulation of inhaled particles in the larynxes of Syrian golden hamsters. Z Versuchstierkd 14:271–276, 1972.

37. Bisconte JC. Kinetic analysis of cellular populations by means of the quantitative radioautography. Int Rev Cytol 57:75–125, 1979.

38. Monticello TM, Morgan KT, Hurtt ME. Unit length as the denominator for quantitation of cell proliferation in nasal epithelia. Toxicol Pathol 18:24–31, 1990.

39. Wells AB. The kinetics of cell proliferation in the tracheobronchial epithelium of rats with and without chronic respiratory disease. Cell Tissue Kinet 3:185–206, 1970.

40. Lamerton LF, Steel GG. Cell population kinetics in normal and malignant tissues. Prog Biophys Mol Biol 18:245–283, 1968.

41. Goldsworthy TL, Morgan KT, Popp JA, Butterworth BE. Guidelines for measuring chemically induced cell proliferation in specific rodent target organs. In Butterworth BE, Slaga TJ (eds): Chemically Induced Cell Proliferation: Implications For Risk Assessment. New York: Alan Liss, 1990 (this volume).
42. Dontenwill W, Chevalier HJ, Harke JP, Lafrenz U, Reznik G, Schneider B. Investigations on the effect of chronic cigarette smoke inhalation in Syrian golden hamsters. J Natl Cancer Inst 51:1781–1832, 1973.
43. Davis BR, Whitehead JK, Gill ME, Lee PN, Butterworth AD, Roe FJC. Response of rat lung to inhaled tobacco smoke with or without prior exposure to 3,4-benzpyrene (BP) given by intratracheal instillation. Br J Cancer 31:469–484, 1975.
44. Bernfeld P, Homburger F, Soto E, Pal KJ. Cigarette smoke inhalation studies in inbred Syrian golden hamsters. J Natl Cancer Inst 63:675–689, 1979.
45. Dalbey WE, Nettesheim P, Griesemer R, Caton JE, Guerin MR. Chronic inhalation of cigarette smoke by F344 rats. J Natl Cancer Inst 64:383–390, 1980.
46. Wehner AP, Dagle GE, Milliman EM, Phelps DW, Carr DB, Decker JR, Filipy RE. Inhalation bioassay of cigarette smoke in rats. Toxicol Appl Pharmacol 61:1–17, 1981.
47. Lam R. Transient epithelial loss in rat larynx after acute exposure to tobacco smoke. Toxicol Lett 6:327–335, 1980.
48. Lewis DJ. The use of horseradish peroxidase to demonstrate degenerate cells in rat larynx after acute tobacco smoke exposure. Toxicol Lett 9:195–199, 1981.
49. Ayres PH, Coggins CRE, Sagartz JW, Burger GT. Induction and regression of histopathology in the rat larynx after acute exposure to smoke from 1R4F cigarettes. Toxicologist 9:139, 1989.
50. Coggins CRE, Lam R, Morgan KT. Chronic inhalation study in rats, using cigarettes containing different amounts of Cytrel tobacco supplement. Toxicology 22:287–296, 1982.
51. Lamb D, Reid L. Mitotic rates, goblet cell increase and histochemical changes in mucus in rat bronchial epithelium during exposure to sulphur dioxide. J Pathol Bacteriol 96:97–111, 1968.
52. Monticello TM, Morgan KT, Everitt JI, Popp JA. Effects of formaldehyde gas on the respiratory tract of rhesus monkeys: Pathology and cell proliferation. Am J Pathol 134: 515–527, 1989.
53. Ura H, Nowak P, Litwin S, Watts P, Bonfil RD, Klein-Szanto AJP. Effects of formaldehyde on normal xenotransplanted human tracheobronchial epithelium. Am J Pathol 134:99–106, 1989.
54. Pardee AB. Biochemical and molecular events regulating cell proliferation. J Pathol 149:1–2, 1986.
55. Loeb LA. Endogenous carcinogenesis: Molecular oncology into the twenty-first century. Cancer Res 49:5489–5496, 1989.
56. Nettesheim P., Klein-Szanto AJP, Marchok AC, Steele VE, Terzaghi M, Topping DC. Studies of neoplastic development in respiratory tract epithelium. Arch Pathol Lab Med 105:1–10, 1981.
57. Steele VE, Nettesheim P. Tumor promotion in respiratory tract carcinogenesis. In Slaga TJ (ed): Mechanisms of Tumor Promotion, vol. 1, Tumor Promotion in Internal Organs. Boca Raton: CRC Press, 1983, pp. 91–105.
58. Kerns WD, Pavkov KL, Donofrio DJ, Gralla EJ, Swenberg JA. Carcinogenicity of formaldehyde in rats and mice after long-term inhalation exposure. Cancer Res 43:4382–4392, 1983.
59. Woutersen RA, van Gardeen-Hoetmet A, Bruijntjes JP, Zwart A, Feron VJ. Nasal tumors in rats after severe injury to the nasal mucosa and prolonged exposure to 10 ppm formaldehyde. J Appl Toxicol 9:39–46, 1989.
60. Chang JCF, Gross EA, Swenberg JA, Barrow CS. Nasal cavity deposition, histopathology and cell proliferation after single or repeated formaldehyde exposures in B6C3F1 mice and F-344 rats. Toxicol Appl Pharmacol 68:161–176, 1983.
61. Swenberg JA, Gross EA, Martin J, Popp JA. Mechanisms of formaldehyde toxicity. In Gibson JE (ed): Formaldehyde Toxicity. New York: Hemisphere Publishing, 1983, pp. 137–147.
62. Casanova M, Heck H d'A. Further studies of the metabolic incorportion and covalent binding of inhaled [³H]- and [14C] formaldehyde in F-344 rats: Effects of glutathione depletion. Toxicol Appl Pharmacol 89:105–121, 1987.
63. Swenberg JA, Richardson FC, Boucheron JA, Deal FH, Belinsky SA, Charbonneau M, Short BG. High-to low-dose extrapolation: Critical determinations involved in the dose response of carcinogenic substances. Environ Health Perspect 76: 57–63, 1987.
64. Ragan DL, Boreiko CJ. Initiation of C3H/10T1/2 cell transformation by formaldehyde. Cancer Lett 13:325–331, 1981.
65. von Hippel PH, Wong KY. Dynamic aspects of native DNA stucture: Kinetics of formaldehyde reaction with calf thymus DNA. J Mol Biol 61: 587–613, 1971.

66. Ma, T-H, Harris MM. Review of the genotoxicity of formaldehyde. Mutat Res 196:37–59, 1988.
67. Lum H, Schwartz LW, Dungworth DL, Tyler WS. A comparative study of cell renewal after exposure to ozone or oxygen. Am Rev Respir Dis 118:335–345, 1978.
68. Wells AB, Lamerton LF. Regenerative response of the rat tracheal epithelium after acute exposure to tobacco smoke: a quantitative study. J Natl Cancer Inst 55:887–891, 1975.
69. Klein-Szanto AJP, Topping DC, Heckman CA, Nettesheim P. Ultrastructural characteristics of carcinogen-induced dysplastic changes in tracheal epithelium. Am J Pathol 98:83–100, 1980.
70. Klein-Szanto AJP, Nettesheim P, Topping DC, Olson AC. Quantitative analysis of disturbed cell maturation in dysplastic lesions of the respiratory tract epithelium. Carcinogenesis 1:1007–1016, 1980.
71. Nettesheim P, Marchok A. Neoplastic development in airway epithelium. Adv Cancer Res 39:1–71, 1983.
72. Monticello TM, Morgan KT. Cell kinetics and characterization of preneoplastic lesions in nasal respiratory epithelium of rats exposed to formaldehyde (abstract). Proceedings of the American Association of Cancer Research 30:195, 1989.
73. Terzaghi-Howe M. Changes in response to, and production of, transforming growth factor type β during neoplastic progression in cultured rat tracheal epithelial cells. Carcinogenesis 10:973–980, 1989.
74. Hubbs AF, Hahn FH, Thomassen DG. Increased resistance to transforming growth factor beta accompanies neoplastic progression of rat trachea epithelial cells. Carcinogenesis 10:1599–1605, 1989.
75. Pitot HC, Goldsworthy T, Moran S. The natural history of carcinogenesis: Implications of experimental carcinogenesis in the genesis of human cancer. J Supramol Cell Biochem 17:133–146, 1981.
76. Hicks RM. Pathological and biochemical aspects of tumor promotion. Carcinogenesis 10:1209–1214, 1983.
77. Barrett JC, Wiseman RW. Cellular and molecular mechanisms of multistep carcinogenesis: Relevance to carcinogen risk assessment. Environ Health Perspect 76:65–70, 1987.
78. Argyris TS. Regeneration and the mechanism of epidermal tumor promotion. CRC Crit Rev Toxicol, 14: 1985.
79. Swenberg JA, Barrow CS, Boreiko CJ, Heck Hd'A, Levine RJ, Morgan KT, Starr TB. Non-linear biological responses to formaldehyde and their implications for carcinogenic risk assessment. Carcinogenesis 4:945–952, 1983.
80. Lutz WK, Maier P. Genotoxic and epigenetic chemical carcinogenesis: one process, different mechanisms. Trends in Pharmacological Sciences 9:322–326, 1988.
81. Keenan KP, Combs JW, McDowell EM. Regeneration of hamster tracheal epithelium after mechanical injury. I. Focal lesions: quantitative morphologic study of cell proliferation. Virchows Arch [B] 41:193–214, 1982.
82. Keenan KP, Combs JW, McDowell EM. Regeneration of hamster tracheal epithelium after mechanical injury. II. Multifocal lesions: Stathmokinetic and autoradiographic studies of cell proliferation. Virchows Arch [B] 41:215–229, 1982.
83. Keenan KP, Combs JW, McDowell EM. Regeneration of hamster tracheal epithelium after mechanical injury. III. Large and small lesions: comparative stathmokinetic and single pulse and continuous thymidine labeling autoradiographic studies. Virchows Arch [B] 41:231–252, 1982.
84. McDowell EM, Becci PJ, Schurch W, Trump BF. The respiratory epithelium. VII. Epidermoid metaplasia of hamster tracheal epithelium during regeneration following mechanical injury. J Natl Cancer Inst 62:995–1008, 1979.
85. Keenan KP, Wilson TS, McDowell EM. Regeneration of hamster tracheal epithelium after mechanical injury. IV. Histochemical immunocytochemical, and ultrastructural studies. Virchows Arch [B] 43:213–240, 1983.
86. Keenan KP, Saffiotti U, Stinson SF, Riggs CW, McDowell EM. Morphological and cytokinetic responses of hamster airways to intralaryngeal or intratracheal cannulation with instillation of saline or ferric oxide particles in saline. Cancer Res 49:1521–1527, 1989.
87. Keenan KP, Saffiotti U, Stinson SF, Riggs CW, McDowell EM. Multifactorial hamster respiratory carcinogenesis with interdependent effects of cannula-induced mucosal wounding, saline, ferric oxide, benzo[a]pyrene and N-methyl-N-nitrosurea. Cancer Res 49:1528–1540, 1989.
88. Wouterson RA, Appelman LM, van Garderen-Hoetmer A, Feron VJ. Inhalation toxicity of acetaldehyde in rats. III. Carcinogenicity study. Toxicology 41:213–231, 1986.
89. Grasso P. Persistent organ damage and cancer production in rats and mice. Arch Toxicol Suppl 11:75–83, 1987.

90. Feron VJ, Wouterson RA. Role of tissue damage in nasal carcinogensis. In Feron VJ, Bosland MC (eds): Nasal Carcinogenesis in Rodents: Relevance to Human hHealth Risk. Wageningen, Netherlands: Pudoc Press, 1989, pp. 76–84.
91. Evans MJ. Cell death and cell renewal in small airways and alveoli. In Witschi H, Nettesheim P (eds): Mechanisms in Respiratory Toxicology, vol. 1. Boca Raton: CRC Press, 1982, pp. 189–218.
92. Moolgavkar SM. Biologically motivated two-stage model for cancer risk assessment. Toxicol Lett 43:139–150, 1988.

Chemically Induced Cell Proliferation:
Implications for Risk Assessment, pages 337-346
©1991 Wiley-Liss, Inc.

Role of Chemically Induced Cell Proliferation in Ethyl Acrylate-Induced Forestomach Carcinogenesis

Burhan I. Ghanayem, R. R. Maronpot, and H. B. Matthews

Ethyl acrylate (EA) is a heavily produced acrylic acid ester used in producing polymers and copolymers, which are utilized for manufacturing latex paint, textiles, paper coatings, dirt release agents, and specialty plastics.

After gavage administration, EA is rapidly absorbed and distributed to all major tissues (1). The highest concentration of EA-derived radioactivity was found in the forestomach, glandular stomach, liver, and kidney, at 4 and 24 hr after dosing (1). Four hours after EA dosing, the protein-bound radioactivity found in the forestomach was four times that detected in the liver. Twenty-four hours after dosing, this protein-bound radioactivity declined in the liver but persisted in the forestomach. Within 24 hr after dosing, approximately 70% of the EA dose was expired as CO_2 and 12% was eliminated in the urine. The three major urinary metabolites of EA were mercapturic acids resulting from the degradation of the glutathione conjugates of EA and acrylic acid (1,2).

Mutagenicity studies in several *Salmonella typhimurium* strains and *Drosophila* indicated that EA is nonmutagenic with or without the addition of metabolic activation systems (3,4). However, EA was positive in a micronucleus test (5).

Acute and chronic toxicity studies suggested that the target of EA toxicity is dependent on the route of EA administration. For example, respiratory alterations were observed in rats exposed to EA vapors (6), while gastric toxicity was observed in rats treated with EA by gavage (7–9). Acute gavage administration of EA caused dose-, concentration-, and time-dependent mucosal and submucosal edema of the forestomach (7). Intraperitoneal or subcutaneous administration of similar EA doses did not produce similar changes (7). These studies suggest that EA-induced toxicity apparently occurs as a result of direct interaction with the forestomach tissue. Furthermore, sulfhydryl-containing agents such as cysteine or cysteamine increased the potential for EA-induced edema while sulfhydryl depletion, either by diethyl malonate or fasting, protected against it. While gavage administration of equimolar methyl or ethyl acrylate doses resulted in similar forestomach lesions, the methyl ester was more potent (8). Acrylic and methacrylic acids, methylmethacrylate, butyl acrylate, and the saturated analogues of ethyl and methyl acrylates essentially had no effect (8). These studies indicated that the structural requirements for developing forestomach lesions are fairly specific and include an intact ester moiety, a double bond, and an unsubstituted β-carbon.

Chronic EA inhalation caused hyperplasia of nasal mucosal cells (10). The epidermis and dermis were the identified targets when EA was applied to the skin (11). Chronic gavage administration of EA (100 or 200 mg EA/kg) to rats and mice caused a dose- and concentration-dependent increase in the incidence of squamous cell papillomas and carcinomas of the forestomach of both sexes of rats and mice (Table 1). No neoplastic lesions were observed at any other site.

Table 1. Incidence of Forestomach Tumors in Male Rats Treated with EA*.

	0%	2% (100 mg/kg)	4% (200 mg/kg)
Squamous cell papillomas	1/50	15/50	29/50
Squamous cell carcinoma	0/50	5/50	15/50
Papilloma or carcinoma	1/50	18/50	36/50

*EA was dissolved in corn oil to allow the administration of 5 ml/kg by gavage.
Data obtained from the National Toxicology Program technical report # 259 (3).

Our studies were designed to investigate the histopathologic effects of acute and prechronic EA administration and the potential to reverse such lesions in the rat forestomach. This work emphasized the role of EA-induced epithelial cell proliferation produced in the forestomach of male F344 rats.

Materials and methods

Chemicals. Ninety-nine percent EA, inhibited with 15–20 ppm of hydroquinone monomethyl ether, was purchased from Aldrich Chemical Company (Milwaukee, WI).

Animals and treatments. Male F344 rats were obtained from Charles Rivers Breeding Laboratories (Wilmington, MA, or Raleigh, NC). Rats were fed NIH 31 diet and water ad libitum in polycarbonate cages in facilities with a relative humidity of 50% ± 10%, temperature of 21–22°C, and a 12 hr dark-light cycle. Rats were housed under these conditions for a minimum of 5 days prior to treatment. All animals were approximately 3- to 4-months-old at the time of treatment.

Single dose-response study. EA was dissolved in corn oil and administered by gavage at a dose volume of 5 ml/kg. Doses of 100, 200, or 400 mg EA/kg were selected to repeat those used in the National Toxicology Program (NTP) chronic study (3) and to provide one higher dose. Control rats received a similar volume of 5 ml corn oil by gavage.

Four hours after dosing, rats were killed, an abdominal incision was made, and the entire stomach was removed. The stomach was dissected free of other tissues, opened across the lesser curvature, and carefully pinned to a piece of cardboard with the mucosa up as shown in Figure 3. Stomachs were rinsed with 0.9% NaCl solution while pinned to the cardboard and carefully dissected into glandular- and forestomachs. Gastric contents were rinsed from the surface of the stomach, then blotted on a filter paper and weighed. Forestomach weight:body weight ratio was calculated and presented as the percent of control.

In order to study the time-course effects of EA, rats were treated with either 5 ml/kg corn oil or 200 mg EA/5 ml corn oil/kg by gavage. Animals were held for 2, 4, 8, or 24 hr. At the end of each holding period, animals were killed and the forestomachs removed and processed as described above.

Effect of two or four EA daily doses. A dose of 200 mg EA/kg, the highest used in the NTP study (3), was administered to rats daily for 2 or 4 consecutive days. Twenty-four hours after the last dose, rats were killed, then stomachs were removed and pinned to a piece of cardboard, washed, and immediately immersed in 10% aqueous buffered neutral formalin. The stomachs were sliced, embedded in paraffin, and stained with hematoxylin/eosin. Microscopic evaluation of coded slides was performed by a pathologist unaware of the dosages given to the treatment groups.

Effect of 14 EA daily doses and recoveries. Five ml/kg corn oil, or 100 or 200 mg EA in 5 ml/kg corn oil, were administered to rats by gavage for 14 consecutive days. Each of the treatment groups was divided into 3 subgroups. A subgroup from each treatment group was killed at 24 hr after the last dose. Subgroups from the corn oil- and the 100 mg/kg-treated groups were killed at 1 and 2 weeks after the last dose. The remaining two subgroups treated with 200 mg EA/kg were killed at 2 and 4 weeks after treatment ceased. Stomachs from each subgroup were processed for microscopic evaluation as described above.

Effect of 90-day EA daily doses and recoveries. Five ml/kg corn oil, or 100 or 200 mg EA in 5 ml/kg corn oil, were administered to rats daily, 5 days per week, for 13 weeks. Representative rats from each treatment group were killed at 24 hr after the last dose, and the stomachs were removed. An interim sacrifice of 5 rats from each group was performed at 8 weeks after the last EA dose. The remaining rats were killed 22 months after the initiation of treatment (a 19-month recovery period). Stomachs were removed and routinely processed as described above, and histopathologic evaluation of hematoxylin/eosin-stained sections was performed by a pathologist unaware of the dosages given to the treatment groups.

Results

Effect of single EA doses. Gavage administration of EA resulted in a dose-dependent mucosal and submucosal edema of the rat forestomach. Data presented in Figure 1 shows a marked increase in the forestomach weight:body weight ratio, which was approximately 2 and 4 times that of control values, within 4 hr after administration of 200 or 400 mg EA/kg, respectively. Vacuolization of the tunica muscularis of the forestomach was also observed by histopathology (not shown). A single gavage dose of 200 mg EA/kg in corn oil was administered to rats, causing a time-dependent increase in the forestomach weight:body weight ratio (Fig. 2). The maximum effect was reached at 8 hr after dosing and declined by 24 hr. The most prominent histopathologic effects were intracellular and intercellular mucosal edema, submucosal edema and inflammation, and vacuolization of the tunica muscularis (not shown). At 24 hr after dosing, forestomach edema was associated with vesicle formation. No epithelial hyperplasia of the forestomach mucosa was detected within 24 hr after a single EA dose (Table 2).

Twenty-four hours after gavage administration of the last of 2 or 4 EA doses, hyperplasia was assessed histopathologically in sections. It was found that EA caused additional severe forestomach lesions including mucosal epithelial cell proliferation (see Table 2). This cell proliferation was more extensive in rats that received 4 daily doses than in those that received 2 daily doses. Glandular stomach lesions such as mucosal and submucosal edema, submucosal inflammation, and superficial mucosal necrosis were also seen in these rats (7).

Two-week studies and recoveries. The effect of EA on the forestomach was apparent on gross examination at necropsy (Fig. 3). Some slightly thickened cream-white mucosal nodules were apparent upon gross examination in rats treated with 100 mg EA/kg/day for 14 days. Microscopic evidence of mucosal hyperplasia and hyperkeratosis was

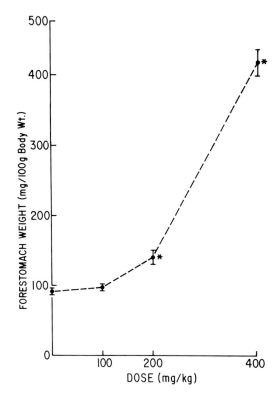

Figure 1. Dose-response (forestomach weight:body weight ratio) determined 4 hr after administration of various EA doses to male rats by gavage. Values are presented as percent of control and are the mean ± SE of a minimum of 5 rats.

present in all rats treated with this dose (Table 3). Changes characterized by mild to moderate uniform thickening of the mucosa were also observed. Generalized moderate to marked papillomatous thickening of mucosa was characterized by confluent raised linear and circular areas of cream-white nodular proliferations with a granular to velvet-like surface texture (Fig. 1). Hair shafts and feed particles were also seen entrapped in the forestomach mucosa of rats treated with the high dose. Rats treated with 200 mg EA/kg had microscopic forestomach lesions that consisted of marked generalized hyperplasia of stratified squamous cell mucosal layer and associated hyperkeratosis (Fig. 4). Thickened mucosa was thrown into folds and papillary projections of epithelium covered by a thick layer of keratin. Areas of mucosal erosion and ulceration were associated with inflammatory cell infiltration of the submucosa (Fig. 4). The severity of EA-induced epithelial cell proliferation of the forestomach mucosa was dose-dependent. Other EA-induced forestomach lesions were also observed, including mucosal and submucosal inflammation and mucosal ulcers. Glandular stomach lesions—observed in rats treated with up to 4 daily doses of EA—were not present in those treated for 14 days (9).

When allowed to recover for 1 week after low EA dosing ceased, rats exhibited a decrease in the incidence and severity of hyperkeratosis and epithelial cell proliferation

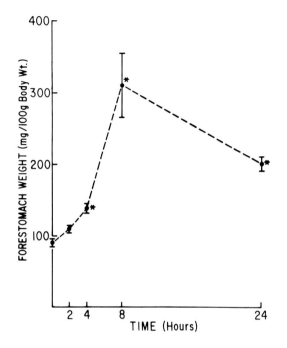

Figure 2. Time-course effect (forestomach weight:body weight ratio) of a 200 mg EA/kg administered to male rats by gavage. Values are presented as percent of control and are the mean ± SE of a minimum of 5 rats.

Table 2. Incidence of Forestomach Hyperplasia in Rats Treated with EA* Daily for One, Two, or Four Days.

Treatment	Hyperplasia incidence
One day	
Corn oil	0/11
200-mg EA/kg	0/8
Two days	
Corn oil	0/11
200-mg EA/kg	8/8
Four days	
Corn oil	0/11
200-mg EA/kg	8/8

*EA was dissolved in corn oil to allow the administration of 5 ml/kg by gavage.

(Table 3). These EA-induced lesions disappeared completely after a 2-week recovery period (Table 3). In contrast, regression of forestomach lesions in rats treated with 200 mg EA/kg was slower. Although most lesions disappeared within 4 weeks after dosing ceased, cell proliferation persisted beyond the 4-week recovery period (Table 3).

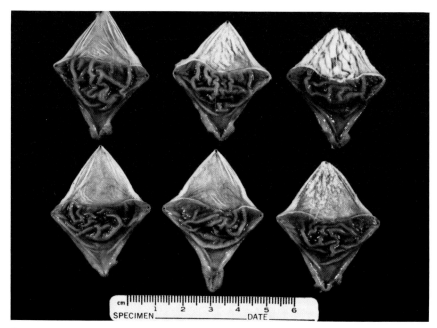

Figure 3. Gross appearance of the mucosal surface of formalin-fixed stomachs from rats treated with (top row, left to right) corn oil, 100 mg EA/kg or 200 mg EA/kg by gavage for 14 consecutive days and killed 24 hr later. Bottom row shows the gross appearance of stomachs from rats treated similarly for 14 consecutive days but sacrificed 14 days after the last dose.

Table 3. Incidence of Forestomach Hyperplasia in Rats Treated With EA* Daily for Two Weeks and Allowed to Recover for Varying Periods.

Treatment	Recovery period	Hyperplasia incidence
Corn oil	None	0/24
	1 week	0/8
	2 weeks	0/8
100-mg EA/kg	None	12/12
	1 week	6/8
	2 weeks	0/8
200-mg EA/kg	None	12/12
	2 weeks	8/8
	4 weeks	8/8

*EA was dissolved in corn oil to allow the administration of 5 ml/kg by gavage.

Thirteen-week studies and recoveries. Treatment of rats with 100 mg EA/kg/day for 5 days per week, for 13 weeks, resulted in a slight thickening of the forestomach mucosa with an occasional elevated focus of white discoloration. At the 200 mg EA/kg/day dose, focal and multifocal nodular proliferations appeared on the forestomach

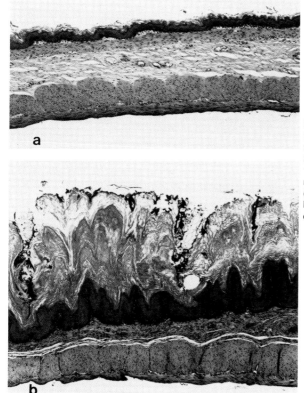

Figure 4. Photomicrographs of forestomachs from male rats treated with corn oil (a) or with 200 mg EA/kg (b) by gavage for 14 days. Corn oil control shows normal rat forestomach. Section (b) shows marked mucosal hyperplasia. Hematoxylin and eosin stain, ×66.

mucosa. These lesions were similar but more localized and less extensive than lesions observed at the end of a 2-week dosing regimen.

Similar microscopic lesions, although more severe than those observed at 2 weeks, were found at the end of 13 weeks of EA dosing (Table 4). Hyperplastic lesions were more localized or focal, with fewer mucosal erosions and ulcers than seen at the end of 2 weeks (Fig. 5). Downgrowths of basal epithelial cells into the submucosa, or acanthosis, were more frequently observed at 13 weeks. In some instances, mechanical displacement of viable mucosal cells into the submucosa was present near healed ulcers.

Discussion

Gavage administration of EA in doses of either 100 or 200 mg/kg/day to F344 rats and B6C3F1 mice for 2 years caused dose- and concentration-dependent increases in the incidence of squamous cell papillomas and carcinomas of the forestomach (Table

Table 4. Incidence of Forestomach Hyperplasia in Rats Treated With EA* Daily for 13 Weeks and Allowed to Recover for Varying Periods.

Treatment	Recovery period	Hyperplasia incidence
Corn oil	None	0/10
	8 weeks	0/5
	19 months	1/18
100-mg EA/kg	None	10/10
	8 weeks	1/5
	19 months	0/12
200-mg EA/kg	None	11/11
	8 weeks	5/5
	19 months	4/15

*EA was dissolved in corn oil to allow the administration of 5 ml/kg by gavage.

1). No neoplastic lesions were seen at other sites. Our early work focused on the characterization of the acute and prechronic toxicity induced by similar doses of EA. These doses caused concentration- and time-dependent mucosal and submucosal edema (7–9). The severity of mucosal hyperplasia of the forestomach, first seen after 2 daily doses of EA, was dose-dependent and increased according to the length of treatment regimen.

Continued repetitive EA dosing for as long as 90 days resulted in profound epithelial cell proliferation of the forestomach. Since the forestomach was the only target organ in the chronic NTP studies, and the only organ affected in the acute and repeat dose studies, this observation suggests that a correlation may exist between continued epithelial cell proliferation and carcinogenicity of the forestomach. However, the relationship between cell proliferation and EA-induced carcinogenicity is not as clear in other organs. For example, long-term EA inhalation caused epithelial cell proliferation of the respiratory passages but no neoplastic lesions (10). Similarly, long-term dermal application of EA caused sustained epithelial cell proliferation of the epidermis but no skin tumors (11). The lack of correlation in these two cases may be the result of EA concentration, the extent of cell proliferation, and the sensitivity and nature of the tissue involved. In the inhalation studies, the highest EA concentration was 75 ppm. In the dermal studies, the maximum EA concentration was 1%; much of that material may have been lost through grooming, evaporation, or contact with cages and bedding. In contrast, the concentration in the NTP gavage studies was 2% for dosages of 100 mg EA/5 ml corn oil/kg, and 4% for a corresponding dose of 200 mg. EA administration by gavage also allows longer contact time of high EA concentrations with the forestomach tissue, with minimal or no loss of EA to evaporation or animal grooming.

We and others hypothesize that marked and prolonged forestomach hyperplasia may have contributed to the carcinogenic effect of a number of chemicals including EA (9,12) and butylated hydroxyanisole (13). The issue of "sustained" cell proliferation appears to be of particular importance. The period for which cell proliferation must be sustained and its universality from one chemical to another and from one tissue to another has yet to be established. Our work has demonstrated that forestomach epithelial cell proliferation continues for as long as EA is administered. However, when administration ceases, recovery begins and is completed with no increase in the incidence of

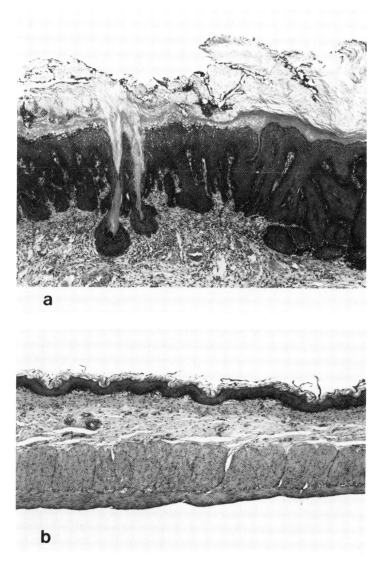

Figure 5. Photomicrographs of forestomachs from male rats treated with with 200 mg EA/kg by gavage for 13 weeks and killed 24 hr after the last dose (a) or 19 months after cessation of dosing (b). (a) shows severe mucosal hyperplasia; (b) shows regression of lesions observed in (a); the forestomach appears normal. Hematoxylin and eosin stain, ×66.

forestomach neoplasia even after 90 daily doses of EA (Table 4). This evidence of reversibility calls for further research to precisely define the time and dose necessary to create sustained cell proliferation and an increased incidence of neoplasia. Furthermore, more work is needed to determine the differences, if any, in the response of various tissues to sustained cell proliferation. In particular, more treatment-stop studies are required to establish the point at which cell proliferation reaches the point of irreversibility.

References

1. Ghanayem BI, Burka LT, Matthews HB. Ethyl acrylate distribution, macromolecular binding, excretion, and metabolism in F344 rats. Fundam Appl Toxicol 9:389–397, 1987.
2. DeBethizy JD, Udinskey JR, Scribner HE, Fredrick CB. The disposition of acrylic acid and ethyl acrylate in male Sprague-Dawley rats. Fundam Appl Toxicol 8:549–561.
3. NTP (National Toxicology Program). Carcinogenesis bioassay of ethyl acrylate. Technical report series #259, publication (NIH) 82-2515. U.S. Department of Health and Human Services, Public Health Service, National Institutes of Health, Research Triangle Park, NC.
4. Waegemaekers THJM, Bensink MPM. Non-mutagenicity of 27 aliphatic acrylate esters in the Salmonella-microsome test. Mutat Res 137:95–102, 1984.
5. Przybojewska B, Dziubaltowska E, Kowalski Z. Genotoxic effects of ethyl acrylate and methyl acrylate in the mouse evaluated by the micronucleus test. Mutat Res 135:189–191, 1984.
6. Silver EH Murphy SD. Potentiation of acrylate ester toxicity by prior treatment with the carboxylesterase inhibitor triorthotolyl phosphate (TOTP). Toxicol Appl Pharmacol 57:208–219, 1981.
7. Ghanayem BI, Maronpot RR, Matthews HB. Ethyl acrylate-induced gastric toxicity I. Effect of single and repetitive dosing. Toxicol Appl Pharmacol 80:323–335, 1985.
8. Ghanayem BI, Maronpot RR, and Matthews HB. Ethyl acrylate-induced gastric toxicity II. Structure-toxicity relationships and mechanism. Toxicol Appl Pharmacol 80:336–344, 1985.
9. Ghanayem BI, Maronpot RR, Matthews HB. Ethyl acrylate-induced gastric toxicity III. Development and recovery of lesions. Toxicol Appl Pharmacol 83:576–583, 1986.
10. Miller RR, Young JT, Kociba RJ, Keyes DG, Bonder KM, Calhoun LL, Ayres JA. Chronic toxicity and oncogenicity bioassay of inhaled ethyl acrylate in Fischer 344 rats and B6C3F1 mice. Drug and Chem Toxicol 8:1–42, 1985.
11. DePass LR, Fowler EH, Meckley DR, Weil CS. Dermal oncogenicity bioassays of acrylic acid, ethyl acrylate, and butyl acrylate. J Toxicol Environ Health 14:115–120, 1984.
12. Ghanayem BI, Maronpot RR, Matthews HB. Association of chemically-induced forestomach cell proliferation and carcinogenesis. Cancer Lett 32:271–278, 1986.
13. Iverson F, Lok E, Rena E, Karpinski K, Clayson DB. A 13-week feeding study of butylated hydroxyanisole: The subsequent regression of the induced lesions in male Fischer F344 rat forestomach epithelium. Toxicology 35:1–11, 1985.

Chemically Induced Cell Proliferation:
Implications for Risk Assessment, pages 347-355
©1991 Wiley-Liss, Inc.

Cell Proliferation and Bladder Tumor Promotion

Samuel M. Cohen and Leon B. Ellwein

That carcinogenesis occurs in multiple stages has been suggested for several decades. Numerous studies done in the 1940s culminated in the two-stage model of initiation and promotion formulated by Berenblum and Shubik (1), the importance of multiple stages and the role of cell proliferation and cell number were later suggested by Nordling (2), and the relationship of time and dose in multistage models was characterized by the mathematical formula of Armitage and Doll (3). Although this formula has worked well for several experimental animal models and many epidemiologic studies of cancer, there have been exceptions. A major difficulty with the Armitage and Doll model is its implicit assumption of constant cell number and proliferation rates during the course of an experiment, assumptions that generally do not hold in high-dose animal experiments (4).

In quantitative risk assessment, several models have been utilized to ascertain possible risk to humans from low-dose exposure—using animal experiments incorporating relatively high-dose, often toxic-level, exposures. In recent years, there has been increasing emphasis on the development of more biologically based risk assessment models than the standard mathematical formulations. These models have taken two different, but complementary, forms. The first is the pharmacokinetic models (5), which attempt to account for species differences in distribution and metabolism of different chemicals to arrive at better dose-response models in terms of dose of the critical metabolite(s) in the target tissue. The second set of models relates the biologic responsiveness of cells to delivered dose and to the development of tumors (6,7). We describe three examples of the latter type of modeling.

Biologic model of carcinogenesis

Approximately 10 years ago, we began to develop a biologic model of carcinogenesis, taking into account the effects of chemicals on both DNA and cell proliferation. This model has been described in detail (7–9), and its basic features are illustrated in Figure 1. We made several fundamental assumptions about the carcinogenic process. The first is that the carcinogenic process results from two sequential events, which we have labeled initiation and transformation. By transformed cells, we mean malignant cells. We include intermediate, benign populations seen in numerous experimental models, such as papillomas and hyperplastic nodules, in the initiated population; they are not considered transformed. A second assumption of the model is that these two critical events occur only in the stem cell population of the target organ. It has been difficult to define "stem cell;" a more appropriate term would be a "susceptible cell population" in the target organ. In layered epithelia, such as the bladder

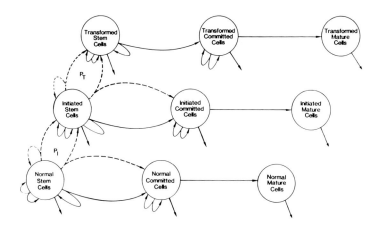

Figure. 1. Diagram represents the biologic model of carcinogenesis originally described by Greenfield et al. (7). The bottom three circles represent the normal differentiation of a tissue. Along the left side are the two stages of carcinogenesis—initiation and transformation. Downward arrows represent cell death, whereas the other arrows represent the combinations of possible results following cell division.

and skin, this population is readily identified as a subset of the basal layer. In other tissues, such as the liver, it is more difficult to define. A third assumption is that the two critical events will not occur and/or will be irreversibly fixed into place without a round of cell division. Fourth, we assume that these events occur in probabilistic fashion; that is, the occurrence of a genetic event during cell division is represented quantitatively as a probability. Obviously, in normal control situations, this probability is very small. Otherwise, tumors would arise rapidly in all organisms and all tissues. The probability may approach zero, but the existence of spontaneous tumors indicates it is not actually zero.

From these assumptions, it is clear that the critical quantitative parameters in carcinogenesis are the number of cells in the normal and initiated susceptible populations, their division rates, and the probabilities of genomic errors during cell division. Some of these parameters can be measured experimentally; others can be inferred from modeling analyses of time and dose response in tumor formation.

We have adopted a simulation approach in our modeling, which can be viewed mathematically as a discrete-time Markov process with time-varying parameters (10). A similar biologic model developed by Moolgavkar and Knudson (6) related initially to the study of human carcinogenesis. They use a closed-form, continuous-time mathematical formulation and emphasized parameter estimation using statistical curve-fitting methods.

N-[4-(5-Nitro-2-furyl)-2-thiazolyl]formamide (FANFT)

FANFT is a potent urinary bladder carcinogen in rats, mice, hamsters, and dogs and is a typical genotoxic carcinogen (11). It is metabolically activated to a reactive electrophile that binds to DNA, and it has proved mutagenic in most short-term assays in which it has been tested. We administered FANFT to male F344 rats at a dose of 0.2% of the diet for various periods of time in a series of experiments and then killed the animals sequentially so that levels of hyperplasia and tumor prevalence could be examined (7). Multiple time points for determination of tumor prevalence provide important information for the accurate assessment of the time course of bladder tumor development. Using these experiments, we were able to show that FANFT has a hyperplastic effect at this dose and that it affects the initiation probability, apparently without increasing the second transformation, probability over background levels.

The dose response of FANFT in male F344 rats was then assessed in a more traditional manner. We administered different doses of the chemical for fixed periods and examined tumor prevalence after 1 and 2 years (12) (Table 1). There was a sharp increase in tumor incidence at doses above 0.01% of the diet, and essentially no tumors appeared even after 2 years at lower doses. This does not mean that an effect is absent at these lower doses, only that with this relatively small number of animals we were unable to detect a significant incidence. The sharp change in the shape of the curve at a dose of approximately 0.01% can be shown to be due to the increased proliferation that occurs in the urothelium at the higher doses of FANFT, as evidenced in Table 1 by the markedly increased labeling index at the higher doses after relatively short periods of FANFT administration. Other experiments have shown DNA interaction even at the lower doses. However, without cell proliferative effects at the lower doses, tumor incidence does not significantly increase. This has obvious implications for low-dose extrapolation of FANFT tumor response (13).

Sodium Saccharin

Saccharin has been shown to induce a significant incidence of bladder cancer in male rats when administered over two generations, that is, when it is administered during gestation and lactation and then to the offspring for the remainder of their life-

Table 1. Effects of Different Doses of FANFT on the Male Rat Urinary Bladder.*

Dose of FANFT (% of diet)	Bladder carcinoma incidence (%)		Labeling index at 10 weeks (% ± SD)
	1 year	2 years	
0.2	100	100	2.02 ± 0.84+
0.1	56	100	2.21 ± 0.74+
0.05	29	87	0.84 ± 0.36+
0.01	0	0	0.11 ± 0.05
0.005	0	0	0.08 ± 0.06
0.001	0	0	0.08 ± 0.06
0.0005	0	0	————
0	0	0	0.10 ± 0.07

*Data are from R. Hasegawa et al. (12).
+Significantly different from controls at $P < 0.05$ by Student's t-test.

spans, up to 2.5 years (14). However, when it is administered beginning after weaning, a small, insignificant incidence of tumors results. In addition, other experiments have demonstrated that if the postweanling male rat is first given an initiating dose of FANFT, N-methyl-N-nitrosourea (MNU), or N-butyl-N-(4-hydroxybutyl)nitrosamine (BBN) and then given saccharin for up to 2 years, a highly significant incidence of tumors results. Also, saccharin administered concurrently with low doses of FANFT (0.005%) acts as a cocarcinogen, and tumors result. The dose used in these experiments has been at 5% of the diet. In dose-response data from two-generation and initiation-promotion studies, no effect has been seen at doses below 3% and 2.5%, respectively.

In extrapolating experimental results to humans, investigators have encountered several problems (14). For one, the male rat appears to be considerably more susceptible than the female rat to the urothelial effects of saccharin. Second, the mouse, hamster, and monkey appear unresponsive to the effects of even extremely high doses of saccharin in the diet. Epidemiologic studies, in addition, do not provide any support for a moderate to high risk of bladder cancer due to saccharin ingestion. The question remains, Is there a small risk for the development of bladder cancer with exposure to saccharin at levels ingested by humans?

In contrast to FANFT, saccharin is not metabolized to a reactive electrophile (it is actually nucleophilic), it does not react with DNA, and it has been shown nongenotoxic in most short-term assays (14). However, when administered in the diet at high doses, there is an increase in urothelial proliferation in the male rat, which begins rapidly after administration begins. The urothelium is normally a mitotically quiescent tissue, with a labeling index of less than 0.1% following a 1-hr pulse of [^{3}H]thymidine. The administration of sodium saccharin at a level of 5% of the diet increases the labeling index 2- to 10-fold. With modeling analyses, we have been able to show that all of the tumorigenic effects of saccharin administration can be explained by the increase in cell proliferation secondary to saccharin administration if one assumes a low, control level of genomic error during each cell division (8,14).

The relationship between cellular activity and genomic error in a target organ is particularly important when one realizes that, in the normal rat, approximately one third of the total lifetime mitoses of the urothelium occur within the first 3 weeks of life. Increased cell proliferation during this early period adequately explains why rats are more susceptible to saccharin-induced tumors when saccharin administration begins at birth than after weaning. The increase in cell proliferation after short periods of administration is dose responsive; no increase in labeling index was observed at doses lower than 2.5% of the diet. This correlates with the dose-related tumor response seen in initiation-promotion studies and in two-generation bioassays.

Unlike DNA-reactive compounds, a dose response for saccharin reactivity is more difficult to ascertain, since DNA adducts are not formed and, therefore, cannot be assayed for. Is there a small, but undetectable increase in cell proliferation at these lower doses, or is a true threshold phenomenon occurring? A knowledge of the mechanism of action of saccharin is needed to distinguish between a lack of sensitivity in detecting increased cell proliferation and a true threshold.

That mechanism remains undefined, but considerable progress has been made in our understanding—enough that a hypothesis of the process in the rat and its implications for human exposure can now be made (14). As indicated above, saccharin does not act by reacting with DNA, and it is now generally accepted that its effects on the urothelium are not due to a contaminant or to calculus formation, as had previously been suggested. In all the above-mentioned long-term bioassays, saccharin was administered in the diet as the sodium salt, the form most widely used in commercial preparations. We compared the short-term effects of other salt forms of saccharin and found that potassium saccharin also increased urothelial proliferation when administered as 5% of the diet, but at significantly lower levels than 5% sodium saccharin. In contrast, calcium saccharin and acid saccharin did not increase proliferative rates. This difference in cell proliferation occurred despite the fact that the urinary concentration of saccharin was similar following the administration of all four forms of saccharin. However, the concentration of several other urinary ions (such as sodium, potassium, and calcium) differed considerably following the administration of the different salt forms; pH, osmolality, and volume also differed.

We recently demonstrated that a silicon-containing precipitate and crystalline material forms in the urine of male rats fed high doses of sodium saccharin, and this is strongly suspected of contributing to the cytotoxicity and regenerative hyperplasia required for the tumorigenic effects of saccharin (14,15). Several aspects of this precipitate and crystal formation are pertinent to the known biology of saccharin in rats and other species.

The normal rat urine, like that of many mammalian species, including humans, contains large numbers of $MgNH_4PO_4$ crystals. These are also present in the urine of rats fed sodium saccharin, as are significant numbers of silicate-containing crystals and large amounts of a silicate-containing precipitate. Others have demonstrated that silicates precipitate in the urine only at appropriate pH. Some studies indicate pH has to be at least 7.0. But in our studies, it appears silicates can form even at a pH of 6.5. In either case, acidifying the urine inhibits the formation of the precipitate and crystals. It has been demonstrated that any treatment that results in acidification of the urine prevents the proliferative effect of saccharin. Rat urine pH is below 6.0 if saccharin is administered as the calcium or acid salt, if NH_4Cl is coadministered, or if sodium saccharin is administered in AIN-76A semisynthetic diet. In any of these cases, urothelial cell proliferation is not seen. Also, formation of this silicate-containing material in the urine requires a protein matrix for its formation.

It is well known that male rat urine contains extremely high levels of protein, particularly $\alpha_{2\mu}$-globulin (16). Female rat urine, although it has considerably less protein than that of male rats because of the near absence of $\alpha_{2\mu}$-globulin, also contains a considerable amount of protein. Nevertheless, this difference in protein profiles could help explain the marked difference in biologic responsiveness of the male and the female rat. We recently demonstrated that saccharin actually binds to urinary proteins (Cohen and Carson, unpublished observations), and the bound protein-saccharin complex may be the material on which the silicate precipitates. Significantly, the major proportion of the saccharin binding to urinary proteins is to $\alpha_{2\mu}$-globulin.

Although these studies have only been performed with sodium saccharin and its related salt forms, similar biologic findings have been observed with the sodium salts of other moderate organic acids, such as ascorbate, glutamate, erythorbate, and citrate (14). A similar mechanism is likely to be operative in all of these situations, since acidification prevents the proliferative and tumorigenic effects of these compounds.

The requirement for urinary pH, and especially the requirement for large amounts of protein, may also help explain the interspecies variations observed so far. There is considerably less protein in mouse and monkey than rat urine, and there do not appear to be significant amounts of $\alpha_{2\mu}$-globulin–like protein in the urine of these species. Similarly, the protein levels of human urine are also considerably lower than in the rat. These mechanistic relationships must be taken into account in extrapolating risk to the human situation. They imply the presence of a threshold phenomenon. The simple use of mathematical expressions to estimate low-dose risk from experimental results at higher doses is clearly inadequate.

2-Aceytlaminofluorene (AAF)

The carcinogen AAF has been studied extensively in several species. In mice, it induces liver and bladder tumors. The enormous data base specifically addressing the concept of low-dose extrapolation includes the "megamouse" study performed by the National Center for Toxicological Research, referred to as the ED_{01} study (17). This study used more than 24,000 female mice administered AAF at various doses for various lengths of time, including groups that were administered the compound for a period of time and then given a control diet for an additional period. However, rather than solving the problem of low-dose extrapolation, it raised additional questions, largely because the dose-response curves for the liver and bladder were different at low doses.

This difference in low-dose responsiveness was originally attributed to a difference in the pharmacokinetics of the compound; more of the compound was thought to be delivered to the liver than to the bladder. However, Beland and his associates recently demonstrated that the relationship between DNA adduct formation and AAF dose as used in the ED_{01} study is linear for both the liver and bladder (18,19). Thus, the difference in tumor response between the liver and bladder cannot be explained simply by pharmacokinetics.

We have examined the ED_{01} study, incorporating AAF mechanistic information, and have shown that both the liver and bladder effects of AAF in the mouse can be explained by our two-event model (13,20). AAF at the doses administered in the ED_{01} study did not increase the rate of proliferation or growth of the liver over the 33-month time course of the experiment. Obviously, AAF had an effect on DNA, since adducts were formed. However, marked decreases have been reported in the metabolism of AAF in foci hepatocytes and in the formation of DNA adducts in the foci ("initiated") hepatocytes. We, therefore, made the assumption that p_I is altered in the liver by AAF, whereas p_T is not. By utilizing a linear relationship between p_I and the AAF dose—based on the linearity of adduct formation—we found that the liver tumor response curves were totally compatible with our two-stage model.

As in the liver, the doses of AAF used in the ED_{01} study produced a linear DNA adduct formation response in the bladder. However, in contrast to the liver, DNA adduct formation would be expected to be essentially similar in normal and initiated urothelial cells, based on the metabolism of AAF. We therefore assumed that both p_I and p_T changed linearly with respect to dose within the dose ranges of the ED_{01} study. Although there was no increased cell proliferation at the lowest doses of AAF evaluated, hyperplasia did occur at doses above 60 ppm. Taking into account the increased cell proliferation at the higher doses interacting with the genotoxic effects on p_I and p_T, we were able to demonstrate that the data were compatible with our two-stage hypothesis. At the lower doses, there was still an effect, but it was not detectable—even with the large number of animals used in the ED_{01} study. The study was designed to detect an increase in incidence of 1% above background; however, at doses below 60 ppm, even at 33 months, incidence is not expected to increase by that much because of the lack of a proliferative response. This gives the appearance of a no-effect level in the bladder, even though DNA adducts are being formed at the lower doses.

The interaction between the effects of cell proliferation (nongenotoxic) and DNA adduct formation (genotoxic) is synergistic. Using computer simulation, we found that after 33 months, bladder tumor prevalence at 150 ppm would be 14% if cell proliferation were the only factor and 6% if genotoxicity were the only mechanism involved. However, if the two effects were both operative, tumor prevalence would reach 100%.

Implications for risk assessment

The above examples clearly show that genotoxic and cell proliferative effects are important in carcinogenesis and that these effects are interactive when both are produced by a given chemical. From these and other analyses, we have postulated a classification of chemical carcinogens (Fig. 2) different from those previously proposed. Chemicals are divided into those interactive with DNA (genotoxic) and those not interactive with DNA (nongenotoxic). Genotoxic compounds are not likely to have a threshold effect. Cell proliferative effects, usually present at the higher doses, will markedly alter the dose-response curve, particularly if there is a lack of cell proliferative effects at lower doses, as seen in the FANFT and AAF bladder carcinoma examples.

Nongenotoxic compounds are divided into those that operate via a cell receptor mechanism, such as phorbol esters, dioxin, and hormones, and those compounds that act by cytotoxicity and consequent regenerative hyperplasia. In both instances, the operative mechanism is an increase in cell proliferation. It remains unclear whether those that operate by a cell receptor mechanism have a threshold effect. However, it is highly likely that those with a cytotoxic mechanism will usually have a threshold below which toxicity, and therefore carcinogenicity, will not occur.

Rather than trying to define chemicals in terms of complete carcinogens, initiators, promoters, etc., we prefer that chemicals be classified as those that are genotoxic, those that act by increasing cell proliferation, and those with both effects. Depending on whether either of these effects relates to the normal and/or initiated cell populations, differences in dose-response curves will result. For example, theoretically, a chemical considered to be a tumor promoter would act by increasing the proliferative rate of initiated cells. In reality, however, most chemicals that do this also increase the proliferation of normal cells. Exposure to such chemicals will result in an increase in tumor incidence if the cell proliferation is sustained for an adequate length of time.

The question arises as to whether any compound that causes increased cell proliferation will eventually be considered a carcinogen. The answer is likely to be no, for a wide variety of reasons. First, the level of increased proliferation may not be adequate to generate a significant incidence of tumors in a group of animals in the time

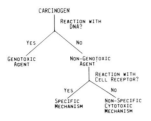

Figure. 2. Diagram represents the proposed classification of chemical carcinogens according to their ability to react directly with DNA or cell receptors. Cell proliferation affects the dose response of all classes of chemical carcinogens. From Cohen and Ellwein (13).

period of a study, usually 2 years. Second, cell proliferation can occur in cells other than stem cells (susceptible cells) in the target tissue. For example, turpentine causes marked proliferation when applied to the skin, but largely in the keratinocytes rather than in the basal cells. In contrast, phorbol esters cause proliferation predominantly of cells in the basal layer, particularly the so-called dark cells. Another major consideration is that the cell proliferation must be sustained for a considerable length of time to result in tumors at a detectable level.

Finally, many agents that cause cell proliferation do so by being cytotoxic. Thus, when administered over a long period of time, they not only stimulate new cell formation but also kill cells. It is a long-sustained imbalance of increased cell proliferation and cell death that provides the opportunity for tumor development. Some chemicals, such as cyclophosphamide, are cytotoxic at high doses and lead to marked increases in cell proliferation without increasing tumor incidence (21). However, when the dose is reduced below the cytotoxic level, tumors result (22). Cyclophosphamide is a well-known genotoxin; in addition to causing cell proliferation in the bladder, it is cytotoxic to bladder tumor cells (23).

Just as the simple paradigm of mutagenesis and carcinogenesis was not adequate to readily classify all chemicals as carcinogens or noncarcinogens, it is likely that cell proliferation will not offer a simple paradigm. However, an understanding of cell proliferation within the carcinogenic process should not only greatly contribute to our knowledge of the mechanism of action of compounds but should also improve our ability to interpret data from high-dose experiments to make them useful in the estimation of low-dose risk.

Acknowledgments

This research was supported by U.S. Public Health Service grants CA32513, CA28015, RR01968, and CA36727 from the National Institutes of Health, grants from the Department of Health, State of Nebraska, and from the International Life Sciences Institute–Nutrition Foundation. We gratefully acknowledge the many contributions of the late Dr. Robert E. Greenfield and the large number of colleagues and technologists who have participated in this research, and we thank Deborah Coleman for her help with the preparation of this manuscript.

References

1. Boutwell RK. Some biological aspects of skin carcinogenesis. Prog Exp Tumor Res 4:207–250, 1964.
2. Nordling CO. A new theory on the cancer-inducing mechanism. Br J Cancer 7:68–72, 1953.

3. Armitage P, Doll R. The age distribution of cancer and a multistage theory of carcinogenesis. Br J Cancer 8:1–12, 1954.

4. Moolgavkar SH. Biologically motivated two-stage model for cancer risk assessment. Toxicol Lett 43:139–150, 1988.

5. Reitz RH, Mendrala AL, Park CN, Andersen ME, Guengerich FP. Incorporation of in vitro enzyme data into the physiologically-based pharmacokinetic (PB-PK) model for methylene chloride: Implications for risk assessment. Toxicol Lett 43:97–116, 1988.

6. Moolgavkar SH, Knudson AG Jr. Mutation and cancer: A model for human carcinogenesis. J Natl Cancer Inst 66:1037–1052, 1981.

7. Greenfield RE, Ellwein LB, Cohen SM. A general probabilistic model of carcinogenesis: Analysis of experimental urinary bladder cancer. Carcinogenesis 5:437–445, 1984.

8. Ellwein LB, Cohen SM. A cellular dynamics model of experimental bladder cancer: Analysis of the effect of sodium saccharin in the rat. Risk Anal 8:215–221, 1988.

9. Ellwein LB, Cohen SM. Comparative analyses of the timing and magnitude of genotoxic and nongenotoxic cellular effects in urinary bladder carcinogenesis. In Travis C (ed): Biologically Based Methods for Cancer Risk Assessment. New York: Plenum Publishing, pp. 181–192, 1989.

10. Howard RA. Markov models. In Dynamic Probabilistic Systems, Vol. 1. New York: John Wiley & Sons, 1971.

11. Cohen SM, Ellwein LB. Cell growth dynamics in long-term bladder carcinogenesis. Toxicol Lett 43:151–173, 1988.

12. Hasegawa R, Cohen SM, St. John M, Cano M, Ellwein LB. Effect of dose on the induction of urothelial proliferation by N-[4-(5-nitro-2-furyl)-2-thiazolyl]formamide and its relationship to bladder carcinogenesis in the rat. Carcinogenesis 7:633–636, 1986.

13. Cohen SM, Ellwein LB. Cell growth dynamics and DNA alterations in carinogenesis. In Moolgavkar SH (ed): Scientific Issues in Quantitative Cancer Risk Assessment. Societal Institute of the Mathematical Sciences, pp. 116–135, 1990.

14. Ellwein LB, Cohen SM. The health risks of saccharin revisited. Crit Rev Toxicol 20:311–326, 1990.

15. Cohen SM, Cano M, Garland EM, Earl RA. Silicate crystals in the urine and bladder epithellium of male rats fed sodium saccharin. Proc Am Assoc Cancer Res 30:204, 1989.

16. Swenberg JA, Short B, Borghoff S, Strasser J, Charbonneau M. The comparative pathobiology of $\alpha_{2\mu}$-globulin nephropathy. Toxicol Appl Pharmacol 97:35–46, 1989.

17. Staffa JA, Mehlman MA (eds): Innovations in Cancer Risk Assessment (ED_{01} Study: Proceedings of a symposium sponsored by the National Center for Toxicology Research, U.S. Food and Drug Administration, and American College of Toxicology. J Environ Pathol Toxicol Oncol, Vol. 3, 1980.

18. Beland FA, Fullerton NF, Kinouchi T, Poirier MC. DNA adduct formation during continuous feeding of 2-acetylaminofluorene at multiple concentrations. IARC Sci Publ 89:175–180, 1988.

19. Beland FA. Metabolic activation of aromatic amine carcinogens in vitro and in vivo. J Univ Occup Environ Health 11 (Suppl):387–397, 1989.

20. Cohen SM, Ellwein LB. Proliferative and genotoxic cellular effects in 2-acetylaminofluorene bladder and liver carcinogenesis. Toxicol Appl Pharmacol 104:79–93, 1990.

21. Cohen SM, Arai M, Jacobs JB, Friedell GH. Induction of papillary tumors and flat carcinoma-in-situ (CIS) of the urinary bladder by cyclophosphamide in male Fischer rats. Proc Am Assoc Cancer Res 20:231, 1979.

22. Schmahl D, Habs M. Carcinogenic action of low-dose cyclophosphamide given orally to Sprague-Dawley rats in a lifetime experiment. Int J Cancer 23:706–712, 1979.

23. Soloway MS. Single and combination chemotherapy for primary murine bladder cancer. Cancer 36:333–340, 1975.

Chemically Induced Cell Proliferation:
Implications for Risk Assessment, pages 357-367
©1991 Wiley-Liss, Inc.

Chemically Induced Cell Proliferation in Carcinogenesis in the Male Rat Kidney

Brian G. Short and James A. Swenberg

Many nongenotoxic nephrocarcinogens are nephrotoxic in the tumorigenic dose range. Among recent findings from two-year bioassays in rodents was a rapidly growing list of chemicals that cause a mild to moderate increase in incidence (up to 25%) of renal adenomas and carcinomas in male, but not female, rats or in mice of either gender. In addition, many of these male rat-specific carcinogens are nephrotoxic in this species and gender, and they manifest as protein droplet nephropathy after acute exposure. The current list of chemicals includes 1,4-dichlorobenzene (1,2), dimethylmethylphosphonate (3), isophorone (4,5), JP-5 jet fuel (6,7), d-limonene (8,9), pentachloroethane (10,11), perchloroethylene (11,12), and unleaded gasoline (13,14).

Protein droplet nephropathy is characterized by accumulation of large hyaline or protein droplets in kidney tubules, representing phagosomal overload of α_{2u}-globulin ($\alpha_{2u}G$) primarily in the second, or P2, segment of the proximal tubule. These chemicals have also been shown to increase the number of granular casts and regenerative tubules, and they accelerate the incidence and severity of the aging rat lesion known as chronic progressive nephrosis (CPN). This gender- and species-specific response has prompted several investigators (15,16) to postulate that $\alpha_{2u}G$ nephropathy causes cytotoxicity such as single-cell necrosis, which induces a restorative hyperplasia in the injured tubule. Although compensatory regeneration is generally regarded as beneficial for the continuing functional and structural integrity of the kidney, excessive or continual regeneration may contribute to carcinogenesis. It has been hypothesized that prolonged elevations in cell turnover in the kidney (15,17) and other organs (18,19) may promote tumors arising from cells previously initiated by environmental or endogenous agents or by cell proliferation itself. Increased proliferation of proximal tubule cells may, therefore, play a pivotal role in neoplasia induced by this group of nephrocarcinogens.

Because unleaded gasoline is an integral part of modern life, its demonstrated carcinogenic potential in the kidney of male rats has drawn considerable attention from the scientific community. Investigative efforts by scientists at the Chemical Industry Institute of Toxicology (CIIT) have focused on an array of biochemical and pathologic aspects of unleaded gasoline–induced nephrotoxicity, genotoxicity, and nephrocarcinogenicity in male rats (16,20–31).

From these as well as other studies (32–35), a clear picture is emerging concerning the relationship of this chemical mixture's nephrotoxicity, cell proliferation and carcinogenicity. Unleaded gasoline may be a model for the group of nephrocarcinogens in male rats; this report will therefore review its effects on $\alpha_{2u}G$ nephropathy, cell proliferation, and tumor promotion. In addition, we shall discuss the effects of 2,2,4-trimethylpentane (TMP), a nephrotoxic, isoparaffinic unleaded gasoline component.

Pathology of nephropathy $\alpha_{2u}G$ nephropathy

In $\alpha_{2u}G$ nephropathy, the most likely cause of cell death in the P2 proximal tubule is lysosomal overload caused by decreased $\alpha_{2u}G$ catabolism or lysosomal dysfunction or both. Lysosomal overload may lead to a release of digestive enzymes into the cytoplasm and impaired autophagy with decreased plasma membrane availability and turnover; this is similar to the condition hypothesized for the toxicity of human Bence Jones proteins in proximal tubules of the rat (36). In any event, the injured cell detaches from the basement membrane and floats downstream, where it collects in granular casts in the thin limb of Henle or exits into the urine. The functional consequences are minimal, since neighboring adjacent cells are rapidly stimulated to divide and replace the lost cell.

Until recently, the effect of age and exposure duration on the severity of unleaded gasoline–induced $\alpha_{2u}G$ nephropathy was unknown. Since liver synthesis of $\alpha_{2u}G$ declines steadily in F344 rats after 150 days (37), whether $\alpha_{2u}G$ nephropathy could be induced in older rats was uncertain. However, in recent studies concentration-related increases in the severity of $\alpha_{2u}G$ nephropathy have been detected, as judged by histochemical stains for $\alpha_{2u}G$ in rats exposed to up to 300 ppm unleaded gasoline or 50 ppm TMP for 48 weeks (29). Compared with earlier time points, however, the severity was diminished, probably reflecting the gradual decline of native $\alpha_{2u}G$ in aging rats. In female rats, $\alpha_{2u}G$ nephropathy was not inducible at any time point.

Chronic cell proliferation

We quantitated site-specific cell proliferation of the various subpopulations of the slowly replicating kidney by autoradiographic methods after using osmotic pumps to administer tritiated thymidine continuously for a week. Perfusion-fixed kidneys were embedded in plastic and stained with Lee's modified basic blue fuchsin, which permitted various cell types to be identified by high-resolution light microscopy (16,28,29). Quantitative cell proliferation studies of the male rat kidney during the last week of a subacute (3-week) inhalation exposure to 2–2000 ppm unleaded gasoline or gavaged TMP (0.2–50 mg/kg) demonstrated maximal, dose-related increases in cell proliferation of the P2 segment of the proximal tubule, located at the site of $\alpha_{2u}G$ accumulation (16).

These results provided incentive for a study to answer a more important question: whether cell turnover is increased in any segments of the proximal tubule (P1, P2, or P3) of male or female rats during chronic exposure to unleaded gasoline or TMP. We also examined the relationship between termination of exposure and reversibility of cell proliferation by measuring cell proliferation at several intervals after the last week of exposure. Again, as in the 3-week studies, increased replication occurred in tubules affected by $\alpha_{2u}G$ nephropathy (Fig. 1). Quantitation of proximal tubule cells undergoing replication demonstrated 4- to 11-fold increases in cell proliferation of the P2 segments of male rats exposed to 300 ppm unleaded gasoline or 50 ppm TMP at all time points (Fig. 2), in contrast to a complete lack of response in female rats (Fig. 3). Smaller but significant increases in cell proliferation occurred in adjacent P3 segment cells. Because they exhibited no cytotoxicity of their own, the P3 cells' proliferative responses probably resulted from stimulatory responses elicited by cytotoxicity in adjacent P2 tubules.

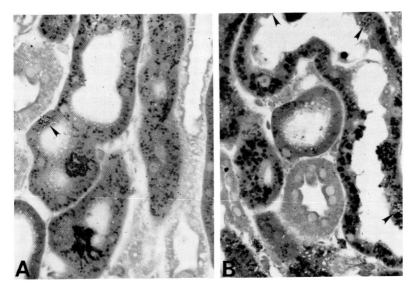

Figure 1. Autoradiography of kidneys of male rats at 22–23 weeks of exposure to 300-ppm unleaded gasoline (UG), with labeling (arrowheads) during the last week of exposure. (A) Control male kidney with few labeled cells and protein droplets. (B) Exposed male kidney with an abundance of labeled cells in protein droplet-filled P2 segments (Lee's methylene blue basic fuchsin, × 320).

Another thought-provoking observation from this study was that proximal tubules in areas of CPN had strikingly high cell turnover rates (Fig. 4), and although the severity and extent of CPN was considered mild, the number of affected tubules in male rats was about 10-fold higher than in female rats. Since chronic unleaded gasoline exposure has been shown to accelerate CPN, it too may contribute a significant portion of proliferating cells that are at increased risk of tumor formation. Reversibility studies indicated that, although cell proliferation was completely reversible at earlier time points, at later time points it was only partially so, despite the complete recovery of protein droplet accumulation. In summary, this was the first study to show the persistence of cell proliferation induced by recurrent cytotoxicity and CPN. The next step was to determine whether similar unleaded gasoline exposure conditions are effective in promoting renal tumor formation in the male rat.

Hydrocarbon promotion study

The most basic model of carcinogenesis consists of two stages: an irreversible initiation stage, followed by a series of reversible promotional steps that result in the formation of a tumor. Experimental animal models of initiation and promotion have been described in skin (38) and several other organs (39,40).

Several investigators have developed initiation-promotion models for the kidney, showing that nephrotoxins can promote renal tumors in rats initiated with *N*-ethyl-*N*-

Cell Proliferation (LI treated/LI control) of
Proximal Tubule Cells of Male Rats Exposed to UG or TMP

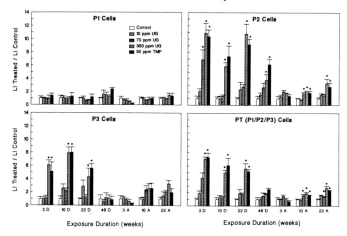

2

Cell Proliferation (LI treated/LI control) of
Proximal Tubule Cells of Female Rats Exposed to UG or TMP

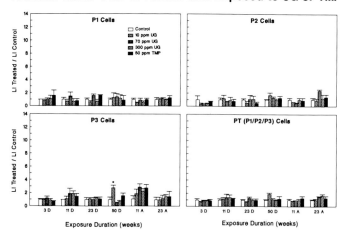

3

Figures 2 and 3. Increases in cell proliferation of P1, P2, P3, and entire proximal tubuie (PT) cells of treated versus control male (3) and female (4) rats at various weeks of exposure. Quantitative autoradiography was performed following continuous thymidine administration *during* (D) the last 7 days of exposure or *after* (A) the last exposure week for 10 days at various exposure intervals. Significantly higher cell proliferation were evident when compared to the exposure interval control ($P < 0.05$) by ANOVA and Newman-Keuls multicomparison tests.

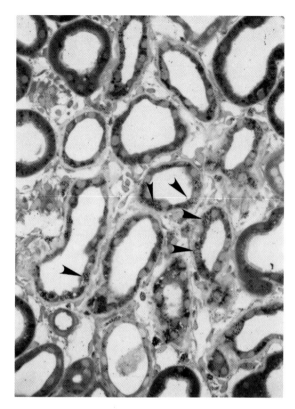

Figure 4. Autoradiographic image of kidney of aged male rat. High magnification of cortical chronic progressive necrosis (CPN) lesion demonstrates constricted tubules surrounded by thick basement membrane and interstitial cells. Note high number of labeled tubular epithelial cells (arrowheads) (Lee's methylene blue basic fuchsin, × 160).

hydroxyethyl-nitrosamine (EHEN) in the drinking water (41,42). The hypothesis was that unleaded gasoline induces renal neoplasia by promoting rather than initiating activity because most assays had shown it to be nongenotoxic (43,44,26). We designed and conducted an extensive hydrocarbon promotion study in male and female rats (Fig. 5) to address the question of unleaded gasoline–induced tumor promotion.

Results of the hydrocarbon promotion study are presented in Tables 1 and 2 for male and female rats, respectively. The number of macroscopic and microscopic renal cell tumors (RCT) was increased in male rats promoted with 50 ppm TMP (4/29) compared with initiation controls (1/29). Total tumor incidence was lower than expected, most likely because we used a lower concentration of EHEN (170 ppm) in the drinking water than previous studies (500 ppm). A clear concentration-related increase in atypical cell foci (ACF) was observed in initiated animals exposed to unleaded gasoline and TMP (Table 1). ACF, also known as dysplastic foci, are small microscopic cortical tubular lesions each comprising one or several enlarged solid or cystic tubules lined by an irregular multilayered epithelium containing large nuclei and basophilic or clear cytoplasm. These foci, based on their phenotypic enzyme expression and morphologic characteristics that are similar to those of tumor cells, are believed to represent preneoplastic precursors to RCT (45,46).

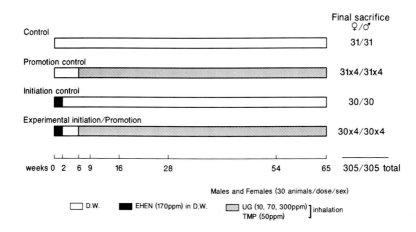

Figure 5. Hydrocarbon promotion study. Experimental design of initiation-promotion study to determine the promoting activity of unleaded gasoline (UG) or 2,2-4-trimethylpentane (TMP) on renal tumorigenesis in male and female rats initiated with ethylhydroxyethylnitrosamine (EHEN).

With this in mind, it was interesting to note that kidneys of female rats in the initiation-promotion groups did not exhibit more microscopic RCT or ACF than did the female initiation controls (Table 2). This study, along with a sequence study to determine the temporal and reversible nature of unleaded gasoline's promotional activity, is discussed in greater detail elsewhere (30).

In summary, unleaded gasoline and TMP demonstrated promotion of EHEN-initiated renal tubule cells to ACF and, less commonly, RCT. It is likely that cell proliferation played a pivotal role in the promotional influence of inhalation exposure to 300 ppm unleaded gasoline and 50 ppm TMP at 48 weeks, since substantial elevations in chronic cell proliferation were observed in male rats exposed to unleaded gasoline and TMP in conditions similar to those of the initiation-promotion study.

Implications for risk assessment

Human beings are widely exposed to chemicals that cause $\alpha_{2u}G$ nephropathy and induce renal tumors in male rats. It is therefore important to assess accurately any risk to human beings exposed to these chemicals. If risk assessment is to be precise enough to allow predictions based on a range of high to low exposures—and in view of what seems to be a species- and gender-specific disease—we must understand the mechanisms involved.

A working hypothesis concerning chemicals that cause $\alpha_{2u}G$ nephropathy and

Table 1. Total Numbers of ACF and RCT in Initiation-Promotion Study of Male Rats Exposed to Unleaded Gasoline (UG), TMP, and EHEN and Sacrificed at 65 Weeks.

Dose (ppm)	N	ACF total number	RCT total number
Control	29	1	0
Promotion control			
10-ppm UG	28	2	0
70-ppm UG	28	3	0
300-ppm UG	30	4	0
50-ppm TMP	30	7	0
Initiation control			
EHEN	29	12	1
Initiation/promotion			
EHEN/10-ppm UG	28	17	0
EHEN/70-ppm UG	27	26	1
EHEN/300-ppm UG	27	54[a]	2
EHEN/50-ppm TMP	29	56[a]	5

[a]Significantly greater compared to initiation control ($P < 0.001$), Newman-Keuls multicomparison test.

Table 2. Total Numbers of ACF and RCT in Initiation-Promotion Study of Female Rats Exposed to Unleaded Gasoline (UG), TMP, and EHEN and Sacrificed at 65 Weeks.

Dose (ppm)	N	ACF total number	RCT total number
Control	28	2	0
Promotion control			
10-ppm UG	29	2	0
70-ppm UG	25	2	0
300-ppm UG	30	1	0
50-ppm TMP	28	1	0
Initiation control			
EHEN	29	18	1
Initiation/promotion			
EHEN/10-ppm UG	29	17	0
EHEN/70-ppm UG	29	17	2
EHEN/300-ppm UG	28	16	2
EHEN/50-ppm TMP	30	17	1

renal cancer states that reversible binding of the chemical to $\alpha_{2u}G$ alters lysosomal catabolism of a poorly digested low-molecular-weight protein to a further reduced state, leading to accumulation of the chemical-$\alpha_{2u}G$ complex in P2 renal epithelial cells, causing lysosomal protein overload and individual cell necrosis. This is followed by cellular regeneration of several portions of the proximal tubule—initially in P2 and P3 segments as long as the rat produces $\alpha_{2u}G$, then progressively including the tubules involved in CPN during aging. Elevated rates of cell proliferation may increase tumor incidence above background rates by increasing the fixation of spontaneously altered DNA into irreversibly initiated cells and by clonally expanding initiated cells in the kidney.

Similar kinds of data are being collected for other chemicals in this group. For example, acute (3-week) exposure of male rats to pentachloroethane and perchloroethylene induces $\alpha_{2u}G$ accumulation, site-specific cytotoxicity, and P2 cell proliferation similar in magnitude to that observed with unleaded gasoline and TMP (11). Cell proliferation data for specific cell types can now be incorporated into the assessment of unleaded gasoline's carcinogenic risk to male rats. For example, such factors as cell proliferation rates averaged over time and the relative numbers of each cell population may be used to determine the relative contribution of proximal tubule cell types (P1, P2, P3) to the pool of proliferating proximal tubule cells during chronic unleaded gasoline exposure. P1, P2, and P3 cells make up about 25, 25, and 50%, respectively, of the proximal tubule cell population. A plot of cell proliferation relative to exposure concentration may be compared to tumor yield at similar exposure concentrations (Fig. 6). The RCT results from the American Petroleum Institute's bioassay on unleaded gasoline may, for example, be compared to cell proliferation results for similar exposure concentrations. The comparison demonstrates strikingly similar curves for proliferation of P2 cells, and to a lesser extent P3 cells, compared to the dose-response curve of RCT yield.

Using preliminary evidence from a quantitative risk-assessment model based on a modification of the Moolgavakar (47) method, proximal tubule cell proliferation data collected for unleaded gasoline were used to model the renal tumor incidence observed in the bioassay (T.B. Starr, personal communication). The weight of evidence from these studies strongly implied that cell proliferation and the associated tumor promotion are the critical links between $\alpha_{2u}G$ nephropathy and renal cancer in male rats.

Risk assessment for human beings is more difficult, expecially in view of the divergent responses of male and female animals to chemical exposure. However, increased human risk is unlikely for several reasons. First, there is no evidence of a human protein that has all the attributes of $\alpha_{2u}G$, including adequate production, binding to the chemical or metabolites, renal filtration, resorption, and lysosomal overload resulting in cytotoxicity. Second, repeated exposure is necessary, since the cytotoxicity is rapidly reversible. In a summary of epidemiologic studies (48), no increased incidence was reported of protein droplet nephropathy or renal cancer from occupational hydrocarbon exposure. It seems, therefore, that chronic hydrocarbon exposure causes cancer in male rats but that unleaded gasoline is not likely to be a carcinogen in human beings.

Acknowledgments

We gratefully acknowledge the technical assistance of Vicki Burnett in the cell proliferation studies. We thank Nancy Youtsey, Don Deyo, and Parker Dodd for their technical assistance in EHEN analysis and Mark Higuchi for operating the inhalation chambers. The generous financial support of the American Petroleum Institute is greatly appreciated.

References

1. National Toxicology Program. Carcinogenesis Studies of 1,4-Dichlorobenzene in F-344/N Rats and B6C3F1 Mice (Gavage Study), NTP Technical Report No. 319. Research Triangle Park: National Toxicology Program, 1987.

Cell Proliferation of Proximal Tubule Segments and Renal Cell Tumors

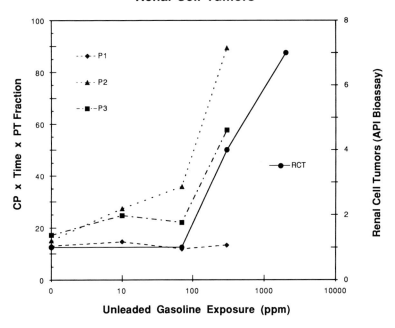

Figure 6. Graph summarizing the dose-response similarity of P2 and P3, but not P1 segment cell replication, observed in male rats during 48 weeks of unleaded gasoline (UG) inhalation exposure, and the number of renal cell tumors (RCT) found in male rats exposed to inhaled UG in a two-year bioassay conducted by the American Petroleum Institute (API). Cell labeling of each segment was averaged over time and multiplied against the estimated ratio of each cell type (P1:P2:P3; 25%:25%:50%) to approximate the total number of replicating cells for each cell type. The chronic bioassay included 60 rats per dose group at 26-month sacrifice time (14).

2. Charbonneau M, Strasser J, Lock EA, Turner MJ, Swenberg JA. 1,4-Dichlorobenzene (1,4-DCB)-induced nephrotoxicity: Similarity with unleaded gasoline (UG)-induced renal effects. In: Bach PA, Lock (eds): Nephrotoxicity: Extrapolation from In Vitro to In Vivo and from Animal to Man. London: Plenum Press, 1989, pp. 557–562.

3. National Toxicology Program. Carcinogenesis Studies of Dimethyl Methylphosphonate in F-344/N Rats and B6C3F1 Mice (Gavage Study), NTP Technical Report No. 323. Research Triangle Park: National Toxicology Program, 1987.

4. National Toxicology Program. Carcinogenesis Studies of Isophorone in F-344/N Rats and B6C3F1 Mice (Gavage Study), NTP Technical Report No. 291. Research Triangle Park: National Toxicology Program, 1987.

5. Strasser JR, Charbonneau M, Borghoff SJ, Turner MJ, Swenberg JA. Renal protein droplet formation in male Fischer 344 rats after isophorone (IPH) treatment. Toxicologist 8:136, 1988.

6. Gaworski CL, MacEwen JD, Vernot EH, Bruner RH, Cowan MJ. Comparison of the subchronic inhalation toxicity of petroleum and oil shale JP-5 jet fuels. In: Mehlman MA (ed): Applied Toxicology of Petroleum Hydrocarbons, vol. 6. Princeton: Princeton Scientific Publishers, 1984, pp. 33–47.

7. Bruner RH. Pathologic findings in laboratory animals exposed to hydrocarbon fuels of military interest. In: Mehlman MA (ed): Renal Effects of Petroleum Hydrocarbons, vol 7. Princeton: Princeton Scientific Publishers, 1984, pp. 133–140.

8. National Toxicology Program. Toxicology and Carcinogenesis Studies of d-Limonene in F-344/N Rats and B6F3F1 Mice (Gavage Study), NTP Technical Report No. 347. Research Triangle Park: National Toxicology Program, 1987.

9. Kanerva RL, Ridder GM, Lefever FR, Alden CL. Comparison of short-term renal effects due to oral administration of decalin or d-limonene in young adult male Fischer-344 rats. Food Chem Toxicol 25:345–353, 1987.

10. National Toxicology Program. Carcinogenesis Bioassay of Pentachloroethane in F-344/N Rats and B6C3F1 Mice (Gavage Study), NTP Technical Report No. 232. Research Triangle Park: National Toxicology Program, 1983.

11. Goldsworthy TL, Lyght O, Burnett VL, Popp JA. Potential role of α_{2u}-globulin, protein droplet accumulation, and cell replication in the renal carcinogenicity of rats exposed to trichloroethylene, perchloroethylene, and pentachloroethane. Toxicol Appl Pharmacol 96:367–379, 1988.

12. National Toxicology Program. Carcinogenesis Bioassay of Tetrachloroethylene (Perchloroethylene) in F-344/N Rats and B6C3F1 Mice (Inhalation Study), NTP Technical Report No. 311. Research Triangle Park: National Toxicology Program, 1986.

13. Halder CA, Warne JM, Hafoum NS. Renal toxicity of gasoline and related petroleum naphthas in male rats. In: Mehlman MA (ed): Renal Effects of Petroleum Hydrocarbons, vol. 7. Princeton: Princeton Scientific Publishers, 1984, pp. 73–88.

14. Kitchen DN. Neoplastic renal effects of unleaded gasoline in Fischer 344 rats. In Mehlman MA (ed): Renal Effects of Petroleum Hydrocarbons, vol 7. Princeton: Princeton Scientific Publishers, 1984, pp. 65–71.

15. Trump BF, Lipsky MM, Jones TW, Heatfield BM, Higginson J, Endicott K, and Hess HB. An evaluation of the significance of experimental hydrocarbon toxicity to man. In Mehlman MA (ed): Renal Effects of Petroleum Hydrocarbons, vol 7. Princeton: Princeton Scientific Publishers, 1984, pp. 272–288.

16. Short BG, Burnett VL, Cox MG, Bus JS, Swenberg JA. Site-specific renal cytotoxicity and cell proliferation in male rats exposed to petroleum hydrocarbons. Lab Invest 57:564-577, 1987.

17. Swenberg JA, Short BG. The influence of cytotoxcity on the induction of tumors. In: Butterworth BE, Slaga T (eds): Nongenotoxic Mechanisms in Carcinogenesis, Banbury Report 25. Cold Spring Harbor, NY: Cold Spring Harbor Laboratory, 1987, pp. 151-164.

18. Argyris TS. Regeneration and the mechanism of epidermal tumor promotion. CRC Crit Rev Toxicol 14:211-258, 1982.

19. Stott WT, Reitz RH, Schumann AM, Watanabe PG. Genetic and nongenetic events in neoplasia. Food Cosmetic Toxicol 19:567–576, 1981.

20. Borghoff SJ, Strasser J, Charbonneau M, Swenberg JA. Analysis of 2,4,4-trimethyl-2-pentanol (TMP-OH) binding to male rat kidney α-globulin and other proteins. Toxicologist 8:135, 1989.

21. Borghoff SJ, Strasser J, Charbonneau M, Swenberg JA. Characteristics of 2,4,4-trimethyl-2-pentanol (TMP-OH) binding to male rat kidney α-globulin and other proteins. Toxicologist 9:79, 1989.

22. Burnett VL, Short BG, Swenberg JA. Localization of α-globulin within protein droplets of male rat kidney: Immunohistochemistry using perfusion-fixed, GMA-embedded tissue sections. J Histochem Cytochem 37:813–818, 1989.

23. Charbonneau M, Lock EA, Strasser J, Cox MG, Turner MJ, Bus JS. 2,2,4-Trimethylpentane-induced nephrotoxicity. I. Metabolic disposition of TMP in male and female Fischer 344 rats. Toxicol Appl Pharmacol 91:171–181, 1987.

24. Charbonneau M, Straser J, Borghoff SJ, Swenberg JA. In vitro hydrolysis of [^{14}C]-α-globulin isolated from male rat kidney. Toxicologist 8:135, 1988.

25. Lock EA, Charbonneau M, Strasser J, Swenberg JA, Bus JS. The reversible binding of a metabolite of 2,2,4-trimethylpentane to a renal protein fraction. Toxicol Appl Pharmacol 91:182–192, 1987.

26. Loury DJ, Smith-Oliver T, Butterworth BE. Assessment of unscheduled DNA synthesis and cell replication in rat kidney cells exposed in vivo or in vitro to unleaded gasoline. Toxicol Appl Pharmacol 75:127–140, 1986.

27. Loury DJ, Goldsworthy TL, Butterworth BE. The value of measuring cell replication as a predictive

index of tissue-specific tumorigenic potential. In: Butterworth BE, Slaga T (eds): Nongenotoxic Mechanisms in Carcinogenesis, Banbury Report 25. Cold Spring Harbor: Cold Spring Harbor Laboratory, 1987, pp. 119–136.

28. Short BG, Burnett VL, Swenberg JA. Histopathology and cell proliferation induced by 2,2,4-trimethylpentane in the male rat kidney. Toxicol Pathol 14:194–203, 1986.

29. Short BG, Burnett VL, Swenberg JA. Elevated proliferation of proximal tubule cells and localization of accumulated α-globulin in F344 rats during chronic exposure to unleaded gasoline or 2,2,4-trimethylpentane. Toxicol Appl Pharmacol 101:414–431, 1989.

30. Short BG, Steinhagen WH, Swenberg JA. Promoting effects of unleaded gasoline and 2,2,4-trimethylpentane on the development of atypical cell foci and renal tubular cell tumors in rats exposed to N-ethyl-N-hydroxyethylnitrosamine. Cancer Res 49:6369–6378, 1989.

31. Swenberg JA, Short BG, Borghoff S, Strasser J, Charbonneau M. The comparative pathobiology of α-globulin nephropathy. Toxicol Appl Pharmacol 97:35–46, 1989.

32. Busey WM, Cockrell BY. Non-neoplastic exposure-related renal lesions in rats following inhalation of unleaded gasoline vapors. In: MA Mehlman (ed): Renal Effects of Petroleum Hydrocarbons, vol 7. Princeton: Princeton Scientific Publishers, 1984, pp. 57–64.

33. Olson MJ, Garg BD, Ramana Murty CV, Roy AK. Accumulation of α-globulin in the renal proximal tubules of male rats exposed to unleaded gasoline. Toxicol Appl Pharmacol 90:43–51, 1987.

34. Olson MJ, Mancini MA, Garg BD, Roy AK. Leupeptin-mediated alteration of renal phagolysosomes: Similarity to hyaline droplet nephropathy of male rats exposed to unleaded gasoline. Toxicol Lett 41:245–254, 1988.

35. Stonnard MD, Phillips PGN, Foster JR, Simpson MG, Lock EA. α-Globulin: Measurements in rat kidney following administration of 2,2,4-trimethylpentane. Toxicol Lett 41:161–168, 1986.

36. Sanders PW, Herrera GA, Galla JH. Human Bence Jones protein toxicity in rat proximal tubule epithelium in vivo. Kidney Int 32:851–861, 1987.

37. Motwani NM, Caron D, Demyan WF, Chatterjee B, Hunter S, Poulik MD, Roy AK. Monoclonal antibodies to α_{2u}-globulin and immunocytofluorometric analysis of α_{2u}-globulin-synthesizing hepatocytes during androgenic induction and aging. J Biol Chem 259:3653–3657, 1984.

38. Berenblum I. The cocarcinogenic action of croton resin. Cancer Res 1:44–48, 1941.

39. Hecker E, Kinz W, Fusenjig NE, Marks F, Thielmann HW (eds): Cocarcinogenesis and Biological Effects of Tumor Promoters, vol. 7, Carcinogenesis—A Comprehensive Survey. New York: Raven Press, 1982, pp. 1–664.

40. Slaga TJ, (ed). Tumor Promotion in Internal Organs, vol. 1, Mechanisms of Tumor Promotion in Internal Organs. Boca Raton: CRC Press, 1983, pp. 1–179.

41. Hiasa Y, Ito N. Experimental induction of renal tumors. CRC Crit Rev Toxicol 17:279–343, 1987.

42. Shirai T, Ohshima M, Maduda A, Tamano S, Ito N. Promotion of 2-(ethylnitrosamino)ethanol-induced renal carcinogenesis in rats by nephrotoxic compounds: Positive response with folic acid, basic lead acetate, and N(3,5-dichlorophenyl)succinimide but not with 2,3-dibromo-1-propanol phosphate. J Natl Cancer Inst 72:477–482, 1984.

43. Conaway CC, Schreiner CA, Cragg ST. Mutagenicity evaluation in petroleum hydrocarbons. In: Mehlman MA (ed): Applied Toxicology of Petroleum Hydrocarbons, vol. 6. Princeton: Princeton Scientific Publishers, 1984, pp. 89–108.

44. Richardson KA, Wilmer JL, Smith-Simpson D, Skopek TR. Assessment of the genotoxic potential of unleaded gasoline and 2,2,4-trimethylpentane in human lymphoblasts in vitro. Toxicol Appl Pharmacol 82:316–322, 1986.

45. Tsuda H, Moore MA, Asamoto M, Satoh K, Tsuchida S, Sato K, Ichihara, A, Ito N. Comparison of the various forms of glutathione S-transferase with glucose-6-phosphate dehydrogenase and γ-glutamyltranspeptidase as markers of preneoplastic and neoplastic lesions in rat kidney induced by N-ethyl-N-hydroxyethylnitrosamine. Jpn J Cancer Res 76:919–929, 1985.

46. Bannasch P. Preneoplastic lesions as end points in carcinogenicity testing. II: Preneoplasia in various non-hepatic tissues. Carcinogenesis 7:849–852, 1986.

47. Moolgavkar SH. Carcinogenesis modeling: From molecular biology to epidemiology. Annu Rev Public Health 7:151–169, 1986.

48. Pitha JV, Hemstreet GP, Asai NR, Petrone RL, Trump BF, Silva FG. Occupational hydrocarbon exposure and renal histopathology. Toxicol Ind Health 3:491–506, 1987.

Chemically Induced Cell Proliferation:
Implications for Risk Assessment, pages 369-388
©1991 Wiley-Liss, Inc.

Evaluation of Cell Proliferation in the Kidneys of Rodents with Bromodeoxyuridine Immunohistochemistry or Tritiated Thymidine Autoradiography after Exposure to Renal Toxins, Tumor Promoters, and Carcinogens

J. M. Ward, C. M. Weghorst, B. A. Diwan, N. Konishi, R. A. Lubet, J. R. Henneman, and D. E. Devor

Carcinogenesis develops in renal and other epithelia through a multistage process (1–5). Whether or not they are involved in genotoxic activities, carcinogens are often organ- and cell-specific toxins that can produce necrotizing and degenerative lesions and death if doses are higher than those that induce tumors (Fig. 1). Tumor promoters are frequently organ-specific toxins (4,6) that also are weak carcinogens for that organ; that is, they cause tumors when administered at relatively high chronic toxic doses and have a long latency period, a process which may be reversible at specific stages (3). Acute effects of genotoxic carcinogens also include DNA damage and repair, adduct formation and clearance, and mutagenesis; cell proliferation also often occurs at higher doses (7,8). In response to these acute effects, tissues regenerate; that is, parenchymal cells or epithelia and such supporting tissues as fibroblasts and blood vessels proliferate at higher than normal levels to repair induced damage especially when it results in cell and tissue loss. Prolonged exposure to the toxin produces chronic changes including various types of cell degeneration, fibrosis, hyperplasia, and cell death, i.e., focal, or individual, cell death. Such a sequence has been described for rat kidney tubular damage caused by toxins (9). Hyperplasia connotes increased "growth" and cell proliferation that is reversible; it may also mean increased numbers of cells per unit area of tissue or regeneration of tissue in an area where cell loss has occurred. Hyperplasia originally was a term used in pathology to indicate microscopic evidence of increased cell proliferation, i.e., increased cellular basophilia, mitotic figures, and numbers of cell layers in a specific anatomical tissue structure.

Chronic tissue damage in rodents and humans usually is associated with hyperplasia and increased levels of cell replication (9,10). In humans, hyperplasia has been inadequately recognized and incompletely documented. Although chronic toxicity is sometimes associated with carcinogenesis (11–20), it does not necessarily lead to tumor formation (21–24). Cumulative toxicity that is usually dose- and time-related can also lead to more acute effects such as focal or diffuse necrosis and death. For carcinogens, early focal putative preneoplastic lesions appear later and can progress into benign tumors, which can become malignant and possibly metastatic (Fig. 1). However, in some systems, including urinary bladder and colon, focal preneoplastic lesions progress directly into malignant lesions (4).

Cells proliferate at a specific rate characteristic for each cell and tissue. When abnormal events such as infections, toxicity, and irradiation interfere with the normal

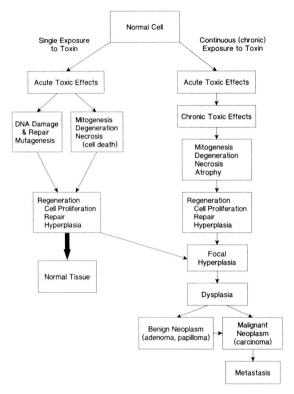

Figure 1. Sequence of events in biological responses to toxins including carcinogens and tumor promoters.

cell cycle, increased rates of cell proliferation may occur to repair tissue damage or as a mitogenic effect of the stimulus. Specific parameters used to determine levels of cell proliferation include the nuclear labeling index (LI), length of the cell cycle, and presence of mitotic figures. The increases or decreases in normal rates of cell replication may affect different stages of the cell cycle (Fig. 2). These stages vary according to sensitivity to carcinogens and toxins (25). For example, S phase is extremely sensitive to carcinogen damage and ultimate carcinogenesis (26). Chemicals which induce hyperplasia by direct effects (mitogenesis) or secondary effects (tissue damage and repair) may also target cells involved in the carcinogenic process including initiated cells (not visible histologically), or cells within focal putative preneoplastic lesions, adenomas, and carcinomas. We have provided evidence that some tumor promoters can target initiated cells or focus cells (27–30). In mouse liver, phenobarbital (PB) appears to target initiated cells since its major promoting effect is to induce many more eosinophilic foci than are found spontaneously or as a result of known initiation (27). Di(2-ethyl-hexyl)phthalate (DEHP), a peroxisomal proliferator, seems to target focus cells because of the increased size of foci found (27). More recently, others have provided similar evidence for PB and another peroxisomal proliferator, WY-14,643, in rats (31).

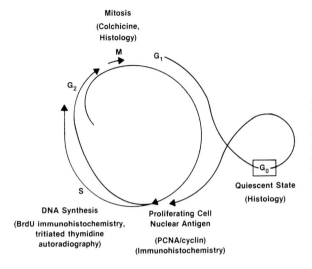

Figure 2. Evaluation of phases of the cell cycle by pathology techniques. Proliferating cell nuclear antigen (PCNA) is detected in G_1 and S phases and DNA synthesis only during S phase. Simplified from Pardee (25).

An increase in normal levels of cell proliferation has implications for carcinogenesis. Mutagenic events may occur more commonly and other damaging activities may be hastened (32). Many naturally occurring human and induced animal tumors are associated with chronic tissue damage (11–13), although information on levels of cell proliferation is limited. Many other chronic processes induced by toxins (21–23) or occurring naturally are not associated with tumor development.

It is the purpose of this chapter to review our work and those of others on rodent renal toxins, carcinogens, and tumor promoters. Methods for evaluating levels of cell proliferation will be reviewed first. We will present information on the renal toxicity, tumor promoting activity, and carcinogenesis of DEHP, and sodium barbital and its metabolites.

Methods for detecting levels of cell proliferation

Determining levels of cell replication in a tissue can be a complex process. Measuring cells in S phase by tritiated thymidine ($[^3H]Tdr$) autoradiography, determining radiolabeled DNA, or using bromodeoxyuridine (BrdU) immunohistochemistry or thymidine kinase biochemistry, has been described (22). Most of these measure the proportion of cells in S phase in a defined time period but do not take into account such important considerations as length of the cell cycle, fraction of cells in G_0 (quiescent state), possible proliferation units, and undifferentiated (stem cells) or differentiated cell types involved. Recently, the monoclonal antibody and immunohistochemical staining techniques for the thymidine analog BrdU have been developed (33–35). A few investigators (22,35) have initially utilized the BrdU nuclear labeling technique to study the role of cellular proliferation in toxicology and carcinogenesis. Several advantages are apparent when using the techniques of BrdU immunohistochemistry compared to those involved in $[^3H]Tdr$ autoradiography. One such advantage is the decreased time needed to recognize S phase–labeled cells. While the time involved in immunostaining BrdU tissue sections can be measured in hours, the exposure time needed for [³H]Tdr auto-radiography can be measured from 1–7 weeks. Secondly, since BrdU is not radioactive, the problems associated with radioactive contamination, waste, and personnel safety are avoided.

The use of BrdU to detect DNA synthesizing cells is not without its negative points. High doses of BrdU have been shown to be mutagenic (36,37) and carcinogenic (38). BrdU also appears to inhibit DNA synthesis, cellular replication (39), differentiation and thymidine uptake in vitro (40). Whether these negative aspects of BrdU exposure are affecting the results generated in recent cell proliferation experiments remains to be addressed. We are currently evaluating the BrdU labeling technique by examining various parameters, including 1) method of administration, 2) route, 3) concentration, and 4) duration of BrdU exposure, and the effect of different fixatives on immunohistochemical staining of BrdU. Steps are also being taken to determine the most accurate methods of quantifying the BrdU–labeled cells, including the number of labeled cells per unit area or per 1000 cells.

Currently, two major methods of BrdU administration are being utilized in this laboratory to evaluate cellular proliferation:

1) Single BrdU injection (pulse dosing): Animals receive a single intraperitoneal injection of BrdU (100 mg/kg, rats; 100 or 200 mg/kg, mice) 1 hr prior to sacrifice. This pulse dose allows us to detect the number of cells synthesizing DNA during a 1-hr window.

2) Continuous dosing with slow-releasing BrdU pellets (Innovative Research of America, Inc., Toledo, OH) or osmotic minipumps (Alza Corp., Palo Alto, CA). A pellet (2.5, 5, 10, 25, or 50 mg) and its pump equivalent implanted sub-cutaneously on the back of each animal releases BrdU over a period of up to 21 days. We therefore can theoretically detect the number of cells that have passed through the S phase until the 21-day exposure period ends. We arbitrarily have designated end points of 4 and 7 days for BrdU continuous exposure. The continuous exposure method was utilized because others (31,41) have shown that, at least with [³H]Tdr autoradiography, it may be nontoxic and more sensitive for detecting chronic low-level increases in levels of DNA synthesis in hepatocytes.

At necropsy, tissues are fixed in either 70% ethanol, Bouins, zinc formalin, or 10% buffered formalin and embedded in paraffin. Sections are hydrolyzed with 4 N HCl for 20 min, rinsed with boric acid-borate buffer (pH 7.6), and digested with 0.01% trypsin (porcine pancreas type II crude, Sigma Chemical Co., St. Louis, MO) for 3 min. These sections are incubated in a 1:200 dilution of a mouse monoclonal antibody to BrdU (Becton Dickinson, Mountain View, CA or Dako Corp., Santa Barbara, CA) and stained with the avidin biotin peroxidase complex (ABC) method using a mouse Vectastain ABC Elite kit (Vector Laboratories, Burlingame, CA) (22,42). Sections are then counterstained with hematoxylin for 2 min. Quantitation of the BrdU-labeled nuclei is performed under light microscopy and expressed as the number of labeled cells per 1000 cells or per mm² of tissue section. It is important to identify the specific cell type studied and not count all other labeled cells in tissues such as fibroblasts, inflammatory cells, and endothelia.

Figure 3 demonstrates the levels of nuclear labeling in the kidneys of rats exposed

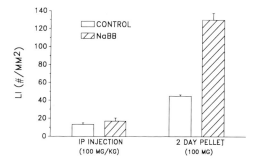

Figure 3. BrdU LI (#/mm^2 of tissue section) of renal cortical tubules comparing a single pulse intraperitoneal injection (200 mg/kg) of BrdU 1 hr prior to sacrifice with a 2-day (48 hr) 100 mg BrdU pellet exposure. Eight-week-old F344/NCr rats sacrificed after 14 days of exposure to sodium barbital (BBNa), 500 ppm in the diet. ABC immunohistochemistry with mouse monoclonal antibodies to BrdU.

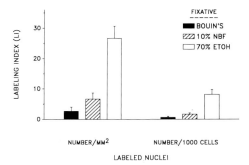

Figure 4. BrdU LI in cortical renal tubules of 6-week-old male B6C3F1 mice receiving a single intraperitoneal injection (200 mg/kg) of BrdU 1 hr prior to sacrifice. Seventy percent ethanol preserves the highest level of BrdU immunoreactivity.

to BrdU by either a single pulse injection or a slow-release pellet. As expected, the levels of labeling are greater in the animals that received the BrdU pellet than in those rats that received a single pulse injection. With either the single pulse dose or continuous exposure techniques, we found that the methods of expressing the number of labeled nuclei as either the number/mm^2 of tissue section or number/1000 cells is not so critical in untreated animals (Fig. 4). The labeling trends remain relatively equal.

Figure 4 shows the effect of different fixatives on the ability to identify BrdU-laden cells. Of the fixatives we evaluated, 70% ethanol with trypsin digestion has proved to be the most advantageous (Fig. 5). Zinc-formalin fixation requires no digestion (data not shown).

We have found potential problems with the use of chronic exposure to BrdU pellets or minipumps (43): The adverse effects of BrdU are dose- and time-related. BrdU appears to be toxic, causing body weight depression with 50 mg pellets in 6-week-old male B6C3F1 mice; high concentrations also inhibit normal rates or changes the pattern of cell replication in small intestine (Fig. 6), liver or kidney (Figs. 7,8); it also may inhibit induced cell proliferation (Fig. 9) and may be mitogenic to some tissues. We are in the process of quantitating these effects. Thus, caution should be used when

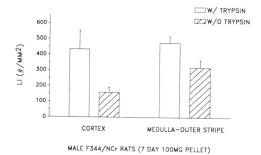

MALE F344/NCr RATS (7 DAY 100MG PELLET)

Figure 5. Trypsinization of tissues increases immunoreactivity of BrdU. Male F344/NCr rats, 6-weeks-old, received a 100 mg BrdU pellet for 7 days.

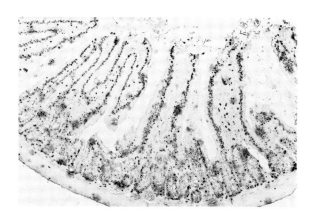

Figure 6. F344 rat small intestine showing abnormal immunolabeling of epithelial nuclei in villi and crypts. Note high LI of villus cell nuclei and relatively low LI of crypt cell nuclei. ABC immunohistochemistry for BrdU, 50 mg pellet BrdU for 4 days, hematoxylin, zinc formalin fixation, ×100.

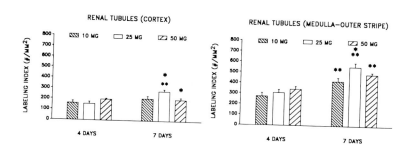

Figure 7. BrdU LI in kidney of 6- to 7-week-old male F344/NCr rat using BrdU pellets of various doses. Note no dose effects at each time period. LI ± SEM. *$P < .05$ vs. Day 4; **$P < .05$ vs. other groups on same day.

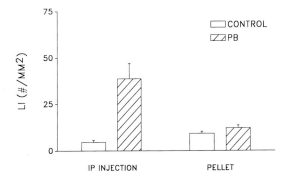

Figure 8. Rat kidney showing high BrdU LI in P3 segment of the proximal tubule (outer stripe of the outer zone of the medulla) (M) and a relatively low LI in cortex (C). ABC immunohistochemistry; 7-day 50 mg BrdU pellet; hematoxylin, zinc formalin fixation; ×100.

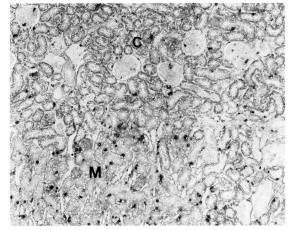

Figure 9. BrdU inhibition of induced hepatocyte proliferation. Six-week-old male F344/NCr rats received dietary phenobarbital (PB) (500 ppm) for 48 hr and during the same time received a 100 mg BrdU pellet. Hepatocyte LI ± SEM.

continuous exposure to BrdU is the basis for determining levels of cell proliferation in any tissue. The chronic exposure to BrdU and/or the ability of the pellets to uniformly release BrdU may be major problems (43). Two- or three-day minipumps may be preferred.

For preliminary studies of rates of cell proliferation in renal tubules, however, we suggest a 4-day exposure to a 10-mg pellet for mature mice and a 50 mg pellet for mature rats. In rats, this dose can provide a nice differentiating effect of a high normal LI in the P3 segment of the proximal tubule (outer stripe of the medulla) versus a lower LI in the cortex (Figs. 7,9).

Renal carcinogens and tumor promoters

Chemicals of diverse classes are renal carcinogens (1). Many have shown genotoxic activity, and the majority are known nephrotoxins. Renal tumor promoters comprise a much shorter list (Table 1) (44–60) and were reviewed by Hiasa and Ito (1). Tumor-promoting activity is usually shown by the ability to amplify or enhance the carcinogenic process. For renal promoters, this activity has usually been demonstrated

Table 1. Examples of Renal Tumor Promoters in Rat Kidney.

Tumor promoter	Reference
p-Aminophenol	44
Acetaminophen	44
β-Cyclodextrin	45
Citrinin	46
Di(2-ethylhexyl)phthalate	47
Diethylacetylurea	48
DL-serine	49
Folic acid	50
Lead acetate	50–52
N-(3,5-dichlorophenyl)succinimide	50,53
Nickel chloride	54
Nicotinamide	55
Nitrilotriacetic acid	56,57
Potassium bromate	58
Sodium barbital	42,59,60
2,2,4-Trimethylpentane	16
Unleaded gasoline	16

by an increase in tumor incidence and not an increase in the numbers or sizes of putative preneoplastic renal tubular cell foci (16,47). The renal carcinogenic process has not been defined as clearly as in the rodent liver (12,61,62); it may therefore be difficult to detect definitive putative preneoplastic tubular lesions, especially in the presence of nephrotoxic lesions and tubular hyperplasia. As noted previously, tumor promoters are commonly weak carcinogens, inducing renal tubular tumors in low incidence after a long latent period, usually more than one year (42). In addition, they are often renal toxins. Tumors induced by nongenotoxic carcinogens are usually of renal tubular origin, while those induced by genotoxic carcinogens are of renal tubular origin or interstitial origin, such as mesenchymal tumors. Sodium barbital (BBNa), a nongenotoxic renal carcinogen, is one exception; it also induces renal pelvic tumors (59,63). Genotoxic carcinogens given chronically may, like nongenotoxic carcinogens, accelerate the carcinogenic process but by other mechanisms. Often, the nongenotoxic tumor promoters are given to rodents at mildly or moderately toxic doses to induce degenerative changes and renal tubular lesions. This toxic effect, caused by the administered chemical or its metabolites, induces tubules and interstitial tissues to regenerate, so they have higher rates of DNA synthesis than do normal tubules. A recently well-documented example of this phenomenon concerns unleaded gasoline (14–16,20). Short et al. (14) proposed that unleaded gasoline produces tumors that arise within the areas of the damaged nephron, such as the P2 segment of the proximal tubule. A similar pathogenesis may be hypothesized for tumor promotion by these nongenotoxic chemicals (16).

Renal tumor-initiating agents

Tumor-initiating agents are potent genotoxic carcinogens used in two-stage carcinogenesis experiments in rats and include N-ethyl-N-hydroxyethylnitrosamine (EHEN) (45,49,51,56,57,61), N-bis(2-hydroxypropyl)nitrosamine (DHPN) (62, Ward and Diwan, unpublished), N-nitrosodiethylamine (DEN) (48,60), streptozotocin (STZ) (53,63), methyl(acetoxymethyl)nitrosamine (59), N-nitroso-dimethylamine (DMN) (46), and N-(4'-fluoro-4-biphenyl)acetamide (52). In mice, we have also used N-nitroso-ethylurea (NEU) transplacentally (23,64). These compounds have been given as single injections or short-term dietary exposures (1–4 weeks) at doses that alone produce low incidences of renal tumors. EHEN appears to be the quickest renal tumor initiator and is used in experiments for 30–52 weeks, but it also causes liver and other tumors (61). DHPN induces renal tubular and mesenchymal tumors from 24–52 weeks and tumors in thyroid, nasal cavity, lung, urinary bladder, and other tissues (62). STZ (50 mg/kg) induces only renal tubular tumors, but also causes diabetes and some deaths from the latter (63). At doses at which these chemicals are used as initiators, renal toxicity is usually not evident. With STZ in rats we found no increase in LI in renal tubules of the rat's outer renal cortex (Fig. 10). Some of the nitrosamines, when given at optimum carcinogenic doses, appear to cause a multifocal tubular hyperplasia that is probably associated with a high LI and preneoplastic lesions.

Sodium barbital (BBNa)

Sodium barbital is a long-acting human sedative hypnotic. It was originally reported to promote intestinal tumors in rats after 1,2-dimethylhydrazine initiation (65), but this has not been confirmed by other investigators (59). Recently, we showed that BBNa was a nephrotoxin as well as a tumor promoter and somewhat weak carcinogen for the rat kidney (42,48,59,60). In mice, BBNa was a renal tumor promoter and liver carcinogen (66), but toxicity data were limited (64). Hydrolysis products of BBNa include diethylacetylurea (DEAU) and 2-ethylbutanoic acid amide (Fig. 11) (48). We studied the nephrotoxic and tumor-promoting activities of BBNa and DEAU (48) using histopathological and BrdU immunohistochemical evaluations. Degenerative renal tubular lesions including vacuolization were seen in the outer cortex after 2 weeks of exposure to BBNa at 500–4000 ppm (Fig. 12). DEAU had similar effects at 500 ppm, the only dose studied. Increased levels of DNA synthesis were seen in areas of degeneration with both compounds (Fig. 13) at this time point and persisted for long periods (Fig. 14–16). At 48 hr after initial dietary exposure, BBNa produced no increase

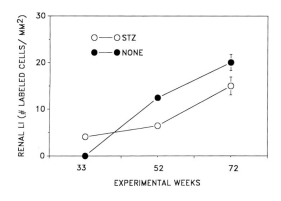

Figure 10. BrdU LI in rat renal cortex after a single intraperitoneal injection (50 mg/kg) of streptozotocin.

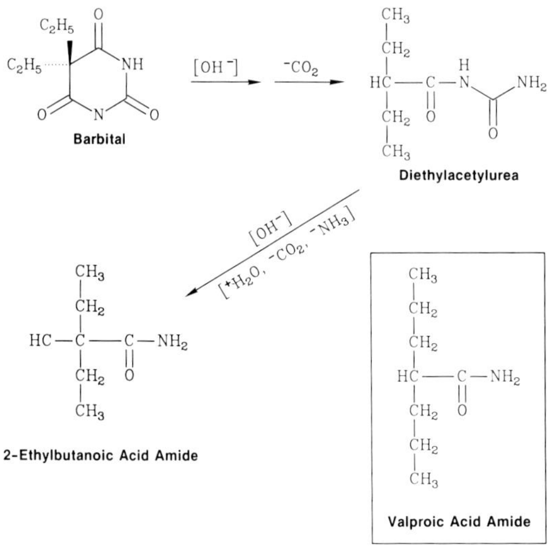

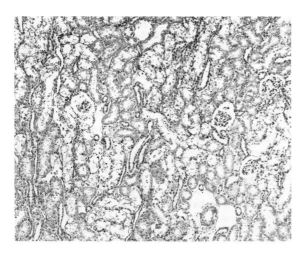

Figure 11. Hydrolysis of 5,5-diethylbarbituric acid (barbital) to DEAU and its further hydrolysis product, 2-ethylbutanoic acid amide (2-EBAA). Note structural similarity with valproic acid amide (VAA).

Figure 12. Rat renal cortex showing pale vacuolated tubules after 14-day exposure to BBNa at 500 ppm. Hematoxylin-eosin staining, ×100.

in LI (Ward JM, unpublished). At 500 ppm and at 14 days, no increase in renal cortical LI was seen using single pulse BrdU, but LI increases were seen with the BrdU pellet (Fig. 3); pulse doses of BrdU or [^{3}H]Tdr in rats receiving 1000 or 4000 ppm did show increases in LI (Fig. 15,16). After 26 weeks, renal toxicity was severe and the entire cortex was involved (Fig. 17). Focal areas of regenerating tubules were associated with both diffuse and focal increases in the LI (Fig. 18). The renal tumors that appeared in

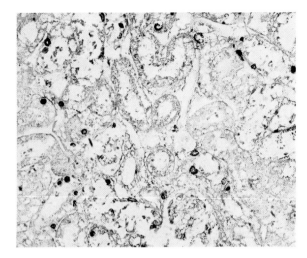

Figure 13. Rat renal cortex with nuclear BrdU labeling (pulse dose) in areas of degenerative lesions after 14 days of BBNa (500 ppm) exposure. ABC immunohistochemistry for BrdU, hematoxylin staining, ×250.

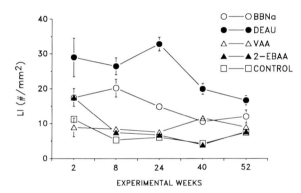

Figure 14. Pulse dosing BrdU renal cortical tubule LI in F344/NCr rats receiving BBNa, its metabolites, DEAU or 2-EBAA or structural analog VAA at 500 ppm in the diet.

rats receiving BBNa were usually small and appeared to arise in periglomerular tubules (63), the sites of BBNa nephrotoxicity (Fig. 19). In a chronic toxicity study of BBNa, after a single-pulse dose of [^{3}H]Tdr, we found that only renal cortical tubules had significantly elevated LI for the entire experimental period while the urinary bladder and liver, also sites susceptible to tumor promotion, did not (Fig. 15). A single-pulse BrdU dose may not be sufficient to detect smaller increases in these latter organs or there may be no increases in LI (67).

DEHP: A special case?

DEHP is an important plasticizer. It is a relatively nontoxic compound with an LD$_{50}$ of 50 mg/kg by gavage in mice (29). In the mouse and rat liver, it is a peroxisomal proliferator and mitogen, and a hepatocarcinogen as demonstrated in 2-year carcinogen

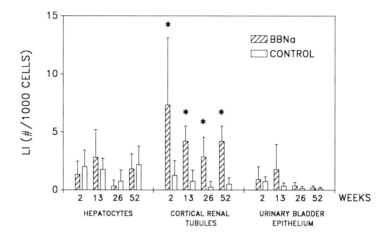

Figure 15. Single-pulse dose [³H]Tdr autoradiography of F344/NCr rat renal cortex, liver and bladder in rats receiving dietary BBNa at 1000 ppm. Adapted from Hagiwara et al. (42).

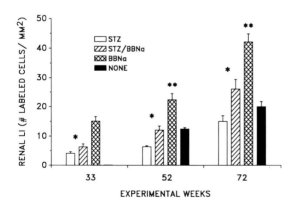

Figure 16. BrdU LI in renal cortex of male F344/NCr rats receiving STZ (50 mg/kg at 6 weeks old), and/or BBNa (4000 ppm in diet) continuously from 8 weeks old. Experimental weeks = weeks after STZ injection. Note: STZ inhibits cell proliferation in rats also exposed to BBNa.

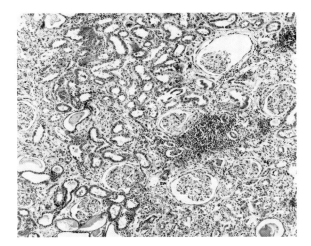

Figure 17. Marked nephrotoxic lesions in male F344/NCr rat after receiving BBNa (4000 ppm) for 72 weeks. Note tubular atrophy and hyperplasia, interstitial fibrosis, and inflammation.

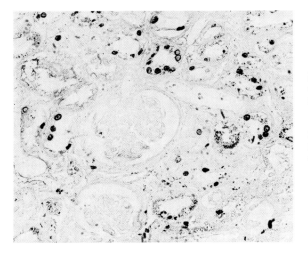

Figure 18. BrdU LI in periglomerular renal cortical tubules of rat after exposure to dietary BBNa (4000 ppm) for 72 weeks. Note granules in tubules and interstitial fibrosis. ABC immunohistochemistry for BrdU; hematoxylin staining ×250.

bioassays (29,68) (Table 2), similar to other peroxisomal proliferators (18,69). In the bioassays, DEHP caused only moderate increases in hepatocellular adenomas and carcinoma incidences, in rats or mice, with few pulmonary metastases or effects on survival. In short-term assays, DEHP has been shown to be a liver tumor promoter in mice but not in rats (29) and a second-stage skin tumor promoter in mice (29,70,71). In the mouse liver, DEHP caused increased rates of expansion of initiated or focus cell clones accompanied by altered morphology (29). DEHP is a renal toxin in mice but is not carcinogenic or tumor-promoting for the mouse kidney (23,68). Several reports, including ours, note that no renal toxicity was seen in rats at 12,000 ppm (29) but a few others report renal lesions that resemble those of aging nephropathy (72). DEHP has been shown to produce in the mouse liver and kidney increased levels of DNA synthesis

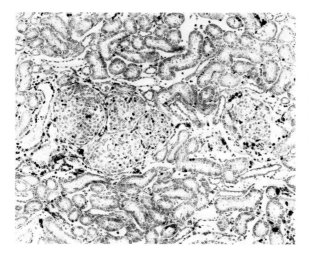

Figure 19. BrdU immunohisto-chemistry showing cell prolif-eration in early tubular adenoma in nephron of rat that received DHPN. Note adjacent regen-erative tubular areas have high LI. Rat received 50 mg BrdU pellet for 4 days prior to sacrifice.

Table 2. Comparison of the Bioeffects of DEHP in Rats and Mice.

Activity	Liver		Kidney	
	Rats	Mice	Rats	Mice
Carcinogen	+ (68)[a]	+ (68)	- (68)	- (68)
Toxin	+ (29,31)	+ (29)	- (29,72)[b]	+ (29)
> Cell proliferation	+ (31)	+ (29)	- [c]	+ (22,23,29)
Tumor promoter	- (29,69)	+ (27–30)	+ (47)	- (23)

[a] Reference number.
[b] Conflicting findings in the literature or definitive data not available.
[c] Ward et al., this review.

which are dose- and time-related (Fig. 20) (22,23,29). DEHP also induces hepatic metallothionein in mice (73). DEHP was demonstrated to be a tumor-promoter for the rat kidney (47) but we could not show elevated levels of renal tubular DNA synthesis in the rat renal cortex after up to 46 weeks of exposure (Fig. 21) using 50 mg BrdU pellets. With frozen sections of kidney, we did not find an increase in renal tubular peroxisomal proliferation (Ward JM, unpublished). It is possible that chronic exposure to the BrdU pellets inhibited DEHP-induced cell proliferation. Peroxisomal prolifera-tion could be readily shown in the livers of the same rats; liver hyperplasia with increased hepatocyte LI was not found (Ward JM, unpublished). Also, adverse histological lesions were not seen in the kidneys of rats given DEHP. We recently found, however, increased tubular pigmentation in these rats. A summary of the contradictory findings are presented in Table 2.

It is interesting to speculate on the contrasting findings regarding DEHP in rats and mice. The pathologic effects of DEHP in livers of both rats and mice are almost identical. Although hepato-carcinogenic activities of DEHP were similar in both species and may be classified as "moderate," most tumors were only found toward the end of

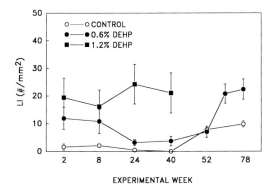

Figure 20. Renal LI in B6C3F1 mice receiving DEHP for periods of up to 78 weeks. Data up to 40 weeks is adopted from Ward et al. (1988) based on pulse dosing of [³H]Tdr and autoradiography. Data from 52–78 weeks is adapted from Konishi et al. (63) and based on pulse dosing of BrdU and immunohistochemistry.

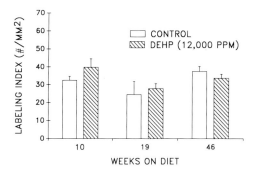

Figure 21. BrdU LI of rat renal cortex after dietary exposure (12,000 ppm) to DEHP for up to 46 weeks. Rats received BrdU 50 mg pellets for 7 days.

the 2-year carcinogenesis bioassay, and tumor-promoting activity was only found in the mouse liver (29,69). DEHP causes peroxisomal proliferation, transient and persistent increases in cell proliferation, lipid peroxidation, and accumulation of lipofuscin in the livers of rats and mice, toxic effects that may be unrelated to those responsible for tumor promotion. We suggest that DEHP targets putative preneoplastic foci of mice for its apparent mitogenic effects and that this is the mechanism of tumor promotion in mouse liver (28). It may be that DEHP acts differently in rats, although another peroxisomal proliferator, WY-14,643, was recently also suggested to target preneoplastic liver foci (67). In the mouse kidney, levels of DNA synthesis are elevated twofold in a dose- and time-related fashion (Fig. 20); nevertheless, renal carcinogenesis or tumor promotion is not evident there (23). At 12,000 ppm of DEHP, renal toxicity is early and severe and a major cause of death in these mice prior to 52 weeks. Mice fed 6000 ppm develop only mild focal renal tubular lesions after several months; these become evident with significant increases in the LI only after 52 weeks. Thus, lack of carcinogenic or tumor-promoting activity may be due to a limited time of enhanced cell replication, i.e., 52 weeks exposure time and 104 weeks, respectively. With continuous exposure to BrdU or [³H]Tdr for 4–7 days, we may be able to detect elevated LI prior to 52 weeks (study in progress).

Aging nephropathy in rats is associated with increased cell replication

We and others have shown that the LI of renal tubules and interstitial components is elevated in rats with naturally occurring aging nephropathy (16,74). Aging nephropathy is a diet-, gender-, and strain-related disease. Degenerative changes in tubules, thickening of tubular basement membranes, and interstitial fibrosis are associated with increased levels of DNA synthesis in tubules and interstitium of cortex and medulla (Fig. 22). These hyperplastic tubules may provide a promoting or copromoting stimulus for nongenotoxic carcinogens. Alternatively, this process may contribute to the low incidence of naturally occurring renal tumors in most strains of rats. A few reports note increased sensitivity of aging rats to renal carcinogens (75), possibly due to the increased levels of DNA synthesis in target cells.

Acknowledgments

Research was funded in part with Federal funds from the Department of Health and Human Services under contract number NO1-CO-74102 with Program Resources, Inc./DynCorp. The content of this publication does not necessarily reflect the views or policies of the Department of Health and Human Services, nor does mention of trade names, commercial products, or organizations imply endorsement by the U.S. Government.

The excellent assistance of Cindy Harris, Kay Scheckles, Shirley Hale, Kathy Breeze, Jennifer Klabansky, Debbie Shores, Debbie Brandenburg, Areitha Smith, Mark Shrader, and Dan Logsdon is gratefully acknowledged.

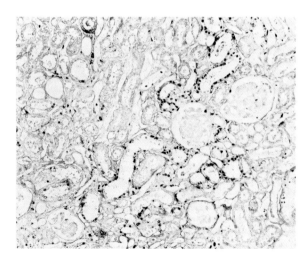

Figure 22. A 52-week-old male F344 rat with early stages of aging nephropathy. Focal high LI is noted. ABC immunohistochemistry; 50 mg BrdU pellet for 4 days, hematoxylin staining, ×100.

References

1. Hiasa Y, Ito N. Experimental induction of renal tumors. Crit Rev Toxicol 17:279–343, 1987.
2. Tsuda H, Hacker HJ, Katayama H, Masui T, Ito N, Bannasch P. Correlative histochemical studies on preneoplastic and neoplastic lesions in the kidney of rats treated with nitrosamines. Virchows Arch[B] 51:385–404, 1986.
3. Pitot HC. Progression: The terminal stage in carcinogenesis. Jpn J Cancer Res 80:599–607, 1989.
4. Ward JM. Pathology of toxic, preneoplastic, and neoplastic lesions. In: Douglas JF (ed): Carcinogenesis and Mutagenesis Testing. Clifton, NJ: Humana Press, 1984, pp 97–130.
5. Ward JM, Reznik G. Refinements of rodent pathology and the pathologist's contribution to evaluation of carcinogenesis bioassays. Prog Exp Tumor Res 26:266–291, 1983.
6. Ward JM, Tsuda H, Tatematsu M, Hagiwara A, Ito N. Hepatotoxicity of agents that enhance formation of focal hepatocellular proliferative lesions (putative preneoplastic foci) in a rapid rat liver bioassay. Fundam Appl Toxicol 12:163–171, 1989.
7. Deal FH, Richardson FC, Swenberg JA. Dose response of hepatocyte replication in rats following continuous exposure to diethylnitrosamine. Cancer Res 49:6985–6988, 1989.
8. Williams GM, Weisburger JH. Chemical carcinogens. In: Klaassen CD, Amdur MO, Doull J (eds): Casarett and Doull's Toxicology, Third edition. New York: MacMillan Co., 1986, pp 99–173.
9. Laurent G, Toubeau G, Heuson-Stiennon JA, Tulkens P, Maldague P. Kidney tissue repair after nephrotoxic injury: Biochemical and morphological characterization. Crit Rev Toxicol 19:147–183, 1988.
10. Lock EA. Studies on the mechanism of nephrotoxicity and nephrocarcinogenicity of halogenated alkenes. Crit Rev Toxicol 19:23–42, 1988.
11. Grasso P. Persistent organ damage and cancer production in rats and mice. Arch Toxicol Suppl 11:75–83, 1987.
12. Clayson DB. Can a mechanistic rationale be provided for non-genotoxic carcinogens identified in rodent bioassays? Mutat Res 221:53–67, 1989.
13. Clayson DB, Nera EA, Lok E. The potential for the use of cell proliferation studies in carcinogen risk assessment. Regul Toxicol Pharmacol 9:284–295, 1989.
14. Short BG, Burnett VL, Cox MG, Bus JS, Swenberg JA. Site-specific renal cytotoxicity and cell proliferation in male rats exposed to petroleum hydrocarbons. Lab Invest 57:564–577, 1987.
15. Short BG, Burnett VL, Swenberg JA. Elevated proliferation of proximal tubule cells and localization of accumulated $\alpha_{2\mu}$-globulin in F344 rats during chronic exposure to unleaded gasoline or 2,2,4-trimethylpentane. Toxicol Appl Pharmacol 101:414–431, 1989.
16. Short BG, Steinhagen WH, Swenberg JA. Promoting effects of unleaded gasoline and 2,2,4-trimethylpentane on the development of atypical cell foci and renal tubular cell tumors in rats exposed to N-ethyl-N-hydroxyethylnitrosamine. Cancer Res 49:6369–6378, 1989.
17. Goldsworthy TL, Lyght O, Burnett VL, Popp JA. Potential role of alpha-$_{2\mu}$-globulin, protein droplet accumulation, and cell replication in the renal carcinogenicity of rats exposed to trichloroethylene, perchloroethylene, and pentachloroethane. Toxicol Appl Pharmacol 96:367–379, 1988.
18. Butterworth BE, Loury DJ, Smith-Oliver T, Cattley RC. The potential role of chemically induced hyperplasia in the carcinogenic activity of the hypolipidemic carcinogens. Toxicol Ind Health 3:129–148, 1987.
19. Butterworth BE, Slaga TJ (eds): Nongenotoxic mechanisms in carcinogenesis. In: Banbury Reports, vol. 25. Cold Spring Harbor, NY: Cold Spring Harbor Laboratory, 1987, pp 397.
20. Swenberg JA, Short B, Borghoff S, Strasser J, Charbonneau M. The comparative pathobiology of $\alpha_{2\mu}$-globulin nephropathy. Toxicol Appl Pharmacol 97:35–46, 1989.
21. Hoel DG, Haseman JK, Hogan MD, Huff J, McConnell EE. The impact of toxicity on carcinogenicity studies: implications for risk assessment. Carcinogenesis 9:2045–2052, 1988.
22. Ward JM, Hagiwara A, Anderson LM, Lindsey K, Diwan BA. The chronic hepatic or renal toxicity of di(2-ethylhexyl)phthalate, acetaminophen, sodium barbital, and phenobarbital in male B6C3F1 mice: Autoradiographic, immunohistochemical, and biochemical evidence for levels of DNA synthesis not associated with carcinogenesis or tumor promotion. Toxicol Appl Pharmacol 96:494–506, 1988.
23. Ward JM, Konishi N, Diwan BA. Renal tubular cell or hepatocyte hyperplasia is not associated with tumor promotion by di(2-ethylhexyl)phthalate in B6C3F1 mice after transplacental initiation with N-nitrosoethylurea. Exp Pathol, in press.

24. Hagiwara A, Ward JM. The chronic hepatotoxic, tumor-promoting, and carcinogenic effects of acetaminophen in male B6C3F1 mice. Fundam Appl Toxicol 7:376–386, 1986.
25. Pardee AB. G₁ events and regulation of cell proliferation. Science 246:603–608, 1989.
26. Kaufmann WK, Rice JM, Wenk ML, Devor D, Kaufman DG. Cell cycle-dependent initiation of hepatocarcinogenesis in rats by methyl(acetoxymethyl)nitrosamine. Cancer Res 47:1263–1266, 1987.
27. Ward JM, Rice JM, Creasia D, Lynch P, Riggs C. Dissimilar patterns of promotion by di(2-ethylhexyl)phthalate and phenobarbital of hepatocellular neoplasia initiated by diethylnitrosamine in B6C3F1 mice. Carcinogenesis 4:1021–1029, 1983.
28. Ward JM, Diwan BA, Lubet RA, Henneman JR, Devor DE. Liver tumor promoters and other mouse liver carcinogens. In Stevenson D, McClain RM, Popp JA, Slaga TJ, Ward JM, Pitot HC (eds): Mouse Liver Carcinogenesis: Mechanisms and Species Comparisons. New York: Wiley-Liss, pp 85–108, 1989.
29. Ward JM, Diwan BA, Ohshima M, Hu H, Schuller HM, Rice JM. Tumor-initiating and promoting activities of di(2-ethylhexyl)-phthalate in vivo and in vitro. Environ Health Perspect 65:279–291, 1986.
30. Ward JM, Ohshima M, Lynch P, Riggs C. Di(2-ethylhexyl)-phthalate but not phenobarbital promotes N-nitrosodiethylamine-initiated hepatocellular proliferative lesions after short-term exposure in male B6C3F1 mice. Cancer Lett 24:49–55, 1984.
31. Marsman DS, Cattley RC, Conway JG, Popp JA. Relationship of hepatic peroxisome proliferation and replicative DNA synthesis to the hepatocarcinogenicity of the peroxisome proliferators di(2-ethylhexyl)phthalate and [4-chloro-6-(2,3-xylidino)-2-pyrimidinylthio]acetic acid (Wy-14,643) in rats. Cancer Res 48:6739–6744, 1988.
32. Ames BN, Gold LS. Dietary carcinogens, environmental pollution, and cancer: Some misconceptions. In: Medical Oncol Tumor Pharmacotherapy, in press.
33. Gratzner HG. Monoclonal antibody to 5-bromo- and 5-iododeoxyuridine: new reagents for detection of DNA replication. Science 218:274–475, 1982.
34. Sugihara H, Hattori T, Fukuda M. Immunohistochemical detection of bromodeoxyuridine in formalin-fixed tissues. Histochemistry 85:193–195, 1986.
35. Tatematsu M, Mutai M, Aoki T, de Camargo JL, Furihata C, Ito N. Proliferation kinetics of pepsinogen altered pyloric gland cells in rats treated with N-methyl-N'-nitro-N-nitrosoguanidine. Carcinogenesis 10:907–911, 1989.
36. Davidson RL, Broeker P, Ashman CR. DNA base sequence changes and sequence specificity of bromodeoxyuridine-induced mutations in mammalian cells. Proc Natl Acad Sci USA 85:4406–4410, 1988.
37. Kaufman ER. Analysis of mutagenesis and sister-chromatid exchanges induced by 5-bromo-2'-deoxyuridine in somatic hybrids derived from Syrian hamster melanoma cells and Chinese hamster ovary cells. Mutat Res 199:68–75, 1988.
38. Napalkov NP, Anisimov VN, Likhachev AJ, Tomatis L. 5-bromodeoxyuridine-induced carcinogenesis and its modification by persistent estrus syndrome, unilateral nephrectomy, and X-irradiation in rats. Cancer Res 49:318–323, 1989.
39. Morris SM, McGarrity LJ, Domon OE, Hinson WG, Kodell RL. Flow cytometric analysis of bromodeoxyuridine-induced inhibition of cell proliferation in the human teratocarcinoma-derived cell line, P3. Environ Mol Mutagen 14:107–114, 1989.
40. Tapscott SJ, Lassar AB, Davis RL, Weintraub H. 5-bromo-2'-deoxyuridine blocks myogenesis by extinguishing expression of MyoD1. Science 245:532–536, 1989.
41. Weghorst CM, Hampton JA, Klaunig JE. Effects of barbiturate compounds on hepatic and renal cell proliferation in the rat. The Toxicologist, 10:718, 1990.
42. Hagiwara A, Diwan BA, Ward JM. Barbital sodium, a tumor promoter for kidney tubules, urinary bladder, and liver of the F344 rat, induces persistent increases in levels of DNA synthesis in renal tubules but not in urinary bladder epithelium or hepatocytes. Fundam Appl Toxicol 13:332–340, 1989.
43. Weghorst CM, Henneman JR, Ward JM. Dose-response to bromodeoxyuridine after continuous exposure in male B6C3F1 mice. J Histochem Cytochem, in press.
44. Kurata Y, Tsuda H, Sakata T, Yamashita T, Ito N. Reciprocal modifying effects of isometic forms of aminophenol on induction of neoplastic lesions in rat liver and kidney initiated by N-ethyl-N-hydroxyethylnitrosamine. Carcinogenesis 8:1281–1285, 1987.
45. Hiasa Y, Ohshima M, Kitahori Y, Konishi N, Fujita T, Yuasa T. β-Cyclodextrin: Promoting effect on the development of renal tubular cell tumors in rats treated with N-ethyl-N-hydroxy-ethylnitrosamine. J Natl Cancer Inst 69:963, 1982.
46. Shinohara Y, Arai M, Hirao K, Sugihara S, Nakanishi K, Tsunoda H, Ito N. Combination effect of

citrinin and other chemicals on rat kidney tumorigenesis. Jpn J Cancer Res 67:147–155, 1976.

47. Kurokawa Y, Takamura N, Matsushima Y, Imazawa T, Hayashi Y. Promoting effect of peroxisome proliferators in two-stage rat renal tumorigenesis. Cancer Lett 43:145–149, 1988.

48. Diwan BA, Nims RW, Ward JM, Hu H, Lubet RA, Rice JM. Tumor promoting activities of ethylphenylacetylurea and diethylacetylurea, the ring hydrolysis products of barbiturate tumor promoters phenobarbital and barbital, in rat liver and kidney initiated by N-nitrosodiethylamine. Carcinogenesis 10:189–194, 1989.

49. Hiasa Y, Enoki N, Kitahori Y, Konishi N, Shimoyama T. DL-serine: Promoting activity on renal tumorigenesis by N-ethyl-N-hydroxyethylnitrosamine in rats. J Natl Cancer Inst 73:297–299, 1984.

50. Shirai T, Ohshima M, Masuda A, Tamano S, Ito N. Promotion of 2-(ethylnitrosamino)ethanol-induced renal carcinogenesis in rats by nephrotoxic compounds: Positive responses with folic acid, basic lead acetate, and N-(3,5-dichlorophenyl)succinimide but not with 2,3-dibromo-1-propanol phosphate. J Natl Cancer Inst 72:477–482, 1984.

51. Hiasa Y, Ohshima M, Kitahori Y, Fujita T, Yuasa T, Miyashiro A. Basic lead acetate: Promoting effect on the development of renal tubular cell tumors in rats treated with N-ethyl-N-hydroxyethylnitrosamine. J Natl Cancer Inst 70:761–765, 1983.

52. Tanner DC, Lipsky MM. Effect of lead acetate on N-(4'-fluoro-4-biphenyl)acetamide-induced renal carcinogenesis in the rat. Carcinogenesis 5:1109–1113, 1984.

53. Shinohara Y, Miyata Y, Murasaki G, Nakanishi K, Yoshimura T, Ito N. Effect of N-(3,5-dichlorophenyl)succinimide on the histological pattern and incidence of kidney tumors induced by streptozotocin in rats. Jpn J Cancer Res 68:397–404, 1977.

54. Kurokawa Y, Matsushima M, Imazawa T, Takamura N, Takahashi M, Hayashi Y. Promoting effect of metal compounds on rat renal tumorigenesis. Journal of American College of Toxicology 4:321–330, 1985.

55. Rosenberg MR, Novicki DL, Jirtle RL, Novotny A, Michalopoulos G. Promoting effect of nicotinamide on the development of renal tubular cell tumors in rats initiated with diethylnitrosamine. Cancer Res 45:809–814, 1985.

56. Hiasa Y, Kitahori Y, Konishi N, Enoki N, Shimoyama T, Miyashiro A. Trisodium nitrilotriacetate monohydrate: promoting effects on the development of renal tubular cell tumors in rats treated with N-ethyl-N-hydroxyethylnitrosamine. J Natl Cancer Inst 72:483–489, 1984.

57. Hiasa Y, Kitahori Y, Konishi N, Shimoyama T. Dose-related effect of trisodium nitrilotriacetate monohydrate on renal tumorigenesis initiated with N-ethyl-N-hydroxyethylnitrosamine in rats. Carcinogenesis 6:907–910, 1985.

58. Kurokawa Y, Aoki S, Imazawa T, Hayashi T, Matsushima Y, Takamura N. Dose-related enhancing effect of potassium bromate on renal tumorigenesis in rats initiated with N-ethyl-N-hydroxyethyl-nitrosamine. Jpn J Cancer Res 76:583–589, 1985.

59. Diwan BA, Ohshima M, Rice JM. Promotion by sodium barbital of renal cortical and transitional cell tumors, but not intestinal tumors, in F344 rats given methyl(acetoxymethyl)-nitrosamine, and lack of effect of phenobarbital, amobarbital, or barbituric acid on development of either renal or intestinal tumors. Carcinogenesis 10:183–188, 1989.

60. Diwan BA, Rice JM, Ohshima M, Ward JM, Dove LF. Comparative tumor-promoting activities of phenobarbital, amobarbital, barbital sodium, and barbituric acid on livers and other organs of male F344/NCr rats following initiation with N-nitrosodiethylamine. J Natl Cancer Inst 74:509–516, 1985.

61. Hiasa Y, Ohshima M, Iwata C, Tanikake T. Histopathological studies on renal tubular cell tumors in rats treated with N-ethyl-N-hydroxyethylnitrosamine. Gann 70:817–820, 1979.

62. Shirai T, Kurata Y, Fukushima S, Ito N. Dose-related induction of lung, thyroid and kidney tumors by N-bis(2-hydroxypropyl)nitrosamine given orally to F344 rats. Jpn J Cancer Res 75:502–507, 1984.

63. Konishi N, Diwan BA, Ward JM. Amelioration of sodium barbital-induced nephropathy and regenerative tubular hyperplasia after a single injection of streptozotocin does not abolish the renal tumor promoting effect of barbital sodium in male F344/NCr rats, Carcinogenesis, in press.

64. Diwan BA, Rice JM, Ohshima M, Wenk ML. Transplacental carcinogenesis by N-nitrosourea in B10.A mice: Effects of postnatal administration of different barbiturates on the incidence and types of tumors. Proceedings of the American Association for Cancer Research 26:137, 1985.

65. Pollard M, Luckert PH. Promotional effect of sodium barbiturate on intestinal tumors induced in rats by dimethylhydrazine. J Natl Cancer Inst 63:1089–1092, 1979.

66. Matsuyama M, Amo H. Promoting effects of long-term administration of barbital on spontaneous hepatic tumorigenesis in B6C3F1 mice. Japan Journal of Hygiene 37:892–896, 1983.

67. Cattley RC, Popp JA. Differences between the promoting activities of the peroxisome proliferator WY-14,643 and phenobarbital in rat liver. Cancer Res. 49:3246–3251, 1989.

68. National Toxicology Program. Carcinogenesis bioassay of di(2-ethylhexyl)phthalate (CAS No. 117-81-7) in F344 rats and B6C3F1 mice (Feed Study). In U.S. Department of Health and Human Services Publication No. (NIH) 82-1773. Bethesda, MD: National Institutes of Health, 1982, pp 127.

69. Popp JA, Garvey LK, Cattley RC. In vivo studies on the mechanism of di(2-ethylhexyl)phthalate carcinogenesis. Toxicol Ind Health 3:151–163, 1987.

70. Diwan BA, Ward JM, Henneman JR, Wenk ML. Effects of short-term exposure to the tumor promoter, 12-O-tetradecanoylphorbol-13-acetate on skin carcinogenesis in SENCAR mice. Cancer Lett 26:177–184, 1985.

71. Diwan BA, Ward JM, Rice JM, Colburn NH, Spangler EF. Tumor-promoting effects of di(2-ethylhexyl)phthalate in JB6 mouse epidermal cells and mouse skin. Carcinogenesis 6:343–347, 1985.

72. Crocker JFS, Safe, SH, Acott P. Effects of chronic phthalate exposure on the kidney. J Toxicol Environ Health 23:433–444, 1988.

73. Waalkes MP, Ward JM. Induction of hepatic metallothionein in male B63C3F1 mice exposed to hepatic tumor promoters: Effects of phenobarbital, acetaminophen, sodium barbital, and di(2-ethylhexyl)phthalate. Toxicol Appl Pharmacol 100:217–226, 1989.

74. Konishi N, Ward JM. Increased levels of DNA synthesis in hyperplastic renal tubules of aging nephropathy in female F344/NCr rats. Vet Pathol 26:6–10, 1989.

75. Reuber MD. Hyperplastic and neoplastic lesions of the kidney in Buffalo rats of varying ages ingesting N-4-(4'-fluorobiphenyl)acetamide. J Natl Cancer Inst 54:427–429, 1975.

Chemically Induced Cell Proliferation:
Implications for Risk Assessment, pages 389-395
©1991 Wiley-Liss, Inc.

Chemically Induced Cell Proliferation in Liver Carcinogenesis

James A. Popp and Daniel S. Marsman

The observation that chronic administration of a specific chemical could result in the appearance of liver tumors in rats was first observed more than 50 years ago (1). Since that time, many chemicals that induce liver tumors in rodents have been identified. Using the data base of the National Toxicology Program, Maronpot and Boorman (2) indicated that 60% of all studies of positive oncogenicity include liver neoplasms in either the rat or mouse. No other organ or tissue has a tumor response rate this high. Chemically induced tumors in any rodent organ generate concern for the chemical's potential effect in exposed human beings. Because the most common positive response in rodents is tumors in the liver, the role of these tumors in predicting potentially serious consequences for exposed human beings has gathered much interest. As a result, tremendous resources have been allocated to develop a better understanding of the mechanisms of hepatocarcinogenicity. But not until we know the mechanisms of tumor induction in the rodent will we be able to judge how relevant a rodent tumor is to predicting human risk.

Research to date has greatly advanced the understanding of chemically induced liver tumors in the rodent. These advances have demonstrated various classes of carcinogens, the importance of metabolic activation, and chemical interaction with cellular macromolecules, particularly DNA. Despite this noteworthy progress, we still do not understand completely the mechanism of action of a single hepatocarcinogen. That cell replication is a key factor in the carcinogenic process is now becoming clear (3). In this chapter we will outline the current understanding of the role of chemically induced hepatocyte proliferation in hepatocarcinogenesis in the rodent.

Hepatocyte proliferation in initiation

Cell proliferation has long been suspected of enhancing the frequency of tumor initiation in many organs (4). Two different mechanisms have been proposed for the role of cell proliferation in enhancing initiation and both are relevant to hepatocarcinogenesis. One suggestion was that cell proliferation enhances initiation by converting chemically induced promutagenic DNA lesions to mutations. In the liver, the concept of cell proliferation as enhancing the rate of initiation has been evaluated in a limited number of experimental studies (5–7). Cayama and colleagues (5) initiated rats with a single dose of a potent direct-acting genotoxic agent, N-methyl-N-nitrosourea (MNU), to cause promutagenic sites in DNA. One initiated group was then subjected to partial hepatectomy as a means of causing enhanced cell proliferation while the second initiated group, the control group, received a sham hepatectomy. The number of initiated cells in the two groups were evaluated by determining the number of γ-glutamyl transpeptidase foci following a growth-selection regimen to cause the expression of initiated cells as foci. The animals with enhanced cell proliferation had 20 times the number of initiated cells (as determined by foci of cellular alteration) compared to the controls, which lacked the proliferative stimulus supplied by the partial hepatectomy. Although this pioneering experiment established hepatocyte proliferation as important in enhancing the initiation process in the liver, it provided limited insight to the mechanism of initiation.

Cell proliferation was proposed to enhance the initiation process by fixing pro-mutagenic events in the DNA, according to this rationale: When a genotoxic carcinogen interacts with DNA, repair processes will begin rapidly to remove the altered DNA base. If the base is repaired before DNA replication, the DNA molecule is not permanently affected. If DNA replication occurs before removal of the altered DNA base, however, then the altered DNA base may be misread, resulting in permanent change or mutation. If this theory is correct, a shortened time interval between DNA injury and DNA replication—limiting the time for repair—would result in higher numbers of initiated cells. Indeed, this concept was demonstrated by administration of a direct DNA-reactive chemical to rats at various times after partial hepatectomy (6). Two-thirds partial hepatectomy was used to induce cell replication in the liver because this procedure synchronizes hepatocytic DNA replication while maximizing the number of hepatocytes entering DNA synthesis. The synchrony of DNA synthesis allowed the experiments to be designed in such a manner that DNA injury was experimentally induced at various times in relation to the peak of DNA replication. Clearly, this and other experimental results demonstrated that initiation is highest when DNA injury has been induced immediately preceding or during the S phase of DNA synthesis (8).

Although, for maximum initiation, the requirement of closely associated DNA injury and hepatocyte replication is best demonstrated by chemicals that react directly with DNA, hepatocyte replication also enhances initiation by chemicals that require metabolic activation. With these chemicals, the time spacing—between partial hepatectomy and administration of the chemical—to achieve maximum initiation—depends on the time required for metabolism. To result in maximum initiation, these chemicals require a longer time interval between their administration and the induced cell proliferation (9,10).

Although studies during the last 15 years have demonstrated clearly that enhanced DNA replication associated with DNA injury resulted in enhanced initiation in the liver, it must be remembered that in the early studies, use of a regenerative stimulus (i.e., partial hepatectomy) was the primary method of inducing hepatocyte proliferation. More recent studies suggested that the concept of enhanced initiation by hepatocyte replication may not be universally true in the liver. As Columbano and colleagues (11) demonstrated recently, additive or augmentative hepatocyte proliferation induced by the administration of mitogenic chemicals did not enhance initiation of the hepatocytes. This reduced initiation seemed not to be caused by any of a variety of possibly confounding factors (11). Demonstrations of equal hepatocyte proliferation and similar DNA binding of the chemical initiator excluded these possibilities as reasons for the observed differences. This suggested the existence of a fundamental difference in either creation or survivability of initiated cells when hepatocyte replication was induced by a mitogenic compared with a regenerative response. However, currently available information does not reveal the mechanistic basis for this difference. Recent work suggests that when the mitogen is removed, foci of cellular alteration believed to arise by clonal expansion of a single initiated cell may regress preferentially (12).

Cell proliferation's second potential role in initiation is one in which forced cell proliferation may yield mutations directly. This concept has received extensive interest (4,13) and has been discussed as a general concept in carcinogenesis (14). A particular spontaneous mutation has many possible origins, including (A) mutagenesis through the action of oxygen-free radicals (15), (B) mutagenesis secondary to spontaneous depurination (16), (C) the infidelity of DNA replication (13), and (D) the possibility of promutagenic "mutator" phenotypes (17). Spontaneous mutation is an attractive hypothesis, but it has no current experimental support in models of hepatocarcinogenesis in rodents. Nevertheless, the concept deserves consideration for explaining the spontaneously initiated cells that occur in rodent livers and, more important, for explaining the carcinogenicity of nongenotoxic carcinogens. Most simply, one may suggest that enhanced hepatocyte replication results in enhanced initiation by fixing an endogenous DNA lesion. If spontaneous DNA injury occurred in the liver, any enhancement of hepatocyte proliferation would increase the probability of fixation of DNA damage. In essence, the concept is the same as the one described in the studies of chemically induced initiation cited above, except that the original DNA injury is a rare "spontaneous" event rather than one caused by administration of an exogenous chemical. Although this concept is difficult to prove because of technical problems in identifying background levels of DNA injury, it is supported by these experimental studies using high doses of initiating agent and by the fact that tumor incidence increases with age.

Hepatocyte proliferation in tumor development

Cell proliferation is important in later stages of tumor development, that is, past the stage of initiation. Indeed, cell proliferation is essential for tumor formation since cancer is a proliferative disease by definition. It is important, however, to look beyond the association of cell proliferation and tumor response and to ask how cell proliferation could preferentially advance the growth and progression of a tumor. First, we consider the role that hepatocyte proliferation has on the development of a tumor in the nonpreneoplastic liver. Second, we consider the effects of chemicals on hepatocyte proliferation in the developing tumor.

Generalized hepatocyte proliferation in tumor development

The relationship between enhanced cell proliferation and tumor development in the target organ has generated extensive discussion (18), particularly concerning hepatocyte proliferation and the development of liver tumors, but the discussions are usually based on incomplete data.

In discussions of a correlation or its absence, the attempt often is to correlate tumors that arose over a prolonged period of exposure with cell proliferation data obtained at a single time point. Unfortunately, the time point examined frequently is an early one (even the first week of chemical administration) preceding the appearance of tumors or any identifiable pretumorous lesion such as hepatic foci of cellular alteration.

Some data are available, however, for comparing liver tumor formation to enhanced hepatocyte replication based on studies in which cell replication was evaluated at multiple time points over the entire time period in which tumors developed (19). In a study from our laboratory, two peroxisomal proliferating agents were selected according to their relative carcinogenicity. The first, di(2-ethylhexyl)phthalate (DEHP), was a weak carcinogen active in only a small number of animals whereas the second, [4-chloro-6-(2,3-xylidino)-2-pyrmidinylthio]acetic acid (Wy-14,643), resulted in a 100% incidence of hepatocellular carcinomas in the animals. Both chemicals caused a comparable enhancement of cell proliferation during the first days of treatment, thus demonstrating noncorrelation between the initial increase in cell proliferation and the chemicals' tumorigenicity. However, when cell proliferation was examined further over a 1-year time course, it became evident that the potent carcinogenic agent (Wy-14,643) caused a persistent elevation of hepatocyte replication while the weak carcinogen, DEHP, did not. In this study with two nongenotoxic agents, therefore, chronic enhancement of hepatocyte proliferation in the liver correlated with the carcinogenic response.

Beyond this example are few other studies in which hepatocyte proliferation has been examined over the entire time course of liver-tumor development. Recent work using the B6C3F1 male mouse suggested that, at least for mice, enhancement of hepatocyte proliferation may not always have predictive value for liver tumorigenicity (20). However, some studies, because of flaws in design and inadequate time-course evaluation, brought conflicting information (21,22), so that we cannot determine currently whether a generalized correlation exists between persistent enhancement of hepatocyte proliferation and tumor development in the liver. Other chemicals, especially those labeled as nongenotoxic, must be examined critically before a general conclusion on correlations can be made.

Since correlations do not prove a cause-and-effect relationship, we cannot conclude, from the demonstration of enhanced cell proliferation alone, that chronic enhancement of cell proliferation is the tumors' cause. Nevertheless, the identification of correlations between chronic enhancement of hepatocyte proliferation and carcinogenicity may be helpful in setting the direction of future mechanistic studies to determine the role of hepatocyte proliferation in liver tumor formation.

Hepatocyte proliferation in the developing tumor

Whether specific chemicals stimulate preferential growth of the altered cells, thereby accounting for the magnitude of the carcinogenic response, is an important question. Two different mechanisms of chemically induced enhancement of cell proliferation may account for the growth of developing neoplasms. First, cell proliferation may be preferentially enhanced in the developing lesion because it is suppressed in the nonneoplastic portion of the liver. Indeed, this is the basis for the rapid appearance of small nodules in the liver of rats subjected to the growth-selection protocol described by Solt and Farber (23), in which a single dose of a carcinogen given to rats acted as the initiating agent. After a period in which the liver recovered from the acute toxic effects of the initiating regimen, the animals were fed 2-acetylaminofluorene (2-AAF) for one week before and one week after partial hepatectomy. Since 2-AAF blocked the proliferative response in the noninitiated but not the initiated hepatocytes, the initiated hepatocytes proliferated preferentially. In this model, the preferential growth of initiated hepatocytes was secondary to the blockage of proliferation of the normal hepatocytes and not a primary effect on the initiated cell. This differential inhibition of cell replication in the livers of rats fed 2-AAF was recently confirmed in an experiment in which the replication rate of cells outside the 2-AAF-induced foci was inhibited 20- to 30-fold (24).

In contrast to the proliferation of hepatocytes inside lesions as a result of differential inhibition, as noted above, it is possible that a direct stimulatory effect may be responsible for the chemical-induced preferential proliferation of hepatocytes in developing lesions. Although no mechanistic examples can yet be identified, data on increased proliferative rates within developing lesions suggest that a direct stimulatory effect may occur with certain chemicals (25–27). One example, in which elevated cell proliferation may be operant, is found in a study comparing the promotional effect of the potent carcinogen Wy-14,643 to the promotional effect of the classic liver tumor promoter phenobarbital (14). Although phenobarbital increased the number of preneoplastic foci observed in initiated livers, it did not cause an increase in the size of these lesions, compared with those of initiation controls. In contrast, Wy-14,643 caused a dramatic increase in the size but not the number of these lesions. These results suggested that, although Wy-14,643 and phenobarbital are both potent promoting agents, they may have fundamentally different modes of action on cell proliferation and the development of tumors. Phenobarbital seemed to be efficient at causing initiated cells to be expressed as small foci but inefficient at causing these lesions to develop further. In contrast, the small number of large foci suggested that Wy-14,643 may be selective but efficient at causing growth due to preferential proliferation of hepatocytes within the lesions. Preliminary data on cell proliferative rates in the developing lesions confirmed that the Wy-14,643–promoted lesions have a high proliferative index (28).

Results of this series of studies strongly suggested that Wy-14,643 has a preferential growth-stimulatory effect on the initiated cells, which results in a rapid increase in lesion size. Chemically altered cell senescence may translate into a preferential growth rate for preneoplastic lesions, and recent work by Bursch and colleagues (29) suggested this may be the operant mechanism in the promotion of lesions by phenobarbital. According to this concept, the increased number of foci observed by Cattley and Popp (14) after administration of phenobarbital was the result of the initiated cells' longer survival.

Understanding the role of preferential chemically induced cell proliferation in lesions may have special significance for the ultimate elucidation of the carcinogenic mechanisms of nongenotoxic carcinogens. Furthermore, application of the two-stage growth-death model for tumors may clarify the role of enhanced cell proliferation and cell loss in the tumor response that follows exposure to nongenotoxic carcinogens (30). Spontaneous initiation is a relatively common event in rat and mouse liver, as evidenced by the high background incidence of liver tumors in several strains of mice and the large number of spontaneous foci of cellular alteration in the livers of rats. Perhaps nongenotoxic chemicals induce tumors by causing the preferential proliferation of spontaneously initiated cells. If this hypothesis proves to be correct, chemically induced cell proliferation could be a central mechanism in the carcinogenic process for at least some agents in the large class of nongenotoxic carcinogens.

Summary

Hepatocyte proliferation has been noted in several stages of the hepatocarcinogenic process. Immediately associated with DNA adducts, hepatocyte proliferation clearly has been shown to enhance initiation. The evidence is strong that enhanced cell proliferation, preceeding DNA repair of endogenous and exogenous lesions, thereby results in the fixation of mutagenic events.

In contrast to the rather well-established role of hepatocyte proliferation in the initiation phase of carcinogenesis, the role of chemically induced hepatocyte proliferation in liver tumor development is supported by sparse information. Although the available data suggest that chronic cell proliferation in the liver may be associated with tumorigenesis, this information is limited to simple correlations and a relatively small number of chemicals. In the carcinogenic process, another aspect of chemically induced cell proliferation would be direct stimulation of the altered hepatocytes to proliferate and develop tumors rapidly. This latter hypothesized activity is the least well characterized and documented for cell proliferation at this time.

Because a quantitative relationship between hepatocyte proliferation and carcinogenic potential has been established for only a few chemicals, general conclusions must await data from correlative studies with other chemicals. Some correlations have been noted, but correlations do not prove cause and effect. The underlying mechanisms of chemically induced cell proliferation must be understood before cause-and-effect relationships between hepatocyte proliferation and enhancement of multiple stages of liver tumor development can be drawn.

References

1. Sasaki T, Yoshida T. Experimentelle Erzeugung des Leberkarzinoms durch Fütterung mit o-Amido-azotoluol. Virchows Arch Pathol Anat 95:175–200, 1935.
2. Maronpot RR, Boorman GA. Interpretation of rodent hepatocellular proliferative alterations and hepatocellular tumors in chemical safety assessment. Toxicol Pathol 10:71–78, 1982.
3. Farber E. Experimental induction of hepatocellular carcinoma as a paradigm for carcinogenesis. Clin Physiol Biochem 5:152–159, 1987.
4. Loeb LA. Endogenous carcinogenesis: Molecular oncology into the twenty-first century—presidential address. Cancer Res 49:5489–5496, 1989.
5. Cayama E, Tsuda H, Sarma DSR, Farber E. Initiation of chemical carcinogenesis requires cell proliferation. Nature 275:60–62, 1978.
6. Kaufmann WK, Rahija RJ, MacKenzie SA, Kaufman DG. Cell cycle-dependent initiation of hepatocarcinogenesis in rats by ($\pm$)-7r,8t-dihydroxy-9t,10t-epoxy-7,8,9,10-tetrahydrobenzo[a]pyrene. Cancer Res 47:3771–3775, 1987.
7. Columbano A, Rajalakshmi S, Sarma DSR. Requirement of cell proliferation for the initiation of liver carcinogenesis as assayed by three different procedures. Cancer Res 41:2079–2083, 1981.
8. Rabes HM, Müller L, Hartmann A, Kerler R, Schuster C. Cell cycle-dependent initiation of adenosine triphosphatase-deficient populations in adult rat liver by a single dose of N-methyl-N-nitrosourea. Cancer Res 46:645–650, 1986.
9. Leonard TB, Lyght O, Popp JA. Dinitrotoluene structure-dependent initiation of hepatocytes in vivo. Carcinogenesis 4:1059–1061, 1983.

10. Tsuda H, Lee G, Farber E. Induction of resistant hepatocytes as a new principle for a possible short-term in vivo test for carcinogens. Cancer Res 40:1157–1164, 1980.

11. Columbano A, Ledda-Columbano GM, Coni P, Pani P. Failure of mitogen-induced cell proliferation to achieve initiation of rat liver carcinogenesis. Carcinogenesis 8:345–347, 1987.

12. Gerbracht U, Brusch W, Kraus P, Putz B, Reinacher M, Timmermann-Trosiener I, Schulte-Hermann R. Effects of hypolipidemic drugs nafenopin and clofibrate on phenotypic expression and cell death (apoptosis in altered foci of rat liver). Carcinogenesis 11:617–624, 1990.

13. Sargentini NJ, Smith KC. Spontaneous mutagenesis: The roles of DNA repair, replication, and recombination. Mutat Res 154:1–27, 1985.

14. Cattley RC, Popp JA. Differences between the promoting activities of the peroxisome proliferator WY-14,643 and phenobarbital in rat liver. Cancer Res 49:3246–3251, 1989.

15. Simic MG, Bergtold DS, Karam LR. Generation of oxy radicals in biosystems. Mutat Res 214:3–12, 1989.

16. Kunkel TA. Mutational specificity of depurination. Proc Natl Acad Sci USA 81:1494–1498, 1984.

17. Glickman BW, Burns PA, Fix DF. Mechanisms of spontaneous mutagenesis: Clues from altered mutational specificity in DNA repair-defective strains. Basic Life Sci 39:259–281, 1986.

18. Ghanayem BI, Maronpot RR, Matthews HB. Association of chemically induced forestomach cell proliferation and carcinogenesis. Cancer Lett 32:271–278, 1986.

19. Marsman DS, Cattley RC, Conway JG, Popp JA. Relationship of hepatic peroxisome proliferation and replicative DNA synthesis to the hepatocarcinogenicity of the peroxisome proliferators di(2-ethylhexyl)-phthalate and [4-chloro-6-(2,3-xylidino)-2-pyrimidinylthio]acetic acid (Wy-14,643) in rats. Cancer Res 48:6739–6744, 1988.

20. Ward JM, Hagiwara A, Anderson LM, Lindsey K, Diwan BA. The chronic hepatic or renal toxicity of di(2-ethylhexyl)phthalate, acetaminophen, sodium barbital, and phenobarbital in male B6C3F1 mice: Autoradiographic, immunohistochemical, and biochemical evidence for levels of DNA synthesis not associated with carcinogenesis or tumor promotion. Toxicol Appl Pharmacol 96:494–506, 1988.

21. Yeldandi AV, Milano M, Subbarao V, Reddy JK, Rao MS. Evaluation of liver cell proliferation during ciprofibrate-induced hepatocarcinogenesis. Cancer Lett 47:21–27, 1989.

22. Smith-Oliver T, Butterworth BE. Correlation of the carcinogenic potential of di(2-ethylhexyl)phthalate (DEHP) with induced hyperplasia rather than with genotoxic activity. Mutat Res 188:21–28, 1987.

23. Solt D, Farber E. New principle for the analysis of chemical carcinogenesis. Nature 263:701–703, 1976.

24. Tatematsu M, Aoki T, Kagawa M, Mera Y, Ito N. Reciprocal relationship between development of glutathione S-transferase positive liver foci and proliferation of surrounding hepatocytes in rats. Carcinogenesis 9:221–225, 1988.

25. Schulte-Hermann R, Ohde G, Schuppler J, Timmermann-Trosiener I. Enhanced proliferation of putative preneoplastic cells in rat liver following treatment with the tumor promoters phenobarbital, hexachlorocyclohexane, steroid compounds, and nafenopin. Cancer Res 41:2556–2562, 1981.

26. Schulte-Hermann R, Schuppler J, Ohde G, Timmermann-Trosiener I. Effect of tumor promoters on proliferation of putative preneoplastic cells in rat liver. Carcinogenesis 7:99–104, 1982.

27. Schulte-Hermann R, Timmermann-Trosiener I, Schuppler J. Promotion of spontaneous preneoplastic cells in rat liver as a possible explanation of tumor production by nonmutagenic compounds. Cancer Res 43:839–844, 1983.

28. Marsman DS, Popp JA. Importance of basophilic hepatocellular foci in the development of hepatic tumors induced by the peroxisome proliferator, WY-14,643. Proc Am Assoc Cancer Res 30:193, 1989.

29. Bursch W, Lauer B, Timmermann-Trosiener I, Barthel G, Schuppler J, Schulte-Hermann R. Controlled death (apoptosis) of normal and putative preneoplastic cells in rat liver following withdrawal of tumor promoters. Carcinogenesis 5:453–458, 1984.

30. Moolgavkar SH. Biologically motivated two-stage model for cancer risk assessment. Toxicol Lett 43:139–150, 1988.

Chemically Induced Cell Proliferation:
Implications for Risk Assessment, pages 397-405
©1991 Wiley-Liss, Inc.

Intermediate Biomarkers and Studies of Cancer Prevention in the Gastrointestinal Tract

Martin Lipkin

Measurements of cell proliferation and differentiation have identified changes in the gastrointestinal tract that are associated with increased susceptibility to gastrointestinal cancer. Early in the development of various precancerous diseases, continued DNA synthesis persists in maturing cells with a delayed onset of normal terminal differentiation. In more advanced stages of precancerous disorders, additional changes occur in the cells as they exhibit progressively increasing degrees of abnormally delayed maturation.

In humans with diseases predisposing to cancer, and in rodents after treatment with chemical carcinogens, among the earliest modifications that develop in gastrointestinal epithelial cells is increased proliferative activity in a basal region of epithelium known as the "proliferative compartment." This hyperproliferation develops in all cancer-prone regions of the gastrointestinal tract that have been studied both in humans and in rodent models—in the esophagus, stomach, and colon. Eventually, excessive numbers of proliferating cells accumulate in the epithelium without undergoing normal maturation (1).

Diseases of the esophagus

In several diseases of the esophagus that lead to increased frequencies of cancer, proliferating epithelial cells in the esophageal basal layer increase in number as the proliferative compartment expands. Barrett's disease of the esophagus leads to a marked increase in the incidence of esophageal cancer, and may account for a large fraction of the esophageal cancer occurring in the United States (2). In this disease, immature epithelial cells accumulate in the esophageal lining and some undergo metaplastic changes; proliferative cells sometimes reach the surface of the esophageal lining as the proliferative compartment expands (3).

A high incidence of esophageal cancer has been found to occur in Linxian, China. Cumulative esophageal cancer death rates have been reported to be as high as 33% for males and 20% for females (4). In this and other high-risk geographic regions, squamous epithelial cells gradually undergo morphologic changes from normal to hyperplasia to dysplasia before the onset of cancer. Precancerous esophageal disease, as studied in Linxian, begins with hyperplasia and dysplasia; the proliferative compartment progressively increases in size and the numbers of proliferative cells markedly increase (5). When esophageal epithelial cells develop increasing degrees of dysplasia and preinvasive carcinoma, the DNA content of individual cells increases along with ploidy.

As normal esophageal squamous epithelial cells undergo differentiation, they express other biomarkers including different molecular species of keratins (6) similar to squamous epidermal cells. However, when these cells become malignant they contain keratin species not present in normal cells (7). They also develop various ectopic tumor-associated antigens including human chorionic gonadotropin, human placental lactogen, α-fetoprotein, carcinoembryonic antigen, and nonspecific cross-reacting antigen (8). These cells also contain lower quantities of surface epidermal growth factor receptors with much higher affinity than normal esophageal cells, as modulation of cell growth is altered during abnormal development.

Diseases of the stomach

Among diseases of the stomach that increase the risk of human gastric cancer, certain characteristic changes occur in the epithelial cells. Increased proliferative activity of these cells is followed by an intermediate stage of abnormal cell differentiation, including metaplasia of the small and large intestinal types and dysplasia. Proliferating epithelial cells fail to differentiate normally as they migrate to the surface of the mucosa, and immature cells line the gastric surface, directly contacting the contents of the stomach.

Thus, in chronic atrophic gastritis, a hyperproliferation of gastric epithelial cells develops as increased numbers of cells replicate and migrate more rapidly than normal to the surface of the epithelial lining where immature epithelial cells are extruded from the surface. In gastric atrophy, the immature proliferative epithelial cell compartment also expands (9).

Recent findings in peptic ulcer disease (10) indicate that proliferation rates of gastric epithelial cells are similar to those of mild gastritis without atrophy and those of minimal gastric atrophy. However, cell proliferation progressively increases with advanced gastric atrophy, reaching a peak in severe atrophy and gastritis as cells that do not terminally differentiate cover the mucosa.

Studies have been conducted in Colombia, South America, of a population with chronic atrophic gastritis and very high incidence of gastric cancer. Three findings were noted: an expansion of the proliferative compartment of epithelial cells; a grossly hyper-proliferative state with excessive numbers of replicating cells in the gastric lining; and a failure of cells to undergo normal maturation (11). Immature cells covered the surface of the stomach and hyperproliferating cells had an abnormal antigen expression.

After surgical resection to treat peptic ulcer disease, individuals may have increased susceptibility to developing gastric cancer in the remaining stomach. Changes that develop in the epithelium after partial gastrectomy include progressive expansion of the proliferative compartment extending to the surface of the stomach and increasing accumulations of abnormally proliferating cells (12).

During development of the abnormal stage of cell differentiation known as metaplasia, which is associated with an increased frequency of stomach cancer, other changes develop in gastric epithelial cells. Intestinal metaplasia increases in the gastric mucosa of patients with cancer at a rate similar to that of individuals with gastric ulcer, suggesting that metaplasia may be a biomarker of precancerous disease. Differences in expression of intestinal enzymes in gastric mucosa have been used to classify metaplastic glands as "complete," or containing all or most small intestinal enzymes, or "incomplete" with fewer enzymes expressed than in normal small intestinal mucosa (13); the latter is considered to more closely resemble dysplasia and carcinoma. In early and more mature metaplasia, the neutral mucin of normal gastric cells is replaced by sialomucin of the small intestine, while advanced metaplasia is manifested by sulphomucins of the colonic type and is considered a marker of dysplasia. In metaplastic gastric epithelium, normal gastric antigens also are lost; in well-differentiated lesions they are replaced by normal intestinal antigens, and in less well-differentiated lesions by embryonic antigens. In chronic atrophic gastritis, hyperproliferating epithelial cells increased the expression of an antigen that is normally decreased in maturing gastric cells.

Diseases of the large intestine

Benign colonic adenomas are believed to represent the intermediate stage between normal colonic epithelial cells and carcinoma; the probability of carcinoma developing in benign colonic adenomas increases directly as adenomas increase in size. In addition to an expansion of the proliferative compartment of epithelial cells in the colonic adenomas of familial polyposis, a complete shift of the entire proliferative region to the surface of the adenomas has been observed (14).

When diseases of the large intestine that lead to increased frequencies of human colorectal cancer are present, smaller expansions of the proliferative compartment have been found through extensive counting of proliferating cells in flat colonic mucosa. This expansion has been observed in familial polyposis, in individuals who have had sporadic adenomas or previous familial and nonfamilial colon cancers, and in ulcerative colitis. Among individuals having colonic carcinomas, the DNA content of flat mucosa cells was increased in the upper third of the colonic crypts, a finding not observed in the colonic mucosa of normal subjects. In patients with ulcerative colitis, it also was possible to identify subpopulations of hyperproliferating cells that expressed an antigen that is normally decreased in maturing cells (15).

Further abnormal properties also have been observed in colonic adenomas: The secretion of the plasminogen activator by tumor promoters will be modulated (16) and the adenomatous epithelial cells will make an abnormal retrograde migration away from the surface of the mucosa deep into the crypts (14), as occurs with malignant cells. However, benign adenomatous epithelial cells do not invade through the basal layer.

During the abnormal development of colonic epithelial cells in precancerous diseases, blood group-related antigens also become modified. Increased expression has been found of Lewis antigens, especially Y and extended Y determinants; the latter, not found in normal colonic mucosa, had a restricted pattern of distribution in normal tissues. LeY expression in polyps was further correlated with histological type and degree of dysplasia. Extended or trifucosyl LeY antigen expression was limited to premalignant adenomatous polyps and was absent from nonpremalignant or hyperplastic polyps. Among the adenomatous polyps, the extended LeY antigen expression tended to correlate with three known parameters of malignant potential: larger polyp size, villous histology, and severe dysplasia. Therefore, the LeY hapten appears to be an oncodevelopmental cancer-associated antigen in the human colon, and extended LeY antigens may be highly specific markers for premalignancy and malignancy (17,18).

Further changes occur in colonic epithelial cells during abnormal differentiation and as neoplasms develop, including the expression of abnormal carbohydrate antigens and morphologic, immunologic, and biochemical modifications in the cells. Modified gene expression also occurs in the hereditary disease *familial polyposis* and in carcinogen-induced and sporadic colonic cancer, as colonic cells undergo abnormal differentiation and develop into adenomas and carcinomas (19-21).

Among modifications in gene expression, the c-*myc* oncogene has been implicated in the processes of normal cell proliferation and differentiation. In normal colonic mucosa, c-*myc* oncogene product was expressed maximally in the normal mid-zone region of differentiating cells, and in dysplastic areas of adenomatous polyp cells. Expression of *ras* gene was found highest in the most differentiated cells in the upper region of normal colonic crypts, and a high level of Ha-*ras* expression appeared to be a marker for a differentiated state of colonic carcinoma cells involving mucin production (22,23). Colonic carcinoma cells also secrete transforming growth factor-alpha (TGF-α) and TGF-β. As with keratinocytes, these may contribute to differentiation of the epithelial cells and an imbalance of these two endogenous growth modifiers to aberrant development of preneoplastic cells.

Thus, as noted in our discussion of the gastrointestinal tract, when diseases that lead to increased frequencies of cancer are present, expanding populations of proliferating epithelial cells are found prior to the development of observable tumors. Throughout the entire gastrointestinal tract, therefore, the cellular proliferation in normal mucosa is comparatively quiescent and fully mature cells are able to develop in order to function, to cover, and to protect the surface of the gastrointestinal tract. Newer studies now show that there are characteristic changes: a lack of terminal differentiation in epithelial cells, modifications of gene expression, and modified responses of the cells to growth factors and tumor promoters that may further contribute to abnormal cell development.

Application of biomarkers to studies of cancer prevention in human subjects

Biomarkers of abnormal gastrointestinal cell proliferation and differentiation may be able to assist in cancer prevention studies (1). Although genetic predisposition contributes to the evolution of gastrointestinal neoplasia, dietary components are believed to have a major influence on the incidence rates of both adenomas and colon cancer among human populations with widely differing cancer frequencies and in different parts of the world. In many studies carried out in animal models, where tumors appear within a short time-frame, studies have indicated that specific dietary factors can inhibit the induction and development of a wide variety of tumors including those arising in the gastrointestinal tract.

Compounds belonging to over 20 different classes of chemicals have potential in chemoprevention; some of these are naturally occurring constituents of food. The chemopreventive agents can be classified in two broad categories (24): inhibitors effective against the formation or activation of tumor initiating agents (i.e., genotoxic agents), or those that work against tumor promoters.

Within the first group are compounds that prevent the formation of carcinogens from precursor substances, that is, ascorbic acid, α-tocopherol and certain plant phenols such as caffeic and ferulic acids; compounds that prevent carcinogenic substances from reaching or reacting with critical target sites in the tissues such as phenols and certain plant flavonoids, flavones, coumarins, and isothiocyanates; and compounds that react with carcinogenic agents by inhibiting the expression of neoplasia, such as retinoids and carotenoids, selenium salts, protease inhibitors, inhibitors of arachadonic acid metabolism, sterols, and a steroid hormone.

Compounds that inhibit tumor promotion include retinoids, protease inhibitors, inhibitors of arachadonic acid metabolism, phenols, agents that increase intracellular cyclic adenosine monophospate (cAMP), and calcium metabolism modulators.

Thus, new rationales for dietary intervention have emerged from epidemiological and animal model studies, and might warrant evaluation in human populations. Epithelial cell proliferation is increased in the colon, stomach, and esophagus before the appearance of tumors in those human subjects with increased susceptibility to gastrointestinal cancer; therefore, the analysis of patterns of gastrointestinal cell proliferation and differentiation were recently considered for possible application in studies of cancer prevention. One example of such an application is found in recent studies involving oral calcium administration to individuals at increased risk for colonic cancer.

Current studies (25–36) have shown a relationship between calcium and hyperproliferation of epithelial cells in human colonic mucosa. Several studies (25–28) have now shown decreased hyperproliferation after supplemental dietary calcium (1250–2000 mg of elemental calcium administered daily for several months). However, proliferation did not change when lower levels of cell replication initially were present (25,29). Studies conducted in vitro showed that increasing levels of calcium decreased the proliferation of normal colonic epithelial cells in the flat mucosa; heterogeneity was observed in familial polyposis cells and loss of response to calcium in advanced stages of adenomas and carcinomas (30–35). In vitro studies also have shown that supplemental calcium provided protection against the damaging effects that bile acids and fatty acids (35), as well as modified histone acetylation (36), have on colonic epithelial cells.

The effects of supplemental dietary calcium on colonic and mammary rodent cells have also been studied (37–54). Supplemental calcium decreased hyperproliferation of colonic epithelial cells when it was induced by deoxycholic acid (37), fatty acids (38), cholic acid (39), and partial enteric resection (40). It also decreased tumor promotion after partial enteric resection and carcinogen administration (41) and administration of the carcinogen azoxymethane (AOM) (43). It decreased hyperproliferation and tumor formation after dietary fat and carcinogen administration (42) and when induced by a low fat diet and AOM (45). It decreased hyperproliferation after a nutritional stress diet low in calcium and vitamin D and high in fat and phospate (44). Further studies showed that calcium decreased colonic tumors when induced by AOM (46), although not DMH (51,52). Calcium reduction of deoxylic acid–induced hyperproliferation was blocked by phosphate (47). ODC was reduced by calcium (48,49) and calcium decreased cholic acid–induced mortality (50). Regarding mammary cells, proliferation was decreased by dietary fat and calcium (53) as was tumor formation (54).

Further intermediate biomarker studies involving polyamine assays in studies of normal and diseased colonic cells indicate that ODC and tyrosine kinase were increased in flat colonic mucosa of individuals with colonic neoplasms, but not in colonic mucosa of normal subjects (55–58). Diallyl sulfide, and guar (a fiber), induced a decrease in ODC activity in various abnormal conditions in rodents (60,61) and beta carotene in humans (59).

Studies of the effects such fibers as wheat bran, psyllium, and guar have on these functions—cell proliferation, levels of fecal mutagens, production of short-chain fatty acids, and polyp formation (62–65)—can also be summarized. Wheat bran (13.15 g fiber) decreased rectal cell proliferation (62), fecal mutagens and secondary bile acids (63), and polyps (65) in human colonic cells; psyllium increased SCFA fermentation compared to cellulose (64). In rodent colonic cells, guar (10%) decreased ODC after DMH administration, but did not decrease tumor level (61); butyrate (12 mM) produced by colonic fermentation of dietary fiber modified histone acetylation, creating less monoacetylated and more di- and triacetylated forms (66).

Some new intermediate biomarkers are now being studied. In rodent colonic cells, the incorporation of bromodeoxyuridine (BrdU) and [^{3}H]thymidine into proliferating cells in S phase produced correlative measurements of cell proliferation (67); after DMH administration the proliferating cell nuclear antigen (PCNA) identified an expanded proliferative compartment (68); also after DMH, enzyme-altered foci were identified (69).

In human colonic cells, the use of Ki-67 labeling index has been found to be a more reliable measure of solid tumor proliferative activity than is tritiated [^{3}H] labeling (70). Amaranthin, a new lectin, has been developed as a marker for epithelial cell differentiation (71). Morphologic changes, including increased goblet cells and deeper and wider crypts, have been found in transitional mucosa (72). In human gastric cells, Le and other antigens have been found to differ in normal and neoplastic mucosa (73).

Thus, measurements of cell proliferation, differentiation, gene structure and expression, and other morphologic measurements in epithelial cells, have begun to serve a new function: They have provided "intermediate biomarkers" in cancer prevention studies that allow investigators to measure early effects of nutritional interventions in cells of both human subjects and animal models. It is anticipated that in future attempts to prevent the development of gastrointestinal cancer, this approach may permit many more nutritional and pharmacologic interventions to be carried out in human subjects than has been possible.

References

1. Lipkin M. Biomarkers of increased susceptibility to gastrointestinal cancer: New application to studies of cancer prevention in human subjects. Perspectives in cancer research. Cancer Res 48:235–245, 1988.
2. Naef AP, Savary M, Ozzello L. Columnar lined lower esophagus: An acquired lesion with malignant predisposition. Report on 140 cases of Barrett's esophagus with 12 adenocarcinoma. J Thorac Cardiovasc Surg 70:826–835, 1975.
3. Herbst JJ, Berenson MM, McCloskey DW, Wiser WC. Cell proliferation in esophageal columnar epithelium (Barrett's esophagus). Gastroenterology 75:683–687, 1978.
4. Li JY. Epidemiology of esophageal cancer in China. NCI Monogr 62:113–120, 1981.
5. Yang G-C, Lipkin M, Yang K, Wang G-Q, Li J-Y, Yang CS, Winawer S, Newmark H, Blot W, Fraumeni JF Jr. Proliferation of esophageal epithelial cells in individuals in Linxian, China. J Natl Cancer Inst 79:1241–1246, 1987.
6. Doran TI, Vidrich A, Sun T-T. Intrinsic and extrinsic regulation of the differentiation of skin, corneal and esophageal epithelial cells. Cell 22:17–25, 1980.
7. Yang K, Lipkin M. AE1 cytokeratin patterns in differentiation states of squamous cell carcinoma of the esophagus. Am J Clin Path, in press.
8. Burg-Kurland CL, Purnell DM, Combs JW, Hillman EA, Harris CC, Trump BF. Immunocytochemical evaluation of human esophageal neoplasms and preneoplastic lesions for β-chorionic gonadotropin,

placental lactogen, α-fetoprotein, carcinoembryonic antigen, and nonspecific cross-reacting antigen. Cancer Res 46:2936–2943, 1986.

9. Deschner E, Winawer SJ, Lipkin M. Patterns of nucleic acid and protein synthesis in normal human gastric mucosa and atrophic gastritis. J Natl Cancer Inst 48:1567–1574, 1972.

10. Sizikov AI, Azykbekov R. Histoautoradiographic study of gastric epithelial DNA synthesis in precancerous lesions of the stomach. Vopr Onkol 27:19–22, 1981.

11. Lipkin M, Correa P, Mikol YB, Higgins PJ, Cuello C, Zarama G, Fontham E, Zavala D. Proliferative and antigenic modifications in epithelial cells in chronic atrophic gastritis. J Natl Cancer Inst 75:613–619, 1985.

12. Offerhaus GJA, van de Stadt J, Samson G, Tytgat GNJ. Cell proliferation kinetics in the gastric remnant. Eur J Cancer Clin Oncol 21:73–79, 1985.

13. Correa P. Chronic gastritis as a cancer precursor. Scand J Gastroenterol 19:131–136, 1984.

14. Lightdale C, Lipkin M, Deschner E. In vivo measurements in familial polyposis: kinetics and location of proliferating cells in colonic adenomas. Cancer Res 42:4280–4283, 1982.

15. Biasco G, Lipkin M, Minarini A, Higgins P, Miglioli M. Proliferative and antigenic properties of the rectal cells in patients with chronic ulcerative colitis. Cancer Res 44:5450–5454, 1984.

16. Friedman E, Gillin S, Lipkin M. 12-O-tetradecanoylphorbol-13-acetate stimulation of DNA synthesis in cultured preneoplastic familial polyposis colonic epithelial cells but not in normal colonic epithelial cells. Cancer Res 44:4078–4086, 1984.

17. Sakamoto J, Furukawa K, Cordon-Cardo C, Yin BWT, Rettig WJ, Oettgen HF, Old LJ, Lloyd KO. Expression of Lewisa, Lewisb, X, and Y blood group antigens in human colonic tumors and normal tissue and in human tumor-derived cell lines. Cancer Res 46:1553–1561, 1986.

18. Kim YS, Yuan M, Itzkowitz SH, Sun QB, Kaizu T, Palekar A, Trump BF, Hakomori S. Expression of LeY and extended LeY blood group-related antigens in human malignant, premalignant, and nonmalignant colonic tissues. Cancer Res 46:5985–5992, 1986.

19. Bodmer WF, Bailey CJ, Bodmer J, Bussey HJR, Ellis A, Gorman P, Lucibello VA, Murday VA, Rider SH, Scambler P, Sheer D, Solomon E, Spurr NK. Localization of the gene for familial adenomatous polyposis on chromosome 5. Nature 328:614–616, 1987.

20. Augenlicht LH, Wahrman MZ, Halsey H, Anderson L, Taylor J and Lipkin M. Expression of cloned sequences in biopsies of human colonic tissue and in colonic carcinoma cells induced to differentiate in vitro. Cancer Res, in press.

21. Vogelstein B, Fearon ER, Hamilton SR, Kern SE, Preisinger AC, Leppert M, Nakamura Y, White R, Alida MM, Bos JL. Genetic alterations during colorectal-tumor development. N Engl J Med 319:525–532, 1988.

22. Chesa PG, Rettig WJ, Melamed MR, Old LJ, Niman HL. Expression of p21 rats in normal and malignant tissues, lack of association with prolifertion and malignancy. Proc Natl Acad Sci USA 84:3234–3238, 1987.

23. Augenlicht LH, Augeron C, Yander G, Laboisse C. Overexpression of ras in mucus-secreting colon carcinoma cells of low tumorigenicity. Cancer Res 47:3763–3765, 1987.

24. Wattenberg LW. Chemoprevention of cancer. Cancer Res 45:1–8, 1985.

25. Lipkin M, Newmark H. Effect of added dietary calcium on colonic epithelial cell proliferation in subjects at high-risk for familial colon cancer. N Engl J Med 313:1381–1384, 1985.

26. Lipkin M, Friedman E, Winawer SJ, Newmark HL. Colonic epithelial cell proliferation in responders and nonresponders to supplemental dietary calcium. Cancer Res 49:248–254, 1989.

27. Rozen P, Fireman Z, Fine N, Wax Y, Ron E. Oral calcium suppresses increased rectal epithelial proliferation of persons at risk of colorectal cancer. Gut 30:650–655, 1989.

28. Isbell G, Hu P-J, Lanza F, Shabot M, Winn R, Rogers R, Hochman L, Michaletz P, Roubein L, Faintuch J, Larso E, Levin B, Wargovich M. Modulation by calcium of colonic mucosal proliferation in patients with sporadic colonic adenomas and carcinomas. Gastroenterology 96:228, 1989.

29. Gregoire RC, Stern HS, Yeung KS, Stadler J, Langley S, Furrer R, Bruce WR. Effect of calcium supplementation on mucosal cell proliferation in high risk patients for colon cancer. Gut 30:376–382, 1989.

30. Buset M, Lipkin M, Winawer S, Swaroop S, Friedman E. Inhibition of human colonic epithelial cell proliferation in vivo and in vitro by calcium. Cancer Res 46:5426–5430, 1986.

31. Appleton GVN, Wheeler EE, Owen RW, Challecombe DN. Intralumenal calcium and colonic cancer: Possible mechanism of action. Gastroenterology 94:10, 1988.

32. Arlow FL, Walczak SM, Majumdar APN. The role of calcium in deoxycholic acid-induced

hyperproliferation of colonic mucosal explants. Gastroenterology 94:12, 1988.

33. Buset M, Lipkin M, Winawer S, Friedman E. Direct and indirect protection of human colonic epithelial cells by calcium. Gastroenterology 92:1334, 1987.

34. Friedman E, Lipkin M, Winawer S, Buset M, Newmark H. Heterogeneity in the response of familial polyposis cells and adenomas to increasing levels of calcium in vitro. Cancer 63:2486–2491, 1989.

35. Buset M, Galand P, Lipkin M, Winawer S, Friedman E. Protection of human colonic epithelial cells from toxicity of biliary and fatty acids by calcium. Gastroenterology 96:66, 1989.

36. Boffa LC, Mariani MR, Newmark H, Lipkin M. Calcium as modulator of nucleosomal histones acetylation in cultured cells. Proc Amer Assn Cancer Res 30:8, 1989.

37. Wargovich MJ, Eng VWS, Newmark HL, Bruce WR. Calcium ameliorates the toxic effects of deoxycholic acid on colonic epithelium. Carcinogenesis 4:1205–1207, 1983.

38. Wargovich MJ, Eng VWS, Newmark HL, Bruce WR. Calcium inhibits the damaging and compensating proliferative effects of fatty acids on mouse colon epithelium. Cancer Lett 23:253–258, 1984.

39. Bird RP, Schneider R, Stamp D, Bruce WR. Effect of dietary calcium and cholic acid on the proliferative indices of murine colonic epithelium. Carcinogenesis 7:1657–1661, 1986.

40. Appleton GVN, Bristol JB, Williamson RCN. Increased dietary calcium and small bowel resection have opposite effects on colonic cell turnover. Br J Surg 73:1018–1021, 1986.

41. Appleton GVN, Davies PW, Bristol JB, Williamson RCN. Inhibition of intestinal carcinogenesis by dietary supplementation with calcium. Br J Surg 74:523–525, 1987.

42. Pence BC, Buddingh F. Inhibition of dietary fat promotion of colon carcinogenesis by supplemental calcium or vitamin D. Proc Amer Assoc Cancer Res 28:154, 1987.

43. Skrypec DJ, Bursey RG. Effect of dietary calcium on azoxymethane-induced intestinal carcinogenesis in male F344 rats fed high fat diets. FASEB J 2:857, 1988.

44. Newmark H, Lipkin M, Maheshwari N. Colonic hyperplasia and hyperproliferation induced by four components of western-style diet. J Natl Cancer Inst, in press.

45. Reshef R, Rozen P, Fireman Z, Fine N, Barzilai M, Shasha S, Shkolnik T. Effect of calcium administration on colonic epithelial cell proliferation in rats during cancer induction by MNNG. Proc Am Assn Cancer Res 30:179, 1989.

46. Wargovich MJ, Allnutt D, Palmer C, Anaya P, Stephens LC. Inhibition of the promotional phase of azoxymethane-induced colon carcinogenesis in the F344 rat by calcium lactate: Effect of simulating 2 human nutrient density levels. Cancer Lett, in press.

47. Hu PJ, Baer AR, Wargovich MJ. Calcium and phosphate: effect of two dietary confounders on colonic epithelial cellular proliferation. Nutr Res 9:545–553, 1989.

48. Arlow FL, Walczak S, Majumdar APN. Attenuation of azoxymethane (AOM)-induced colonic mucosal ornithine decarboxylase (ODC) and tyrosine kinase (TYR-K) activity by calcium in rats. Gastroenterology 96:14, 1989.

49. Baer AR, Wargovich MJ. Dietary calcium and vitamin D inhibit colonic ornithine decarboxylase (ODC) activity induced by bile acids. FASEB J:469, 1989.

50. Cohen BI, Mosbach EM, McSherry CK, Matoba N, Stenger RJ. Dietary calcium ameliorates cholic acid toxicity in a hamster model of cholelithiasis. Gastroenterology 58:586, 1989.

51. Karkara M, Patrick PC, Glauert HP. Effect of dietary calcium and vitamin D on colon tumors induced by 1,2-dimethylhydrazine in Fischer-344 rats. FASEB J:469, 1989.

52. Kaup SM, Behling AR, Choquette LL, Greger JL. Colon tumor development in DMH-initiated rats fed varying levels of calcium and butterfat. FASEB J:469, 1989.

53. Zhang L, Bruce WR, Bird RP. Proliferative activity of murine mammary epithelium as affected by dietary fat and calcium. Cancer Res 47:4905–4508, 1987.

54. Jacobson EA, James KA, Russell R, Newmark HL, Carroll KK. Effects of dietary fat, calcium, and vitamin D on growth and mammary tumorigenesis induced by 7,12-dimethylbenz[a]anthracene in female Sprague Dawley rats. Cancer Res 49:6300–6303, 1989.

55. Baer AR, Lambert M, Wargovich MJ. Ornithine decarboxylase. Heterogeneity of enzymatic activity in colorectal neoplasia. Gastroenterology 96:21, 1989.

56. Colarian J, Arlow F, Calzada R, Luk GD, Majumdar APN. Differential activation of ornithine decarboxylase (ODC) and tyrosine kinase (TYR-K) in the rectal mucosa of patients with hyperplastic (HP) and adenomatous polyps. Gastroenterology 9:93, 1989.

57. McGarrity TJ, Peiffer LP, Pegg AE. Mucosal ornithine decarboxylase activity and polyamine content as markers for colonic polyps. Gastroenterology 96:334, 1989.

58 Elitsur Y, Mehta R, Theiss HW, Luk GD. Ornithine decarboxylase (ODC) activity and polyamine levels in normal and cancerous human colonocytes. Gastroenterology 96:139, 1989.

59. Phillips RW, Willis MS, Luk GD, Mehta R, Kikendall JW, Bowen PE, Maydonovitch CL, Andrada F, Wong RK. Beta-carotene normalizes rectal mucosal ornithine decarboxylase activity in patients with colon carcinoma. Gastroenterology 96:391, 1989.

60. Baer AR, Anaya P, Wargovich MJ. Effect of organosulfur compounds on induction of colonic ornithine decarboxylase activity by initiating or promoting agents in the mouse. Gastroenterology 96:21, 1989.

61. Klurfeld D, Adamson I, Kritchevsky D. Ornithine decarboxylase (ODC) activity in colonic mucosa: Modulation by dietary fiber. FASEB J III:943, 1989.

62. Alberts D, Buller W, Einspahr J, Rees-McGee S, Ramanujuan P, Aickin W, Earnest D, Phelps J, Pethigal P, Ritenbaugh C, Atwood J, Wilbur L, Meyskens F. Dietary wheat bran (WB) fiber supplementation significantly reduces [^{3}H]thymidine crypt organ labeling index (LI) in rectal mucosal biopsies from patients with resected colorectal cancers. Proc Am Assn Can Res 30, 1989.

63. Reddy BS, Engle A, Katsifis S, Simi B, Bartram P. Biochemical epidemiology of colon cancer. Effect of type of dietary fiber on stool mutagens and bile acids. FASEB J III:943, 1989.

64. Haynes SR, Lupton JR. The effects of cellulose and psyllium supplementation on short-chain fatty acid profiles in healthy females. FASEB J III:1069, 1989.

65. DeCosse JJ, Miller H, Lesser MH. Effect of wheat fiber and vitamin C and E on rectal polyps in patients with familial adenomatous polyposis. J Natl Cancer Inst 81:1290–1297, 1989.

66. Lupton JR, Boffa LC, Newmark H, Lipkin M. Dietary fiber induced modulation of butyrate level in rat colon leads to hyperacetylation of nucleosomal histone in colonic epithelial cells. FACEB J III:1069, 1989.

67. Isbell G, Hu P-J, Lynch P, Roubein L, Katz R, Cafferty S, Patel S, Wargovich MJ. A comparison of tritiated thymidine autoradiography and bromodeoxyuridine immunoperoxidase techniques for measuring epithelial proliferation in the human colon. Gastroenterology 96:228, 1989.

68. Yamada K, Yoshitake K, Ahnen DJ. Proliferating cell nuclear antigen (PCNA) expression detects expansion of the proliferative compartment in carcinogen treated colonic mucosa in the rat. Gastroenterology 96:555, 1989.

69. Pretlow TP, Barrow BJ, O'Riordan MA, Stellato TA, Pretlow TG. Colons of carcinogen-treated F344 rats have enzyme-altered foci. Proc Amer Assoc Can Res 30: 1989.

70. Deshmukh P, Ramsay L, Garewal H. Ki-67 labeling index is a more reliable measure of solid tumor proliferative activity than tritiated thymidine [^{3}H]labeling. Proc Am Assn Can Res 30:287, 1989.

71. Rinderle SJ, Goldstein IJ, Luk GD, Resau J, Rigot WL, Boland CR. Development of a new lectin amaranthin (ACA) as a marker for epithelial cell differentiation in the human colon. Gastroenterology 96:417, 1989.

72. Lawson MJ, White L, Coyle P, Butler RN, RobertsThomson IC, Conyers RAJ. Proliferative and enzyme activity in transitional mucosa adjacent to colonic cancer. Gastroenterology 96:290, 1989.

73. Sakamoto J, Watanabe T, Tokumaru T, Morimoto T, Akiyama S, Takagi H, Ueda R, Nakazato H. Antigens of normal gastric tissues and gastric cancers markers of gastric mucosal cell differentiation and gastric carcinoma subsets. Proc Amer Assoc Cancer Res 30:353, 1989.

Chemically Induced Cell Proliferation:
Implications for Risk Assessment, pages 407-416
©1991 Wiley-Liss, Inc.

Role of Hepatocyte Proliferation in α-Hexachlorocyclohexane and Phenobarbital Tumor Promotion in B6C3F1 Mice

Joseph C. Siglin, Christopher M. Weghorst, and James E. Klaunig

Chemical carcinogenesis in the rodent liver is a multistage process that involves the sequential transformation of normal cells into malignant cells (1–4). At least three distinct stages—initiation, promotion and progression—can be identified in this process by using various histological and histochemical techniques (3). Initiation involves the interaction of a genotoxic carcinogen or reactive metabolite with cellular DNA to produce an irreversibly altered cell (5). Tumor promotion is the selective proliferation of the initiated cell by intrinsic factors (i.e., hormones and growth factors) or such extrinsic factors as toxic chemicals or other agents (3,4). In the rodent liver, the promotion stage results in the formation of demonstrable lesions, hepatocellular foci, which appear as discrete islands of phenotypically altered hepatocytes (6). The third stage, progression, is thought to involve the advancement of preneoplastic foci to the neoplastic stage of cancer (adenoma or carcinoma) (3,4). All three stages of tumorigenesis may be influenced by chemical carcinogens.

A number of chemicals that are not directly mutagenic have been found to induce hepatic cancer in rodents (7–11). The mechanism(s) by which these compounds cause liver cancer are not known; however, a common characteristic of many is the ability to induce cell proliferation in the rodent liver (12). The proliferative stimulus provided by these chemicals may induce hepatic neoplasia through one of two mechanisms. First, the rapid and sustained induction of cell proliferation may result in the decreased fidelity of cellular DNA, producing an increased incidence of potentially critical DNA mutations (13). This rapid induction of cell proliferation may overwhelm normal cellular DNA repair mechanisms, eventually resulting in irreversibly altered cells. Alternatively, the nonmutagenic carcinogens may be acting as tumor promoters, producing hepatic cancer through the selective proliferation of previously initiated cells (11).

In our present research, we examined this latter possibility by assessing the role of cell proliferation in murine hepatic tumorigenesis induced by two nongenotoxic hepatic carcinogens, α-hexachlorocyclohexane (HCH) and phenobarbital (PB). Although neither compound exhibits any direct mutagenic activity, both HCH and PB have been shown to induce hepatocyte proliferation in the rodent liver and to promote the formation of hepatic tumors (6,8,11,12,15–19). Our investigation consisted of two phases. In the first, the hepatic tumor-promoting ability of these compounds was evaluated in the diethylnitrosamine (DENA)-initiated infant B6C3F1 mouse. In the second phase, we assessed the potential influence of short-term HCH and PB treatment on the induction of hepatocyte proliferation in noninitiated and DENA-initiated infant B6C3F1 mice. The initiated infant mouse was selected for the present research since this model has been shown to be highly sensitive to the induction of cancer following a single carcinogen treatment (20–22).

Materials and methods

Chemicals. We purchased DENA (Eastman Kodak Co., Rochester, NY), PB (Sigma Chemical Co., St. Louis. MO), and HCH (Aldrich Chemical Co., Milwaukee, WI). These chemicals were obtained in the highest available purities (99%+).

Animals. C3H male and C57Bl/6 female mice were obtained from Charles River Laboratories, Inc., Kingston, NY, and bred to produce B6C3F1 hybrid offspring. All mice received Certified Purina Rodent Chow #5002 (Ralston Purina Co., St. Louis, MO) and fresh drinking water ad libitum.

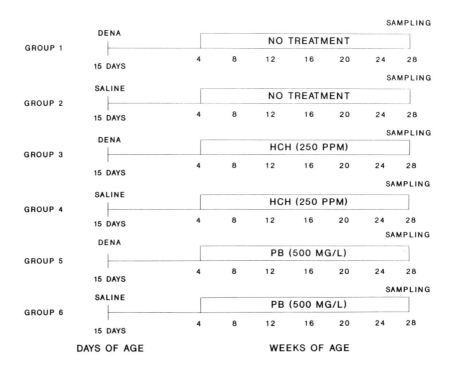

Figure 1. Experimental protocol for the evaluation of the hepatic tumor-promoting ability of PB and HCH in 15-day-old DENA-initiated B6C3F1 mice. Fifteen male and 15 female B6C3F1 mice were randomly assigned to each group. Mice were treated with either DENA (5 μg/g bw) (Groups 1,3, and 5) or saline (0.1 ml) (Groups 2,4, and 6) at 15 days of age. At 30 days of age, mice in Groups 3 and 4 received HCH (250 ppm) in their laboratory chow for 24 weeks while those in Groups 5 and 6 received PB (500 mg/l) in their drinking water for 24 weeks. Mice in Groups 1 and 2 received control diet and deionized drinking water. All mice were sampled at 28 weeks of age as described in the text.

Experiment 1

Fifteen-day-old mice were randomly distributed into six experimental groups (Fig. 1). Each group consisted of 15 male and 15 female B6C3F1 mice. Mice in Groups 1, 3, and 5 received a single intraperitoneal (i.p.) injection of DENA (5 µg/g body weight) in saline at 15 days of age. Similarly, mice in groups 2, 4, and 6 received a single i.p. injection of only saline at 15 days of age. At weaning (28 days of age), mice in Groups 3 and 4 received HCH in the diet (250 ppm), while mice in Groups 5 and 6 received PB in the drinking water (500 mg/l). Mice from Groups 1 and 2 were given deionized water and untreated basal diet throughout the study. At 24 weeks postweaning (28 weeks old), all mice were killed by carbon dioxide asphyxiation, weighed, and necropsied. Livers were removed, weighed, and examined for grossly visible lesions. Each liver was cut into 2-mm-thick slices, fixed in 10% phosphate-buffered formalin, embedded in paraffin, and sectioned. Hematoxylin and eosin (HE)-stained liver sections were subsequently examined by light microscopy and hepatic lesions were classified according to criteria previously defined (23–25). Statistical comparisons were subsequently performed using Fisher's exact test, one-way analysis of variance (ANOVA), and Scheffe's post hoc test.

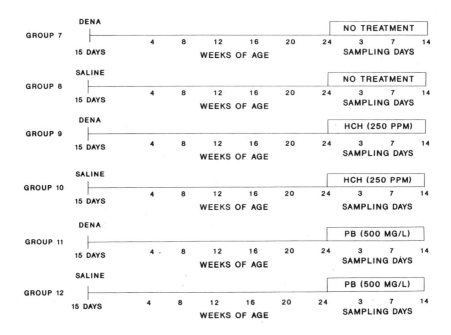

Figure 2. Experimental protocol for evaluation of hepatic DNA synthesis in B6C3F1 male and female mice. Mice were treated with DENA (5 µg/g bw) or saline (0.1 ml) at 15 days of age. Beginning at 24-weeks-old, mice were exposed to HCH in the diet (250 ppm), PB in the drinking water (500 mg/l), or no treatment. Osmotic mini-pumps containing [3H]thymidine were implanted in mice at the start of exposure and mice were sampled at 3, 7, or 14 days thereafter.

Experiment 2

In the second phase of the study, we assessed the responsiveness of preneoplastic hepatocellular foci in male and female B6C3F1 mice to HCH-or PB-induced DNA synthesis (Fig. 2). For this experiment, 15-day-old male and female mice were divided into six groups; each group had nine male and nine female mice. Mice in Groups 7, 9, and 11 each received a single i.p. injection of DENA (5 μg/g body weight) in saline at 15 days old, while mice in Groups 8, 10, and 12 received saline alone. Beginning at 24 weeks of age, mice in Groups 9 and 10 received HCH in the diet (250 ppm), while mice in Groups 11 and 12 received PB in the drinking water (500 mg/l). Mice in Groups 7 and 8 were maintained on deionized drinking water and untreated basal diet throughout the study. At the start of exposure, all mice in Groups 7–12 were implanted with osmotic minipumps (Model 2002, Alza Corp., Palo Alto, CA) containing [³H]thymidine (50 Ci/mmol; 1 μCi/ml) for evaluation of hepatic DNA synthesis. After 3, 7, and 14 days of exposure, 3 male and 3 female mice from each group were killed and necropsied. Livers were removed, weighed, cut into 2-mm slices, and fixed in 10% phosphate-buffered formalin. Deparaffinized tissue sections were dipped in NTB2 photographic emulsion (Eastman Kodak Co., Rochester, NY), exposed at 15°C for 5 weeks, developed, and then stained with HE. In these autoradiographs, the percentage of hepatocytes undergoing DNA synthesis was determined by counting the number of labeled and unlabeled hepatocytes. A minimum of 1,000 cells per area of interest were counted. DNA synthesis was assessed in hepatocellular foci and in the normal surrounding liver.

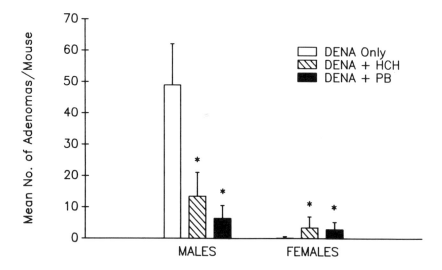

Figure 3. Effect of chronic HCH and PB treatment on hepatic tumorigenesis in non-initiated and DENA-initiated infant B6C3F1 mice. A value statistically different from respective DENA-only treatment group is indicated by an * (*P* < 0.05).

Statistical comparisons were subsequently performed using ANOVA and Scheffe's post hoc test (26).

Results

Figure 3 illustrates the results from Experiment 1. Hepatic foci or adenomas were not observed in untreated mice or in mice treated with HCH or PB alone. In contrast, hepatic foci and adenomas were seen in male and female mice receiving DENA only, DENA plus HCH, and DENA plus PB. The number of hepatic adenomas in male mice was increased in comparison to similarly treated female mice for all DENA treatments. Female mice receiving DENA plus HCH or DENA plus PB showed a significant increase in the incidence and multiplicity of hepatic adenomas, compared to females receiving DENA only. Male mice treated with DENA plus HCH or DENA plus PB showed a significant decrease in hepatic adenoma multiplicity compared with males receiving DENA only. No differences were observed for either gender in the incidence or multiplicity of hepatic foci in the DENA only–, DENA plus HCH–, or DENA plus PB–treated mice (data not shown).

In Experiment 2, DENA treatment (5 μg/g body weight) at 15 days of age produced hepatocellular foci in both male and female B6C3F1 mice. The foci and normal surrounding liver were subsequently evaluated for their responsiveness to the mitogenic stimulus of HCH and PB to determine if the gender-dependent difference

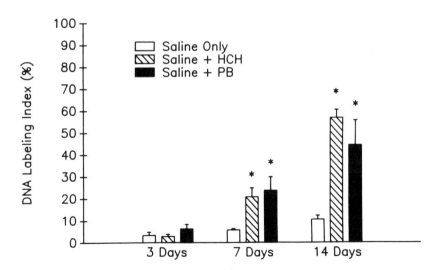

Figure 4. Hepatocyte DNA synthetic activity in noninitiated male B6C3F1 mice following short-term treatment with HCH, PB, or no treatment. A value statistically different from respective control (saline only) is indicated by an * ($P < 0.05$).

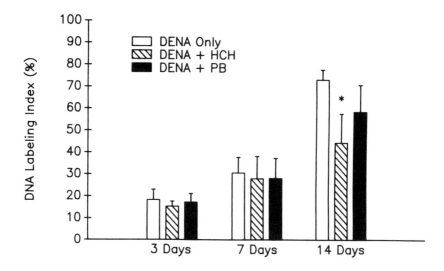

Figure 5. Hepatocyte DNA synthetic activity in DENA-initiated infant B6C3F1 male mice following short-term treatment with HCH, PB, or no treatment. A value statistically different from respective control (DENA only) is indicated by an * (P < 0.05).

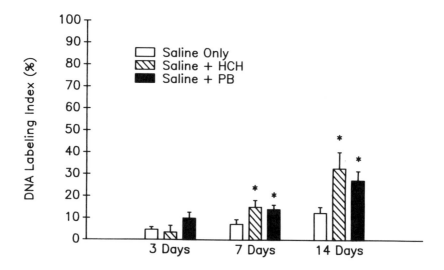

Figure 6. Hepatocyte DNA synthetic activity in noninitiated female B6C3F1 mice following short-term treatment with HCH, PB, or no treatment. A value statistically different from respective control (saline only) is indicated by an * (P < 0.05).

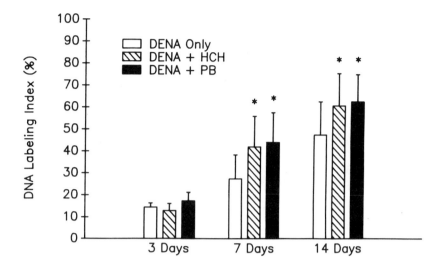

Figure 7. Hepatocyte DNA synthetic activity in DENA-initiated infant B6C3F1 female mice following short-term treatment with HCH, PB, or no treatment. A value statistically different from respective control (DENA only) is indicated by an * (P < 0.05).

in hepatic tumorigenesis seen with these compounds (observed in Experiment 1) correlated with their ability to induce DNA synthesis in preneoplastic hepatocellular foci. The results of Experiment 2 are presented in Figures 4–7. Figure 4 shows DNA labeling indices for male mice injected with saline and then treated with either HCH in the diet (250 ppm) or PB in the drinking water (500 mg/l). After 3 days of treatment, no significant differences were seen in the labeling indices of these three male groups. However, after 7 and 14 days of treatment, a significant elevation in hepatocyte DNA synthetic activity was observed in males receiving either HCH or PB compared to untreated (saline-only–treated) males. HCH-treated males were observed to have a fourfold and fivefold increase in hepatocyte DNA synthesis following 7 and 14 days of treatment, respectively. The DNA labeling index remained approximately four times higher in PB-treated males than in untreated males following both 7 and 14 days of exposure. DNA labeling indices for male mice initiated with DENA and then given HCH, PB, or no treatment are shown in Figure 5. DNA synthetic activity in the hepatocellular foci of HCH- and PB-treated males was comparable to that of untreated (DENA-only–treated) males following 3 and 7 days of exposure. After 14 days of treatment, the DNA labeling index in foci of HCH-treated males was significantly decreased compared to that in untreated males, while the DNA labeling index for foci in PB-treated males was lower than in untreated males, but not statistically different. DNA labeling indices for female mice injected with saline and then given either HCH, PB, or no treatment are shown in Figure 6.

Results for these female groups were similar to those described for males injected with saline and then given HCH, PB, or no treatment. However, the increase in hepatocyte DNA synthesis in females treated with HCH or PB for 7 and 14 days was of a lower magnitude than that observed for similarly treated male mice. After 7 days of promoter treatment, DNA synthesis in the HCH- and PB-treated females was approximately two times higher than that of untreated (saline-only–treated) females. After 14 days of promoter exposure, hepatocyte DNA synthesis in PB-treated females remained approximately two times higher than in untreated females, while the labeling index for HCH-treated females was further elevated, i.e., approximately three times higher than in untreated females. DNA labeling indices for female mice initiated with DENA and then given either HCH, PB, or no treatment are shown in Figure 7. After 3 days of treatment, no significant differences in hepatocyte DNA synthesis were observed in the hepatocellular foci of these groups. However, after 7 and 14 days of treatment, DNA labeling indices for foci of HCH- and PB-treated females were significantly increased compared to those of untreated (DENA-only–treated) females. At the 7-day sampling period, a 1.5-fold increase in DNA synthetic activity was seen in hepatocellular foci of females receiving HCH or PB. After 14 days of promoter treatment, labeling indices for foci of both HCH- and PB-treated females were approximately 1.3 times higher than that for untreated females.

Discussion

Previous investigations by our group and others using the DENA-initiated infant B6C3F1 mouse have shown that chronic exposure to liver tumor promoters inhibited hepatic tumorigenesis in male mice, while promoting hepatic tumor formation in female mice (9,10,15,16,18,19). In the present study, chronic HCH and PB exposure resulted in a similar gender-based difference in hepatic tumor formation in 15-day-old DENA-initiated B6C3F1 mice. Exposure to PB or HCH decreased the number of hepatic adenomas in male B6C3F1 mice compared to male mice receiving DENA only. In contrast, chronic PB or HCH treatment of female B6C3F1 mice promoted hepatic adenoma formation compared to female mice that received DENA only. The means by which these compounds inhibit or promote hepatic tumorigenesis in DENA-initiated infant male and female mice remains unclear. However, it is apparent that hepatocellular foci induced by DENA treatment in 15-day-old male and female mice respond differently to the induction of DNA synthesis by HCH and PB. Exposure stimulated DNA synthesis in female mice, but failed in male mice. PB and HCH exposure enhanced DNA synthetic activity in the liver of foci-free male and female mice, and in the normal surrounding liver of foci-containing male and female B6C3F1 mice, PB and HCH. This indicates that after short-term treatment, the normal hepatocytes remained responsive to the proliferative stimulus of these two liver tumor promoters. Based on these findings, it is clear that the ability of PB and HCH to stimulate DNA synthesis in hepatocellular foci of the B6C3F1 mice correlated with the ability of these compounds to promote or inhibit hepatic tumorigenesis. This suggests that foci produced in DENA-initiated infant male and female B6C3F1 mice may possess essential differences in their ability to respond to the proliferative effects of tumor promoters such as PB and HCH. Treatment of infant mice with initiating carcinogens such as DENA may result in different populations of initiated cells in the different genders. These initiated cells may give rise to a different population of hepatocellular foci possessing differing susceptibilities to tumor promotion. Four types of DENA-generated hepatocellular preoplastic cells may be postulated based upon the present results: 1) cells possessing the ability to advance to neoplasia irrespective of treatment with extrinsic tumor promoters; 2) cells advancing to neoplasia only under the direct influence of a promoting agent; 3) cells refractory to the influence of the promoter and thus dormant; and 4) cells that may, through direct interaction with the promoter, regress to the normal phenotype. DENA-generated preoplastic hepatocellular foci generated in the rat by DENA treatment have been shown to exhibit variable alterations in enzyme activity (27). These findings and the results of the present research support the hypothesis for the existence of different types of preoplastic cells induced by DENA treatment. Furthermore, it is now apparent that in the 15-day-old DENA-initiated B6C3F1 mouse, the ability of HCH and PB to promote hepatic tumorigenesis in females or inhibit males is in direct association with the ability of these compounds to induce DNA synthesis in hepatocellular foci. Together, these results suggest a causal relationship between the ability of nongenotoxic carcinogens to induce cell proliferation with their ability to promote or inhibit tumor formation in the mouse liver.

References

1. Farber E. Ethionine carcinogenesis. Adv Cancer Res 7:383–474, 1963.
2. Farber E, Camaron R. The sequential analysis of cancer development. Adv Cancer Res 31:125–226, 1980.
3. Schulte-Hermann R. Tumor promotion in the liver. Arch Toxicol 57:147–158, 1985.
4. Schulte-Hermann R. Initiation and promotion in hepatocarcinogenesis. Arch Toxicol 60:179–181, 1987.
5. Miller EC, Miller JA. Mechanisms of chemical carcinogenesis. Cancer 47:1055–1064, 1981.
6. Schulte-Hermann R, Timmermann-Trosiener I, Schuppler J. Response of liver foci in rats to hepatic tumor promoters. Toxicol Pathol 10:63–70, 1982.
7. Uchida E, Hirono I. Effect of phenobarbital on the induction of liver and lung tumors by dimethylnitrosamine. Jpn J Cancer Res 70:639–644, 1979.
8. Diwan BA, Rice JM, Ohshima M, Ward JM. Interstrain differences in susceptibility to liver carcinogenesis initiated by N-nitrosodiethylamine and its promotion by phenobarbital in C57Bl/6NCr, C3H/HeNCrmtv, and DBA/2NCr mice. Carcinogenesis 7:215–220, 1986.
9. Klaunig JE, Weghorst CM, Pereira MA. Effect of the age of B6C3F1 mice on phenobarbital promotion of diethylnitrosamine-initiated liver tumors. Toxicol Appl Pharmacol 90:79–85, 1987.
10. Klaunig JE, Pereir MA, Ruch RJ, Weghorst CM. Dose-response relationship of diethylnitrosamine-initiated tumors in neonatal Balb/c mice: Effect of phenobarbital promotion. Toxicol Pathol 16:381–385, 1988.
11. Schulte-Hermann R, Schuppler J, Ohde G, Timmermann-Trosiener I. Effect of tumor promoters on proliferation of putative preneoplastic cells in rat liver. Carcinogenesis 7:99–104, 1982.
12. Schulte-Hermann R, Parzefall W. Failure to discriminate initiation from promotion of liver tumors in a long-term study with the phenobarbital-type promoter α-hexachlorocyclohexane and the role of sustained stimulation of hepatic growth and monooxygenases. Cancer Res 41:4140–4146, 1981.
13. Schulte-Hermann R, Schuppler J, Timmermann-Trosiener I, Ohde G, Bursch W, Berger H. The role of growth of normal and preneoplastic cell populations for tumor promotion in rat liver. Environ Health Perspect 50:185–194, 1983.
14. Schroter C, Parzefall W, Schroter H, Schulte-Hermann R. Dose-Response studies on the effects of α, β and γ-hexachlorocyclohexane on putative preneoplastic foci, monooxygenases, and growth in rat liver. Cancer Res 47:80–88, 1987.
15. Diwan BA, Rice JM, Ward JM, Ohshima M, Lynch PH. Inhibition by phenobarbital and lack of effect

of amobarbital on the development of liver tumors induced by N-nitrosodiethylamine in juvenile B6C3F1 mice. Cancer Lett 23:223–234, 1984.

16. Klaunig JE, Weghorst CM, Pereira MA. Effect of phenobarbital on diethylnitrosamine and dimethylnitrosamine induced hepatocellular tumors in male B6C3F1 mice. Cancer Lett 42:133–139, 1988.

17. Pereira MA, Knutsen GL, Herren-Freund SA. Effect of subsequent treatment of chloroform or phenobarbital on the incidence of liver and lung tumors in initiated by ethylnitrosourea in 15 day old mice. Carcinogenesis 6:203–207, 1984.

18. Pereira MA, Klaunig JE, Herren-Freund SL, Ruch RJ. Effect of phenobarbital on the development of liver tumors in juvenile and adult mice. J Natl Cancer Inst 77:449–452, 1986.

19. Weghorst CM, Klaunig JE. Phenobarbital promotion in diethylnitrosamine-initiated infant B6C3F1 mice: Influence of gender. Carcinogenesis 10:609–612, 1989.

20. Vesselinovitch SD, Rao KVN, Mihailovich N, Rice JM, Lombard S. Development of broad spectrum of tumors by ethylnitrosourea in mice and the modifying role of age, sex, and strain. Cancer Res 34:2530–2538, 1974.

21. Vesselinovitch SD. Certain aspects of hepatocarcinogenesis in the infant mouse model. Toxicol Pathol 15:221–228, 1987.

22. Vesselinovitch SD, Mihailovich N. Kinetics of diethylnitrosamine hepatocarcinogenesis in the infant mouse. Cancer Res 43:4253–4259, 1983.

23. Frith CH, Ward JM. A morphologic classification of proliferative and neoplastic lesions in mice. J Environ Pathol Toxicol 3:329–351, 1979.

24. Lipsky MM, Hinton DE, Klaunig JE. Biology of hepatocellular neoplasia in the mouse. I. Histogenesis of safrole-induced hepatocellular carcinoma. J Natl Cancer Inst 67:365–376, 1981.

25. Ward JM. Morphology of potential preneoplastic hepatocyte lesions and liver tumors in mice and a comparison with other species. In: Popp JA (ed): Mouse Liver Neoplasia: Current Perspectives. Hemisphere, Washington, DC., 1984, pp. 1–26.

26. Gad S, Weil CS. Statistics and Experimental Design for Toxicologists. Telford Press, New Jersey, 1986.

27. Pitot HC, Barnsness L, Goldsworthy T, Kitagawa T. Biochemical characterization of stages of hepatocarcinogenesis after a single dose of diethylnitrosamine. Nature 271:456–458, 1978.

Chemically Induced Cell Proliferation:
Implications for Risk Assessment, pages 417-428
©1991 Wiley-Liss, Inc.

Control of 1,2-Dimethylhydrazine–Induced Crypt Hyperplasia by Natural-Killer Cells and Its Relevance to Carcinogenesis

Gabriel G. Altmann and Peeyush K. Lala

We have examined the effects of chronic doses of 1,2-dimethylhydrazine (DMH) on the various parts of the small intestine in young-adult male Wistar rats (1,2) and on the duodenum in young-adult male CD1 mice (3). The resultant crypt hyperplasia and concomitant expansion of the mitotic pool of crypt cells were quantitated by histometry, according to methods worked out earlier (4–6). These measurements were made at various time points during the chronic treatment as well as after various DMH dosages, and after elimination or activation of the host natural-killer (NK) cell population. These results together with some new data have identified a central role of NK cells in the containment of hyperplasia, along with possible mechanisms that may permit progression of hyperplasia to neoplasia. An overview of this work and its relevance to chemical carcinogenesis is presented here.

Conclusions from the rat model

Young-adult Wistar male rats received 25 mg/kg DMH subcutaneously twice a week for 3 months; then the dose was halved to 25 mg/kg once a week. The latter dose was administered for 3 additional months, that is, the total treatment time was 6 months. Sacrifice was at 1-month intervals, with histologic samples taken from the duodenum, jejunum, and upper, middle, and lower ileum. Crypt cells and mitotic cells were each counted in representative crypt sections. In our experience, these absolute cell numbers are sensitive and reliable measures of crypt size and mitotic activity (4–6).

In all samples, crypt size increased gradually during the first 3 months, then transiently dropped to near control levels after the DMH dose was halved by less-frequent administration. This drop amounted to a nearly complete disappearance of hyperplasia, and will be referred to henceforth as "regression." Crypt size after a month started to increase again, but at a slower rate that was in proportion to the lowered DMH dose. The rate of increase in crypt size was thus proportional to the level of the DMH dose, whereas the extent of the (short-lasting) regression of the hyperplasia exceeded the extent of the decrease in the DMH dose level. Additional, host-related factors were therefore assumed to play a role in the countering of hyperplasia that made up the regression phase (see below).

The mitotic number changed in proportion to crypt size, that is, the ratio of the two values, or mitotic index, remained constant. In other words, the relative durations of mitosis and interphase in the cell cycle remained essentially unaltered during the DMH treatment. This finding indicates that both the hyperplasia and its regression took place in the cycling pool of the crypt cells.

If average cell cycle parameters remain constant, an increase in mitotic number may mean an increased recruitment of reserve stem cells into the cycle or an increased number of differentiative (terminal) divisions in a fraction of the cycling cells. Since reserve stem cells are not present in the epithelium of the small intestine (7), the latter effect was assumed. This would mean that a fraction of the population of cycling cells underwent more than the usual three terminal divisions before differentiating into nonmitotic, functional cells. Thus, these cells had a changed mitotic pattern, and their number as well as their extra number of mitoses could be calculated using cell kinetic considerations (2).

Carcinogens are believed to act primarily at the stem cell level, where they bring about minor genetic alterations (8,9). It was assumed that the progeny of these altered stem cells constituted the altered cycling population in the crypts and therefore the source of the crypt hyperplasia. The computed number of these altered cells was shown to increase linearly during the first 3 months of DMH treatment; it then dropped to near zero (regression) after the DMH dose was halved and then started to rise again linearly at half the previous rate (Fig. 1).

The mechanism that allows altered cycling cells to be produced may be envisaged as a result of genetic alterations in a fraction of the stem cells. The progeny of these stem cells—which we may refer to as altered transit, or cycling, cells—were thus seen to accumulate in a manner dependent on the DMH dose and were also seen to regress to a number close to zero when the DMH dose was halved (Fig. 1). This regression was clearly due to more than just the lowering of the DMH dose. We hypothesized (2) that a lowering of the DMH dose may have allowed a partial recovery of the natural host cellular defense mechanism(s) (e.g., NK cells, which may exert a containing role on the altered cycling cells of the crypt). We confirmed this hypothesis in a mouse model (3), as summarized below.

Conclusions from the mouse model

Young-adult male CD1 mice were used. The effects of DMH were evaluated on the duodenum (3). Various DMH doses were used: 30 mg/kg/week (medium dose), 60 mg/kg/week (high dose), and 100 mg/kg/week (very high dose); all these doses were administered for 4–20 weeks. Crypt hyperplasia in the mouse was quite extensive within 1 month of the beginning of treatment (15–30% after the medium dose); its extent appeared to be primarily dependent on DMH dose rather than on treatment duration. Treatment for longer than 1 month did not increase the hyperplasia. The very high dose produced 42% hyperplasia, which was enhanced to 54% after concomitant intraperitoneal administration of anti–asialo GM-1 antibody (αAGM-1) for 1 week. Similarly, some enhancement of hyperplasia was observed when the medium and the high doses were supplemented with αAGM-1. This antibody selectively eliminates the NK cells (10). The enhancement of hyperplasia indicated the involvement of the NK cells in controlling hyperplasia. This, however, could not be demonstrated conclusively in these experiments because, by using the standard ^{51}Cr-release assay with ^{51}Cr-labeled YAC-1 lymphoma targets, DMH itself was found to suppress NK activity of host splenocytes (3).

The proof for the role of the NK cells came from study of the regression phase (Fig. 2) combined with a selective depletion of host NK activity in vivo. After the medium-level DMH dose was halved (to 15 mg/kg/week), crypt hyperplasia completely disappeared, and crypt size (Fig. 2, top) and mitotic number (Fig. 2, bottom) returned to normal (control) values. It did not seem to make a difference whether we took the samples 2 or 5 weeks after halving the DMH dose. When the DMH half-dose was repeatedly supplemented with αAGM-1, the regression did not take place either in total crypt (Fig. 2, top) or mitotic (Fig. 2, bottom) cell number. This treatment totally abolished host NK activity, and crypt hyperplasia remained at the level induced by the former medium-level DMH dose (Fig. 2). Since depletion of NK cells prevented the regression, it must have been caused by host NK cells. The αAGM-1 by itself did not cause any hyperplasia in control animals.

After it was observed that elimination of the NK cells restored hyperplasia, activation of these cells was attempted by administering polyinosinic-polycytidylic acid (poly I:C) to DMH-treated mice (Fig. 2). This compound augments NK activity by stimulating interferon production (11). Poly I:C treatment caused a marked reduction of crypt size (Fig. 2, top) and mitotic number (Fig. 2, bottom) in DMH-treated mice, whereas it produced no such reduction in control animals.

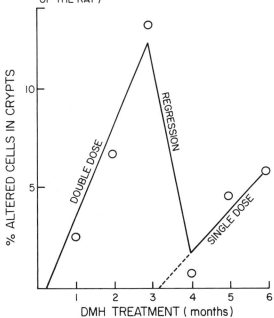

NUMBER OF ALTERED CELLS IN CRYPTS
(POOLED FOR THE WHOLE SMALL INTESTINE OF THE RAT)

Figure 1. Number of altered cells, in the form of percentage (circles) (calculated from data in ref. 2), plotted against the length of chronic DMH treatment. The dose of DMH was 25 mg/kg twice a week during the first 3 months and 25 mg/kg once a week during the next 3 months. A linear increase in number of altered cells occurred during both dose periods (coefficient of variation, 0.9–1 for the two lines of best fit), with a drop to near zero between the two periods. This drop is referred to as regression. Since regression exceeded that which would be expected on the basis of the dose change alone, it was proposed that host defenses came into play.

The above experiments, employing an elimination or an activation of NK cells, indicated that the crypts of DMH-treated mice contained a sizable population of NK sensitive cells. These cells then are the altered cells that had been postulated, on the basis of kinetic considerations, to be present in the hyperplastic crypts. Thus, they express NK target structures and in all probability represent the cycling progeny of the genetically altered stem cells (Fig. 3).

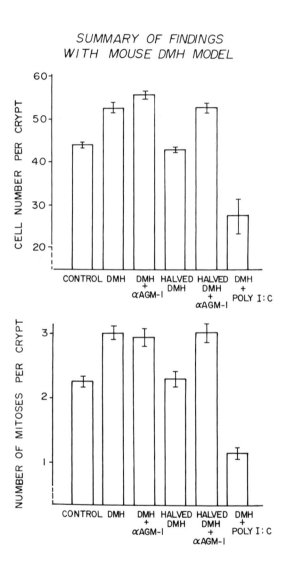

SUMMARY OF FINDINGS
WITH MOUSE DMH MODEL

Figure 2. Summary of results of histometric measurements in mice in experiments described in reference 3: (top) mean number of crypt cells (±SEM) per representative crypt; (bottom) mean mitotic number (±SEM) per representative crypt. Both values were increased significantly over control with DMH given chronically at 30 mg/kg/week. Further but minor increase in crypt size and maintenance of the increase in mitoses was seen when DMH was supplemented by intraperitoneal αAGM-1 for 2 or 5 weeks. When the halved DMH dose was supplemented with αAGM-1, the regression did not take place: the crypt cell number and the mitotic number remained at the levels corresponding to the 30 mg/kg/week dose of DMH. Since αAGM-1 is specific in eliminating the NK cell population, regression was caused by the NK cells. When DMH was supplemented with poly I:C for 5 days, crypt cell number and mitotic number decreased markedly, to about half the control value. Poly I:C activates NK cells, which in this experiment then eliminated most cells carrying NK target structures. Such cells were probably numerous in the crypts in this set of experiments. That sizable crypts remained indicates that normal cells not sensitive to NK cells were present.

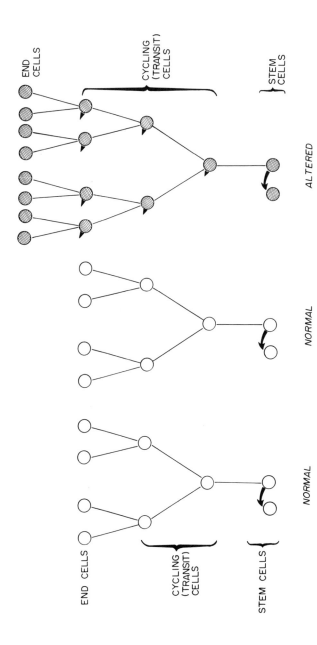

Figure 3. Our present concept of DMH-induced crypt hyperplasia is illustrated. The crypts would contain normal and altered stem cells. Statistically, all stem cell division would yield one daughter cell that remains a stem cell and one transit cell. The transit cells normally undergo about two more terminal divisions and then differentiate into non-mitotic, functional cells. The altered transit cells—that is, the progeny of the altered stem cells—undergo more than the normal number of terminal divisions. The progeny express NK cell target structures (illustrated as triangles) and cause hyperplasia as long as NK activity is inhibited. Since altered stem cells apparently escape killing by NK cells, they may not express the target structures or they may be in a secluded microenvironment not accessible to NK cells.

Further results on the role of the NK cells

If the NK cells eliminate all the altered stem cells as well as the altered proliferative transit cells after the hyperplasia regresses, there should be no memory left of the previous initiation and of the former presence of altered cells. On the other hand, if some or all of the altered stem cells escape elimination by the NK cells and only the transit cells are eliminated, the hyperplasia would be revived by the elimination of NK cells at any time after regression is produced. Indeed, this was observed in a study initiated recently in our laboratory (in progress). The administration of the medium DMH dose (30 mg/kg/week) was stopped at 2 months. The mice were then left without treatment for 1 month, during which time the crypts regressed to normal size and mitotic activity. At the end of this 1-month period, αAGM-1 was administered every 2 days for 1 week. Hyperplasia and mitotic number returned to the level seen with the medium DMH dose (Fig. 4). This indicated the survival of the altered stem cells for at least 1 month. This would mean that either the altered stem cells are not direct targets of the NK cells or they are in a protective microenvironment not accessible to the NK cells.

Histologic examination showed large, solitary lymphoid-type cells in the crypts of DMH-treated mice (3,12). They were seen in close proximity to cells of the lower and middle crypt, where the transit cells are present. They were not seen as a rule in the crypt base, where the stem cells are located. These large lymphoid cells may represent NK cells that migrate into the crypts to eliminate the target cells. This question is being examined further by immunocytochemical methods.

Implications concerning the promotion phase of carcinogenesis

Our results so far indicate that the early phase of DMH carcinogenesis involves production of altered stem cells (initiation) by DMH and that these stem cells in turn produce a progeny of altered transit cells, which become targets of the NK cells. The NK cells, on the other hand, are themselves inactivated by the DMH. This may allow a survival of the initiated cells and their progeny, allowing the DMH to exert its promoting action. A few carcinogens have been shown to suppress NK activity (13–15); such suppression by DMH was shown in our recent work (3). In the experiment in which crypt hyperplasia was made to recur by the administration of αAGM-1 (Fig. 4), the antibody could theoretically be viewed as a promoter. In the intestinal model of carcinogenesis, a promoter may thus need only to inactivate NK cells, as innate mitogenic influences probably are present in the tissue. Until now, the mitogenic nature of promoters has been emphasized as a most important property since it ensures the growth of the initiated cell population (16,17). There is some evidence that phorbol esters, which have been emphasized so far for their mitogenic influence, also exert a suppressing effect on NK activity (18).

In the stage of DMH carcinogenesis we examined for regression (first 12–16 weeks), the crypt hyperplasia was fully reversible. According to Richards (19), in later stages of carcinogenesis, hyperplasia can no longer be reversed by stopping the DMH administration. There is a possibility that in this later stage, host NK cells may be inhibited by another mechanism such as the production of prostaglandin E_2 (PGE$_2$), similar to that observed in the tumor-bearing host (20). Furthermore, it was shown that chronic administration of indomethacin to block PGE_2 synthesis revived host NK activity and halted tumor progression and metastasis (21). In the phase of DMH carcinogenesis we have examined so far, indomethacin was found to be ineffective for reviving NK activity and preventing crypt hyperplasia (unpublished data). It remains to be tested whether indomethacin is effective in the late promotion phase, when the crypts no longer regress spontaneously. It is possible, then, that in the intestinal model, like in the skin (22), the promotion phase has more than one stage.

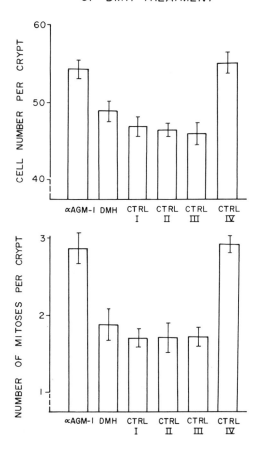

EFFECT OF αAGM-1
AFTER INTERRUPTION
OF DMH TREATMENT

Figure 4. Preliminary results (values ±SEM) are shown. The mice received DMH at 30 mg/kg/week for 2 months; then the treatment was stopped. A month later, αAGM-1 alone was administered intraperitoneally every 2 days for 1 week. Crypt size (top) and mitotic number (bottom) increased to the level corresponding to the chronic DMH dose. Resumption of DMH administration (second column) increased both values over control, but only to a slight degree. Control I (CTRL I) represents a group treated with DMH for 2 months, the treatment then stopped for 1 month, at which time the animals were killed. Control II represents sham controls, injected with the vehicle only for 2 months, after which no further treatment was given. Control III represents DMH-untreated animals that received only αAGM-1 for 1 week. Control IV represents a group that was maintained on the chronic DMH dose at the time of killing.

Implications concerning the progression of hyperplasia to dysplasia and neoplasia

Under chronic DMH administration, the stage of adenoma and adenocarcinoma is reached within 9 months. Most tumors occur in the colon, but the duodenum and jejunum may show a reasonable yield, especially with the higher DMH doses (23–25). In current DMH protocols, about a 1- or 2-month period of chronic DMH administration is regarded as a period of initiation (26). The next 5 or 6 months are regarded as a period of "promotion." The animals do not receive the carcinogen during this period, and tumors develop within about 1 year. Just one treatment with DMH or a related compound is also sufficient to provide some tumor yield (reviewed in ref. 27). Progression can thus take place spontaneously. It is possible that the main requirement during this period is suppression of NK activity, which may take place through various mechanisms, including PGE_2 production. An alternative hypothesis would be that some or all of the altered stem cells undergo a gradual spontaneous change toward the neoplastic genome, so that tumors may develop at locations not accessible to the NK cells.

It has been a consistent observation that adenomas and adenocarcinomas occur at hyperplastic sites (28–30), but the transition from the hyperplasia to neoplastic cells is not fully understood. In our rat model, a few adenomas and adenocarcinomas appeared within 6 months, all located in the duodeno-jejunal region. The level of crypt hyperplasia was highest at the tumor sites. All parameters of hyperplasia were substantially increased here within the otherwise normal-looking tissue surrounding the tumors (1). Thus, crypt cell number, mitotic number, and average nucleolar size were increased above controls by 18, 36 and 71%, respectively, whereas in the nontumorous tissue these values were 10, 22, and 29% above control as a part of the generalized hyperplasia due to the DMH treatment. It appeared that by some as-yet-unknown mechanism, tumor sites and highly hyperplastic sites were interrelated.

Generally, neoplasia is probably a result of several series of mutations, or "hits," which after several stages lead to the neoplastic genome (31,32). This multi-hit theory of cancer development may explain some of the findings with the DMH model of carcinogenesis. The first hit would generate the altered stem cells. This would be recognizable morphologically as the ensuing hyperplasia caused by the progeny of these cells. It is likely that in this altered cell population, the genome is more predisposed to further hits than elsewhere, since progression usually takes place in areas of hyperplasia. The second series of genetic hits would occur either as a result of spontaneous mutation or as an effect of mutagens contained in the diet. Morphologically, this would be recognized as atypical and dysplastic crypts in which a part of the cell population does not follow the normal regulatory signals and accumulates at unusual locations in the stream of normal cells migrating to the villi. In this stage, a shift of [³H]thymidine-labeled mitotic cells toward the crypt apex would be seen (33,34), or microadenomas would be present in various parts of the crypts (25,35).

We have preliminarily tested the validity of the multi-hit theory using our model of carcinogenesis. If the dysplastic stage is a result of further mutations, feeding mutagens to the DMH-treated mice might bring about this stage relatively early. Therefore, in four mice kept on DMH treatment for 2 months we supplemented the diet for the last 2 weeks with 2-aminofluorene; that supplementation was immediately preceded by a single gastric instillation of 20-methylcholanthrene (40 mg/kg) dissolved in corn oil. This protocol was based on the report that after pretreatment of mice with 20-methylcholanthrene, 2-aminofluorene becomes mutagenic to small intestinal epithelial cells (36). Two of the four animals, after the 2 weeks of 2-aminofluorene, displayed several microadenomas with some regularity in the lower duodenal crypts (Fig. 5–8). The microadenomas contained small basophilic cells very different in appearance from the columnar cells of the crypts. Controls that received only DMH or only DMH plus 2-aminofluorene (i.e., no 20-methylcholanthrene) did not show changes other than hyperplasia.

Conclusion

The role of NK cells in eliminating certain primary tumors and their metastases is reasonably well established (e.g., refs. 37–41). The role of these cells in carcinogenesis,

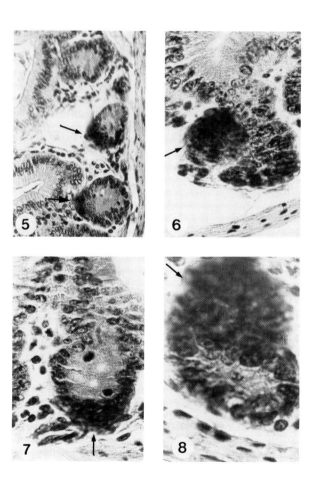

Figure 5–8. Histologic sections from the lower duodenum stained with periodic acid–Schiff and hematoxylin. The mice received regular DMH treatment for 2 months. In addition, they received 2-a m i n o f l u o r e n e (0.05%) in their diet during the last 2 weeks. Prior to the inclusion of 2-aminofluorene in the diet, the small intestinal epithelium was sensitized to this mutagen by a single, intragastric dose of 20-methylcholanthrene. Microadenomas (arrows) occurred with some regularity at various locations in the crypts. The microadenomas appear as darkish masses because they contain small basophilic cells very different from the normal columnar crypt cells. (Magnifications: Fig. 5, ×370; Fig. 6, × 790; Fig. 7, × 830; Fig. 8, ×1030.)

however, has remained unknown; the few experiments addressing this question were indecisive because the carcinogens themselves suppressed NK activity (e.g., refs. 13–15). Our studies employing depletion and stimulation of NK cells permitted a rigorous testing of the role of these cells in the early events of DMH carcinogenesis.

The finding that the NK cell–mediated control becomes effective early in carcinogenesis has important implications for the entire process of carcinogenesis. Most importantly, it implies that the fraction of altered cells in the hyperplastic crypts express NK target structures and therefore are likely to be lysed by the NK cells unless NK activity is suppressed. A most important requirement for a promoter, then, is to suppress NK activity. Such a suppressing mechanism is probably present endogenously in the intestine in the form of bile acids, which are known to elevate PGE_2 levels (42). PGE_2, in turn, is inhibitory to NK cells (41). Thus, autochthonous promotion in the intestine is possible.

The further events in carcinogenesis probably correspond to events predictable by the multi-hit theory of cancer and would involve spontaneous mutations or action of environmental mutagens on the altered cell population in which the genome is probably predisposed to some degree of further changes. In this respect our preliminary experiment with a mutagen in the diet is relevant. After only 2 weeks of this diet in mice treated for 2 months with DMH, unexpectedly high numbers of microadenomas appeared in part of the upper small intestine. It is likely (but still to be tested) that some such adenomas would become neoplastic under longer influence of the mutagen or perhaps other mutagens.

A general implication of the present work would be that carcinogenesis can be interrupted very early by stimulation of host NK cells. Immunoprevention of cancer may thus be possible following exposure to carcinogens.

Acknowledgments

This work was supported by grants from the Cancer Research Society of Canada (G.G.A.) and the National Cancer Institute of Canada (P.K.L.). The authors are grateful to L. A. Schembri for his expert technical assistance.

References

1. Snow AD, Altmann GG. A morphometric study of the rat duodenal epithelium during the initial six months of 1,2-dimethylhydrazine carcinogenesis. Cancer Res 43:4838–4849, 1983.
2. Altmann GG, Snow AD. Effects of 1,2-dimethylhydrazine on the number of epithelial cells present in the villi, crypts and mitotic pool along the rat small intestine. Cancer Res 44:5522–5531, 1984.
3. Altmann GG, Parhar RS, Lala PK. Hyperplasia of mouse duodenal crypts and its control by NK cells during the initial phase of DMH carcinogenesis. Int J Cancer, 1990.
4. Altmann GG, Leblond CP. Factors influencing villus size in the small intestine of adult rats as revealed by transposition of intestinal segments. Am J Anat 127:15–36, 1970.
5. Altmann GG. Influence of bile and pancreatic secretions on the size of the villi of the small intestine in the rat. Am J Anat 132:167–178, 1971.
6. Altmann GG. Influence of starvation and refeeding on mucosal size and epithelial renewal in the rat small intestine. Am J Anat 133:391–400, 1972.

7. Cheng H, Leblond CP. Origin, differentiation, and renewal of the four main epithelial cell types in the mouse small intestine. I. Columnar cell. Am J Anat 141:461–480, 1974.
8. Miller EC, Miller JA. Searches for ultimate chemical carcinogens and their reactions with cellular macromolecules. Cancer 47:2327–2345, 1981.
9. Potten CS. Clonogenic, stem and carcinogen-target cells in small intestine. Scand J Gastroenterol Suppl 104:3–14, 1984.
10. Kasai M, Yoneda T, Habu S, Maruyama Y, Okumura K, Tokunaga T. In vivo effect of anti-asialo GM1 antibody on natural killer activity. Nature 291:334–335, 1981.
11. Oehler JR, Herberman RB. Natural killer cell-mediated cytotoxicity in rats. III. Effects of immunopharmacologic treatments on natural reactivity and on reactivity augmented by polyinosinic-polycytidylic acid. Int J Cancer 21:221–229, 1978.
12. Altmann GG, Parhar RS, Lala PK. Accumulation of altered crypt cells and their sensitivity to NK cells during early DMH carcinogenesis in the murine duodenum. Proceedings of 32nd annual meeting of the Canadian Federation of Biological Societies, University of Calgary, June 14–17, 1989, 1989; p 142.
13. Gorelik E, Herberman RB. Inhibition of the activity of mouse natural killer cells by urethane. J Natl Cancer Inst 66:543–548, 1981.
14. Ehrlich R, Efrati M, Malatzky E, Shochat L, Bar-Eyal A, Witz IP. Natural host defence during oncogenesis. NK activity and dimethylbenzanthracene carcinogenesis. Int J Cancer 31:67–73, 1983.
15. Kalland T, Forsberg JG. 3-Methylocholanthrene transiently inhibits the lytic step of mouse natural killer cells. J Natl Cancer Inst 72:385–390, 1983.
16. Becker FF. Recent concepts of initiation and promotion in carcinogenesis. Am J Pathol 105:3–9, 1981.
17. Friedman EA. A multistage model for human colon carcinoma development from tissue culture studies. Prog Clin Biol Res 186:175–186, 1985.
18. Tanaka K, Chang KSS. Modulation of natural killer sensitivity of murine trophoblast cells by tumor promoter and interferon. Int J Cancer 29:315–321, 1982.
19. Richards TC. Changes in crypt cell populations of mouse colon during recovery from treatment with 1,2-dimethylhydrazine. J Natl Cancer Inst 66:907–912, 1981.
20. Parhar RS, Lala PK. Changes in the host natural killer cell population in mice during tumor development. II. The mechanism of suppression of NK activity. Cell Immunol 93:265–279, 1985.
21. Lala PK, Parhar RS, Singh P. Indomethacin therapy abrogates the prostaglandin-mediated suppression of natural killer activity in tumor-bearing mice and prevents tumor metastasis. Cell Immunol 99:108–118, 1986.
22. Slaga TJ. Host factors in the susceptibility of mice to tumour initiating and promoting agents. In: Turusov V, Montesano R (eds): Modulators of Experimental Carcinogenesis. Lyons: International Agency for Research on Cancer, 1983, pp. 257–273.
23. Wiebecke B, Key U, Lohrs U, Eder M. Morphological and autoradiographical investigations on experimental carcinogenesis and polyp development in the intestinal tract of rats and mice. Virchows Arch [A] 360:179–193, 1973.
24. Chang WWL. Histogenesis of symmetrical 1,2-dimethylhydrazine–induced neoplasms of the colon in the mouse. J Natl Cancer Inst 60:1405–1418, 1978.
25. Sunter JP. Experimental carcinogenesis and cancer in the rodent gut. In: Appleton DR, Sunter JP, Watson AJ (eds): Cell proliferation in the gastrointestinal tract. London: Pitman Medical, 1980, pp. 255–277.
26. Temple NJ, El Khatib SM. Effect of high fat and nutrient depleted diets on colon tumor formation in mice. Cancer Lett 37:109–114, 1987.
27. Nigro ND. Animal model for colorectal cancer. Prog Clin Biol Res 186:161–173, 1985.
28. Williamson RC, Bauer FL, Terpstra OT, Ross JS, Malt RA. Contrasting effects of subtotal enteric bypass, enterectomy and colectomy on azoxy methane–induced intestinal carcinogenesis. Cancer Res 40:538–543, 1980.
29. Williamson RC, Rainey JB. The relationship between intestinal hyperplasia and carcinogenesis. Scand J Gastroenterol Suppl 104:57–76, 1984.
30. Rainey JB, Davies PW, Williamson RC. Effect of hypothermia on intestinal adaptation and carcinogenesis in the rat. Br J Cancer 55:265–268, 1987.
31. Peto R. Detection of risk of cancer to man. Proc R Soc Lond [Biol] 205:111–120, 1979.
32. Dix D, Cohen P, Flannery J. On the role of aging in cancer incidence. J Theor Biol 83:163–173, 1980.
33. Lipkin M. Phase 1 and phase 2 proliferative lesions of colonic epithelial cells in diseases leading to colonic cancer. Cancer 34:878–888, 1974.

34. Lipkin M, Deschner E. Early proliferative changes in intestinal cells. Cancer Res 36:2665–2668, 1976.
35. Wright N, Alison M. The Biology of Epithelial Cell Populations. Oxford: Clarendon Press, 1984, pp. 805–841.
36. Fouarge M, Mercier M, Poncelet F. Liver, kidney and small-intestine microsomal-mediated mutagenicity of carcinogenic aromatic amines. Mutat Res 125:23–31, 1984.
37. Greenberg AH, Green M. Non-adaptive rejection of small tumour inocula as a model of immune surveillance. Nature 264:356–359, 1976.
38. Haller O, Hansson M, Kiessling R, Wigzell H. Role of non-conventional natural killer cells in resistance against syngeneic tumour cells in vivo. Nature 270:609–611, 1977.
39. Hanna N, Fidler I. Role of natural killer cells in the destruction of circulating tumor emboli. J Natl Cancer Inst 65:801–809, 1980.
40. Riccardi C, Santoni T, Barlozzari T, Pucetti P, Herberman RB. In vivo natural reactivity of mice against tumor cells. Int J Cancer 25:475–486, 1980.
41. Lala PK. PGE_2-mediated inactivation of potentially tumoricidal effector cells of the host during tumor development. Relevance to metastasis and immunotherapy. In: Abraham S (ed): Carcinogenesis and Dietary Fat. Boston: Kluwer Academic Publishers, 1989, pp. 219–232.
42. Narisawa T, Takahashi M, Niwa M, Fukaura Y, Wakizaka A. Involvement of prostaglandin E_2 in bile acid–caused promotion of colon carcinogenesis and anti-promotion by the cyclooxygenase inhibitor indomethacin. Jpn J Cancer Res 78:791–798, 1984.

Chemically Induced Cell Proliferation:
Implications for Risk Assessment, pages 429-438
©1991 Wiley-Liss, Inc.

Biochemical Basis of Allylamine-Induced Aortic Smooth Muscle Cell Proliferation

Lydia R. Cox and Kenneth S. Ramos

The pathways that govern normal cellular growth and differentiation, as well as those that guide pathologic progression, have been the focus of intense research in recent years. A number of unrelated medical disorders such as rheumatoid arthritis, pulmonary fibrosis, cancer, and atherosclerosis are characterized by uncontrolled cellular proliferation. Thus, it is likely that common pathways are associated with the deregulation of cell proliferation in these disparate conditions. Our laboratory is particularly interested in the processes by which chemical exposure alters vascular cell function and modulates smooth muscle cell differentiation and growth. A chemically induced disease state that resembles naturally occurring atherosclerosis presents a useful model in which to study the cellular and molecular alterations associated with enhanced proliferation of vascular smooth muscle cells.

Medial smooth muscle cells of the normal adult aorta are primarily in a quiescent state of growth (1) and are specialized for contraction (2). The contractile state of these cells within the normal blood vessel wall is considered a functional extreme in the phenotypic spectrum (2). Under the influence of various stimuli, they may modulate toward a different functional extreme characterized by enhanced synthetic or proliferative activity. Cells in the synthetic state are not specialized for contraction but are distinguished by their ability to migrate, proliferate, and synthesize and secrete extracellular matrix components (2). Phenotypic modulation of smooth muscle cells occurs during various physiologic processes, including fetal and postnatal development (3), regeneration and repair of blood vessels (2), and myometrial development during pregnancy (3). Such phenotypic changes are reversible and occur as functional adaptations during normal growth and development.

Modulation of the smooth muscle cell phenotype is also an early event in the pathogenesis of atherosclerosis (2,4). Unlike the normal growth and development process, phenotypic modulation during progressive pathologic conditions may not be fully reversible. The cellular signals that mediate the modulation of smooth muscle cells from a contractile to synthetic phenotype, either in normal development or in diseased states, are not yet known.

The structural and compositional changes within the vascular wall characteristic of the atherosclerotic process are of a progressive nature (5,6). In its earliest stages, atherosclerosis is characterized by focal intimal thickenings, lesions that primarily consist of smooth muscle cells. Macrophages, extracellular matrix components, and intra- and extracellular lipids accumulate within the intima as the lesion advances. Intimal thickenings may progress to fibrous plaques as a function of age. Fibrous lesions contain a larger number of smooth muscle cells as well as macrophages and other leukocytic cells, necrotic debris, and cholesterol; the deposition of collagen, elastin, and proteoglycans is also increased. The proliferation of smooth muscle cells and accumulation of extracellular matrix components within the lesion contribute to occlusion of the vessel lumen. Advanced lesions can become calcified or hemorrhage. Thrombosis may develop, resulting in myocardial or cerebral infarction. The majority of deaths due to cardiovascular disease are attributed to end-organ infarction, the major clinical sequela of atherosclerosis.

The mechanisms by which atherosclerosis is initiated remain unclear. Epidemiologic and experimental evidence have, however, identified risk factors that influence its rate of development. Both primary and secondary risk factors have been defined based on their causal relationship to the development of atherosclerotic lesions (6). Primary risk factors, those which directly influence the rate of atherogenesis, include abnormalities in plasma lipoprotein metabolism, hypertension, diabetes, and smoking. Secondary risk factors do not directly affect atherogenesis, but may modify primary risk factors; these include dietary excess, obesity, and coronary-prone behavior (type A personality). Although the presence of one risk factor may be sufficient to accelerate the atherogenic process, the presence of several may potentiate lesion development.

Epidemiologic evidence linking smoking to the development of atherosclerosis and other cardiovascular disorders is reinforced by pathologic data that demonstrate that smoking initiates, aggravates, and/or accelerates lesion formation (7,8). Smoke contains many substances which potentially influence the atherogenic process, including nicotine, carbon monoxide, cadmium, carbon disulfide, and benzo[a]pyrene. Nicotine, for example, can stimulate DNA synthesis in arterial smooth muscle cells in vitro (9). Carbon monoxide may directly damage endothelial cells or increase cell permeability (6,9), allowing blood constituents to interact with underlying vascular components. Administration of a single component of tobacco smoke, benzo[a]pyrene, can result in the formation of vascular lesions (10). Unlike other primary risk factors, smoking may not only accelerate the formation of vascular lesions but initiate their development as well.

Chemical exposure from other sources may also initiate or accelerate lesion development. Epidemiologic evidence has established a correlation between occupational and environmental exposure to chemicals and the development of atherosclerosis (11,12). Experimental studies have also established a link between exposure to chemicals and the development of vascular lesions. Chronic administration of p-hydrazinobenzoic acid, a constituent of the cultivated mushroom *Agaricus bisporus*, results in the formation of vascular lesions in mice (13) which are characterized by loss of intimal integrity, smooth muscle cell proliferation, and necrosis. Aortic smooth muscle cell hyperplasia is also induced by T-2 toxin, a mycotoxin isolated from several *Fusarium* species (14). Acute and subchronic administration of T-2 toxin to rats also damages endothelial cells and results in the accumulation of basement membrane–like material in the intima. Subchronic exposure to allylamine, an aliphatic amine utilized in various industrial processes, results in smooth muscle cell proliferation and fibrosis in the coronary arteries and aorta of various animal species (15,16). Focal vascular lesions characterized by extensive smooth muscle cell proliferation are also noted in several animal species upon administration of carcinogenic polycyclic aromatic hydrocarbons such as benzo[a]pyrene (10) and dimethylbenz[a]anthracene (10,17).

The deleterious effects of these chemicals are not always limited to the cardiovascular system. T-2 toxin has been shown to produce malignant tumors in the gastrointestinal tract, pancreas, and pituitary (14). Thus, the toxicologic profile of these chemicals may be complicated by multiple target organ effects. The lack of target organ specificity may limit their usefulness as tools to investigate chemically induced cardiovascular toxicity. In contrast, allylamine is considered a specific cardiovascular toxicant when administered by a variety of methods in a number of animal species. Gross lesions are evident in the myocardium, aorta, and coronary arteries of animals exposed subchronically to allylamine (15,16). As in naturally occurring atherosclerosis, vascular lesions are characterized by smooth muscle cell proliferation and fibrosis. Interestingly, the characteristic lipid accumulation found in human atherosclerosis is not observed in allylamine-induced vascular injury without supplemental dietary cholesterol (15). The specificity of allylamine-induced target organ toxicity—and the similarity between allylamine-induced vascular lesions and naturally occurring atherosclerosis—make allylamine a useful tool to investigate chemically induced vascular injury.

Allylamine (CH_2=CH-CH_2-NH_2) is a primary, unsaturated aliphatic amine utilized in the vulcanization of rubber and in the organic synthesis of pharmaceuticals (18). Although the mechanism(s) by which allylamine produces its target organ toxicity has (have) yet to be fully elucidated, the site-specific bioactivation of allylamine to its aldehyde, acrolein (CH_2=CH-CHO), is a prerequisite for the manifestation of vascular toxicity (19,20). Conversion of allylamine to acrolein is catalyzed by benzylamine oxidase, a copper-containing amine oxidase found primarily in vascular tissue (20). Acute cytotoxicity studies show that acrolein is an extremely reactive compound that alters the thiol status of target cells, inactivates a variety of sulfhydryl-dependent enzymes, and binds covalently to cellular nucleophilic centers (21–23). Hydrogen peroxide, which is also formed in this oxidative deamination process, may promote peroxidative injury through the formation of hydroxyl radicals (24). Acrolein can also be converted via NADPH-dependent microsomal enzymes to glycidaldehyde, a potent mutagen and carcinogen (21).

In these studies, an experimental model that incorporates features of both in vivo and in vitro systems has been utilized to investigate chemically induced vascular injury. Allylamine was chosen as a prototypical toxin because of its unusual vascular selectivity. As the manifestation of vascular lesions upon exposure to allylamine may be dependent upon mitogenic and chemotactic signals released from blood constituents and neighboring cell types, an in vivo dosing regimen was utilized to induce vascular injury (25–27).

Materials and methods

Male Sprague-Dawley rats weighing 175–200 g were gavaged with allylamine hydrochloride (pH 7.0, 70 mg/kg) or tap water daily for 20 days. At the end of the dosing regimen, thoracic aortae were excised and the vascular smooth muscle cells were isolated and grown in culture (25–27). Functional and biochemical assessments were conducted in vitro to facilitate the investigation of cellular and molecular mechanisms involved in the expression of vascular injury.

Previous studies have shown that subchronic exposure to allylamine affected, either directly or indirectly, ^{32}P incorporation into various components of the phosphoinositide cycle and resulted in a decreased turnover (27). These alterations may be directly associated with changes in the proliferative potential of smooth muscle cells upon allylamine exposure. The present studies were designed to further investigate the association between allylamine-induced alterations in phosphoinositide turnover and smooth muscle cell phenotype. Pharmacologic manipulation of phosphoinositide metabolism was accomplished by incubation of cultures with dibutyryl cAMP (db cAMP; 0.2 mM) and theophylline (0.1 mM), or neomycin (1.25 mM), for 72 or 24 hr, respectively. The concentrations utilized in this study have been reported to produce alterations in the phosphoinositide/inositol phosphate profiles of mammalian cells (28,29). At the end of the desired exposure periods, cultures were processed for further analyses.

To assess the proliferative capability of the cells, treated cultures were labeled with 5 µCi/ml [methyl-^3H]thymidine triphosphate for 1 hr and processed according to the method of Palmberg et al. (30). After labeling, cultures were rinsed with a balanced salt solution and the cellular protein was precipitated with trichloroacetic acid (5%). Protein was collected, pelleted, and then digested in 0.1 N NaOH overnight. Digested samples were counted by liquid scintillation and standardized for protein content.

Inositol phosphates were labeled in treated cultures by incubation with 10 µCi/ml [^3H]myoinositol for 48 hr. Lithium chloride (10 mM) was added for the last 24 hr to enhance the inositol phosphate signal. An additional incubation with unlabeled myoinositol (10 mM; 1.5 hr) followed the labeling period. Cellular proteins were precipitated with trichloroacetic acid (5%) and washed with three volumes of dimethyl ether. Samples were processed through a 1 ml Dowex formate column and the inositol phosphates were eluted with a series of buffers containing increasing concentrations of formate according to the procedure described by Berridge et al. (31). ^{32}P-labeled standards were coeluted with samples, which were then counted by liquid scintillation. Incorporation into each inositol phosphate was standardized to the total amount of radioactivity recovered from the column.

Thymidine labeling was analyzed by the Mann-Whitney U-test. Incorporation into inositol phosphates was compared using Student's t-test. The 0.05 level of probability was accepted as significant. Values shown in Table 1 represent the mean ± SEM.

Results

Increased levels of the intracellular messenger cAMP have been shown to specifically inhibit phosphoinositide kinase activity in vascular smooth muscle cells (32). At the end of the 72-hr exposure to db cAMP and theophylline, cultures were assessed for morphologic changes and processed for [^3H]thymidine and [^3H]myoinositol labeling studies. The morphology of db cAMP–treated cells was strikingly different from those exposed to vehicle control (25). Cells obtained from allylamine-treated animals became more elongated and spindle-shaped upon exposure to db cAMP and theophylline. A dramatic inhibition of [^3H]thymidine uptake into cells treated with db cAMP and theophylline was also observed (Table 1). This inhibition in DNA synthesis correlated with a decrease in incorporation into the inositol phosphates (Fig. 1).

Table 1. DNA Synthesis in Smooth Muscle Cells from Allylamine-treated Rats.[a]

| | [3H]Thymidine incorporation (cpm/ug cellular protein) | |
Group	Vehicle	Treatment
db cAMP + theophylline	1560 ± 87	27 + 7*
Neomycin	1570 ± 250	1480 ± 190

[a]Smooth muscle cells cultured from allylamine-treated animals were exposed in vitro to db cAMP (0.2 mM) and theophylline (0.1 mM), or neomycin (1.25 mM), for 72 or 24 hr, respectively. Cells were labeled with 5 μCi/ml [3H]thymidine triphosphate for 1 hr and processed to determine incorporation into DNA. Values represent the mean ± SEM (n = 4–5).
*Significantly different from respective vehicle, $P < 0.05$.

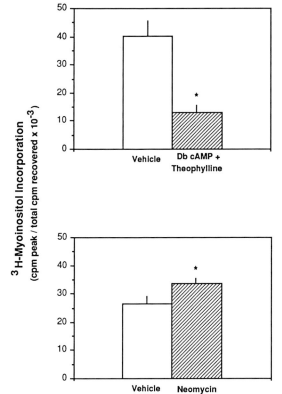

Figure 1. Inositol phosphate profile of smooth muscle cells cultured from allylamine-treated rats and exposed in vitro to dibutyryl cAMP and theophylline or neomycin. Smooth muscle cells isolated from allylamine-treated animals were exposed to dibutyryl cAMP (0.2 mM) and theophylline (0.1 mM) or neomycin (1.25 mM), for 72 or 24 hr, respectively. Cultures were labeled with [3H]myoinositol for 48 hr and then processed for inositol phosphate analysis. Results are expressed as counts per minute (cpm) per peak standardized by the total cpm recovered from the column × 10⁻³. Values represent the mean ± SEM (n = 2–5). *Significantly different from vehicle, $P < 0.05$.

The effects of neomycin were also evaluated because of its ability to bind to phosphoinositide 4-phosphate and phosphoinositide 4,5-bisphosphate, thus preventing their hydrolysis by phospholipase C and inhibiting the production of inositol phosphates (29). At the end of a 24-hr exposure to neomycin, morphologic observations were made and cultures were processed for [^{3}H]thymidine and [^{3}H]myoinositol labeling studies. In contrast to cells treated in vitro with db cAMP and theophylline, morphologic changes were not observed in cells treated with neomycin (results not shown). Consistent with these observations, no alterations in [^{3}H]thymidine labeling were observed in neomycin-treated cultures (Table 1). The lack of morphologic alterations or changes in DNA synthesis upon exposure to neomycin was unexpected, based on the reported effects of this compound. Incorporation into inositol phosphates was significantly increased in cultures treated with neomycin (Fig. 1). The increase in labeling of total inositol phosphates was attributed to an increase of myoinositol incorporation into inositol 1-phosphate specifically.

Discussion

Previous work from our laboratory has detailed alterations in the morphology, function, and biochemistry of aortic smooth muscle cells cultured from rats dosed with allylamine hydrochloride (25–27). Cells isolated from control animals were elongated and exhibited an extensive network of myofilaments. Consistent with these differentiated features, smooth muscle cells cultured from control animals contracted in response to pharmacologic stimuli, while cells isolated from allylamine-treated animals did not respond. Cells from treated animals were rounded and characterized by numerous ribosomes and rough endoplasmic reticulum; they also displayed an enhanced ability to synthesize DNA and collagen over cells from control rats. Allylamine-induced alterations in the proliferative potential of aortic smooth muscle cells were seen in both primary and secondary cultures.

The enhanced mitogenic responsiveness observed in synthetic smooth muscle cells from allylamine-treated animals has been the focus of additional studies in our laboratory. Although many important steps between mitogen binding to a receptor and mitosis have been identified, our work has focused upon the phosphoinositide signaling system responsible for the transduction of mitogenic signals across the plasma membrane. Alterations in this signaling system have been observed in spontaneously hypertensive rats, both in transformed, highly proliferative cells (28,33) as well as in smooth muscle cells exhibiting altered growth potential (34). The transduction of mitogenic signals via phosphoinositide hydrolysis relies upon a bifurcating pathway to regulate a cascade of intracellular events. The water-soluble inositol phosphate products mobilize intracellular stores of calcium, while diacylglycerol, a lipid-soluble product, activates protein kinase C (35). The pharmacologic manipulation of phosphoinositide metabolism in the present studies has focused upon inositol phosphate production. The data obtained will be discussed in the context of additional experiments which have investigated protein kinase C activation.

The pharmacologic manipulation of phosphoinositide metabolism by exposure to db cAMP and theophylline resulted in the modulation of the smooth muscle phenotype in cells obtained from allylamine-treated animals, as judged by changes in morphology, DNA synthesis, and inositol phosphate production. In contrast, previous studies have shown that incorporation into inositol phosphates was not altered in smooth muscle cells obtained from control animals upon exposure to db cAMP and theophylline (27). These data suggest that the elevation of cAMP selectively inhibits phosphoinositide hydrolysis in cells from allylamine-treated animals. The sustained elevation of intracellular levels of cAMP may mediate the modulation of smooth muscle cells from a proliferative state towards a more contractile phenotype. In this regard, previous studies have demonstrated that exposure to db cAMP and theophylline can inhibit mitosis and promote the maintenance of contractile features of smooth muscle cells in vitro (36). Exposure to the cyclooxygenase product prostacyclin, which is known to stimulate adenylate cyclase, has been shown to inhibit DNA synthesis in cultures of smooth muscle cells obtained from atherosclerotic human aortae (37). Although these data present an intriguing association between cAMP levels and the phenotypic state of vascular smooth muscle cells, the exact role of cAMP as a regulatory factor in phospho-inositide metabolism and phenotypic modulation has yet to be determined.

Neomycin exposure, in contrast, did not inhibit phosphoinositide hydrolysis in vascular smooth muscle cells. Incorporation of ^{32}P into inositol 1-phosphate increased upon exposure to neomycin, an effect not associated with alterations in morphology or proliferative capability. The actions of neomycin on phosphoinositide metabolism and second messenger formation may vary according to experimental conditions and cell type (38,39).

Previous work from our laboratory has demonstrated that incorporation into phosphatidic acid, the phosphorylated product of diacylglycerol, was significantly lower in cells obtained from allylamine-treated animals in comparison to controls (27). This difference may reflect an alteration in the fate of diacylglycerol upon subchronic exposure to allylamine. Changes in the level of intracellular second messengers may be significant in the expression of an altered phenotype. Since diacylglycerol is extremely short-lived and therefore difficult to measure under most experimental conditions, studies were designed to investigate protein kinase C activation by pharmacologic manipulation of enzymatic activity. A 24-hr exposure to sphingosine (125–500 ng/ml), an inhibitor of protein kinase C activity, was shown to suppress serum-induced DNA synthesis in cells cultured from allylamine-treated animals (27). Proliferation of smooth muscle cells in the synthetic state induced by allylamine appears, therefore, to be a protein kinase C–dependent process. In contrast, sphingosine did not inhibit DNA synthesis in cells from control animals. These data suggest that mitogenic responsiveness in smooth muscle cells from control animals is much less dependent upon the activation of protein kinase C.

Treatment of cells from control animals with 12-O-tetradecanoylphorbol-13-acetate (TPA; 1–100 ng/ml) for 24 hr resulted in an increase in proliferative activity (27). Activation of protein kinase C by TPA, therefore, enhanced the overall mitogenic responsiveness of control cells. In contrast, exposure of cells from allylamine-treated animals to low concentrations of TPA inhibited thymidine uptake. Prolonged exposure of a protein kinase C activator such as TPA might result in the down-regulation of protein kinase C activity, particularly in cells with high basal activity (40).

Conclusion

The data suggest that allylamine-induced alterations in the turnover of phosphoinositides and activity of protein kinase C are associated with a modulation of the smooth muscle phenotype towards a synthetic state. This phenotypic modulation is expressed in both primary and secondary culture (27). The stability of these phenotypic changes suggests they may be heritable, and that allylamine is producing alterations at the genetic level.

The interpretation of these data is consistent with the monoclonal theory of atherogenesis, as first proposed by Benditt and Benditt (41). Based on the monotypism of glucose-6-phosphate dehydrogenase enzymes found in the smooth muscle cells of individual atherosclerotic lesions, the theory proposes that these cells are the progeny of a single, altered smooth muscle cell. The monoclonal nature of atherosclerotic lesions underscores their similarity to benign neoplastic growth in smooth muscle cell tumors or leiomyomas of the uterus. The sequence of events culminating in focal smooth muscle cell hyperplasia may actually be analogous to the initiation-promotion phases of carcinogenesis (17). Upon exposure to a mutagenic agent, for example, smooth muscle cells may exist in a genetically altered state in the vasculature. Lesion development is likely to be dependent upon exposure to growth-promoting factors which will enable altered cells to proliferate. Alternatively, mutations could induce constitutive production of growth factors within smooth muscle cells, resulting in autocrine stimulation and smooth muscle cell hyperplasia (42).

Since mutational activation of cellular oncogenes has been associated with altered cell growth in many types of human cancer (43), an analogous situation may exist in the smooth muscle cell growth associated with atherogenesis. Recent evidence has shown that DNA isolated from human atherosclerotic plaques is capable of transforming NIH 3T3 cells and producing tumors in nude mice (44). The positive response in this gene transfer assay indicates that oncogene(s) may be activated within the cells of human atherosclerotic plaques. The development of human neoplasms has also been linked to the mutational inactivation of genes known as anti-oncogenes or tumor suppressor genes (45). Atherosclerotic lesion development may also be associated with the mutational inactivation of genes that regulate growth within the vasculature, although no evidence in support of this concept has yet been found. Characterization of the cellular and molecular mechanisms by which chemicals may induce vascular injury is of great potential significance.

Acknowledgments

This research was supported in part by National Institute of Environmental Health Sciences grant ES 04849.

References

1. Clowes AW, Reidy MA, Clowes MM. Kinetics of cellular proliferation after arterial injury. I. Smooth muscle growth in the absence of endothelium. Lab Invest 49:327–332.
2. Campbell GR, Campbell JH. Smooth muscle phenotypic changes in arterial wall homeostasis: Implications for the pathogenesis of atherosclerosis. Exp Mol Pathol 42:139–162.
3. Campbell GR, Chamley-Campbell JH. The cellular pathobiology of atherosclerosis. Pathology 13:423–440.
4. Sjolund M, Madsen K, van der Mark K, Thyberg J. Phenotypic modulation in primary cultures of smooth muscle cells from rat aorta. Differentiation 32:173–180.
5. Ross R. The pathogenesis of atherosclerosis—an update. N Engl J Med 314:488–500.
6. Grundy SM. Atherosclerosis: Pathology, pathogenesis, and role of risk factors. Dis Mon 29:1–58.

7. United States Department of Health, Education and Welfare, Report of the Surgeon General. Smoking and Health. Washington, D.C.: Government Printing Office, 1979.
8. Paffenbarger RS, Hyde RT, Wing AL, Hseih C. Cigarette smoking and cardiovascular diseases. IARC Sci Publ 74:45–60.
9. Thyberg J. Effects of nicotine on phenotypic modulation and initiation of DNA synthesis in cultured arterial smooth muscle cells. Virchows Arch [B] 52:25–32.
10. Albert RE, Vanderlaan M, Burns FJ, Nishizumi M. Effect of carcinogens on chicken atherosclerosis. Cancer Res 37:2232–2235.
11. Kurppa K, Hietanen E, Klockars M, Partinen M, Rantanen J, Rossemaa T, Viikari J. Chemical exposures at work and cardiovascular morbidity. Scand J Work Environ Health 10:381–388.
12. Levine RJ. Dinitrotoluene: Human atherogen, carcinogen, neither, or both? Chemical Industry Institute of Toxicology (CIIT) Activities 7:2–5.
13. McManus BM, Toth B, Patil KD. Aortic rupture and aortic smooth muscle tumors in mice: Induction by *p*-hydrazinobenzoic acid hydrochloride of the cultivated mushroom *Agaricus bisporus*. Lab Invest 57:78–85.
14. Yarom R, Sherman Y, Bergmannm F, Sintov A, Berman LD. T-2 toxin effect on rat aorta: Cellular changes in vivo and growth of smooth muscle ells in vitro. Exp Mol Pathol 47:143–153.
15. Lalich JJ. Coronary artery hyalinosis in rats fed allylamine. Exp Mol Pathol 10:14–26.
16. Boor PJ, Moslen MT, Reynolds ES. Allylamine cardiotoxicity: I. Sequence of pathologic events. Toxicol Appl Pharmacol 50:581–592.
17. Majesky MW, Reidy MA, Benditt RP, Juchau MR. Focal smooth muscle proliferation in the aortic intima produced by an initiation-promotion sequence. Proc Natl Acad Sci USA 82:3450–3454.
18. Boor PJ, Hysmith RM. Allylamine cardiovascular toxicity. Toxicology 44:129–145.
19. Nelson TJ, Boor PJ. Allylamine cardiotoxicity IV: Metabolism to acrolein by cardiovascular tissue. Biochem Pharmacol 31:509–514.
20. Ramos K, Grossman SL, Cox LR. Allylamine-induced vascular toxicity in vitro: Prevention by semicarbazide-sensitive amine oxidase inhibitors. Toxicol Appl Pharmacol 95:61–71.
21. Beauchamp RO Jr, Andjelkovich DA, Kligerman AD, Morgan KT, d'A Heck H. A critical review of the literature on acrolein toxicity. CRC Crit Rev in Toxicol 14:309–380.
22. Cox LR, Ramos K. Acrolein-induced alterations in total non-protein thiol content in cultured rat aortic endothelial and smooth muscle cells. The Pharmacologist 28:183.
23. Ramos K, Cox LR. Primary cultures of rat aortic endothelial and smooth muscle cells: I. An in vitro model to study xenobiotic-induced vascular cytotoxicity. In Vitro Cell Dev Biol 23:288–296.
24. DiGuiseppi J, Fridovich I. The toxicology of molecular oxygen. Crit Rev Toxicology 12:495–504.
25. Cox LR, Murphy SK, Ramos K. Morphologic modulation of vascular smooth muscle cells upon subchronic exposure to allylamine: Reversal by dibutyryl cyclic adenosine monophosphate. In Vitro Toxicology 1:183–187.
26. Cox LR, Ramos K. Allylamine-induced phenotypic modulation of aortic smooth muscle cells. J Exp Pathol 71:11–18, 1989.
27. Cox LR, Murphy SK, Ramos K. Modulation of phosphoinositide metabolism in aortic smooth muscle cells by allylamine. Exp Mol Pathol, in press.
28. Lockwood AH, Borislow S, Lazarus A, Murphy SK, Pendergast M. Cellular signal transduction and the reversal of malignancy. J Cell Biochem 237–255.
29. Carney DJ, Scott DL, Gordon EA, LaBele EF. Phosphoinositides in mitogenesis: Neomycin inhibits thrombin-stimulated phosphoinositide turnover and initiation of cell proliferation. Cell 42:477–488.
30. Palmberg L, Sjolund M, Thyberg J. Phenotype modulation in primary cultures of arterial smooth muscle cells: Regulation of the cytoskeleton and activation of synthetic activities. Differentiation 29:275–283.
31. Berridge MJ, Dawson RMC, Downes PC, Helsop JP, Irvine RF. Changes in the levels of inositol phosphates after agonist dependent hydrolysis of membrane phosphoinositides. Biochem J 212:473–482.
32. Doctrow SR, Lowenstein JM. Inhibition of phosphatidylinositol kinase in vascular smooth muscle membranes by adenosine and related compounds. Biochem Pharmacol 36:2255–2262.
33. Sugimoto Y, Whitman M, Cantley LC, Erikson RL. Evidence that Rous sarcoma virus transforming gene product phosphorylates phosphatidylinositol and diacylglycerol. Proc Natl Acad Sci USA 81:2117–2121.
34. Heagerty AM, Ollerenshaw JD, Swales JD. Abnormal vascular phosphoinositide hydrolysis in the spontaneously hypertensive rat. Br J Pharmacol 89:803–807.

35. Berridge MJ. Inositol trisphosphate and diacylglycerol as second messengers. Biochem J 220:345–360.
36. Chamley JH, Campbell GR. Trophic influences of sympathetic nerves and cyclic AMP on differentiation and proliferation of isolated smooth muscle cells in culture. Cell Tissue Res 161:497–510.
37. Orekhov AN, Tertov VV, Mazurov AV, Andreeva ER, Repin VS, Smirnov VN. Regression of atherosclerosis in cell culture: Effects of stable prostacyclin analogues. Drug Development Research 9:189–201.
38. Hughes BP, Auld AM, Barritt GJ. Evidence that neomycin inhibits plasma membrane Ca^{+2} inflow in isolated hepatocytes. Biochem Pharmacol 37:1357–1361.
39. Hagiwara M, Inagaki M, Kanamura K, Ohta H, Hidaka H. Inhibitory effects of aminoglycosides on renal protein phosphorylation by protein kinase C. J Pharmacol Exp Ther 244:355–360.
40. Kariya K, Kawahara Y, Tsuda T, Fukuzaki H, Takai Y. Possible involvement of protein kinase C in platelet-derived growth factor-stimulated DNA synthesis in vascular smooth muscle cells. Atherosclerosis 63:251–255.
41. Benditt EP, Benditt JM. Evidence for a monoclonal origin of human atherosclerotic plaques. Proc Natl Acad Sci USA 70:1753–1756.
42. Hoshi H, Kan M, Chen JK, McKeehan WL. Comparative endocrinology-paracrinology-autocrinology of human adult large vessel endothelial and smooth muscle cells. In Vitro Cell Dev Biol 24:309–324.
43. Land H, Parada LF, Weinberg RA. Cellular oncogenes and multistep carcinogenesis. Science 222:771–778.
44. Penn A, Garte SJ, Warren L, Nesta D, Mindich B. Transforming gene in human atherosclerotic plaque DNA. Proc Natl Acad Sci USA 83:7951–7955.
45. Sager R. Tumor suppressor genes: The puzzle and the promise. Science 246:1406–1412.

Chemically Induced Cell Proliferation:
Implications for Risk Assessment, pages 439-444
©1991 Wiley-Liss, Inc.

Role of Iron in Cell Proliferation and Tumorigenesis

*Claus-Peter Siegers, Dirk Bumann, Hans-Dieter Trepkau,
Beate Schadwinkel, and Gustav Baretton*

Iron is known to have stimulatory effects on cell proliferation (1,2); little data, however, exist concerning the influence of iron on tumor growth. Cocarcinogenic effects of iron ions have been observed—in the form of an increased yield of lung tumors—following repeated intratracheal instillation of ferric oxide given together with benzo[a]pyrene or diethylnitrosamine (3,4). Large dose subcutaneous (s.c.) or intramuscular application of iron-dextrane and certain other polysaccharide iron complexes were able to induce local sarcomas (5,6). Nothing, however, is known about the influence of dietary iron in initiating and promoting tumor development in the gastrointestinal tract. We therefore studied the effect of iron-enriched diets on intestinal tumorigenesis following 1,2-dimethylhydrazine (DMH) treatment in mice. We also studied the influence of iron or the iron-complexing agent deferrioxamine on cell growth in an established human colon carcinoma cell line, Caco-2.

Method

Tumor incidence in vivo

Male NMRI mice weighing 26–28 g were distributed randomly into control and experimental groups of 20 animals each. Iron-enriched diets (0.5–3.5% Fe-fumarate; AltrominR pellets) were fed daily and 20 mg/kg DMH given by s.c. application once weekly for 10 weeks; controls received DMH and were fed a normal diet of AltrominR pellets. In a second series of experiments, mice received the iron-enriched diet of 3.5% Fe-fumarate between week 11 and 20, i.e., following the 10-week DMH treatment period; controls received the normal diet. After 20 weeks the mice were killed, and organs were excised and inspected macroscopically for tumors; tumors were found exclusively in the distal colon and rectum. As preparation for histomorphological examination, the colon and rectum were divided into proximal, medial, and distal segments, and the detected tumors were classified.

Estimation of total iron in liver and colon

Total iron concentrations were measured in the livers and proximal colonic mucosa 4 weeks after feeding the iron-enriched diets or at the end of the 20-week observation period using a reagent kit commercially available from Boehringer, Mannheim, West Germany.

Cell culture experiments

The human colon carcinoma cell line Caco-2 was cultured in Dulbecco's minimum essential medium (4.5 g/L glucose) supplemented with 5% bovine serum albumin, glutamine, amino acids (Eagle's minimum essential medium), Hepes, and 125000 U penicillin/12.5 mg streptomycine per 500 ml medium. The cells were seeded in 24-well tissue culture plates and trypsinized before being counted. Fe(III) chloride or deferrioxamine (Desferal, Ciba-Geigy, Basel) were added to the medium 24 hr after seeding; the cells were counted 24–96 hr later.

Tumour incidence

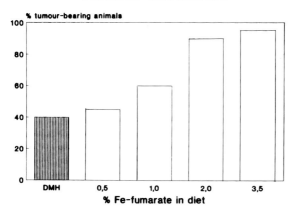

Figure 1. Influence of iron-enriched diets on tumor incidence following DMH-treatment.

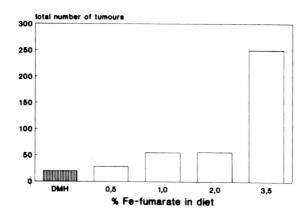

Results

Iron-enriched diets caused a concentration-dependent increase in tumor rate (Fig. 1,2); threshold concentration for this effect was 1.0% Fe-fumarate in the diet. The cotumorigenic effect of iron was seen in both schedules of administration, i.e., simultaneously with the carcinogen DMH or in the carcinogen-free treatment period (weeks 11–20) (see Table 1). An influence of iron ions on the microsomal and cytosolic enzymes DMH-demethylase and alcohol dehydrogenase involved in the bioactivation of DMH to the ultimate carcinogen was excluded (7). A regimen of iron-enriched diets resulted in a concentration-dependent accumulation of iron in the liver and colon after 4 weeks (Fig. 3). At the end of the 20-week observation period, iron content was still enhanced in the liver but not in the colon (data not shown).

In Caco-2, the administration of up to 3 mg/L Fe(III) chloride caused a concentration-dependent stimulation of cell growth (Fig. 4), i.e., higher concentrations were inhibitory. Fe(III) salts were ineffective in this respect (data not shown). In comparison, the iron-complexing agent deferrioxamine markedly depressed cell growth

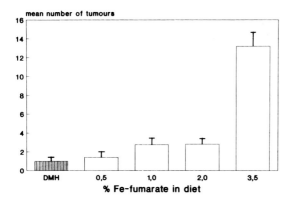

Figure 2. Influence of iron-enriched diets on tumor incidence following DMH treatment.

Table 1. Tumor Incidence in the Distal Colon and Rectum of Mice Treated with DMH

Group	Number of tumor-bearing animals	Mean number of tumors	Total number of tumors
1. DMH 20	13/19	2.4 ± 0.6	45
2. DMH 20 + Fe-fumarate simultaneously	18/19	13.2 ±15.*	>250
3. DMH 20	11/18	6.9 ± 1.9	130
4. DMH 20 + Fe-fumarate (week 11–20)	17/18	15.7 ± 1.6**	>280

Mice in groups 1 and 3 were treated with 20 mg/kg DMH subcutaneously weekly for 10 weeks. Group 2: Fe-fumarate (3.5%) simultaneously with DMH. Group 4: Fe-fumarate (3.5%) following DMH treatment period (week 11–20).
$*P < 0.05$ compared to group I, $**P < 0.05$ compared to group II

in the Caco-2 cell line (Fig. 5). This effect of Fe(III) ions was not observed in a renal epithelial cell line (LLC-PK$_1$) or a human hepatoma cell line (Hep G2) (data not shown). We concluded that iron promotes intestinal tumorigenesis by stimulating cell proliferation; this effect seems to be selective for tumor cells. The effect of iron on cell growth is explained by its essential presence in the enzyme ribonucleotide-reductase, which represents a significant factor in DNA synthesis (8).

Discussion

The essential role of iron in cell growth has been previously described. Iacopetta and coworkers (9) found a good correlation between the number of transferrin

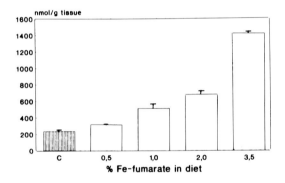

Figure 3. Influence of iron-enriched diets on total iron concentrations in liver and colon after 4 weeks.

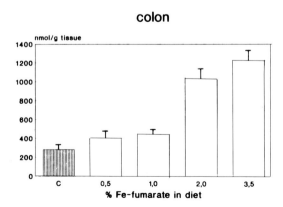

receptors and the iron uptake by nine leukemic cell lines. When monoclonal antibodies block the transferrin receptors of human T-lymphocytes, the result is an arrest of the cell cycle in the S phase; continuous inhibition is followed by cell death (10). Moreover, the iron-complexing agent deferrioxamine is known as a potent inhibitor of DNA synthesis and cell proliferation, as demonstrated in Hela cells (11), human lymphocytes (12–14), leukemic cell lines (15), and human neuroblastoma-derived cell lines (16).

Iron is also known to activate oxygen and to stimulate lipoperoxidative processes (17). Reactive oxygen species seem to be involved in cell proliferation and tumor promotion (18). Thus, the effects of iron seen in our in vivo and in vitro models may also be based on inducing an oxidative stress in the colonic mucosa.

An important role of iron metabolism and storage has been suggested for human cancer risk assessment. A higher risk for primary liver cell carcinoma was observed in

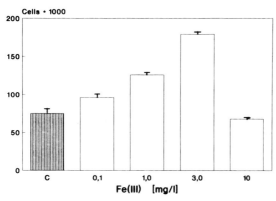

Figure 4. Effect of Fe(III) chloride on cell growth of an established human colon carcinoma cell line, Caco-2.

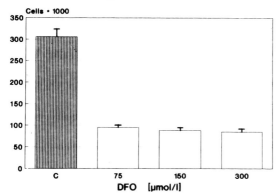

Figure 5. Effect of the iron-complexing deferrioxamine (DFO) on cell growth of an established human colon carcinoma cell line, Caco-2.

patients with idiopathic hemochromatosis (19), and an increased incidence of tumors of the colon and urinary bladder was found in the epidemiological study of Stevens and coworkers (20) in correlation to parameters of iron storage and metabolism. Finally, it has been proposed that withholding iron may prove to be a mechanism of defense against infection and neoplasia (21,22).

References

1. Forsbeck K, Nielsen K. The dynamic morphology of the transferrin-transferrin receptor system in leukaemia/lymphoma cell lines and its relation to iron metabolism and cell proliferation. Scandinavian Journal of Haematology 35:145–154, 1985.
2. Laskey J, Wess I, Schulman HM, Ponka P. Evidence that transferrin supports cell proliferation by supplying DNA synthesis. Exp Cell Res 176:87–95, 1988.
3. Saffiotti U, Cefis F, Kolb H. A method for the experimental induction of bronchogenic carcinoma. Cancer Res 28:104–124, 1968.
4. Saffiotti U, Montesano R, Sellakumar AR, Cefis F, Kaufman DG. Respiratory tract carcinogenesis in hamsters induced by different numbers of administrations of benza[a]pyrene and ferric oxide. Cancer Res 32:1073–1081, 1972.
5. Richmond HG. Induction of sarcoma in the rat by iron dextran complex. Br Med J 1:947–949, 1959.
6. Haddow A, Horning ES. On the carcinogenicity of an iron-dextran complex. J Natl Cancer Inst 24:139–147, 1960.
7. Siegers CP, Bumann D, Baretton G, Younes M. Dietary iron enhances the tumor rate in dimethylhydrazine-induced colon carcinogenesis in mice. Cancer Lett 41:251–256, 1988.
8. Reichard P, Ehrenberg A. Ribonucleotide reductase - a radical enzyme. Science 221:514–519, 1983.
9. Iacopetta BJ, Morgan EH, Yeok CGT. Transferrin receptors and iron uptake during euthyroid cell development. Biochem Biophys Acta 687:204–210, 1982.
10. Trowbridge IS, Lopez F. Monoclonal antibody to transferrin receptor blocks transferrin binding and inhibits human tumor cell growth in vitro. Proc Natl Acad Sci 79:1175–1179, 1982.
11. Robbins E, Pederson T. Iron, its intracellular localization and possible role in cell devision. Proc Natl Acad Sci USA 66:1244–1251, 1970.
12. Hoffbrand AV, Ganeskaguru K, Hooton JWL, Tattersall MHN. Effect of iron deficiency and deferrioxamine on DNA-synthesis in human cells. Br J Haematol 33:517–526, 1976.
13. Lederman MH, Cohen A, Lee JWW, Freedman MH, Gelfand EW. Deferrioxamine: a reversible S-phase inhibitor of human lymphocyte proliferation. Blood 64:748–753, 1984.
14. Bowern N, Ranshaw IA, Badenoch-Jones P, Doherty PC. Effect of an iron chelating agent on lymphocyte proliferation. Australian Journal of Experimental Biology and Medical Sciences 62:743–754, 1984.
15. Foa P, Maiolo AT, Lombardi L, Villa L, Polli EE. Inhibition of proliferation of human leukaemic cell populations by deferrioxamine. Scand J Haematol 36:107–110, 1986.
16. Blatt J, Stitley S. Antineuroblastoma activity of deferrioxamine in human cell lines. Cancer Res 47:1749–1750, 1987.
17. Aust SD, Svingen BA. The role of iron in enzymatic lipid peroxidation. In Pryor WA (ed): Free Radicals in Biology Vol. 5. New York: Academic Press, 1982, pp. 29–64.
18. Perera MIR, Betschart JM, Virji MA, Katyal SL, Shinozuka H. Free radical injury and liver tumor promotion. Toxicol Pathol 15:51–59, 1987.
19. Niederaus C, Fischer R, Sonnenberg A, Stremmel W, Trampisch HJ, Strohmeyer G. Survival and causes of death in cirrhotic and noncirrhotic patients with primary hemochromatosis. N Engl J Med 313:1256–1262, 1985.
20. Stevens RS, Jones DY, Micozzi MS, Taylor PR. Body iron stores and the risk of cancer. N Engl J Med 319:1047–1052, 1988.
21. Weinberg ED. Iron in neoplastic disease. Nutr Cancer 4:223–233, 1983.
22. Weinberg ED. Iron withholding: a defense against infection and neoplasia. Physiol Rev 64:65–102, 1984.

Chemically Induced Cell Proliferation:
Implications for Risk Assessment, pages 445-455
©1991 Wiley-Liss, Inc.

Proliferation Kinetics and Development of Pepsinogen-altered Pyloric Gland Cells in the Glandular Stomach of Rats Treated with Chemicals

Masae Tatematsu, Tomoyuki Shirai, Kumiko Ogawa,
Makoto Asamoto, and Nobuyuki Ito

The effectiveness of medium-term in vivo screening tests for liver and bladder carcinogens and promoters is based on the tests' ability to identify and quantitate putative preneoplastic changes (1,2). Until recently, however, we had no adequate in vivo intermediate-term screening test for gastric carcinogens and promoters because no comparable marker was available for putative preneoplastic changes in the stomach. Such a test is particulaly needed because the induction of gastric cancer is a long-term process (3).

The ability to identify preneoplastic lesions in investigations of gastric carcinogenesis therefore had high priority. Of the three pepsinogen isozymes—Pg 1, Pg 3, and Pg 4—which have been separated from the pyloric mucosa by polyacrylamide-gel electrophoresis (4), Pg 1 is known to disappear or decrease preferentially in areas of pyloric mucosa during the early stages of N-methyl-N'-nitro-N-nitrosoguanidine (MNNG)-induced gastric carcinogenesis and before morphologically distinct preneoplastic histologic changes appear (5,6). This altered pepsinogen isozyme pattern has also been observed consistently in gastric tumors (7). More recent immunohistochemical studies have demonstrated individual pyloric glands low in Pg 1 (thus termed Pg-1–altered pyloric glands, PAPG) after MNNG-treatment (8), and these studies have revealed that cells of the pyloric-gland cell type within gastric tumors contain little or no Pg 1 (9). In addition, induction of PAPG was found to depend on dose of MNNG administered, and PAPG numbers increased with time (8,9). The susceptibility of different rat strains to induction of gastric carcinomas by MNNG also correlated with their susceptibility to induction of PAPG (10). The evidence is strong, therefore, that PAPG detected immunohistochemically may be considered putative preneoplastic lesions in the glandular stomach of rats.

Theoretically, preneoplastic or neoplastic populations should present some degree of autonomy with regard to proliferation. To learn whether PAPG demonstrate any such alteration in cell division kinetics, Experiment 1 was performed using the immunohistochemical approach of bromodeoxyuridine (BrdU) incorporation. In addition, the efficacy of PAPG as end-point marker lesions for use in medium-term screening of gastric carcinogens and gastric promoters was assessed. After initiation with MNNG, test chemicals were administered for 14 weeks along with sodium chloride as an enhancing cofactor (11). Seventeen chemicals were investigated for their influence on PAPG development with the Experiment 2 protocol.

Materials and Methods

Experiment 1

Animals and chemicals. Forty-five male WKY/NCrj rats (Charles River Japan, Kanagawa) were housed in plastic cages with hardwood chips, in an air-conditioned room, and a 12-hr light/12-hr dark cycle. The animals were given food (Oriental MF, Oriental Yeast Co., Tokyo) and water ad libitum. They were divided into MNNG-treated and control groups, all being allowed free access to the diet. From 7 weeks of age, 25 rats in the MNNG-treated group were given drinking water containing 100 µg/ml MNNG (Aldrich Chemical Co., Milwaukee, WI) for 10 weeks, then returned to normal tap water, and killed at week 12.

For quantitative analysis of proliferating cells in pyloric mucosa, 5 rats from each group received an intraperitoneal injection of BrdU, 100 mg/kg of body weight, 1 hr before they were killed. For quantitative analysis of the migration of pyloric gland cells, cumulative labeling with BrdU was done. Five rats from each group were given BrdU by Alzet miniosmotic pump, model 2001 (Alza Corp., Palo Alto, CA) continuously for 4, 7, or 10 days before death. Osmotic minipumps, delivering 120 µg BrdU per hour, were implanted subcutaneously in the animals' backs. Immediately upon sacrifice, the excised stomachs were fixed in sublimated formaldehyde (12) and cut into approximately 8 strips that were processed, embedded in paraffin, and sectioned routinely.

Double immunohistochemistry. Immunogold-silver staining (IGSS) (13) was used to detect BrdU incorporated into DNA (14,15). Before immunostaining the sections were treated with Lugol's iodine, and all traces of iodine were removed with 2.5% sodium thiosulfate. Then sections were treated with 4 N HCl for 20 min at 37°C, neutralized with 0.2 M boric acid-borate buffer at pH 7.6, and incubated with 0.04% actinase (Kaken Kagaku, Tokyo) for 3 min at 37°C. Tissue sections were initially treated with mouse monoclonal antibody against BrdU (Becton Dickinson, Mountain View, CA) and then with colloidal gold-labeled goat immunoglobulin (IgG) against mouse IgG (Janssen, Olen, Belgium). Gold particles were subsequently revealed by the silver precipitation reaction. The avidin-biotin-peroxidase complex (ABC) method (16) was used to demonstrate binding of antibodies against Pg 1 in the pyloric mucosa. Anti-Pg 1 serum was prepared as described previously (17). Sections were treated with rabbit anti-rat Pg 1 IgG, biotin-labeled goat anti-rabbit IgG, and ABC (Vectastain ABC kit, PK 4001, Vector Laboratories, Burlingame, CA). Sites of peroxidase binding were determined by the diaminobenzidine method of Graham and Karnofsky (18).

For double immunostaining, sections were stained first for BrdU using the IGSS method, with primary antibody diluted at 1:100 and then processed for Pg 1 binding by the ABC method using primary antibody diluted at 1:4000. The sections were counterstained with hematoxylin for microscopic examination. As a negative control for the specificity of anti-BrdU and anti-Pg 1 antibodies, preimmune mouse and rabbit sera were used, respectively, instead of anti-BrdU mouse IgG and anti-Pg 1 rabbit IgG.

Immunohistochemical analysis. Pyloric mucosa is composed of pyloric columns consisting of a gastric pit, an isthmus (generative cell zone), and a basal pyloric gland (19). The cells that stain particularly strongly for Pg 1 immunohistochemically appear as normal pyloric gland cells close to the lamina muscularis mucosa. PAPG staining weakly or negatively for Pg 1 were diagnosed on the basis of location in this same basal zone. Since PAPG were previously demonstrated in both altered pyloric mucosa consisting of hyperplastic or atrophied tissue, or both, and in normal-looking pyloric mucosa (8–10). Therefore, only the latter was analyzed in this investigation to maintain comparability with results obtained from normal, nontreated groups and avoid the influence of degenerative change. Percentages of flash- and cumulative BrdU-labeled normal (2000 normal pyloric gland cells were sampled) and Pg 1-altered pyloric gland cells (1000 Pg 1-altered pyloric gland cells were sampled) were calculated from each animal analyzed. Numbers of flash-labeled cells per pyloric column in a total of 200 pyloric columns were also calculated for each animal. For statistical analysis of labeling indices, the two-tailed t-test was applied to establish significant differences.

Experiment 2

    Chemicals. Commercial chemicals used were of the purest grade available, and they were obtained as follows: 9,10-dimethyl-1,2-benzanthracene (DMBA), sodium cholate (Na-C), sodium tauroglycocholate (Na-TGC), sodium deoxycholate (Na-DC), and sodium taurocholate (Na-TC) from Wako Pure Chemical Industries, Osaka; *N*-nitroso-*N*-methylurea (MNU) and lithocholic acid (LCA) from Sigma Chemical Co., St. Louis, MO; *N*-ethyl-*N'*-nitronitrosoguanidine (ENNG), catechol, and chenodeoxycholic acid (CDCA) from Aldrich Chemical Co., Milwaukee, WI; 3'-methyl-4-dimethyl-aminoazobenzene (3'-Me-DAB), MNNG, and sodium glycocholate (Na-GC) from Tokyo Kasei Kogyo Co., Tokyo; *N*-butyl-*N*-(4-hydroxybutyl)nitrosamine (BBN) from Izumi Chemical Co., Yokohama; phenobarbital from Iwai Seiyaku Co., Tokyo; and 4-nitroquinoline-1-oxide (4-NQO) and dihydroxy-di-*N*-propylnitrosamine (DHPN) from Nacalai Tesque, Kyoto.

    Animals. Two hundred seventy male WKY/NCrj rats were housed in the same living conditions and fed the same diet as the animals in Experiment 1 (The experimental

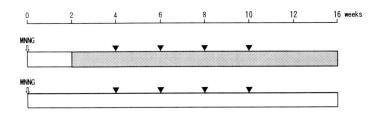

Figure 1. Experimental design of the medium-term bioassay for gastric carcinogens and promoters using PAPG as the end-point lesions. MNNG, single intragastric intubation of 160 mg/kg body weight; □, basal diet; ■, test chemical administration; ▼, saturated sodium chloride solution, 1 ml/rat intragastrically.

Table 1. Bromodeoxyuridine Flash-Labeling Indices

	Labeled cells/ pyloric column[a]	Labeled pyloric gland cells/ 100 pyloric gland cells
No. of animals	5	5
Pyloric column		
Control group	2.2 ± 0.6[b,c]	0.1 ± 0.1[d]
MNNG-treated group		
Without PAPG[e]	2.4 ± 0.6[c]	0.2 ± 0.1[d]
With PAPG[f]	3.9 ± 1.0	1.7 ± 0.5

[a] Number of labeled cells per isthmus associated with normal pyloric glands only or glands containing PAPG.
[b] Mean ± standard deviation.
[c] Significantly different from PAPG at $P < 0.05$.
[d] Significantly different from PAPG at $P < 0.01$.
[e] Normal-appearing pyloric gland with high Pg-1 content.
[f] Containing pepsinogen 1-altered pyloric gland.

protocol is shown in Fig. 1). The animals were divided into two groups, and the first was given a single dose of 160 mg/kg of body weight MNNG as a solution in dimethylsulfoxide by intragastric intubation (i.g.). After two weeks on the basal diet, they received one of the test compounds in drinking water or by i.g. for 14 weeks, at the concentrations given in Table 1. In addition, 1 ml of saturated sodium chloride solution was given by i.g. once each week at weeks 4, 6, 8, and 10. Group 2 was treated the same way as Group 1 but without test chemical administration. Animals were killed at the end of week 16, the stomachs fixed in sublimated formalin, and cut into about 8 strips which were embedded in paraffin.

Immunohistochemical staining for Pg 1. Immunohistochemical testing for Pg 1 was performed as for Experiment 1. The numbers of PAPG per 1 cm of mucosal length were calculated by counting lesions in all stomach strips. The length of pyloric mucosa analyzed on histologic slides was measured with a general-purpose, color-image processor (Olympus Model VIP-21C, Olympus Co., Tokyo).

Results

Experiment 1

Double immunohistochemical analysis of Pg 1 and BrdU. In the controls (Fig. 2A), pyloric gland cells stained strongly for Pg 1 immunohistochemical features and mitoses were observed only in the isthmus region. PAPG (Fig. 2B) were found in otherwise normal-appearing pyloric mucosa in rats treated with MNNG, at a frequency of 3.8 ± 1.1 (mean ± S.D. at 10 weeks, n = 5) and 4.1 ± 0.6 (at 12 weeks, n = 20) per 100 pyloric glands. Mitoses were found in the isthmus and also in PAPG, although rarely.

Flash-labeling indices at week 12 are summarized in Table 2. Double Pg 1 and BrdU immunohistochemical analysis of pyloric mucosa taken from control animals killed 60 min after one injection of BrdU showed that the labeled epithelial cells were confined to a zone several cells wide, at the isthmus region with almost no Pg 1 content,

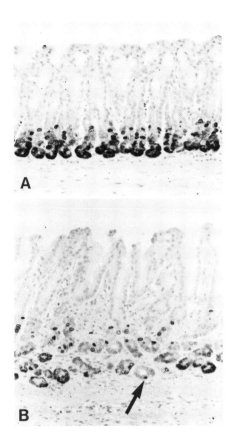

Figure 2. (A) Results of double immunohisto-chemical staining for BrdU incorporation and Pg 1 in pyloric mucosa of control rats 60 min after a single injection of label. Labeled cells are confined to the isthmus region. ×150. (B) Double immu-nohistochemical staining for BrdU and Pg 1 in pyloric mucosa of a rat treated with MNNG 60 min after single injection of BrdU. Labeled cells are primarily confined to the isthmus but some cells in PAPG (arrow) also demonstrate BrdU incor-poration. ×200.

and that normal Pg 1-positive pyloric gland cells demonstrated no BrdU incorporation (Fig. 2A). In the MNNG-treated group, however, an appreciable number of PAPG cells were positive (Fig. 2B). The number of labeled cells per pyloric column containing PAPG was also significantly higher ($P < 0.05$) than the respective figure for columns containing only normal Pg 1-positive pyloric glands.

Sequential changes in labeling indices of pyloric gland cells brought about by continuous BrdU administration for 4, 7, and 10 days in control and MNNG-treated groups are summarized in Figure 3. In controls, after 4 days of continuous BrdU administration all gastric pit epithelial cells and pyloric gland cells in the upper one-third of the pyloric gland with high Pg 1 content were labeled. By the seventh day of con-tinuous labeling, 60% of the cells with high Pg 1 content showed incorporation of BrdU. Unlabeled pyloric gland cells with high Pg 1 content were located only in the lower one-third of the glands. After 10 days of continuous BrdU administration, about 20% of the pyloric gland cells with high Pg 1 content located at the bottom of the gland were still not labeled. Although no differences were evident between the MNNG-treated group and controls in labeling index and location of labeled cells of pyloric glands with high

Table 2. Numbers of Pg 1-Altered Pyloric Glands in Pyloric Mucosa

Treatment	Dose (%)	Route	No. of animals	No. of PAPG/ pyloric mucosa (cm) mean ± SD
Gastric carcinogen				
MNNG	0.005	W[a]	14	7.04 ± 1.61[b]
ENNG	0.005	W	12	6.48 ± 1.62[b]
MNU	0.04	W	12	7.01 ± 2.42[b]
4-NQO	1 mg twice weekly	IG	13	3.41 ± 1.13[d]
Catechol	0.8	D	14	3.69 ± 0.70[b]
Nongastric carcinogen				
DHPN	0.1	W	14	1.92 ± 1.03
DMBA	0.01	D	13	1.96 ± 1.22
Phenobarbital	0.05	D	10	1.98 ± 0.95
3'-Me-DAB	0.06	D	15	2.86 ± 0.58
BBN	0.05	W	14	2.85 ± 0.99
Bile acids				
Sodium taurocholate (Na-Tc)	0.25	D	14	4.09 ± 1.34[b]
Sodium glycocholate (Na-Gc)	0.3	D	15	3.78 ± 1.31[c]
Sodium cholate (Na-C)	0.3	D	17	3.72 ± 0.73[b]
Sodium tauroglycocholate (Na-TGC)	0.3	D	18	2.87 ± 1.29
Sodium deoxycholate (Na-DC)	0.3	D	15	2.82 ± 1.03
Chenodeoxycholic acid (CDCA)	0.1	D	15	2.78 ± 1.08
Lithocholic acid (LCA)	0.5	D	16	2.01 ± 0.50
Control	–	–	15	2.57 ± 0.53

[a] D, in diet; W, in drinking water; IG, intragastric administration.
[b] Significantly different from control at $P < 0.001$.
[c] Significantly different from control at $P < 0.01$.
[d] Significantly different from control at $P < 0.05$.

Pg 1 content, different cell kinetics were apparent in cells of PAPG induced by MNNG. After 4 days of cumulative labeling with BrdU, cells in the upper half of the PAPG were labeled, and by the seventh day of continuous labeling about 90% of the PAPG cells demonstrated BrdU incorporation. Almost 100% of cells comprising PAPG were labeled after 10 days of continuous BrdU labeling. The labeling indices of PAPG cells were therefore significantly higher than those of pyloric gland cells with high Pg 1 content at days 4 ($P < 0.02$), 7 ($P < 0.001$), and 10 ($P < 0.01$). Because renewal of the pyloric gland cells occurs by a pipeline system (19), the life span of pyloric gland cells with high Pg 1 content in control and MNNG-treated groups was estimated to be 11–13 days. Although the calculation is complicated by the fact that cells in PAPG themselves demonstrated mitotic activity, continuous labeling was found to reduce their estimated life span considerably, to 6–8 days.

Experiment 2

Pyloric mucosa in each of the groups consisted of normal areas as well as regions of mucosal hyperplasia and atrophy. PAPG were easily distinguished immunohistochemically from pyloric glands with high Pg 1 content. The compounds tested in this experiment were tentatively classified into three groups: gastric carcinogens, nongastric

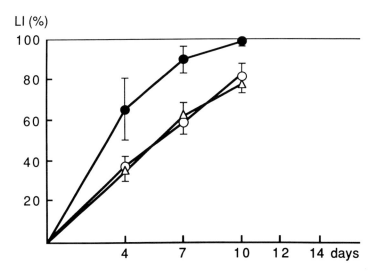

Figure 3. Percentage of labeled pyloric glandular cells, plotted against period of cumulative labeling; ●, labeling index (LI) of PAPG in the experimental group; ○, LI of normal-looking pyloric glands with high Pg 1 content in the experimental group; △, LI of phloric glands in controls; bar, standard deviation. Each point estimated from data for 5 animals.

carcinogens, and bile acids. The gastric carcinogens—MNNG, ENNG, MNU, 4-NQO, and catechol—all exerted potent enhancing effects on the development of PAPG ($P <$ 0.05–0.001). Nongastric carcinogens were without significant influence, but three— Na-TC, Na-GC, and Na-C—of seven bile acids were associated with clear increases in PAPG numbers. Quantitative data for PAPG are summarized in Table 1.

Discussion

Since Pg 1 has been proposed as a negative marker for detection of preneoplastic changes in gastric epithelium during the early phase of gastric carcinogenesis, it is important to distinguish Pg 1 decreases in preneoplastic lesions from those in degenerate, immature, or regenerating gastric epithelium. Any stimulus, carcinogenic or toxic, that increases the proliferative activity of gastric mucosa and thus increases the number of cells in S phase might result in reduced Pg 1 production. In this study, to avoid the toxic effects of MNNG on gastric mucosa, PAPG cell kinetics were investigated only 2 weeks after carcinogen withdrawal. A second reason for the timing was that the presence of a carcinogen might influence the PAPG cell kinetics (20).

Increased rates of cell generation and labeled cells per pyloric column in normal-appearing pyloric mucosa treated with MNNG have been reported by Deschner et al. (21) and Wilson and MaCartney (22). In our experiment, the fact that the number of flash-labeled cells per pyloric column containing PAPG was significantly ($P < 0.05$) higher than that number for pyloric columns with only normal pyloric glands suggests that the elevated labeling index of pyloric mucosa treated with MNNG might be caused by changes in the PAPG-containing columns.

Continuous labeling with BrdU clearly indicated that the cells of normal pyloric glands and of PAPG are derived from the germinative cells in the isthmus region and that they undergo a downward migration (6,19). Continuous labeling revealed cell turnover in PAPG to be about 5 days faster than that of pyloric gland cells with high Pg 1 content. Thus, in addition to increased proliferation, life span was reduced.

In our previous work (6,23), we proposed a hypothesis for the relationship between Pg 1 biochemical changes and stomach carcinogenesis, based on life span of pyloric gland cells as estimated by pulse labeling and sequential appearance of gastric lesions. We suggested that administration of MNNG alters stem cells and that the newly generated, altered pyloric gland cells demonstrated change in gene expression for Pg 1. A few preneoplastic stem cells with altered genes involved in carcinogenesis would be expected to be produced by MNNG, either through altered stem germ cells or directly from normal stem cells. Neoplastic germ cells may arise from preneoplastic germ cells in the pyloric mucosa. The theoretical "altered pyloric gland cells" discussed in our previous work seem equivalent, therefore, to the PAPG demonstrated in the current study using immunohistochemical staining by Pg 1. Although PAPG are not distinguishable from surrounding pyloric glands solely on the basis of morphologic changes, their component cells differ from surrounding pyloric gland cells in proliferation kinetics, which suggests they should be considered preneoplastic changes in stomach carcinogenesis.

Use of PAPG as end-point lesions for medium-term in vivo screening of gastric carcinogens and promoters demands conditions that allow their rapid development. Rapid production of PAPG after MNNG initiation has been observed under the influence of strong gastric carcinogens, but a relatively long period is required for the effects of promoters to become apparent (24). In the design of in vivo medium-term bioassay protocols, choosing a suitable experimental period is important; if the period is too short, weak gastric carcinogens and gastric promoters may not be detected. Na-TC is considered to be a weak gastric promoter (25,26), but the administration of sodium chloride during Na-TC treatment promoted PAPG development significantly after only 12 weeks. Thus, we proposed the experimental model (Experiment 2) to consist of four components: (a) PAPG as the end-point marker, (b) a single dose of MNNG (160 mg/kg of body weight) as the initiator, (c) test-chemical administration for 14 weeks, and (d) administration of saturated sodium chloride solution during test-chemical exposure.

Of the carcinogens tested in the system, all the generally recognized nongastric carcinogens including DHPN (27,28), DMBA (29), phenobarbital (30,31), 3'-Me-DAB (31,32), and BBN (33), lacked enhancing activity for PAPG development. However, the potent gastric carcinogens MNNG (3), ENNG (34), MNU (35), 4-NQO (36,37), and catechol (38) were all positive in terms of increases in the numbers of PAPG in this assay system. Among seven bile acids tested, Na-TC (25,26), Na-Gc, and Na-C also demonstrated enhancing effects. Further studies are required to confirm whether the latter two bile acids are true promoters of gastric cancers.

Since promoters and some carcinogens are nonmutagenic, our current findings suggested that the medium-term in vivo system used has advantages over other short-term in vitro bacterial systems. The gastric carcinogen catechol (38) and the promoter Na-TC (25,26) were, for example, detected as positive by our system, but they generally lacked mutagenic activity in in vitro bacterial mutagenesis assays (39). A combination of mutagenicity testing and our system might be appropriate for accurate assessment.

Conclusion

The cell kinetics of pepsinogen 1-altered pyloric glands with low Pg 1 content were analyzed using double immunohistochemical staining for BrdU incorporation and Pg 1. After administration of 100 μg/ml MNNG in the drinking water to male WKY/NCrj rats for 10 weeks, treatment was terminated and the animals killed 2 weeks later. BrdU was given either as a single intraperitoneal injection (100 mg/kg of body weight) 1 hr before sacrifice or continuously by osmotic minipump (120 μg/hr) for 4, 7, and 10 days before killing. IGSS was used to detect BrdU, and the ABC method was adapted to demonstrate Pg 1. PAPG were found only in the MNNG-treated group. The numbers of labeled cells in the pyloric columns containing PAPG were elevated ($P < 0.05$) over normal values. After continuous BrdU administration, the life span of cells comprising PAPG was estimated to be 6–8 days whereas that of normal pyloric gland cells was 11–13 days. Thus, the data indicated that PAPG cells are characterized by altered proliferation kinetics, which suggested their preneoplastic nature and involvement in gastric carcinogenesis.

These findings were supported by the results of a second study in which 270 male WKY/NCrj rats were treated first with a single dose of MNNG (160 mg/kg of body weight) and starting two weeks later, were administered 1 of 5 gastric carcinogens, 5 nongastric carcinogens, or 7 bile acids for 14 weeks. Analyses of pyloric-mucosa sections for PAPG after the animals' sacrifice at week 16 revealed more lesions produced by the 5 gastric carcinogens and 3 of the 7 bile acids. None of the nongastric carcinogens exerted any significant modification of PAPG induction. These results strongly suggested that this experimental model would be useful for detecting gastric carcinogens as well as promoters of gastric carcinogens in a relatively short time period.

Acknowledgments

This research was supported in part by Grants-in-Aid for Cancer Research from the Ministry of Education, Science and Culture, the Ministry of Health and Welfare of Japan, and the Society for Promotion of Pathology of Nagoya.

References

1. Ito N, Tatematsu M, Nakanishi K, Hasegawa R, Takano T, Imaida K, Ogiso T. The effects of various chemicals on the development of hyperplastic liver nodules in hepatectomized rats treated with N-nitroso-diethylamine or N-2-fluorenylacetamide. Gann 71:832–842, 1980.
2. Fukushima S, Hagiwara A, Ogiso T, Shibata M, Ito N. Promoting effects of various chemicals in rat urinary bladder carcinogenesis initiated by N-nitroso-N-butyl-(4-hydroxybutyl)amine. Food Chem Toxicol 21:59–68, 1983.

3. Sugimura T, Fujimura S. Tumour production in glandular stomach of rats by N-methyl-N'-nitrosoguanidine. Nature 216:943–944, 1967.

4. Furihata C, Kawachi T, Sugimura T. Premature induction of pepsinogen in developing rat gastric mucosa by hormones. Biochem Biophys Res Commun 47:705–711, 1972.

5. Furihata C, Sasajima K, Kazama S, Kogure T, Kawachi T, Sugimura T, Tatematsu M, Takahashi M. Changes in pepsinogen isozymes in stomach carcinogenesis induced in rats by N-methyl-N'-nitro-N-nitrosoguanidine. J Natl Cancer Inst 55:925–930, 1975.

6. Tatematsu M, Saito D, Furihata C, Miyata Y, Nakatsuka T, Ito N, Sugimura T. Initial DNA damage and heritable permanent change in pepsinogen isoenzyme pattern in the pyloric mucosa of rats after short-term administration of N-methyl-N'-nitro-N-nitrosoguanidine. J Natl Cancer Inst 64:775–781, 1980.

7. Tatematsu M, Furihata C, Hirose M, Shirai T, Ito N, Nakajima Y, Sugimura T. Changes in pepsinogen isozymes in stomach cancer induced in Wistar rats by N-methyl-N'-nitro-N-nitrosoguanidine and in transplantable gastric carcinoma (SG2B). J Natl Cancer Inst 58:1709–1716, 1977.

8. Tatematsu M, Furihata C, Mera T, Shirai T, Matsushima T, Ito N. Immunohistochemical demonstration of induction of pyloric glands with low pepsinogen 1 (Pg 1) content in rat stomach by N-methyl-N'nitro-N-nitrosoguanidine. Gann 77:238–243, 1986.

9. Tatematsu M, Furihata C, Katsuyama T, Mera Y, Inoue T, Matsushima T, Ito N. Immunohistochemical demonstration of pyloric gland type cells with low pepsinogen isozyme 1 (Pg 1) in preneoplastic and neoplastic tissues of the stomach of rats treated with N-methyl-N'-nitro-N-nitrosoguanidine. J Natl Cancer Inst 78:771-777, 1987.

10. Tatematsu M, Aoki T, Inoue T, Mutai M, Furihata C, Ito N. Coefficient induction of pepsinogen 1-decreased pyloric glands and gastric cancers in five different strains of rats treated with N-methyl-N'-nitro-N-nitrosoguanidine. Carcinogenesis 9:495–498, 1988.

11. Tatematsu M, Mutai M, Inoue K, Ozaki K, Furihata C, Ito N. Synergism between sodium chloride and sodium taurocholate and development of pepsinogen-altered pyloric glands: Relevance to a medium-term bioassay system for gastric carcinogens and promoters in rats. Jpn J Cancer Res 80:1035–1040, 1989.

12. Meuwissen SGM, Mullink H, Bosma A, Gals G, Defize J, Flipse M, Westerveld BD, Tas M, Brakke J, Kreuning J, Eriksson AW, Meyer CJLM. Immunocytochemical localization of pepsinogens I and II in the human stomach. In: Kreuning J, Samloff IM, Rotter JI, Eriksson AW (eds): Pepsinogens in Man; Clinical and Genetic Advances. Aalsmeer: Mur-Kostveroren, 1984, pp. 123–130.

13. Holgate CS, Jackson P, Cowen PN, Bird CC. Immunogold-silver staining: New method of immunostaining with enhanced sensitivity. J Histochem Cytochem 31:938–944, 1983.

14. Sugihara H, Hattori T, Fukuda M. Immunohistochemical detection of bromodeoxyuridine in formalin-fixed tissue. J Histochem Cytochem 29:193–195, 1986.

15. Achutte B, Reynders MMJ, Bosman FT, Blijham GH. Effect of tissue fixation on anti-bromodeoxyuridine immunohistochemistry. J Histochem Cytochem 35:1343–1345, 1987.

16. Hsu SM, Raine L, Fanger H. Use of avidin-biotin-peroxidase complex (ABC) in immunoperoxidase techniques: A comparison between ABC and unlabelled antibody (PAP) procedures. J Histochem Cytochem 29:577–580, 1981.

17. Furihata C, Saito D, Fujiki H, Kanai Y, Matsushima T, Sugimura T. Purification and characterization of pepsinogens and a unique pepsin from rat stomach. Eur J Biochem 105:43–50, 1980.

18. Graham RC Jr, Karnofsky MJ. The early stage of absorption of injected horseradish peroxidase in the proximal convoluted tubules of mouse kidney: Ultrastructural cytochemistry by a new technique. J Histochem Cytochem 14:291–302, 1966.

19. Hattori T, Fujita S. Tritiated thymidine autoradiographic study of cell migration and renewal in the pyloric mucosa of golden hamsters. Cell Tissue Res 175:49–57, 1976.

20. Zedeck MS, Grab DJ, Sternberg SS. Differences in the acute response of the various segments of rat intestine to treatment with the intestinal carcinogen methylazoxymethanol. Cancer Res 37:32–36, 1977.

21. Deschner EE, Tamura K, Bralow P. Sequential histopathology and cell kinetic changes in rat pyloric mucosa during gastric carcinogenesis induced by N-methyl-N'nitro-N-nitrosoguanidine. J Natl Cancer Inst 63:171–179, 1979.

22. Wilson NW, Macartney C. A comparison of in vitro and in vivo gastric mucosal cell kinetics. Lab Invest 58:459–465, 1988.

23. Tatematsu M, Furihata C, Katsuyama T, Hasegawa R, Nakanowatari J, Saito D, Takahashi M, Matsushita T, Ito N. Independent induction of intestinal metaplasia and gastric cancer in rats treated with N-methyl-N'-nitro-N-nitrosoguanidine. Cancer Res 43:1335–1341, 1983.

24. Tatematsu M, Aoki T, Asamoto M, Furihata C, Ito N. Enhancing effects of N-ethyl-N'-nitro-N-nitrosoguanidine and sodium taurocholate on development of pepsinogen 1 decreased pyloric glands in rats initiated with N-methyl-N'nitro-N-nitrosoguanidine. Jpn J Cancer Res 78:312–316, 1987.

25. Salmon RJ, Laurence M, Thierry JP. Effect of taurocholic acid feeding on methyl-nitro-N-nitrosoguanidine induced gastric tumors. Cancer Lett 22:315–320, 1984.

26. Kobori O, Shimizu T, Maeda M, Atomi Y, Watanabe J, Shoji M, Morioka Y. Enhancing effect of bile and bile acid on stomach tumorigenesis induced by N-methyl-N'-nitro-N-nitrosoguanidine in Wistar rats. J Natl Cancer Inst 73:853–861, 1984.

27. Hiasa Y, Kitahori Y, Konishi N, Shimoyama T, Lin J-C. Sex differential and dose dependence of phenobarbital promoting activity in N-bis(2-hydroxypropyl)nitrosamine-initiated thyroid tumorigenesis in rats. Cancer Res 45:4087, 1985.

28. Shirai T, Masuda A, Imaida K, Ogiso T, Ito N. Effects of phenobarbital and carbazole on carcinogenesis of the lung, thyroid, kidney, and bladder of rats pretreated with N-bis(2-hydroxypropyl)nitrosamine. Jpn J Cancer Res 79:460, 1988.

29. Shirai T, Fukushima S, Ikawa E, Tagawa Y, Ito N. Induction of prostate carcinoma in situ at high incidence in F344 rats by a combination of 3,2-dimethyl-4-aminobiphenyl and ethinyl estradiol. Cancer Res 46:6423, 1986.

30. Peraino C, Fry RJM, Staffeldt E, Kisieleski WE. Effects of varying the exposure to phenobarbital on its enhancement of 2-acetylaminofluorene-induced hepatic tumorigenesis in rats. Cancer Res 33:2701–2705, 1973.

31. Kitagawa T, Sugano H. Enhancing effect of phenobarbital on the development of enzyme-altered islands and hepatocellular carcinomas initiated by 3'-methyl-4(dimethylamino)azobenzene or diethylnitrosamine. Gann 69:679–687, 1978.

32. Giese LA, Clayton CC, Miller EC, Brauman CA. Effect of certain diets on hepatic tumor formation due to 3'-methyl-p-dimethylaminoazobenzene. Cancer Res 6:679–684, 1946.

33. Ito N, Arai M, Sugihara S, Hirao K, Makiura S, Matayoshi K, Denda A. Experimental urinary bladder tumors induced by N-butyl-N-(4-hydroxybutyl)nitrosamine. Gann Monograph 17:367–381, 1975.

34. Sugimura T, Kawachi T. Experimental stomach cancer. In: Busch H (ed): Methods in Cancer Research New York: Academic Press, 1973, pp. 245–308.

35. Hirota N, Aonuma T, Yamada S, Kawai T, Saito K, Yokoyama T. Selective induction of glandular stomach carcinoma in F344 rats by N-methyl-N-nitrosourea. Jpn J Cancer Res 78:634–638, 1987.

36. Takahashi M, Saito H, Effect of 4-nitroquinoline 1-oxide with alkylbenzenesulfonate on gastric carcinogenesis in rats. In: Morris HP, Yoshiota T (eds): Gann Monograph. Tokyo: Maruzem, 1970, pp. 241–261.

37. Tatematsu M, Takahashi M, Fukushima S, Hananouchi M, Shirai T. Effects in rats of sodium chloride on experimental gastric cancers induced by N-methyl-N'-nitro-N-nitrosoguanidine or 4-nitroquinoline-1-oxide. J Natl Cancer Res 55:101–106, 1975.

38. Hirose M, Kurata Y, Tsuda H, Fukushima S, Ito N. Catechol strongly enhances rat stomach carcinogenesis: A possible new environmental stomach carcinogen. Jpn J Cancer Res 78:1144–1149, 1987.

39. Silverman SJ, Andrews AW. Bile acids: Co-mutagenic activity in the Salmonella-mammalian-microsome mutagenicity test: Brief communication. J Natl Cancer Inst 59:1557–1559, 1977.

Chemically Induced Cell Proliferation:
Implications for Risk Assessment, pages 457-467
©1991 Wiley-Liss, Inc.

Chemically Induced Cell Proliferation as a Predictive Assay for Potential Carcinogenicity

Byron E. Butterworth

Carcinogenesis is a complex process involving sequential mutations in growth regulatory genes and subsequent clonal expansion of the resulting preneoplastic or neoplastic cells (1,2). One difficulty in detecting chemical carcinogens is that the latency period for disease development is very long; approximately 20 years will pass from the beginning of smoking to measurable cigarette-induced lung cancer. In rodent models, test agents must often be administered over the lifetime of the animal (approximately two years) before visible chemically induced tumors are observed (3). Bioassays to evaluate the carcinogenic activity of a chemical in rodents can take from three to four years and cost up to one million dollars. Consequently, there is a need for short-term predictive assays to estimate potential carcinogenic activity of chemicals to which people are or will be exposed. The underlying principle for any such test must be that the biological activity measured in cultured cells or specific tissues is reflective of key events in the carcinogenic process (4).

The terms *initiation, promotion,* and *progression* have been used to describe various steps in the carcinogenic process, and assays that could measure these activities would be candidates for short-term predictive tests. These events are difficult to define rigorously because they are so highly dependent on the particular experimental model and species under study. For example, a chemical might be called a promoter because it accelerates tumor formation in the two-stage mouse skin painting carcinogenesis model, but the same chemical may exhibit no activity with the exact same protocol when tested on a different strain of mouse (5).

Genotoxicity as a predictive assay for potential carcinogenicity

Initiation events refer to mutations in or altered expression of normal cellular growth control genes resulting in active oncogenes and/or inactivated tumor suppressor genes. The term *initiation* is normally used very generally because so little is actually known about the events that occur in this stage of carcinogenesis, and because it is often impossible to identify which of the many genetic and cellular alterations present in neoplastic cells occurred in the initiation phase. For example, in the initiation portion of initiation/promotion protocols, animals are treated with a single dose of a potent mutagen such as benzo[a]pyrene or diethylnitrosamine, resulting in potential mutations in hundreds of different growth control genes, at thousands of different sites, in millions of different cells. Nevertheless, understanding a toxicant's mode of action is often valuable in toxicological evaluations, even if our understanding does not include its mechanism of action.

Evidence indicates that DNA-reactive chemicals are often carcinogenic in target tissues that are the site of mutagenic activity (6). This observation is the basis for a variety of predictive assays designed to detect those genotoxic carcinogens whose primary biologic activity is direct alteration of the information encoded in the DNA. Such alterations may be point mutations, insertions, deletions, or changes in chromosome structure or number. Chemicals exhibiting such activity are called genotoxicants and can usually be identified by assays that measure reactivity with the DNA, induction of mutations, induction of DNA repair, or cytogenetic effects. The first short-term test that was proposed and validated for use in predicting potential carcinogenicity is the Salmonella/microsome mutagenicity assay, or Ames test, which quantitates chemically induced reversion mutations in specially engineered strains of bacteria (7). Other assays have been developed in bacterial or mammalian cell cultures supplemented with a metabolic activation system, or in the intact animal (8–10). The development of these predictive tests is one of the greatest successes in modern toxicology. Assays such as the Ames test are conducted worldwide every year to identify potential carcinogens. Most corporations now consider the profile of genotoxic activity when developing compounds; rarely is a new product marketed and later shown to be a mutagenic carcinogen.

Nongenotoxic carcinogens

Nongenotoxic chemicals are those whose parent compounds or metabolites lack DNA reactivity or for which direct chromosome-altering effects is not a primary biologic activity. Various classification schemes of genotoxic and nongenotoxic carcinogens as well as many different subclasses of agents have been described (4,11–13). It is important to further define the mechanisms by which these agents act, because the term *nongenotoxic* is too general to be of value. For example, the potent liver tumor promoter 2,3,7,8-tetrachlorodibenzo-p-dioxin (TCDD), appears to be acting at vanishingly low doses through specific cellular receptors (14). In contrast, bladder tumors produced by saccharin are associated with sustained hyperplasia and proliferation seen only at massive doses of the chemical (15). Thus, questions of mechanism, predictive assays, and risk assessment models are probably not the same for these two agents, although both are nongenotoxic carcinogens.

Chemically induced cell proliferation in carcinogenesis

Theoretical basis of short-term tests

Mutagenic activity is an effective predictor of carcinogenic activity because mutations in growth control genes are one step in carcinogenesis. This is supported by the observation that mutagenic chemicals are often carcinogenic and by the identification of oncogenes in rodent and human tumors (7,16–20).

Predictive assays for the nongenotoxic carcinogens must be based on the mechanisms by which they act in the animal (21–24). A common biologic activity for many of the nongenotoxic carcinogens is that of chemically induced cell proliferation (4). The theoretical basis for induced cell proliferation as a predictive assay is: first, the process of cell proliferation can in itself result in mutagenic events; and second, clonal growth of preneoplastic cells increases the target population of those cells that need only one or two further mutations to become fully malignant. Direct and secondary alterations in growth control that are related to induced cell proliferation may provide a selective growth advantage for preneoplastic cells. In contrast to mutagens, the action of most chemicals that alter growth control can be reversible to some point and continuous application over extended periods is often required for carcinogenic activity to occur (25). This suggests that for these agents, altered growth control may play the critical role in tumor formation.

Chemical induction of cell proliferation

There are numerous ways that chemicals might induce a mitogenic response, including: interacting with cellular receptors and growth factors; causing cell death and subsequent regenerative growth; interrupting tissue growth control mechanisms such as cell-to-cell communication; and inhibiting programmed cell death or apoptosis (26,27). In general, there appear to be two broad classes of cell proliferation-inducing chemicals: those that are directly mitogenic and those that are cytotoxic and cause regenerative growth (28).

Phenobarbital, α-hexachlorocyclohexane, and the peroxisomal-proliferating liver carcinogens are mitogenic and induce an increase in liver size that is sustained as long as the compound is continually administered (29–33). Cell proliferation occurs during the first few days of treatment, but then returns to baseline levels. However, under conditions of continued exposure to such agents, rates of cell turnover are dramatically increased in developing preneoplastic foci (34).

Other nongenotoxic carcinogens such as furan, chloroform, carbon tetrachloride, and methapyrilene are cytotoxic and under bioassay conditions induce a sustained regenerative hyperplasia to replace dead cells, with increases in the labeling index (LI) of up to two orders of magnitude in the target organ relative to controls (35–39). Some compounds such as [4-chloro-6-(2,3-xylidino)-2-pyrimidinylthio]acetic acid (Wy-14,643) induce multiple effects, producing liver hyperplasia, a sustained elevation in cell turnover, and altered growth control in preneoplastic foci (40).

There are numerous roles that cell replication may play in the carcinogenic process (1,41). Enhanced replication increases the frequency of spontaneous mutations and the probability of converting DNA adducts into mutations before they can be repaired (3,42–45). The mutation or altered expression of oncogenes and growth control proteins are strongly implicated in cancer (18,20,41,46,47). The chance for an initiating event is enhanced during replication because while these genes are being transcribed, the DNA is unwound and its exposure and susceptibility to endogenous and exogenous carcinogen-induced DNA damage is increased, even though DNA repair may be enhanced in these regions as well (48–51).

Additionally, tumor promotion and progression are associated with a sustained induction of cell replication (52,53). The multistep process of carcinogenesis involves the clonal expansion of initiated or altered cells (1,41). Those compounds that alter growth control and cause preferential growth and elevated cell turnover of initiated cells will greatly increase the target size of those cells that need only a few further genetic alterations to become cancerous (3,34,40,54).

Nongenotoxic complete carcinogens

There is a misconception that only DNA-reactive compounds can effect all the changes necessary to produce tumors by themselves and be classified as so-called complete carcinogens. In fact, under the chronic, lifetime maximum tolerated dose (MTD) regimen typically used for cancer bioassays, nongenotoxic agents will often yield tumors as a result of those extreme conditions (55,56). The myriad of examples in this volume illustrate the importance of dealing with this fact. Induced cell proliferation, as we have discussed, is associated with both initiation and promotion events.

A compound that only induces spontaneous tumor growth must be called a complete carcinogen, even though the agent's primary activity may only have been tumor promotion. For example, spontaneous foci of preneoplastic cells can increase with time in the rat livers because of intrinsic factors and natural mutagenic insults and without any chemical exposure (57). Chemicals that alter growth control when administered over the animal's lifetime may cause these foci to accelerate tumor formation (29,54,58). Mice that have undergone partial hepatectomy and have not been treated with any chemicals will have liver regrowth with a concomitant increase in tumor formation (59). The incidence of spontaneous mammary gland carcinoma in control female F344 rats is 2.1% at 104 weeks, but rises to 11.2% in life-span studies (140-146 weeks) (60). Nongenotoxic chemicals that increase the cell turnover rate in that tissue may shorten the time in which spontaneous tumors appear (3).

Comparison of predictive assays based on mutagenicity versus induced cell proliferation

Analysis based on the plus/minus approach

The perception that carcinogenic potential could be predicted with a two-day Ames test instead of a two-year bioassay has produced a revolution affecting both the fields of genetic toxicology and experimental carcinogenesis. Among mutagenesis researchers, the concern no longer focuses on the implications of germ cell mutations and has turned instead to identifying potential carcinogens. Mutational assays have been redefined as short-term tests for carcinogens. The atmosphere surrounding genetic toxicology was often that if a chemical had produced any tumors in any species, in any target organ, at any dose, by any mechanism, that carcinogenic outcome was given a "plus" or positive-response label. The implied goal for any proposed short-term test was, then, to achieve a positive response with that chemical. A plus in any mutagenicity assay was often automatically assumed to be the complete reason why the chemical was carcinogenic. If a negative response was observed, further mutagenicity tests or variations of those tests were often conducted until the desired positive response was seen. However, as more validation studies were conducted, it became clear that there was a wide variety of apparently nongenotoxic carcinogens for which there were no predictive assays. For example, in a recent National Toxicology Program/National Cancer Institute (NTP/NCI) study of 73 chemicals, over half of the carcinogens tested were negative in the Ames test (19).

Table 1 illustrates analysis of data primarily from the NTP/NCI study using the traditional plus/minus evaluation. Given that chemical carcinogenesis is such a complex, multistep process and that short-term bacterial and cell culture tests differ in so many important ways from the intact animal (or in human beings), it is amazing that the short-term mutagenicity tests are as accurate as they are. For example, positive predictivity of the Ames test (percentage of Ames-positive chemicals that prove to be carcinogenic in a rodent model), has always been high and in the range of 80–95% (7,16,17,19). Most mutagens are carcinogens. However, the Ames test cannot be expected to detect agents that are acting primarily through a nongenotoxic mechanism. In the NTP/NCI study, the negative predictivity of the Ames test (percentage of chemicals that were Ames negative, that were proven later to be noncarcinogenic in a rodent model) was only 51%, presumably because many nongenotoxic carcinogens were included in the chemicals examined (19). A positive Ames test is strongly indicative of carcinogenic potential. A negative Ames test suggests that the compound is probably not a genotoxic carcinogen, but provides no information concerning whether it may or may not be a nongenotoxic carcinogen.

The selected examples presented in Table 1 reveal three general classes of carcinogens. First are potent nongenotoxic carcinogens such as TCDD that may act through various specific mechanisms; they may, for instance, interact with cellular receptors to alter growth control and allow the preferential expansion of preneoplastic or initiated cells. Second are the classical genotoxic carcinogens such as 1,2- dibromo-3-chloropropane that appear to act primarily by inducing mutations. Third are the nongenotoxic carcinogens typified by tris(2-ethylhexyl)phosphate that require massive doses in excess of 500 mg/kg/day to produce tumors. Often, the mode of action for these kinds of chemicals appears to be the induction of organ specific toxicity and subsequent cell proliferation.

Table 1. Short-term Test Results for Selected Carcinogens.

Carcinogen[1]	Dose mg/kg/day	Ames	Mou lym	Chrom aberr	Sce
TCDD	0.00001	–	–	–	–
Polybrominated biphenyl mix	0.2	–	–	–	–
Recerpine	0.2	–	–	–	–
1,2-Dibromo-3-chloropropane	0.3	+	+	+	+
Cytembena	3.0	+	+	+	+
1,2-Dibromomethane	4.0	+	+	+	+
Tris(2-ethylhexyl)phosphate	707	–	–	–	–
Cinnamyl anthranilate	1188	–	+	–	–
Di(2-ethylhexyl)adipate	1609	–	–	+	?
Saccharin	3000	–	?	–	–

[1]Reported short-term test results with selected carcinogens (Tennant et al., 1987; Ellwein and Cohen, 1990). Column headings are Ames: Salmonella/microsome test; Mou lym: L5178Y mouse lymphoma mutagenicity assay; Chrom Aberr: induction of chromosome abberations in Chinese hamster ovary cells; and Sce: induction of sister chromatid exchanges in Chinese hamster ovary cells.

Databases

A substantial number of validation assays have been conducted with mutagenicity assays so that investigators have an idea as to the carcinogen classes that might accurately be detected by a given mutagenicity assay (7,16,17,19). In contrast, it is not yet possible to use induced cell proliferation as a predictive assay for carcinogenic potential for either the cytotoxic or mitogenic carcinogens because there is no quantitative database that defines the extent and duration of induced cell proliferation to carcinogenic activity under bioassay conditions (28). This same lack of quantitative information also prevents any realistic assessment of the relevance of tumors produced in this manner to potential effects in human beings. While some information is available in relating proliferation to carcinogenic potential (61–63), most of the data in the current literature was not obtained under bioassay conditions. Until recently, no rigorous experimental guidelines were in place to allow new information to be analyzed as a cohesive database (64).

Bioassay conditions

For whole animal genotoxicity assays, the use of massive doses of the test chemical, different routes of administration than were used in the carcinogenicity bioassays (including intraperitoneal injection), and even assessment of activity in tissues that are not the target for cancer, still serve as overall indicators of potential genotoxicity (10). In contrast, simplistic plus/minus versus carcinogen/noncarcinogen comparisons—with disregard for bioassay conditions, target organ specificity, and quantitative dose-response relationships—will be inappropriate in assessing the predictive potential of induced cell proliferation. The carcinogenic activity of mutagens might be considered an intrinsic property of the chemical and will be dependent on the dose delivered to the target tissue. In contrast, a growing body of evidence indicates that the carcinogenic activity of the cytotoxic non–DNA-reactive carcinogens secondary to induced cell proliferation in the target tissue and is, therefore, conditional on doses high enough to produce cell proliferation or other promoting stimuli.

In building a database to correlate the extent and duration of chemically induced proliferation to carcinogenic activity, original bioassay conditions must be duplicated to the extent possible. Changing the route of administration or even the vehicle can have dramatic effects on cell proliferation and the resulting tumor response (65). For example, if chloroform is administered to female mice in corn oil by gavage, then cytotoxicity, cell proliferation, and, eventually, cancer are observed in the liver. If the same amount of chloroform is administered on a daily basis in the drinking water, then neither cytotoxicity, increased cell proliferation, nor cancer are seen (38,39).

Quantitative versus qualitative data

Table 2 illustrates the traditional approach in validating mutagenic short-term tests. Any information about dose-response relationships; species-, sex-, or target organ-specificity; or preneoplastic lesions is discarded in favor of columns of plus/minus comparisons. In fact, more detailed information is needed, not less. Different amounts of cell proliferation may be required to produce tumors in different tissues and test species. We have observed slight, transient increases in cell proliferation with some noncarcinogens. Thus, the simplistic plus/minus comparisons as shown in Table 2 will have to be replaced with quantitative relationships when relating cell proliferation and cancer. The following nongenotoxic carcinogens have been shown to produce a sustained increase in the labeling index (LI) over controls under bioassay conditions in the appropriate target tissue: Wy-14,643 yields a tenfold increase over controls in the LI in the male rat liver; unleaded gasoline yields a fivefold increase over controls in the LI in the female mouse liver; and furan yields a tenfold increase in the LI over controls in the male rat liver (37,40,65). The complexity of these relationships is so great that it may be some time before a sufficiently large cell proliferation database has been generated and our understanding of these processes is sufficient to serve as the basis for either required testing for potential carcinogenicity or new risk assessment models.

Specificity

Of additional concern with the NTP/NCI database was the observation that some of the mutagenicity assays exhibited a low specificity, showing a positive response for many noncarcinogens (19). This problem tends to be a property of particular assays, suggesting that both the underlying basis for this behavior and the criteria for declaring a result positive may need to be re-examined for those proposed short-term tests.

Much remains to be learned about the role of induced cell proliferation in the carcinogenic process and the additional factors that may be important to more completely understand these phenomena. For example, while the basal cells in the small intestine turn over at a rapid rate, this tissue is not very susceptible to tumor formation and more research will be required to understand why. Cell proliferation produced by different types of agents is not equally effective in producing preneoplastic foci in

Table 2. Mutagenicity/carcinogenicity Data.

Compound[1]	Ames test	Carcinogenicity
2-Biphenylamine HCL	Positive 10 mg/plate with activation	Female mouse circulatory system 386 mg/kg/day
1,2-Dibromo-3-chloropropane	Positive 0.3 mg/plate with activation 0.3 mg/kg/day	Multiple organs male and female mouse and rat
Caprolactam	Negative 10,000 mg/plate	No induced tumors 1931 mg/kg/day
Traditional analysis		
2-Biphenylamine HCL	+	+
1,2-Dibromo-3-chloropropane	+	+
Caprolactam	−	−

[1]Data from Tennant et al., 1987.

experimental carcinogenesis models (66). Some mitogenic stimuli will affect cells in preneoplastic foci differently than in surrounding normal cells (34). Induced cell proliferation cannot always be equated with tumor induction. Many noncarcinogens produce a mild hyperplasia or transient increase in cell turnover that is apparently insufficient for detectable tumor formation (61). Nevertheless, in many cases knowledge of chemically induced tissue-specific cell proliferation and its relationship to tumor induction can be critical information in choosing new chemicals for development, selecting doses for cancer bioassays, and assessing potential risk to humans.

Examination of mutagenic and mitogenic activity in concert

It is also important to recognize that even though a compound may be a weak mutagen, other biologic activity of the molecule may be more important in tumor induction. In fact, both mutagenic and mitogenic activity should be considered when evaluating any carcinogen. Studies with the highly mutagenic, tobacco-specific nitrosamine 4-(N-methyl-N-nitrosamino)-1-(3-pyridyl)-1-butanone (NNK) indicate that a quantitative understanding of both promutagenic DNA adducts and cell proliferation secondary to toxicity are required to account for the site-specific nature of malignant tumor formation within the rat nose (67). Knowledge of cytotoxicity and cell proliferation, as well as the dose delivered to the target cells as assessed by DNA adduct formation, provides far more realistic risk assessment calculations than just considering the administered dose of chemical (67–70).

A weight-of-evidence approach should be used to determine the extent to which a compound should be classified as genotoxic or might better fit into a nongenotoxic carcinogen category. Such an approach might include examination of constituents on the molecule that would suggest DNA reactivity, overall results from cell culture assays, activity in the whole animal, dose- and target organ-specificity, histopathological evaluation of tumor development, and other potential mechanisms of carcinogenicity such as induced cell proliferation.

References

1. Pitot HC. Fundamentals of Oncology. New York: Marcel Dekker, 1986.
2. Stanbridge JE. Identifying tumor suppressor genes in human colorectal cancer. Science 247:12–13, 1990.
3. Swenberg JA, Short BG. In Butterworth BE, Slaga TJ (eds): Nongenotoxic Mechanisms in Carcinogenesis. Banbury Report 25. Cold Spring Harbor, New York: Cold Spring Harbor Laboratory, 1987, p. 151.
4. Butterworth BE. Considerations of both genotoxic and nongenotoxic mechanisms in predicting carcinogenic potential. Mutat Res, in press, 1990.
5. Fischer SM, Baldwin JK, Jasheway DW, Patrick KE Cameron GS. Phorbol eser induction of 8-lipoxigenase in inbred SENCAR (SSIN) but not C57Bl/6J mice correlated with hyperplasia, edema, and oxidant generation but not ornithine decarboxylase induction. Cancer Res 48:658–664, 1988.
6. Miller EC, Miller JA. Searches for ultimate chemical carcinogens and their reactions with cellular macromolecules. Cancer 47:2327, 1981.
7. McCann J, Choi E, Yamasaki E, Ames BN. Detection of carcinogens as mutagens in the Salmonella/microsome test: Assay of 300 chemicals. Proc Natl Acad Sci USA 72:5135, 1975.
8. Hsie AW, O'Neill JP, McElheny VK (eds): Mammalian Cell Mutagenesis: The Maturation of Test Systems, Banbury Report 2. Cold Spring Harbor, New York: Cold Spring Harbor Laboratory, 1979.

9. Bridges BA, Butterworth BE, Weinstein IB (eds): Indicators of Genotoxic Exposure, Banbury Report 13. Cold Spring Harbor, New York: Cold Spring Harbor Laboratory, 1982.
10. Ashby J, de Serres FJ, Shelby MD, Margolin BH, Ishidote M, Becking GC (eds): Evaluation of Short-Term Tests for Carcinogens Report of the International Programme on Chemical Safety's Collaborative Study on In Vivo Assays. Cambridge: Cambridge University Press, 1988.
11. Weisburger JH, Williams GM. Carcinogen testing: current problems and new approaches. Science 214:401–407, 1981.
12. Weisburger JH, Williams GM. The decision-point approach for systematic carcinogen testing. Food and Cosmetic Toxicology 19:561–566, 1981.
13. Williams GM, Weisburger JH. Carcinogen risk assessment. Science 221:6, 1983.
14. Poland A, Kimbrough RD (eds): Biological mechanisms of dioxin action. Banbury Report 18. Cold Spring Harbor, New York: Cold Spring Harbor Laboratory, 1984.
15. Ellwein LB, Cohen SM. Critical Reviews in Toxicology, in press.
16. Purchase IFH, Longstaff E, Ashby J, Styles JA, Anderson D, Lefevre PA, Westwood FR. An evaluation of 6 short-term tests for detecting organic chemical carcinogens, Br J Cancer 37:873–958, 1978.
17. Sugimura T, Sato S, Nagao S, Yahagi T, Matsushima T, Seino Y, Takeuchi N, Kawachi T. Overlapping of carcinogens and mutagens. In Magee PN, et al. (ed): Fundamental in Cancer Prevention. Tokyo: University of Tokyo Press, Baltimore: University Park Press, 1976, pp. 191–215.
18. Land H, Parada LF, Weinberg R. Cellular oncogenes and multistep carcinogenesis. Science, 222:771–778, 1983.
19. Tennant RW, Margolin BH, Shelby MD, Zeiger E, Hasman JK, Spalding J, Caspary W, Resnick M, Stasiewicz S, Anderson B, Minor R. Prediction of chemical carcinogenicity in rodents from in vitro genetic toxicity assays. Science 236:933–941, 1987.
20. Reynolds SH, Stowers JS, Patterson RM, Maronpot RR, Aaronson SA, Anderson M. Activated oncogenes in B6C3F1 mouse liver tumors: Implications for risk assessment. Science 237:1309–1316, 1987.
21. ICPEMC. Mutagenesis testing as an approach to carcinogenesis. Mutat Res 99:73–91, 1982.
22. ICPEMC. Report of ICPEMC task group 5 on the differentiation between genotoxic and non-genotoxic carcinogens. Mutat Res 133:1–49, 1984.
23. ICPEMC. The need for biological risk assessment in reaching decisions about carcinogens. Mutat Res 185:243–269, 1987.
24. ICPEMC. Can a mechanistic rationale be provided for non-genotoxic carcinogens identified in rodent bioassays? Mutat Res 221: 53–67, 1989.
25. Goldsworthy TL, Hanigan MH, Pitot HC. Models of hepatocarcinogenesis in the rat—contrasts and comparisons. Crit Rev Toxicol 17:61–89, 1986.
26. Bursch W, Lauer B, Timmermann-Trosiener I, Barthel G, Schuppler J, Schulte-Hermann R. Controlled death (apoptosis) of normal and putative preneoplastic cells in rat liver following withdrawal of tumor promoters. Carcinogenesis 5:453–458, 1984.
27. Lutz WK, Maier P. Genotoxic and epigenetic chemical carcinogenesis: one process, different mechanisms. Trends Pharmacol Sci 9:322–326, 1988.
28. Loury DJ, Goldsworthy TL, Butterworth BE. The value of measuring cell replication as a predictive index of tissue-specific tumorigenic potential. In Butterworth BE, Slaga TJ (eds): Nongenotoxic Mechanisms in Carcinogenesis. Banbury Report 25. Cold Spring Harbor, New York: Cold Spring Harbor Laboratory, 1987a, pp. 119–136.
29. Schulte-Hermann R, Schuppler J, Ohde G, Bursch W, Timmermann-Trosiener I. Phenobarbital and other liver tumor promoters. In Nicholini C (ed): Chemical Carcinogenesis. New York: Plenum Press, 1982, pp. 231–260.
30. Schulte-Hermann R, Schuppler J, Timmerman-Trosiener I, Ohde G, Bursch W, Berger H. The role of growth of normal and preneoplastic cell populations for tumor promotion in rat liver. Environ Health Perspect 50:185–194, 1983.
31. Schroter C, Parzefall W, Schroter H, Schulte-Hermann R. Dose-response studies on the effects of α-, β-, and γ-hexachlorocyclohexane on putative preneoplastic foci, monooxygenases, and growth in rat liver. Cancer Res 47:80–88, 1987.
32. Schulte-Hermann R, Oschs H, Bursch W, Parzefall W. Quantitative structure-activity studies on effects of sixteen different steroids on growth and monooxygenases of rat liver. Cancer Res 48:2462–2468, 1988.

33. Conway JG, Cattley RC, Popp JA, Butterworth BE. Possible mechanisms in hepatocarcinogenesis by the peroxisome proliferator di(2-ethylhexyl)phthalate. Drug Metab Rev. 21:65–102, 1990.
34. Cattley RC, Popp JA. Differences between the promoting activities of the peroxisome proliferator Wy-14,643 and phenobarbital in rat liver. Cancer Res 49:3246–3521, 1989.
35. Mirsalis JC. Genotoxicity, toxicity and carcinogenicity of the antihistamine methapyrilene. Mutat Res 185:309–317, 1987.
36. Doolittle DJ, Muller G, Scribner HE. The relationship between hepatotoxicity and induction of replicative DNA synthesis following single or multiple doses of carbon tetrachloride. J Toxicol Environ Health 22:63–78, 1987.
37. Wilson DM, Goldsworthy TL, Popp JA, Butterworth BE. Evaluation of genotoxicity, cytotoxicity, and cell proliferation in hepatocytes from rats and mice treated with furan. Proceedings of the American Association for Cancer Research 31:103, 1990.
38. Corley RA, Mendrala AL, Smith FA, Staats DA, Gargas ML, Conolly RB, Andersen ME, Reitz RH. Development of a physiologically-based pharmacokinetic model for chloroform. Toxicol Appl Pharmacol 103:512–527, 1990.
39. Reitz RH, Menrala AL, Corley RA, Quast JF, Gargas ML, Andersen ME, Statts DA, Conolly RB. Estimating the risk of liver cancer associated with human exposures to chloroform. Toxicol Appl Pharmacol, in press.
40. Marsman DS, Cattley RC, Conway JG, Popp JA. Relationship of hepatic peroxisome proliferation and replicative DNA synthesis to the hepatocarcinogenicity of the peroxisome proliferators di(2-ethylhexyl)phthalate and [4-chloro-6-(2,3-xylidino)-2-pyrimidinylthio]acetic acid (Wy-14,643) in rats. Cancer Res 48:6739–6744, 1988.
41. Farber E, Sarma DSR. Biology of disease. Lab Invest 56:4–22, 1987.
42. Craddock VM. Cell proliferation and experimental liver cancer. In Cameron HM, Linsell CA, Warwick GP (eds): Liver Cell Cancer. Amsterdam: Elsevier/North Holland Biomedical Press, 1976, pp. 153–201.
43. Columbano A, Rajalakshmi S, Sarma DSR. Requirement of all proliferation for the initiation of liver carcinogenesis as assayed by three different procedures. Cancer Res 41:2079–2083, 1981.
44. Stott WT, Reitz RH, Schumann AM, Watanabe PG. Genetic and nongenetic events in neoplasia. Food and Cosmetic Toxicology 19:567–576, 1981.
45. Allegretta M, Nicklas JA, Siram S, Albertini RJ. T cells responsive to myelin basic protein in patients with multiple sclerosis. Science 247:718–721, 1990.
46. Stewart TA, Pattengale PK, Leder P. Spontaneous mammary adenocarcinomas in transgenic mice that carry and express MTV/myc fusion genes. Cell 38:627–637, 1984.
47. Adams JM, Harris AW, Pinkert CA, Corcoran LM, Alexander WS, Cory S, Palmiter RD, Brinster RL. The c-myc oncogene driven by immunoglobulin enhancers induces lymphoid malignancy in transgenic mice. Nature 318:533–538, 1985.
48. Bailey A, Saliba D, Miller DM. A marked increase in sensitivity to carcinogenesis is associated with induced protooncogene expression without DNA synthesis. Proceedings of the American Association for Cancer Research 30:183, 1989.
49. Coni P, Bigone FA, Pichiri G, Ledda-Columbano GM, Columbano A, Rao PM, Rajalakshmi S, Sarma DSR. Studies on the kinetics of expression of cell cycle dependent proto-oncogenes during mitogen-induced liver cell proliferation. Cancer Lett 47:115–119, 1989.
50. Braun L, Mead JE, Panzica M, Mikumo R, Bell GL, Fausto N. Transforming growth factor beta mRNA increases during liver regeneration: A possible paracrine mechanism of growth regulation. Proc Natl Acad Sci USA 85:1539–1543, 1988.
51. Mead JE, Fausto N. Transforming growth factor alpha may be a physiological regulator of liver regeneration by means of an autocrine mechanism. Proc Natl Acad Sci USA 86:1558–1562, 1989.
52. Slaga TJ (ed): Mechanisms of Tumor Promotion, vols. 1–4, Boca Raton: CRC Press, Inc., 1983–1984.
53. Argyris TS. Epidermal tumor promotion by damage in the skin of mice. In Slaga TJ, et al. (eds): Skin Carcinogenesis: Mechanisms and Human Relevance. New York: Alan R. Liss, Inc., 1989, pp 63–80.
54. Pitot HC, Sirica AE. The stages of initiation and promotion in hepatic carcinogenesis. Biochim Biophys Acta 605:191, 1980.
55. Butterworth BE, Slaga TJ (eds): Nongenotoxic Mechanisms in Carcinogenesis. Banbury Report 25. Cold Spring Harbor, New York: Cold Spring Harbor Laboratory, 1987, pp. 397.
56. Iversen OH, (ed): Theories of Carcinogenesis. Washington, DC: Hemisphere Publishing Corp., 1988, pp. 327.

57. Popp JA, Scortichini BH, Garvey LH. Quantitative evaluation of hepatic foci of cellular alteration occuring spontaneously in Fischer-344 rats. Fundam Appl Toxicol 5:314–319, 1985.
58. Cattley RC, Marsman DS, Popp JA. Effect of age on the carcinogenicity of the peroxisome proliferator Wy-14,643 in rats. Proceedings of the American Association for Cancer Research 31:151, 1990.
59. Newberne PM, Clark AJ. Promotion of liver tumors in B6C3F1 mice by partial hepatectomy or dietary choline deficiency. The Toxicologist 2:63–64, 1982.
60. Solleveld HA, Haseman JK, McConnell EE. Natural history of body weigh gain, survival, and neoplasia in the F344 rat. Journal of the National Cancer Institute 72:929, 1984.
61. Ward JM, Hagiwara A, Anderson LM, Linsey K, Diwan BA. The chronic hepatic or renal toxicity of di(2-ethylhexyl)phthalate, acetaminophen, sodium barbital, and phenobarbital in male B6C3F1 mice: Autoradiographic, immunohistochemical, and biochemical evidence for levels of DNA synthesis not associated with carcinogenesis or tumor promotion. Toxicol Appl Pharmacol 96:494–506, 1988.
62. Mirsalis JC. In vivo measurement of unscheduled DNA synthesis and S-phase synthesis as an indicator of hepatocarcinogenesis in rodents. Cell Biol Toxicol 3:165–173, 1987.
63. Mirsalis JC, Tyron CK, Steinmetz KL, Loh EK, Hamilton CM, Bakke JP, Spalding JW. Measurement of unscheduled DNA synthesis and S-phase synthesis in rodent hepatocytes following in vivo treatment: Testing of 24 compounds. Environ Mol Mutagen 14:155–164, 1989.
64. Goldsworthy TL, Morgan KT, Popp, JA, Butterworth BE. Guidelines for measuring chemically induced cell proliferation in specific rodent target organs. In Butterworth BE, Slaga TJ (eds): Chemically-Induced Cell Proliferation: Implications for Risk Assessment, 1990.
65. Goldsworthy TL, Sprankle CS, Strasser J, Butterworth BE. Induction of cell replication in male and female mouse livers after inhalation exposure to unleaded gasoline: potential role in tumor formation. J Toxicol Environ Health, in press.
66. Ledda-Columbano GM, Columbano A, Curto M, Ennas MG, Coni P, Sarma DSR, Pani P. Further evidence that mitogen-induced cell proliferation does not support the formation of enzyme-altered islands in rat liver by carcinogens. Carcinogenesis 10:847–850, 1989.
67. Belinsky SA, Walker VE, Maronpot RR, Swenberg JA, Anderson MW. Molecular dosimetry of DNA adduct formation and cell toxicity in rat nasal mucosa following exposure to the tobacco specific nitrosanime 4-(N-methyl-N-nitrosamino)-1-(3-pyridyl)-1-butanone and their relationship to induction of neoplasia. Cancer Res 47:6058–6065, 1987.
68. Hoel DG, Kaplan NL, Anderson MW. Implications of nonlinear kinetics on risk estimation in carcinogenesis. Science 219:1032–1037, 1983.
69. Casanova M, Deyo D, Heck H. Covalent binding of inhaled formaldehyde to DNA in the nasal mucosa of Fischer 344 rats: Analysis of formaldehyde and DNA by high-performance liquid chromatography and provisional pharmacokinetic interpretation. Fundam Appl Toxicol 12:397–417, 1989.
70. Starr TB. Quantitative cancer risk estimation for formaldehyde. In Feron VJ, Bosland MC (eds): Nasal Carcinogenesis in Rodents. Pudoc Wageningen, 1989, pp. 179–184.

Chemically Induced Cell Proliferation:
Implications for Risk Assessment, pages 469-479
©1991 Wiley-Liss, Inc.

The Role of Somatic Mutations and Cell Replication Kinetics in Quantitative Cancer Risk Assessment

Suresh H. Moolgavkar and E. Georg Luebeck

Although somatic mutations, broadly defined as heritable alterations of the genome, appear to be central in carcinogenesis, it is now a widely accepted fact that cell replication kinetics also play an important role by affecting mutation rates and sizes of critical cell populations. Thus, cell replication kinetics should be explicitly incorporated into quantitative models of cancer risk assessment. A two-stage carcinogenesis model that explicitly considers cell replication kinetics was developed approximately 10 years ago by Moolgavkar and colleagues and shown to be consistent with a large body of epidemiologic and experimental data (1–4).

Much attention has been focused recently on the quantitative analysis of enzyme-altered foci in rodent hepatocarcinogenesis experiments. These foci are believed to represent clones of premalignant cells and provide some of the best quantitative data on the interplay of somatic mutations and cell proliferation in carcinogenesis (5–7). Considerable effort has been expended in quantifying the number and size distribution of these enzyme-altered foci. Yet, no systematic analyses of this data have been undertaken beyond the application of techniques (8,9) originally proposed by Druckrey (10) for the analysis of malignant tumors. In this paper, we will summarize a method for the analysis of altered hepatic foci that is based on the two-stage carcinogenesis model and illustrate it through an experiment in which rats were administered *N*-nitrosomorpholine (NNM) at various concentrations in their drinking water.

The model and some of its consequences

The model has two features: a) transition of target stem cells into cancer cells via an intermediate stage in two steps that are rate-limiting, irreversible, and hereditary at the cellular level; and b) growth and differentiation of normal target and intermediate or initiated cells. Within the context of chemical carcinogenesis, the two rate-limiting steps represent "initiation" and "progression," with clonal expansion of intermediate cells representing "promotion." This model, which is a generalization of Knidson's recessive oncogenesis model (11), is consistent with a large body of experimental and epidemiologic data (2). Some of the consequences of the model are obvious upon reflection. Clearly, the model provides a natural framework for the initiation-promotion-initiation (IPI) protocol (2,12). The first administration of initiator creates some initiated cells, then promotion expands the clones of those cells and creates a large pool ready for malignant conversion by the second dose of initiator. The number of intermediate or enzyme-altered foci depends upon both the rate of initiation and the growth kinetics of initiated cells. Thus, if there is a certain spontaneous background rate of initiation, it is impossible to determine from the number of foci alone whether or not an agent is an initiator in treated animals. Indeed, in any population undergoing a birth-death process, the probability that the population will become extinct is non-zero. If the rate of cell division and cell death are α and β, respectively, then the asymptotic probability that the clone generated by a cell becomes extinct is β/α. These ideas will be more fully developed below. It can also be shown within the framework of the model that if an agent affects the size distribution of intermediate foci then it must have either promoting or antipromoting activity.

We will use this model to analyze altered hepatic foci after administration of a chemical agent. Specifically, we are interested in answering the following questions: Is the agent an initiator or a promoter? How do initiation and promotion depend upon the agent dose? Are there reasonable definitions of the agent's initiating and promoting potencies?

To address these questions, the biologic model must be translated into mathematical form and its parameters estimated from data using some statistical procedure such as maximizing the likelihood. The mathematical and statistical details have appeared elsewhere (13,14), and these technicalities need not concern us here. However, we would like to point out here that the mathematical model yields expressions for the number of altered foci and the size distribution of these foci in terms of the number of cells in each focus. On the other hand, the data are obtained in terms of the number of transections in a two-dimensional slice of the liver, and the diameter of these transections in micrometers. Thus, in order to relate the two, we must make an assumption regarding the diameter of a typical hepatocyte and use stereological methods to translate three-dimensional into two-dimensional quantities, or vice versa. In the example presented below, we have assumed that the average hepatocyte has a radius of 12 μm. Wicksell's formula was used to translate the three-dimensional quantities generated by the mathematical model into two-dimensional quantities for data-fitting by the method of maximum likelihood. Details of the procedure are given elsewhere (14).

The objectives of the analysis are to estimate the rate of initiation and the net rate of intermediate cell proliferation as functions of the dose of agent under consideration. However, more can be learned as is illustrated by an application of the method to ATPase-deficient foci in the livers of rats exposed to NNM in their drinking water.

An example

We have applied some of these ideas to this study of ATPase-deficient foci in the livers of rats exposed to NNM in their drinking water, and are grateful to Dr. Michael Schwarz of the German Cancer Research Center for making the data for this study available to us. A total 162 animals were administered NNM in their drinking water at various concentrations (0, 0.1, 1,5, 10, 20, 40 parts per million) starting at 14 weeks old. Animals were sacrificed at different ages, and their livers examined for ATPase-deficient foci. Table 1 shows the number of animals in each dose group, the total number of ATPase-deficient transections observed, and the range of ages at which animals in each of the dose groups were sacrificed. The analysis presented is based on transections with diameters between 120 and 1,000 μm.

The results of our analysis are presented in Figures 1 through 5. Figure 1 shows

Table 1. Details of NNM Experiment.

Dose (parts per million)	Number of animals	Total number of transsections	Range of treatment times (in days)
0	36	84	112–686
0.1	30	114	225–686
1.0	23	123	217–616
5.0	17	217	210–441
10.0	18	217	204–364
20.0	19	345	196–399
40.0	19	554	84–217
TOTAL	162	1654	

the rate of initiation per cubic centimeter of liver and the net growth rate of ATPase-deficient foci $(\alpha-\beta)$ as functions of the dose of NNM. The best-fitting regression lines through the points are also shown. We suggest that initiation and promotion potencies be defined by the ratio of the slope and the intercept of the appropriate regression line. Potencies defined in this way measure the proportionate increase over background of the rates of initiation and promotion. Based on the regression lines in Figure 1, the initiation potency of NNM is 0.392 ppm (per part per million) and the promotion potency is 0.044 ppm. Note that these potencies depend upon the units used for measurement of dose. Our analysis thus indicates that NNM is a strong initiator and a weak promoter. However, we must caution the reader against inferring from this statement that the initiating activity of NNM is more important than the promoting activity insofar as carcinogenesis is concerned. In fact, the mean number of initiated cells is an exponential function of $\alpha-\beta$, and thus the effect of $\alpha-\beta$ ultimately dominates. If the dose-response curves for initiation and promotion are not linear, then, of course, the problem of defining potencies is more difficult. A single summary index of activity is therefore not very meaningful. If there is a threshold for promotion, then the concept of potency must be given more careful thought. In the NNM data set analyzed here, there does not appear to be evidence of a threshold.

Figure 2 shows the actual and mean number of transections per square centimeter observed in the different dose groups and the expected number generated by the model using the estimated parameters.

The value of $(\alpha-\beta)$ ranges from nearly 0.0054 per cell per day in the control group to about 0.021 per cell per day in the 40 ppm dose group. These values correspond to approximate doubling times of 128 and 33 days, respectively. During the estimation procedure, we also obtain estimates of β/α. From the estimates of $(\alpha-\beta)$ in each of the dose groups and of β/α, estimates of the rate of cell division, as shown by α, can be obtained. These estimates range from about 0.5 per cell per day, corresponding to an average cell cycle time of about 2 days in the lowest dose groups, to about 2.00 per cell per day, corresponding to an average cell cycle time of about 12 hr in the highest dose group. This latter figure is almost certainly too fast for mammalian cells, indicating that these data cannot be used to obtain accurate estimates of α. One of the reasons is that estimates of α are very sensitive to estimates of β/α: a 1% change in β/α leads to a 100%

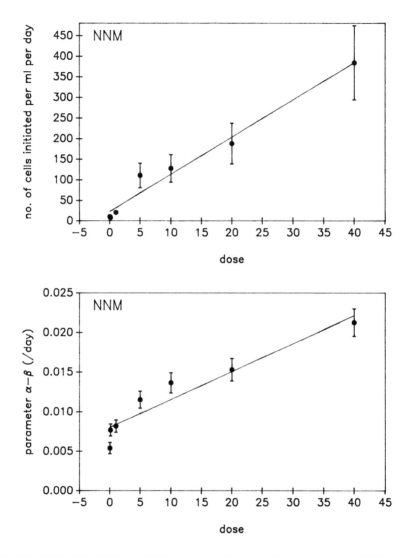

Figure 1. Parameter estimates (and 95% confidence intervals) plotted against dose of NNM in parts per million. The parameter (α–β) is the net rate of growth of altered cells.

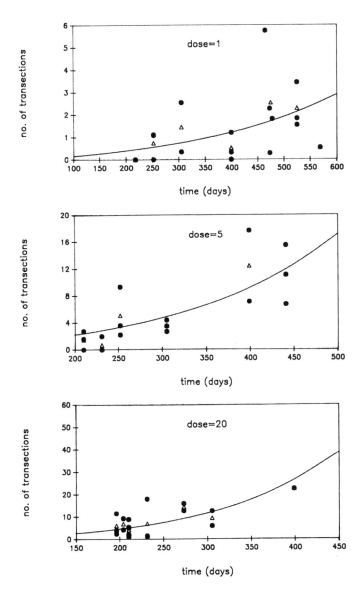

Figure 2. Number of transections per square centimeter of liver plotted against time on treatment for 3 different dose groups. The filled circles represent actual observations. For example, in dose group 5 ppm, there were two animals killed after 400 days on treatment. One of these had 16 transections and the other 6 per square centimeter of liver. The open triangles represent the mean of the observations at that time point.

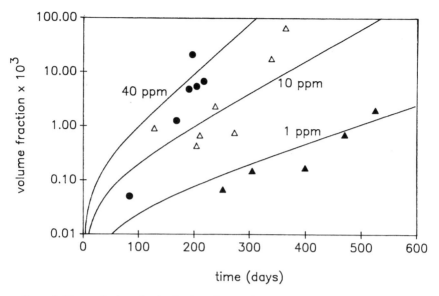

Figure 3. Observed volume fraction for three doses and model predicted volume fraction as a function of time on treatment. For observed volume fractions: filled circles dose group 40 ppm; open triangles 10 ppm; filled triangles 1 ppm. Note the rather substantial outlier in the 40 ppm group at about 100 days. However, measurements of observed volume fractions are rather imprecise.

change in α. Estimates of α are also highly dependent on assumptions regarding the radius of the altered cell. Ideally, it would be helpful if the experimentalist could measure α directly as a function of dose.

The estimated parameters can be used in the model to generate volume fractions occupied by altered foci in the different dose groups and at different times. Figure 3 shows the model-generated volume fractions and the observed volume fractions at three different doses. The agreement between the two is quite good, although there is a rather substantial outlier in the 40 ppm group.

The upper panel of Figure 4 shows the total number of nonextinct (visible and invisible) foci per cubic centimeter expected at various times for various dose groups. The lower panel of Figure 4 shows the density function for the distribution of sizes of foci with radii larger than 60 μm at a time 300 days after the start of the experiment. Note the shift to larger sizes with increasing dose. Figure 5 shows the expected number of detectable foci, that is, those with diameters larger than 120 μm generated by the model; compare these with numbers generated by the reconstructive methods of Fullman and Saltykov. Comparison with the upper panel of Figure 4 shows that there are a large number of undetectable foci.

The rate of initiation ranges from roughly 10–384 per day per cubic centimeter. These estimates of initiation rates depend upon assumptions about cell size and are sensitive to small changes in estimates of β/α and must, therefore, be accepted with caution.

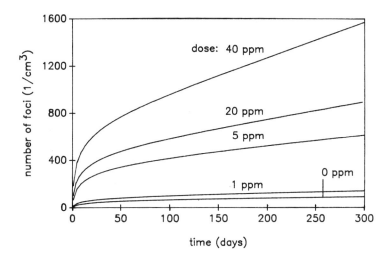

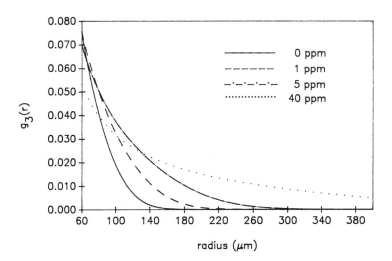

Figure 4. Upper panel: Number of altered foci per cubic centimeter of liver generated by the model plotted against time on treatment for 5 dose groups. Lower panel: The density function (truncated at 60 μm) of the distribution of radii of foci after 300 days on treatment.

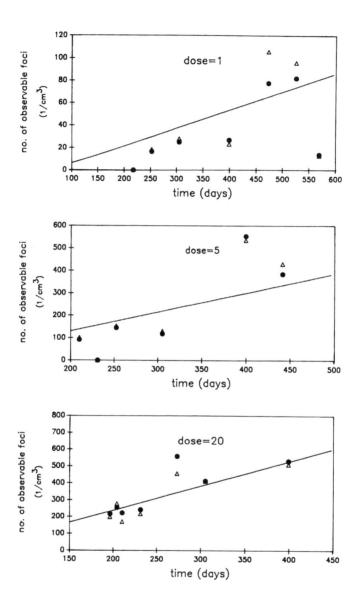

Figure 5. Expected number of observable foci (radii larger than 60 μm) generated by the model compared with numbers generated by the reconstructive methods of Saltykov (triangles) and of Fullman (filled circles) as modified by Nychka et al. (17).

Discussion

In this paper we have sketched a method for the analysis of altered foci in hepatocarcinogenesis experiments. This method utilizes all the information that is available and is therefore preferred to methods that use only single measures of response such as the volume fraction of altered cells or the mean size of altered foci. In addition, the role of dose and time can be studied simultaneously.

Of the parameters estimated, the net growth rate $(\alpha-\beta)$ of foci is independent of assumptions regarding mean cell size. This is intuitively clear because $(\alpha-\beta)$ determines the doubling time of altered foci, and this time depends only on the volume of the foci and not on the exact number of cells in the foci. In contrast, the estimate of the initiation rate depends upon the assumed cell size. The initiation potency as defined here, however, is independent of assumptions regarding cell size. We recall that, if cell death is important, then simply counting up the number of altered foci is not a good measure of initiation frequency because a larger number of initiated cells never develop into foci. There is also a great deal of uncertainty associated with the usual stereological methods used for counting foci.

With $(\alpha-\beta)$ and β/α estimated, it is of course possible to compute α and β. However, there are two problems: (1) β/α depends upon assumptions regarding cell size; (2) small changes in β/α make rather large differences in the estimates of α and β. Any estimate of α must be accepted with caution, that is, the available data are not equal to the task of accurately estimating α and β. It would be preferable to measure α (or equivalently, the average cell cycle time) directly.

We have proposed working definitions of initiation and promotion potencies. Another definition has recently been proposed by Pitot et al. (15). The advantage of our approach is that we use all the available data to define these important quantities, whereas Pitot et al. base their definitions on summary indices such as total number of foci in three dimensions and volume fraction. In particular, their definition of initiation potency overlooks the fact that a large fraction of initiated cells may never give risk to recognizable foci. Furthermore, their definitions depend upon the time at which the observations are made, while ours are theoretically independent of time. The great virtue of their approach is its simplicity, while our analysis requires a great deal of computation. We suspect that the two methods would yield comparable results, if not in absolute values, at least in relative ordering of the chemical agents examined.

The range of values in the upper panel of Figure 1 indicates that on average between 10 (in the 0 dose group) and 384 (in the 40 ppm dose group) initiated cells are generated per day per cubic centimeter of liver. These numbers translate, respectively, to 3,650 and 140,610 initiated cells per year. In comparison, the model predicts approximately 100 and 1,760 nonextinct foci per cubic centimeter at 1 year in dose groups 0 and 40, respectively. Thus, the vast majority of initiated cells do not generate foci. In any tissue in growth equilibrium, cell division rates must be approximated by cell death rates, so any initiated cell must have almost as great a probability of dying as of dividing. Our estimate of β/α, which is very close to 1, is a mathematical reflection of this fact. Schulte-Hermann and colleagues (16) have shown that apoptosis may play an important role during promotion in the liver. Although estimates of initiation rates must be accepted with caution, our general conclusion that a large fraction of initiated cells die without giving rise to visible foci remains true.

Several biologists have expressed skepticism regarding this conclusion, so it is worthwhile to examine it in some detail. As we have pointed out, there is experimental evidence of cell death in altered foci. Also, as we have explained, cell death rate must be close to the cell division rate or the foci would grow explosively. When an initiated cell is created, unless it is subject to very different biological imperatives than those observed in foci, it must divide or die with the same rate constants that hold for cells in foci, as must each of the daughter cells. As the clone grows in size, the probability of extinction of the entire clone decreases. In other words, if the inferred kinetics of division and death that apply to foci are also true when the focus is born as a single cell, then a large number of initiated cells simply die without giving rise to visible foci. As noted above, the probability of this occurring is β/α.

Assuming identical rates of initiation, the total number of altered cells depends only upon $\alpha-\beta$ and not upon α and β individually. However, the distribution of altered cells in foci of different sizes depends upon both α and β. For a fixed $\alpha-\beta$, a large value of α, that is, a large cell division rate and a correspondingly large cell death rate, leads to a small number of large foci, while a small value of α leads the altered cells to pile up in a large number of small foci. This behavior may explain the observations contrasting some peroxisome proliferators (small number of large foci) and phenobarbital (large number of small foci) as promoters.

Admittedly, the simple biological model on which this analysis is based makes a number of assumptions. First, there is considerable evidence of heterogeneity of growth rates among the altered foci. We are unable to take explicit account of this and therefore our parameters $(\alpha-\beta)$ should be thought of as averages. Second, the growth rate of an individual focus probably changes with time but in order to keep the computations tractable we have assumed that the growth rate is constant. Finally, initiated cells are not synonymous with ATPase-deficient or enzyme-altered cells. Had we used some other enzyme marker for foci, we could have arrived at somewhat different results. However, until a marker for initiated cells is discovered, we must be content to use surrogates. Our analysis here therefore refers strictly only to ATPase-deficient, not initiated, cells. Despite these rather obvious and unavoidable deficiencies of the method, we believe that we obtain reasonable results based on all the available information.

As the example of NNM illustrates, most carcinogenic chemicals probably exhibit both initiating and promoting activities. A detailed study of the initiating and promoting activities as functions of dose is the first step in a rational approach to quantitative cancer risk assessment.

Acknowledgments

Supported by PHS grant CA-47658 from the National Cancer Institute.

References

1.　Moolgavkar SH, Venzon DJ. Two-event models for carcinogenesis: Incidence curves for childhood and adult tumors. Mathematical Biosciences 47:55–77, 1979.

2. Moolgavkar SH, Knudson AG. Mutation and cancer: A model for human carcinogenesis. J Natl Cancer Inst 66:1037–1052, 1981.

3. Moolgavkar SH, Dewanji A, Venzon DJ. A stochastic two-stage model for cancer risk assessment. I. The hazard function and the probability of tumor. Risk Anal 8:383–392, 1988.

4. Moolgavkar SH, Cross FT, Luebeck G, Dagle GE. A two-mutation model for radon-induced lung tumors in rats. Radiation Res 121:28–37, 1990.

5. Emmelot P, Scherer E. The first relevant cell stage in rat liver carcinogenesis: A quantitative approach. Biochim Biophys Acta 605:247–304, 1980.

6. Goldsworthy TL, Hanigan MH, Pitot HC. Models of hepatocarcinogenesis in the rat—contrasts and comparisons. Crit Rev Toxicol 17:16–89, 1986.

7. Goldfarb S, Pugh TD. Enzyme histochemical phenotypes in primary hepatocellular carcinomas. Cancer Res 41:2092–2095, 1981.

8. Kunz HW, Tennekes HA, Port RD, Schwarz M, Lorke D, Schaude G. Quantitative aspects of chemical carcinogenesis and tumor promotion in liver. Environ Health Perspect 50:113–122, 1983.

9. Schwarz M, Pearson D, Buchman A, Kunz W. The use of enzyme-altered foci for risk assessment of hepatocarcinogenesis. In Travis CC (ed): Biologically Based Methods for Cancer Risk Assessment. NATO ASI Series, Series A: Life Sciences Vol 159, New York: Plenum Press, 1989, pp 31–39.

10. Druckrey H. Quantitative aspects in chemical carcinogenesis. In Truhaut R (ed): Potential Carcinogenic Hazards from Drugs. UICC Monographs Series Vol 7, New York: Springer-Verlag, 1967, pp 60–78.

11. Knudson AG. Mutation and cancer: Statistical study of retinoblastoma. Proceedings of the National Academy of Sciences, USA 68:820–823, 1971.

12. Potter VR. A new protocol and its rationale for the study of initiation and promotion of carcinogens in rat liver. Carcinogenesis 2:1375–1379, 1981.

13. Dewanji A, Venzon DJ, Moolgavkar SH. A stochastic twostage model for cancer risk assessment. II. The number and size of premalignant clones. Risk Anal 9:179–187, 1979.

14. Moolgavkar SH, Luebeck EG, de Gunst M, Port RE, Schwarz M. Quantitative analysis of enzyme-altered foci in rat hepatocarcinogenesis experiments. Carcinogenesis, in press.

15. Pitot HC, Goldsworthy TL, Moran S, Kennan W, Glauert HP, Maronpot RR, Campbell HA. A method to quantitate the relative initiating and promoting potencies of hepatocarcinogenic agents in their dose-response relationships to altered hepatic foci. Carcinogenesis 8:1491–1499, 1987.

16. Schulte-Hermann R, Parzefall W, Bursch W, Timmermann-Trosiener I. Hepatocarcinogenesis by non-genotoxic compounds. In Travis CC (ed): Biologically Based Methods for Cancer Risk Assessment. NATO ASI series, Series A: Life Sciences Vol 159, New York: Plenum Press, 1989, pp 155–163.

17. Nychka D, Pugh TD, King JH, Koen H, Wahba G, Chover J, Goldfarb S. Optimal use of sampled tissue sections for estimating the number of hepatocellular foci. Cancer Res 44:178–183, 1984.

Chemically Induced Cell Proliferation:
Implications for Risk Assessment, pages 481-499
©1991 Wiley-Liss, Inc.

Incorporating Cell Proliferation in Quantitative Cancer Risk Assessment: Approaches, Issues, and Uncertainties

Chao Chen and William Farland

Although the Armitage-Doll multistage model (1) fits some selected human cancer incidence data, the biologic underpinnings of the model have been criticized because the model fails to account for the rate of cell proliferation in the process of tumorigenesis, namely, the clonal growth of preneoplastic cells. If clonal growth is part of the tumorigenic process, then its rate may be a rate-limiting step for tumor formation. Therefore, cell proliferation should be included in any tumor growth model from which a dose-response model is developed. A two-event model proposed by Moolgavkar and colleagues (2,3) has attracted great attention because it incorporates clonal expansion of initiated cells.

In the traditional, multistage construct of carcinogenesis, proliferation of initiated cells is a major factor in tumor formation. An excellent review of the initiation and promotion concept in hepatocarcinogenesis is given in Pitot and Sirica (4). There is some evidence that a chemical with only an initiation capability may not induce a significant increase of malignant tumors unless the chemically induced initiated cells can be stimulated to proliferate either by the chemical itself or its reactive metabolites, or by the host condition (5). On the other hand, if a chemical has only cell proliferation potential, its tumorigenic effect would not be manifested unless spontaneously or chemically induced initiated cells already exist. The tumor incidence rate in animals exposed to a chemical having only proliferation potential would depend on the number of spontaneous initiated cells in the exposed animals: those with more such cells would obviously show more tumor response. Therefore, the effects of initiation and promotion must be explicitly incorporated in a cancer dose-response model if it is to approximate reality. Although cell proliferation has many competing mechanisms, the process is characterized by an increase of mitotic rate, a decrease of cell loss rate, or both. This concept is used to construct a mathematical tumor growth model that incorporates explicitly the mitotic rates of initiated and malignant cells (see section describing Model 2).

Three mathematical models incorporating cell proliferation of initiated cells are discussed as possible approaches for dose-response modeling: (1) a two-event model proposed by Moolgavkar and colleagues (2,3); (2) a two-event model that incorporates explicitly mitotic rates of initiated and malignant cells; and (3) Neyman and Scott's one-hit and two-stage model (6) which distinguishes between the primary (first generation)

The views expressed in this paper are those of the authors and do not necessarily reflect the views and policies of the U.S. Environmental Protection Agency.

initiated cells and their daughter cells. Evidence supporting each model and data required for model construction are described.

In this paper, we use the second model to construct a biologically based dose-response model that incorporates data taken from dinitrotoluene (DNT) studies. The objectives are twofold: (1) to highlight the role of mitotic information in quantitative cancer risk assessment, and (2) to identify and discuss issues and uncertainties when an attempt is made to incorporate available biological information in dose-response modeling. Data from DNT studies are used as an example to stimulate discussion of issues and uncertainties in this process. In the last decade, researchers at the Chemical Industry Institute of Toxicology (CIIT) have conducted numerous studies on technical grade DNT (TDNT: 76.49% 2,4-DNT, 18.83% 2,6-DNT) and its two principal isomers, and have generated data which may be used to construct a biologically based dose-response model.

Mathematical tumor growth models

The importance of incorporating cell proliferation in a tumor growth model was recognized as early as three decades ago by Armitage and Doll (7), who considered a two-stage model of carcinogenesis and assumed that the growth of initiated cells follows a deterministic growth function. Rigorous stochastic modeling was first developed by Neyman (8,9), Kendal (10), Neyman and Scott (6), and Moolgavkar and colleagues (2,3). Except for Neyman and Scott (6), all of these studies investigated essentially the same model, i.e., the two-stage model incorporating clonal expansion of initiated cells.

In this paper, we propose a two-event (or two-stage) model that explicitly incorporates mitotic rate as a parameter (Model 2). The mathematical formulation of the model is presented in Appendix A. Two other mathematical tumor growth models that incorporate cell proliferation are also discussed as possible bases for developing dose-response models. We present these different models to stimulate interaction between quantitative risk assessors and research biologists and to encourage generation of data useful for quantitative risk assessment.

Model 1: Moolgavkar model

In addition to that presented in publications by Moolgavkar and his colleagues (2,3), the most direct support of the Moolgavkar model comes from initiation-promotion and initiation-promotion-initiation studies showing that initiation, promotion, and progression are crucial steps in tumor formation. Although the actual number of steps of carcinogenesis may exceed the number of steps postulated in the model, it should not prevent the researcher from building a model on some of these steps that are observable or estimable from laboratory data. The Moolgavkar model assumes that a normal (target) cell must undergo at least two critical events—initiation and progression—before it reaches a malignant stage. The clonal expansion of initiated cells increases the probability of malignant transformation. The schematic representation of the model is as follows:

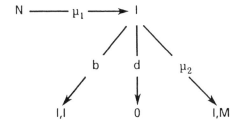

The paradigm indicates that an initiated cell can give birth to another initiated cell with rate b, it can die with rate d, and it can give birth to an initiated cell and a malignant cell with rate μ_2. The induction of initiated cells from target cells (N) is assumed to follow a Poisson process. The target cells may consist of stem cells and/or differentiated cells. If the target cells consist of two or more subpopulations of cells, the transition rate μ_1 is assumed to be the weighted mean of the transition rates from each of the subpopulations. The rates b and d control the growth of initiation cells. Since the birth and death of malignant cells are not considered, the model implicitly assumes that once an initiated cell is transformed into a malignant cell, it becomes a malignant tumor with a probability of 1.

The parameters μ_1, b, d, and μ_2 can be estimated from information on the number and size of induced preneoplastic and neoplastic lesions, as demonstrated in the following DNT example. However, if possible, it is always desirable to measure these parameters directly from laboratory experiments rather than estimating them indirectly from alternative data.

Model 2: A modified two-event model

The biologic justification for the model is the same as that for the Moolgavkar model. However, this model differs from the Moolgavkar model in two respects: (1) the mitotic rates of initiated cells and malignant cells are explicitly considered in the model by assuming that the times to mitosis for these cells are random variables following some probability distribution, and (2) the birth-death process of malignant cells is considered. In this paper, we consider only the case where time to mitosis is a random variable with exponential distribution. The more general case, in which extensive computation is required, will be presented elsewhere. This model is consistent with the observation of tumors in nodules or tumors in tumors as described in Farber and Sarma (11) and Pugh and Goldfarb (12). The schematic view of the model is as follows:

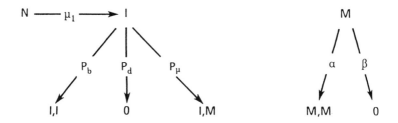

Under Model 2, the lifetime of initiated cells is assumed to be a random variable following exponential distribution. At the end of cell lifetime, an initiated cell divides into two initiated cells with probability P_b, disappears (cell loss) with probability P_d, or divides into an initiated cell and a malignant cell with probability P_μ. Similarly, at the end of the cell's lifetime, a malignant cell either divides into two malignant cells with probability α, or disappears (cell loss) with probability β. For convenience, the term "time to mitosis" is used as a synonym of cell lifetime and the term "mitotic rate" as the reciprocal of mean cell lifetime, even though these interpretations are more restrictive than the general interpretations of the model.

Note that parameters P_b, P_d, and P_μ are the probabilities (not rates) that each of the three mutually exclusive events will occur with a total probability of 1 at the end of an initiated cell's life. The difference between rate and probability is that rate represents an amount of change over time in terms of days or months, while the probability is dimensionless and represents the proportion of times a specific event will occur. For instance, a birth rate of 0.5 per day is equivalent to one birth every two days, while a probability of birth $(P_b) = 0.5$ suggests a 50% probability that an initiated cell will give rise to two daughter initiated cells after cell division. Similarly, α and β are probabilities with a sum equal to one. This model requires information on mitosis of initiated cells and malignant cells. The model can be simplified by assuming that a tumor is formed upon the occurrence of a single malignant cell, an assumption made in the Moolgavkar model. If such an assumption is made, the data required for Model 2 are not greater than that required for Model 1 when mitotic information on initiated cells is available. In fact, if the mitotic rate for initiated cells is known, there are fewer parameters to be estimated than with the Moolgavkar model because, under Model 2, the sum of P_b, P_d, and P_μ equals 1; thus, only two parameters (rather than three) need to be estimated.

Model 3: Neyman-Scott model

Neyman and Scott (6) developed a model to answer questions raised by their colleagues at the University of California at Berkeley who were studying the question of whether urethane carcinogenesis involves one or more than one stage. After the two-event model failed to adequately fit the urethane data given to them by their colleagues, Neyman and Scott proposed an alternative model. While the reasons used by Neyman and Scott for rejecting their original two-stage or two-event model are not convincing, their alternative model seems biologically plausible. The schematic representation of the model is given below.

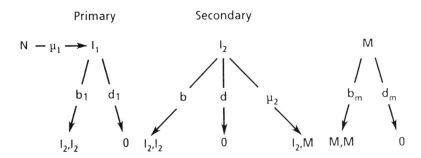

Mathematically, this model says that a primary initiated cell differs from its daughter or secondary initiated cells with respect to its ability to give birth to malignant cells. Neyman and Scott assume that only the secondary—not the primary—initiated cells can produce malignant cells. This seems to be consistent with the postulation that a promoter such as TPA, which can increase the mitotic rate for the initiated cells, might also cause some genetic alteration such as gene amplification which is necessary for tumor formation (13). Since a promoter does more than just increase the frequency of cell division, primary initiated cells may differ from their daughter cells; therefore, they should differ in their ability to be transformed into malignant cells. These differences have a profound effect on the rate of tumor formation because the number of primary initiated cells depends on the initiation potential, while the number of secondary initiated cells depends on the proliferation potential of a carcinogen. The biological plausibility of the Neyman-Scott model should be investigated further. In addition to the necessary data, this two-event model also requires information on the production rate from primary initiated cells to the secondary initiated cells. Further research is needed to determine how this information can be obtained.

DNT as an example

DNT is used as an example to stimulate discussion of issues, problems, and data gaps that may arise when one attempts to incorporate cell proliferation into quantitative risk estimation. Although it may be postulated that some isomers of DNT cause initiated cells to proliferate, there is no direct measurement of the increase of mitosis due to DNT exposure. Therefore, an indirect estimation of cell growth must be employed. In this paper, the average number of gamma glutamyl transferase positive (GGT^+) foci per liver is used to estimate some of the parameters in Model 2 and to construct a dose-response model for DNT. These calculations assume that GGT^+ foci represent the preneoplastic lesions of hepatocellular carcinomas. The number of detectable foci depends on both the initiating and promoting potential of DNT; however, the size of the foci depends only on the promoting potential of DNT.

Data base

TDNT is a potent hepatocarcinogen in rats, while its largest component, 2,4-DNT, is weakly hepatocarcinogenic or nonhepatocarcinogenic when tested alone. Both 2,4-DNT and 2,6-DNT have foci-enhancing activity in animals that have been previously administered diethylnitrosamine (DEN) as an initiator. Since only 2,6-DNT among the six DNT isomers tested was found to have demonstrable initiation activity, the promoting activity of DNT isomers is considered to be an important determinant of TDNT carcinogenicity, presumably acting by inducing proliferation in liver cells initiated by 2,6-DNT. Table 1 shows that the study performed by the Chemical Industry Institute of Toxicology (CIIT) (14) which had a larger 2,6-DNT concentration in the TDNT mixture than did the National Cancer Institute (NCI) study (15) produced much higher liver tumor incidence. The difference in these two studies raised speculation concerning which component of TDNT is responsible for tumor production and led to a series of subsequent studies. Table 2 shows the initiation potential of DNT isomers that are the components of TDNT; each of the isomers was tested as an initiator in an initiation-promotion protocol. Table 3 shows the promotion activities of 2,4-DNT and 2,6-DNT in animals initiated by a single dose of DEN (150 mg/kg). Table 4 presents GGT$^+$ foci/cm^3 in F344) male rats following 0, 0.7, and 3.5 mg/kg/day of 2,6-DNT in the NIH diet. The study was conducted to investigate the effect of diets on 2,6-DNT hepatocellular carcinogenesis. Only data on NIH diets are reproduced here because they provide a data base for modeling cancer risk and comparing the results in the NCI study.

Construction of a 2,6-DNT dose-response model

Model 2 will be used to construct a dose-response model. Although data in Tables 2 and 3 have demonstrated that 2,6-DNT has both initiation and promotion effects, these data are not sufficient to determine parameters of initiation and promotion in the model. Because of the lack of such data, this example should not be considered as a quantitative risk assessment for DNT. The purpose of this example is to demonstrate the types of data that are required to construct a biologically based dose-response model and to highlight problems and issues associated with this effort.

Table 1. Incidences of hepatocellular carcinomas in F344 male rats in the NCI[15] and CIIT[14] DNT bioassays.[a]

	Study duration (weeks)	Total TDNT	Dose (mg/kg/d) 2,4-DNT content	2,6-DNT content	Tumor study incidence
NCI[15]	104	0	0	0	0/70 (0%)
	104	14	13.3	0.7	3/48 (6%)
CIIT[14]	104	0	0	0	1/120 (1%)
	104	3.5	2.68	0.66	10/130 (8%)
	104	14	10.7	2.6	98/128 (77%)
	55[a]	35	26.8	6.6	32/40 (80%)

[a] Animals were killed at 55 weeks because of high mortality.

Table 2. Initiation potential of DNT isomers[a]

Treatment	GGT+ foci/cm^2
Control	0.20
2,4-DNT	0.20
2,6-DNT	4.04
2,5-DNT	0.28
3,5-DNT	0.53
3,4-DNT	0.74
2,3-DNT	0.76

[a]A single dose of DNT (75 mg/kg) was given to animals 12 hours after two-third liver hepatectomy (16). Growth selection of altered cells to foci was achieved by use of carbon tetrachloride and 2-acetyl-aminofluorene.

Table 3. Promotion activities in animals given 2,4-DNT and 2,6-DNT in the diet for 12 weeks following initiation by a single dose of DEN.

Number	Treatment	GGT+ foci/cm^3
1	DEN, 150 mg/kg, ip	0
2	2,4-DNT alone, 27 mg/kg/d	0
3	2,6-DNT alone, 14 mg/kg/d	571
4	Treatments No. 1 and No. 2	546
5	Treatments No. 1 and No. 3	867

Estimation of parameters. Except for the probabilities P_b, P_d, and P_μ, all the other parameters to be estimated below have the unit per cell per day. Although Table 2 provides evidence that 2,6-DNT is the only isomer with demonstrable initiation activity, the data cannot be used to estimate the initiation rate, μ_1, because they are given in terms of foci per cross-section area (cm^2), not per volume (cm^3). To calculate foci per volume, the researcher would need information not available to us on size distribution of foci. Using the observed number of foci per liver and the expected number of foci predicted by equation B-1 in Appendix B, we can estimate parameters μ_1, P_b, and P_d, assuming that a focus becomes detectable when it contains 10 or more cells, i.e., m = 10 in equation B-1. This is consistent with the assumption used in the laboratory when these foci were counted (18). Note that in this calculation, b and d represent birth and death rates for an initiated cell; they are not the same parameters used in Model 2. In these calculations, liver volume is assumed to be 10 cm^3; thus, the number of foci per liver is 10 times those presented in Table 4. The number of normal hepatocytes per liver, which is assumed to be the target cell population, is calculated by the formula

$$N(t) = N_0 \exp\{ \frac{\rho}{\zeta}[1\text{-}\exp(- \zeta t)]\}$$

where $N_0 = 142 \times 10^6, \zeta = 3.93 \times 10^{-2}$, and $\rho = 0.118$.

While it may be biologically more reasonable to assume that only a subset of hepatocytes is the primary target population, the assumption will not change the prediction

Table 4. Average GGT+ Foci/cm3 in Animals Exposed to 2,6-DNT in NIH Diet for Different Durations (17)[a]

	Months after exposure began		
Dose (mg/kg/d)	3	6	12
0	6	9	55
0.7	15	106	250
3.5	63	321	a

[a] Livers exhibited multiple foci, neoplastic nodules (6 of 10), and hepatocellular carcinomas (6 of 10). The presence of these latter lesions did not allow for accurate quantitation of foci in these livers.

of cancer risk because a decrease of N is compensated by an increased estimate of μ_1. The parameters of this equation are estimated on the basis of the number of hepatocytes in Wistar rats as presented by Altman and Dittmer (19). When t is large, N(t) approaches the maximum value of about $2,850 \times 10^6$ cells. The calculation and data used to estimate the parameters can be found in Chen and Moini (20).

Although actual data for the calculation are not available, there is sufficient evidence to indicate that initiation and cell growth are dose-dependent. In this example, we assume that the initiation rate is linearly dependent on dose D, while the growth rate b depends on dose D through the equation $b(D) = 1-exp[-(a_0 + a_1 \times D)]$. When the birth rate is small, b(D) is almost linearly related to the dose. This mathematical form is selected because it prevents b from exceeding 1, since it does not seem biologically reasonable to estimate in vivo a cell division time of less than 24 hrs based on our knowledge of mitotic rate in most tissues. To reduce the number of parameters that must be estimated, we have assumed that the death rate, d_0, for the initiated cells is not dependent on dose. The resulting parameter estimates (calculated by the least squares method) are as follows:

$$\mu_1(D) = 7.30 \times 10^{-9} + 1.52 \times 10^{-9} \times D$$

$$b(D) = 1-exp[-(7.60 \times 10^{-2} + 4.74 \times 10^{-2} \times D)]$$

where D is 2,6-DNT dose in mg/kg/day, and $d_0 = 7.00 \times 10^{-2}$.

Table 5 shows the predicted and observed number of foci under each dose-time category in Table 4. Except for the control group at 182 days, the equation appears to fit the data very well.

To use Model 2, the parameter λ (mitotic rate) must be estimated. From b(D) and d_0 above, we note that the ratio of birth to death in the control group is about 0.52/0.48. Since $P\mu$ is very small in comparison to P_b and P_d, it is reasonable to assume that $P_b = 0.52$ and $P_d = 1-P_b-P_\mu \cong 0.48$. Therefore, the approximate mitotic rate λ can be obtained from b(D) using the relationship $b(D) = \lambda(D)P_b$ as follows:

$$\lambda(D) = 1-exp[-(0.15 + 0.09 \times D)].$$

It should be noted that if the mitotic rate is available, the above calculations are not necessary.

Table 5. Observed and predicted number of foci per liver.

		Foci/Liver	
Time (dY)	Dose (mg/kg/d)	Observed	Predicted
91	0	60	75
182	0	90	220
365	0	550	519
91	0.65	150	286
182	0.65	1060	994
365	0.65	2500	2487
91	3.25	630	961
182	3.25	3210	3099

Table 6. Incidence of hepatocellular carcinomas in male F344 rats one year after exposure to TDNT and its two major isomers (18).

Dose treatment	(mg/kg/d)	Tumor incidence
Control	0	0/20 (0%)
2,4-DNT	27	0/20 (0%)
2,6-DNT	7	18/20 (90%)
TDNT	35	9/19 (47%)

To estimate the parameters P_μ, the relative magnitude of birth and death rates of malignant cells is assumed to be 0.90/0.10. In addition to providing information on foci (Table 4), the study by Goldsworthy et al. (17) provides information on production of hepatocellular carcinomas. This response can be used to estimate P_μ. Except for the highest dosed group (3.5 mg/kg/day at 12 months) which showed 60% (6 of 10 animals per group) of the animals with hepatocellular carcinomas, no other groups showed any carcinomas in the liver. These data, and the observation (Table 6) by Leonard et al. (18) that when male F344 rats were fed 7 mg/kg/day of 2,6-DNT for one year, 90% (18 of 20) developed hepatocellular carcinomas, are used to estimate P_μ, along with the other parameters that have already been estimated from foci data.

The model always overpredicts cancer risk at low doses when P_μ is assumed to be independent of dose. Therefore, it is reasonable to assume that P_μ is dose-dependent. Assuming that P_μ is linearly related to dose, the resultant estimate of P_μ is:

$$P_\mu(D) = 5.88 \times 10^{-12} + 3.09 \times 10^{-8} \times D.$$

Using these estimated parameters, we can predict the cancer risk due to 2,6-DNT. Table 7 shows the observed and predicted incidences of carcinomas over time.

Figure 1 shows that cancer response increases much more rapidly with time when animals are exposed at higher doses than when exposed at lower doses. At low doses, the probability of cancer over time increases slowly. However, at 2.5 mg/kg/day, the probability of cancer increases sharply with time. It can be demonstrated (not shown here) that this phenomenon is due to an increase of mitotic rates for initiated cells; for

Table 7. Observed and predicted incidence rates of hepatocellular carcinomas in animals exposed to different dose levels of 2,6-DNT.

Dose (mg/kg/d)	Observed[a]/Predicted time (days)			
	91	182	365	728
0	0/0	0/0	0/0	0/0
0.7	0/0	0/0	0/0.01	NA/0.25
3.5	0/0.003	0/0.02	0.6/0.52	NA/1.00
7	NA/0.014	NA/0.13	0.90/0.99	NA/1.00

[a]The observed incidence rates for the first three dosed groups are taken from Tables 4; those in the highest dose group are taken from Table 6. NA = not available.

corresponding doses of 0.5 and 2.5 mg/kg/day, those rates are respectively 0.177 and 0.312 per day. This example suggests that if the carcinogen increases the mitotic rate, then the dose-response relationship can be very nonlinear, as shown in Figure 2. Figure 3 compares predicted cancer risks at low doses between Model 2 and the linearized multistage model, a default procedure that is currently being recommended by the U.S. Environmental Protection Agency for cancer risk assessment in the absence of a biological or mechanistic rationale for selecting an alternative model (21). In addition to the predicted cancer risk calculated by using the linearized multistage model, the maximum likelihood estimate for that model is also given in Figure 3. The predictions

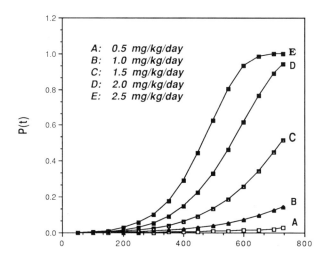

Time, t days

Figure 1. Predicted cancer risk, P(t), by time t in animals exposed to different 2,6-DNT dosages.

by both Model 2 and the maximum likelihood estimate for the linearized multistage model are very similar at and below the observed dose range; however, as expected, the risk calculated by this procedure is much greater than that predicted by Model 2 using a low dose.

Prediction of cancer risk due to TDNT exposure. It would seem reasonable to expect that the tumor response in animals exposed to TDNT is much greater than that in animals exposed only to the 2,6-DNT fraction contained in the TDNT because 2,4-DNT also has been shown to have proliferation induction potential (Table 3). However, this expectation is not supported by model prediction or by actual observation demonstrated by studies of Leonard et al. (18) (Table 6), in which animals exposed to 7 mg/kg/day of 2,6-DNT alone showed significantly greater tumor response (90% vs. 47%) than did those exposed to 35 mg/kg/day of TDNT, which contains the same amount (7 mg/kg/day) of 2,6-DNT. It seems that tumor response in the TDNT-treated animals can be predicted solely on the basis of its 2,6-DNT content, as indicated when the TDNT tumor incidence data in Table 1 is compared with the 2,6-DNT-based predictions in Table 7. One can postulate that 2,4-DNT does not increase the probability of tumor formation because Pμ depends only on 2,6-DNT, not 2,4-DNT, and perhaps because some genetic alteration in initiated cells is induced by 2,6-DNT but not by 2,4-DNT promotion. However, predicting the risk for TDNT from the 2,6-DNT fraction may be artifactual because an inappropriate enzyme marker is used to identify preneoplastic lesions.

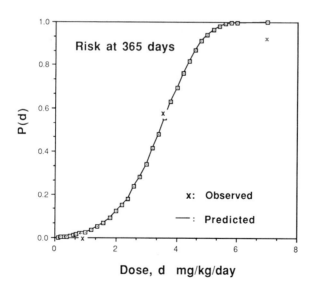

Figure 2. Observed and predicted lifetime (365 days) cancer risk, P_d, over a dose range of 2,6-DNT.

Discussion of issues, uncertainties, and data gaps stimulated by the DNT example

In the DNT example, we have used 2,6-DNT–induced GGT⁺ foci as preneo-plastic lesions to estimate initiation and cell growth parameters and to construct a biologically based dose-response model for 2,6-DNT. The model seems to suggest that the tumor incidence due to TDNT exposure mainly comes from the carcinogenic action of 2,6-DNT. However, this may not be the case if the presence of the GGT⁺ phenotype is a necessary but not sufficient condition for an island to be preneoplastic. For instance, if preneoplastic lesions require the presence of both GGT⁺ and adenosine triphosphatase (ATPase) abnormalities, then the use of foci with GGT⁺ alone as a marker would have inflated the actual number of preneoplastic lesions and possibly led to an over-estima-tion of initiation and cell growth rates. If data on combinations of various enzyme markers are available, our model can be used to test the hypothesis that foci with a certain combination of enzyme markers are preneoplastic lesions. Similar studies are reported by Dr. Pitot in these proceedings. However, to achieve such a goal with a reasonable degree of confidence, one would need direct laboratory measurement of mitotic rates for cells with different enzyme markers, rather than an estimate taken indirectly from foci data, as we have done in this example.

One perceived advantage of using a model that incorporates cell proliferation for risk assessment is that it can be used to adjust for differences in background tumor rates among species. This adjustment is possible because both initiation and cell proliferation

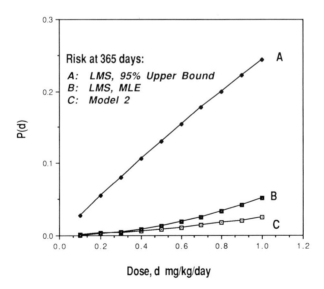

Figure 3. Comparison of predicted cancer risks due to 2,6-DNT exposure, calculated by Model 2 and the linearized multistage (LMS) model.

are explicitly incorporated in the model as parameters. However, DNT serves as an example to caution us that more information is needed before this advantage can be exploited. Although 2,4-DNT shows a promoting effect on DEN-induced initiated cells (Table 3), it may not promote either 2,6-DNT-induced or the spontaneously induced initiated cells in B6C3F$_1$ mice because no liver tumors were observed in the NCI mouse study. This suggests that, when assessing a promoter that induces proliferation in initiated cells in an initiation-promotion protocol in animals, one cannot always extrapolate from animals to humans by assuming that the chemical will promote the spontaneously induced initiated cells in humans. Thus, if a compound is considered a "pure" promoter, it is important to determine whether or not it promotes spontaneously induced initiated cells. The importance of determining the mechanism of tumor induction between chemically induced and spontaneously induced tumors has been recognized in studies (22) in which activated oncogenes in mouse liver tumors were examined and compared between two treatment groups. Since 2,4-DNT does not appear to contribute toward tumor induction of TDNT, it should be determined whether or not 2,4-DNT promotes 2,6-DNT–induced initiated cells and whether 2,4-DNT can transform these initiated cells into malignant cells. No data are available to answer this question.

From this example, one can see that if information on mitosis of preneoplastic (and preferably neoplastic also) lesions is available, cell growth parameters can be better estimated. In addition to mitotic information, number and size distribution of preneoplastic lesions and, preferably, of neoplastic lesions as well, are useful for constructing a biologically based dose-response model.

Discussion

Despite competing mechanisms for cell proliferation, from a modeler's view the process is adequately characterized by data relating to the increase of mitotic rate or the decrease of cell loss or both. The most direct measurement of cell proliferation is mitosis; this greatly simplifies the need to develop different mathematic models for different mechanisms of cell proliferation. However, this does not imply that the basic mechanism studies are not useful for modeling. The understanding of basic mechanisms of cell proliferation is crucial for risk extrapolation from animals to humans—the ultimate goal of risk assessment. Furthermore, understanding the mechanisms of cell proliferation may help us learn to estimate the relationship between dose and mitotic rate.

For most bioassays, the observed end points are the incidences of tumors. This experimental system is not statistically efficient for dose-response modeling because it requires a large number of animals to detect tumor response at low doses. On the other hand, the effect of the dose at the cellular level is statistically more powerful because there are many times more cells than animals. Therefore, a dose-response model constructed on the basis of cellular dynamics would be not only biologically more meaningful but also statistically more efficient. To construct a biologically based dose-response model, it is important to know the precise relationship between dose and various cellular dynamic/growth rates, such as rates of initiation and mitoses.

In this paper, we assume that in the initiated cell population the cell lifetime (or more restrictively, time to mitosis) follows an exponential distribution; this assumption needs further investigation. Laboratory and statistical procedures for estimating the distribution of cell lifetimes need to be developed.

Conceptually, we should continue to seek the tumor's observable preneoplastic precursor lesions, e.g., preneoplastic nodules. If these data are available, they would provide a larger sample of cells or lesions than does a population of animals. A specific example in the liver would be to observe foci, nodules, and carcinomas. Data useful for this approach of dose-response modeling include information on the number of preneoplastic and neoplastic lesions per animal and their size distribution over time. For DNT, we have only the incidence rates of nodules, i.e., proportion of animals with nodules; data on nodules per animal are not available. A procedure using the sequential data on preneoplastic and neoplastic lesions to construct a dose-response model is given by Chen and Moini (20). The advantage of this approach is that, when rate of formation of the first-stage preneoplastic lesions such as foci can be measured, it is not necessary to assume cell independence, a factor which is required by the three models discussed in this paper. Instead, the independence of preneoplastic lesions, which presumably is biologically more reasonable, is assumed.

Continued innovative thought and data collection will be necessary to further develop biologically based dose-response models for carcinogenesis. The use of existing data sets and the development of alternative models based on them should stimulate discussion between biologists and biostatisticians which will be necessary to reach this goal.

Appendix A. Derivation of model 2

Assumptions

1. The number of normal (target) cells $N(t)$ (N cells) is deterministic in time t.
2. The number of initiated cells produced by N cells is a Poisson process with a production rate $\mu_1(t)N(t)$, where $\mu_1(t)$ is the rate of initiation for an N cell.
3. Each primary (first generation) initiated cell may generate a clone by cell division. At end of cell life, an initiated cell may give birth to two daughter cells with probability P_b, die with probability P_d, or give birth to an initiated cell and a malignant cell with probability P_μ. Assume that the life length for an initiated cell has a probability density function $f_1(t)$.
4. At the end of cell life, each malignant cell either divides into two malignant cells with probability α, or dies with probability β. Assume that the life length for a malignant cell has a probability density function $f_2(t)$.
5. All cells go through the same process independently.

Derivation of tumor incidence rate

Let $Y(t)$, $Z(t)$ be random variables representing, respectively, the number of initiated cells and malignant cells, at time t. Let $\phi(t) = \phi(y, z|t)$ be the probability-generating function (pgf) of $[Y(t), Z(t)]$ given that the process starts with a single initiated cell and no malignant cell at time $t = 0$, i.e., $Y(0) = 1, Z(0) = 0$. Let $\Theta(t)$ be the pgf of $Z(t)$ given that the process starts with a single malignant cell at $t = 0$. By considering whether or not a cell life terminates, and if it terminates, all the possible events following the termination, it can be shown (23) that the functions ϕ and Θ satisfy the following equations:

$$\phi(t) = y[1-F_1(t)] + \int_0^t [P_b\phi^2(t-s) + P_d + P_\mu\phi(t-s)\,\Theta(t-s)]dF_1(s), \quad \text{(A-1)}$$

where

$$\phi(0) = y, \, F_1(s) = \int_0^s f_1(x)dx,$$

and

$$\Theta(t) = z[1-F_2(t)] + \int_0^t [\alpha\Theta^2(t-s) + \beta]dF_2(s), \quad \text{(A-2)}$$

where

$$\Theta(0) = z, \, F_2(s) = \int_0^s f_2(x)dx.$$

Assume that the lifetime distribution for initiated cells and malignant cells are respectively given by

$$F_1(t) = 1 - \exp(-\lambda t), \lambda > 0,$$

and

$$F_2(t) = 1 - \exp(-\gamma t), \gamma > 0.$$

Note that the mean cell lifetimes are now $1/\lambda$ for initiated cells, and $1/\gamma$ for malignant cells. For instance, if t is time in days and $\lambda = 0.2$, then the mean lifetime for initiated cells is 5 days. Substituting these distribution functions into Equations A-1 and A-2, we have

$$\phi(t) = y\exp(-\lambda t) + \lambda \int_0^t [P_b\phi^2(t-s) + P_d + P_\mu\phi(t-s)\,\Theta(t-s)]\exp(-\lambda s)ds \quad \text{(A-3)}$$

and

$$\Theta(t) = z\exp(-\gamma t) + \gamma \int_0^t [\alpha\Theta^2(t-s) + \beta]\exp(-\gamma s)ds. \quad \text{(A-4)}$$

Multiplying $\exp(\lambda t)$ to both sides of Equation A-3, changing variable $\tau = t - s$, and differentiating, we have

$$\frac{d}{dt}\phi(t) = \lambda[P_b\phi^2(t) - \phi(+) + P_d + P_\mu\phi(t)\,\Theta(t)]. \quad \text{(A-5)}$$

Similarly, Equation A-4 is equivalent to

$$\frac{d}{dt}\Theta(t) = \gamma[\alpha\Theta^2(t) - \Theta(t) + \beta]. \quad \text{(A-6)}$$

Equation A-5 is a Riccati equation with nonconstant coefficient. The analytic solution is difficult to obtain. However, if we assume, as does the Moolgavkar model, that a malignant tumor cell does not undergo the birth and death process, then $\Theta(t) = z$, and the analytic solution is readily obtainable (see a more general case below).

Equation A-6 is a Riccati equation with constant coefficients and is recognized as a homogeneous birth-death process. The solution is readily found to be

$$\Theta(t) = \frac{B(t) + [1 - B(t) - A(t)]z}{1 - A(t)z}$$

where
$$B(t) = \frac{1 - exp(gt)}{1 - r exp(gt)}, g = \gamma(\alpha - \beta), \alpha \neq \beta, \text{ and } r = \alpha/\beta.$$

$B(t)$ is the probability of extinction. We shall need the probability of nonextinction $q(t) = 1 - B(t)$ in the derivation of probability of tumor.

Note that under our proposed model, when a malignant cell is born within a clone starting from a primary initiated cell, this malignant cell can die or form a small malignant island within the clone. (This is consistent with the observation of tumors within a nodule described by Pugh and Goldfarb (12). Since a nodule can become a malignant tumor only when there is at least one nonextinct malignant cell (or a malignant island), we introduce a random variable, $W(t)$, the number of nonextinct malignant islands (originated from a first-generation malignant cell some time before t) at time t, for a process starting with a single initiated cell at time $t = 0$. For a process starting with a single initiated cell, at most one nodule can be formed, and thus $W(t)$ is the number of nonextinct malignant tumors within a nodule that originates from an initiated cell.

To calculate probability of cancer at time t, we have to define what constitutes a cancer tumor. A cancer tumor can be defined as a clone that contains a certain number of nonextinct malignant islands, $W(t)$. In this paper, we assume that a cancer tumor is formed at time t when at least one of these malignant islands survives at that time. Let $\Psi(t) = \Psi(y, w|t)$ be the pgf of $[Y(t), W(t)]$ given that the process starts with a single initiated cell at $t = 0$. Ψ satisfies the following integral equation:

$$\Psi(t) = y exp(-\lambda t) + \int_0^t \{P_b \Psi^2(t\text{-}s) + P_d + P_\mu[1 - (1 - w)q(t\text{-}s)\psi(t\text{-}s)]\}exp(-\lambda s)ds$$
(A-7)

$$\Psi(0) = y.$$

Using the same operations as in converting Equation A-3 to Equation A-5, we have

$$\frac{d}{dt}\Psi(t) = \lambda\{P_b\Psi^2(t) - \Psi(t) + P_d + P_\mu[1 - (1 - w)q(t)]\Psi(t)\}$$
(A-8)

where
$$q(t) = 1 - B(t) = \frac{exp(gt)(1 - r)}{1 - r exp(gt)}.$$

The function $q(t)$ has a limiting value, $q_0 = \lim_{t \to \infty} q(t) = 1 - \frac{\beta}{\alpha}$

Incorporating the Poisson process of producing initiated cells from N-cells as described in assumption 2, let $\Pi(t, t_0) = \Pi(y, w|t, t_0)$ be the pgf of $[Y(t), W(t)]$, given $N(t), Y(t_0) = 0$ and $W(t_0) = 0$. Then, it is well-known (see for example, Moolgavkar and Venzon (2) that $\Pi(t, t_0)$ is given by

$$\Pi(t,t_0) = \exp\{ \int_{t_0}^{t} \mu_1(s)N(s)[\psi(t-s)-1]ds\} \tag{A-9}$$

The hazard function of the tumor is given by

$$\eta(t,t_0) = -\frac{d}{dt}\log \Pi(1,0|t,t_0) = -\int_{t_o}^{t}\mu_1(s)N(s)\frac{d}{dt}\psi(1,0|\ t-s)ds. \tag{A-10}$$

In general, $\Psi(1,0|t-s)$ must be calculated numerically from Equation A-8. However, when the limiting value q_0 is substituted in place of $q(t)$, an exact solution of Ψ can be obtained as follows:

$$\psi(y,w|t-s) = \frac{y_1-y_2 \left(\frac{y-y_1}{y-y_2}\right) \exp[\ \lambda P_b(y_1-y_2)(t-s)]}{1-\left(\frac{y-y_1}{y-y_2}\right) \exp[\ \lambda P_b(y_1-y_2)(t-s)]} \tag{A-11}$$

where $y_1 < y_2$ are two real roots of the equation

$$P_b X^2 - \{1-P_\mu[1-(1-w)q_0]\}X + P_d = 0 \tag{A-12}$$

Therefore, $\Psi(1,0|t-s)$ is obtained by substituting $y = 1$ and $w = 0$ in Equation A-11 and Equation A-12. Equations A-10 and A-11 are used in the DNT calculation.

Appendix B. Expected number of detectable foci

Assume that an initiated cell is subject to homogeneous birth-death processes with birth and death rates given respectively by b and d, $b \neq d$. By the theory of birth and death processes, it can be shown (20,24) that the probability that a nonextinct focus, born at $t = 0$, contains m or more cells at time t is

$$D_m(t) = [1-P_0(t)][A(t)]^{m-1},$$

where

$$P_0(t) = \Gamma(t), A(t) = r\Gamma(t),$$

and

$$\Gamma(t) = \frac{1-exp(\delta t)}{1-rexp(\delta t)} ; \delta = \text{b-d and } r = {}^b/_d, \quad b \neq d.$$

If it is assumed that a focus become detectable when its size is equal to or greater than m cells, then the expected number of detectable foci at time t is given by

$$F(t) = \int_0^t \mu_1 N(s) D_m(t-s) ds. \tag{B-1}$$

This formula involves parameters μ_1, b, and d. Equation B-1 is used to estimate parameters μ_1, b, and d, and then to derive parameters λ, P_b, P_d, in the DNT example.

Acknowledgments

We are grateful to Drs. J. Popp and T. Goldsworthy of CIIT, and to Drs. D. Krewski and J. Zielinski of Canada Health and Welfare, for their reviews and suggestions.

References

1. Armitage P, Doll R. The age-distribution of cancer and a multi-stage theory of carcinogenesis. Br J Cancer 8:1–12, 1954.
2. Moolgavkar S, Venzon D. Two-event models for carcinogenesis: incidence curves for childhood and adult tumors. Math Biosci 47:55–77, 1979.
3. Moolgavkar S, Knudson A. Mutation and cancer: A model for human carcinogenesis. J Natl Cancer Inst 66:1037–1052, 1981.
4. Pitot H, Sirica A. The stages of initiation and promotion in hepatocarcinogenesis. Biochim Biophys Acta 605:191–215, 1980.
5. Laib R, Klein K, Bolt H. The rat liver foci bioassay: I. Age-dependence of induction by vinyl chloride of the ATPase-deficient foci. Carcinogenesis 6(1):65–68, 1985.
6. Neyman J, Scott E. Statistical aspect of the problem of carcinogenesis. Proceedings of the Fifth Berkeley Symposium on Mathematical Statistics and Probability, vol. 4. Univ. of California Press, 1967, pp 745–776.
7. Armitage P, Doll R. A two stage theory of carcinogenesis in relation to the age distribution of human cancers. Br J Cancer 11:161–169, 1957.
8. Neyman J. A two–step mutation theory of carcinogenesis. In U.S. National Institutes of Health, 1958.
9. Neyman J. A two-step mutation theory of carcinogenesis. Bull Inst Int Stat 38:123–135, 1961.
10. Kendall D. Birth-and-death processes, and the theory of carcinogenesis. Biometrika 47:13–21, 1960.
11. Farber E, Sarma D. Hepartocarcinogenesis: A dynamic cellular perspective. Lab Invest 56:4–22, 1987.
12. Pugh T, Goldfarb S. Quantitative histochemical and autoradiographic studies of hepatocarcinogenesis in rats fed 2-acetylaminofluorene followed by phenobarbital. Cancer Res 38:4450–4457, 1978.
13. Hollstein M, Yamasaki H. Understanding multi-stage carcinogenesis at the molecular level: notes on recent progress. In Travis, C (ed): Biologically Based Methods for Cancer Risk Assessment. New York: Plenum Publishing Co., 1989.
14. Chemical Industry Institute of Toxicology. Final Report, 104-Week Chronic Toxicity Study in Rats. Project No. 2010-101, Hazelton Laboratories, Inc., 1982.
15. Bioassay of 2,4-dinitrotoluene for possible carcinogenicity. National Cancer Institute Publication. NIH 78-1360, Washington, DC: Government Printing Office, 1978.
16. Popp J, Leonard T. The hepatocarcinogenicity of dinitrotoluenes. In Riskert, DE (ed): Toxicity of Nitroaromatic Compounds. New York: Hemisphere Publishing Corp, 1985, pp. 53–60.
17. Goldsworthy T, Hamm T, Rickert D, Popp J. The effect of diet on 2,6-dinitrotoluene hepatocarcinogenesis. Carcinogenesis 7:1909–1915, 1986.
18. Leonard T, Lyght O, Popp J. Dinitrotoluene structure-dependent initiation of hepatocytes in vivo. Carcinogenesis 4(8):1059–1061, 1987.
19. Altman P., Dittmer D. Biological Data Book, 2nd ed, vol 1. Bethesda, Maryland: Federation of American Societies of Experimental Biology, 1972.

20. Chen C, Moini A. Cancer dose-response models incorporating clonal expansion. In Moolgavkar S (ed): Scientific Issues in Quantitative Cancer Risk Assessment. Boston: Birkhauser Publishing Company, 1990, pp 153–175.
21. U.S. Environmental Protection Agency. Guidelines for carcinogen risk assessment. Federal Register 51(185):33992–34003, Washington, DC: US Government Printing House, September 24, 1986.
22. Reynolds S, Stowers S, Patterson R, Maronpot R, Aaronson S, Anderson M. Activated oncogenes in B6C3F1 mouse liver tumors: implications for risk assessment. Science 237:1309–1316, 1987.
23. Mode C. Multitype Branching Processes: Theory and Applications. New York: American Elsevier Company, 1971.
24. Dewanji A, Venzon D, Moolgavkar S. A stochastic two-stage model for cancer risk assessment: II. The number and size of premalignant clones. Risk Anal 9(2):179–189, 1989.

Chemically Induced Cell Proliferation:
Implications for Risk Assessment, pages 501-516
©1991 Wiley-Liss, Inc.

The Relationship Between Carcinogenic Potency and Maximum Tolerated Dose is Similar for Mutagens and Nonmutagens

Gay Goodman, Alexander Shlyakhter, and Richard Wilson

Correlations between carcinogenic potency (β or $1/TD_{50}$) and acute toxicity (LD_{50}) and between carcinogenic potency and maximum tolerated dose (MTD) have been described by several authors (1–5). The correlations have been attributed in part to a bias inherent in the carcinogenicity bioassay, namely, that the carcinogenic potencies of chemicals that are highly toxic and only weakly carcinogenic cannot be measured, since any such chemical would not produce excess tumors in the typically 50–100 experimental animals receiving it at the MTD (3). But a chemical at the opposite end of the spectrum, one highly carcinogenic relative to its MTD, could certainly be identified under the same bioassay conditions. If a chemical of the latter type were to produce tumors in 100% of the study animals at all doses tested (typically MTD, MTD/2, and MTD/4), its carcinogenic potency could not be determined using standard methods. However, potency could be estimated under these circumstances by incorporating time-until-tumor data, or another bioassay could be run at lower doses.

In fact, such chemicals are only rarely identified, most likely because few exist. Their absence from the data base amounts to evidence that carcinogenicity in the rodent bioassay is tied, presumably biologically, to toxicity (4). Given this observation, along with data on biochemical mechanisms of DNA damage and repair, Ames and co-workers (6,7) and others (8) suggested that for both genotoxic and nongenotoxic chemicals, toxic effects mediate the carcinogenicity observed in rodent bioassays.

Of the 928 chemicals (with Chemical Abstracts numbers) tested in long-term mouse or rat carcinogenicity bioassays and listed in the Carcinogenic Potency Data Base (CPDB) (9–11), we count 435 (280 for mice and 251 for rats) that have demonstrated carcinogenic potency at $P < 0.01$ (two-tailed test) in at least one target site; this is in general agreement with Gold et al.(12). We have arbitrarily chosen $P < 0.1$ as a cutoff for statistical significance; 521 of the 928 chemicals fall into this category (353 for mice and 318 for rats). Analysis in this report has been performed on subsets (explained below) of those chemicals defined by TD_{50} values significant at $P < 0.1$, $P < 0.05$, $P < 0.025$, or $P < 0.01$.

In lifetime rodent bioassays, chemicals are tested at the highest possible dose to maximize the probability that a significant site-specific excess of tumors will appear. The problem with testing at doses near the MTD is that some toxic effects may be inevitable. Indeed, as the bulk of papers presented in this symposium would indicate, it might be that many chemicals are carcinogenic at high doses primarily because of some mechanism related to their toxicity, hypothesized to be the result of cell death, oxygen-radical release, and cell proliferation (7,8,13). For several nongenotoxic chemicals, the evidence suggests that tumorigenesis occurs only when the dose is high enough to produce quantifiable toxicity at the tumor target site; saccharin induction of bladder tumors in male rats is a notable example (14).

Do genotoxic chemicals cause cancer at high doses because they are genotoxic or because they are toxic? Since local toxicity at one or more sites is a probable consequence of dosing near the MTD, there may be synergistic effects due to toxicity (and consequent cell proliferation), even for chemicals that are carcinogenic *primarily* through genotoxicity. We approach the problem by asking whether the relationship between carcinogenic potency and MTD is weaker for mutagenic than for nonmutagenic agents. The maximum dose administered (MaxD) in a bioassay is usually fixed at the MTD; it consequently may be used as a surrogate for the MTD (2,5). In the work reported here, we addressed whether the TD_{50} has a different dependence on MaxD and on LD_{50} for mutagenic carcinogens than for nonmutagenic carcinogens. We also looked at the relationship between TD_{50} and MaxD in *Salmonella* mutagens as a function of the lowest effective dose (LED) for mutagenicity.

Methods

Two sets of chemicals were studied. The first comprised 222 chemicals tested by the National Cancer Institute/National Toxicology Program (NCI/NTP) and tabulated according to "structural alerts" (S/A) and mutagenicity (M) to *Salmonella* by Ashby and Tennant (15). Chemicals positive for both S/A and M were designated by Ashby and Tennant as +/+, chemicals negative for S/A and M were designated as –/–, and so forth. For concordant chemicals, i.e. those designated +/+ or –/–, we followed Ashby and Tennant's classification scheme. For the nonconcordant (+/– or –/+) chemicals, we made an assignment of mutagenicity or nonmutagenicity on the basis of (a) mutagenicity in *Salmonella* tests not considered by Ashby and Tennant, (b) mutagenicity in other bacterial systems, or (c) mutagenicity in some eukaryotic in vitro test, using *IARC Monographs Supplement 6* as a reference (16). If positive for S/A and untested for mutagenicity, a chemical was classified as mutagenic. In this manner, we categorized 117 chemicals as nonmutagens and 100 as mutagens; the remaining 5 could not be categorized.

The second set consisted of 245 chemicals that had tested positive for mutagenicity in various *Salmonella* strains, and for which quantitative information (i.e., revertant colonies at each dose level) was available. All data were from studies published by Zeiger and associates (17–19). From these data we estimated, for each chemical, the LED in each test, and we took the geometric mean of the LEDs over all tests. The chemicals were divided into three groups according to mean LED: low (LED <10 mg), intermediate (10 mg ≤ LED <100 mg), and high (LED ≥ 100 mg).

The minimum TD_{50}s at a given level of statistical significance were taken from the CPDB of Gold and colleagues (9–11). (For the NCI/NTP chemicals, the experiments yielding the appropriate minimum TD_{50} values were not necessarily those performed by the NCI/NTP. Note that "NCI/NTP dataset" here refers to the CPDB tabulation of all pertinent experimental results for these NCI/NTP chemicals and does not imply that the data came exclusively from NCI/NTP experiments.) Data from combined sites (tumor-bearing animals, abbreviated by Gold and co-workers as tba or

TBA) were ignored. Data were obtained separately for mice and rats. Gender was ignored. Only oral and inhalation routes were considered. If the tumor incidence in the control group for a given site exceeded 60%, the TD_{50} at that site was disregarded. The TD_{50} values were chosen to satisfy a given statistical significance criterion: $P < 0.01$, $P < 0.025$, $P < 0.05$, or $P < 0.1$. We shall refer to the data selected according to these significance criteria as sets A, B, C, and D, respectively. Minimum LD_{50}s were obtained from the *Registry of Toxic Effects of Chemical Substances* (20); only oral and inhalation routes were allowed. The designated MaxD is the highest dose in the same experiment from which the minimum TD_{50} was derived.

Tests for similarity

A dummy-variable method was used to test the null hypothesis that a pair of regression lines are coincident. The datasets are combined and linear regression is performed for the model:

$$y = b_0 + b_1 x + c_1 \delta + c_2 \delta x,$$

where $\delta = 0$ for the first dataset and $\delta = 1$ for the second. A t-test is made of the probability that the coefficients c_1 and c_2 are significantly different from zero. (SAS software was used to compute the statistical parameters.)

If the sample variances s^1_2 and s^2_2 for datasets 1 and 2 are assumed to have χ^2 distributions, then for comparison of the two variances, an F test may be performed to determine the confidence with which we can reject the null hypothesis, $H_0:(\sigma_1^2 = \sigma_2^2)$, in favor of the alternative hypothesis, $H_1:(\sigma_1^2 \neq \sigma_2^2)$, where σ^2 is the underlying variance. The ratio s_1^2/s_2^2 is compared to the F statistic computed given the number of chemicals n_1 and n_2 in datasets 1 and 2.

The observed value r of the correlation coefficient ρ may be transformed to a new, approximately normal variable z_r, defined by

$$z_r = \frac{1}{2}[\ln(1 + r) - \ln(1 - r)].$$

For comparison of two values r_1 and r_2 obtained from independent samples of size n_1 and n_2, the variable Z is defined as

$$Z = \frac{z_1 - z_2}{\sigma_z},$$

where σ_z is the standard error of the difference between z_1 and z_2:

$$\sigma_z = \sqrt{\frac{1}{n_1 - 3} + \frac{1}{n_2 - 3}}.$$

Z is evaluated in terms of a standard normal distribution, yielding the probability that the null hypothesis, $H_0:(\rho_1 = \rho_2)$, is true (21).

Simulation

It has been argued by Rieth and Starr (22) that since the range of MaxDs "spans over six orders of magnitude," whereas the possible range of finite and significantly non-zero single-dose values of carcinogenic potency β at a given MaxD is, according to Bernstein et al., confined to a 30-fold range around 1/MaxD (2), then a high degree of correlation between β and MaxD is inevitable. This line of reasoning leads to a specific, answerable question: Is the relationship between β and MaxD stronger than what would be observed if the measured potency were randomly selected from the possible values that could arise under a given set of experimental constraints?

To examine the degree to which the quantitative relationship between β and MTD is an artifactual consequence of the bioassay conditions, we have simulated a simplified bioassay based on the complete experiments in the NCI/NTP datasets described above. Before performing the simulations, we calculated a carcinogenic potency based on partial data from the bioassay as follows. For each experiment that had provided a minimum TD_{50} value under the particular selection criterion (A, B, C, or D), we noted the control group tumor incidence a_0, the maximum tumor incidence a_m, and the total number of animals n_0 and n_m in the control and MaxD groups, respectively. A carcinogenic potency based on this pseudo single-dose experiment was calculated as

$$\beta = \ln \left[\frac{1-(a_0/n_0)}{1-(a_m/n_m)} \right]$$

(Note that this is the same formula for potency used by Bernstein et al. [2] in their simulation of the results of single-dose bioassays.) This value for β was plotted against 1/MaxD, and linear regression analysis was performed.

To simulate the pseudo single-dose experiment, a_m was allowed to take discrete integer values between $(a_0 + 1)/n_0$ and $(n_m - 1)/n_m$. The probability distribution of a_m was assumed to be uniform, and a value was chosen at random for calculation of carcinogenic potency according to the equation cited above. Note that no test for statistical significance was performed during this random selection process, and therefore the lowest values of simulated potencies would be expected to be lower than what would actually be allowed, at least at the higher significance levels (sets A and B). The method for calculating the statistical significance of TD_{50} values in the CPDB reflects the fact that the experiments are multidose rather than single dose (23). Using maximum-likelihood estimators, it allows for the significance of a dose trend even when the maximum number of total tumors is not by itself statistically significant at a given confidence level (24). Since it is not a small task to translate the TD_{50} significance criterion into a lower limit on potency in a single-dose experiment, we have elected to perform our analysis at this time without such an added restriction; a future report will deal with this problem (Shlyakhter, Goodman and Wilson, unpublished data).

Results

For the NCI/NTP data, $1/TD_{50}$ versus 1/MaxD is plotted in Figure 1 and

$1/TD_{50}$ versus $1/LD_{50}$ is plotted in Figure 2 for mice and for rats and using different symbols for mutagenic and nonmutagenic chemicals. Data taken at the two extremes of statistical significance, sets A and D ($P < 0.01$ and $P < 0.1$), are plotted for the MaxD data. One level ($P < 0.025$) is plotted for the LD_{50} data. At higher statistical significance (i.e., $P < 0.01$), the comparison of LD_{50} datasets is less meaningful, since the number of points is so small (especially for the rat nonmutagens) that the sample is unlikely to be representative. Similarly, in the high-LED group of the Zeiger data, the small number of points sets a limit on the statistical significance level worth examining. Using $P < 0.025$ as the cutoff for the Zeiger mutagens, $1/TD_{50}$ versus $1/MaxD$ is plotted for mice and for rats if Figure 3, with different symbols for the low-, intermediate-, and high-LED groups. Table 1 shows the results of obtaining the least squares fit to the normal-error linear-regression model

$$\log(1/TD_{50})_i = b_0 + b_1 \cdot \log x_i + \varepsilon_i,$$

where x is $1/MaxD$ or $1/LD_{50}$. The slope ($\pm SD$), zero intercept ($\pm SD$), observed correlation coefficient, number of points, and sample variance are given for each plot.

The slopes for mutagenic and nonmutagenic chemicals (NCI/NTP data, MaxD and LD_{50}) and for chemicals with low, intermediate, and high LEDs (Zeiger's *Salmonella* mutagens, MaxD) were compared (Table 2). All pairwise comparisons based on the MaxD resulted in failure to reject the null hypothesis of equal slopes (with $\geq 90\%$ confidence), with the exception of the mouse dataset A, where it is rejected with 99.5% confidence. For the comparisons based on LD_{50}, the null hypothesis is rejected for the rat dataset (99.9% confidence). In both cases for which the slopes were significantly different, the intercepts also differed significantly (>99% confidence). Examination of the LD_{50} data (Fig. 2) suggests that a linear model may not be appropriate for the mutagenic chemicals.

Comparison of sample variances (s_2) between mutagens and nonmutagens and between pairs of LED groups is also shown in Table 2. In every case, the variance for the mutagens is greater than the variance for the nonmutagens. The sample variances based on the MaxD are significantly different for the most stringently selected mouse data, set A (90% confidence) and for all rat datasets: set A (90% confidence) and sets B, C, and D (95% confidence). Sample variances based on the LD_{50} were not significantly different. Pairwise comparison between LED groups reveals no significant difference ($\geq 90\%$ confidence).

For completeness, in Table 2 we also give a comparison of observed correlation coefficients for mutagens/nonmutagens and low/medium/high LED groups, although we think this is less informative than the comparison of sample variances. (The degree of correlation for a given sample may be high even when the variance is large, and for two samples with equal correlation coefficients, the variances might be quite different.) We found that in every case in which there was a significant difference in sample variances, there was also a significant difference in correlation coefficients. In two cases in which no significant difference in sample variances occurred, there was nevertheless a significant difference in correlation coefficients: the mutagen/nonmutagen comparison for mouse dataset D and the medium/high LED comparison for mice.

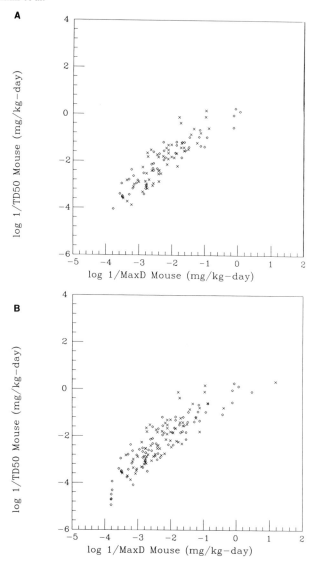

Figure 1. Log-log plot of $1/TD_{50}$ versus $1/MaxD$ for NCI/NTP chemicals tested in mice (A and B) and rats (C and D). ×, mutagens; ◇, nonmutagens. A and C, TD_{50} significant at $P < 0.01$; B and D, TD_{50} significant at $P < 0.1$. See text for details.

TD_{50} significance level: Effect on variance

As the significance level for selection of the minimum TD_{50} value is lowered, the sample variance increases. All comparisons were tested for significance at the 90%

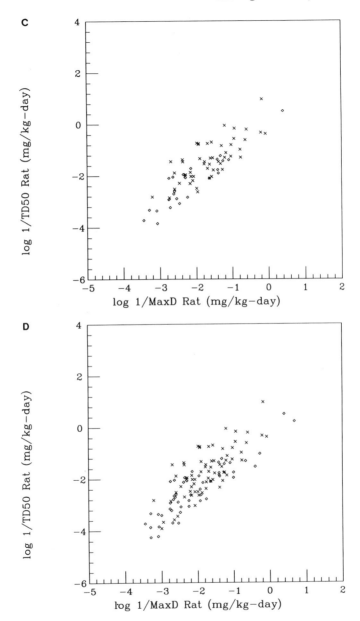

confidence level or higher. The variances differ significantly for the nonmutagens tested in mice (99% confidence) and the mutagens tested in rats (95% confidence) between the most stringently selected dataset (A) and the other three sets, but the variances of these

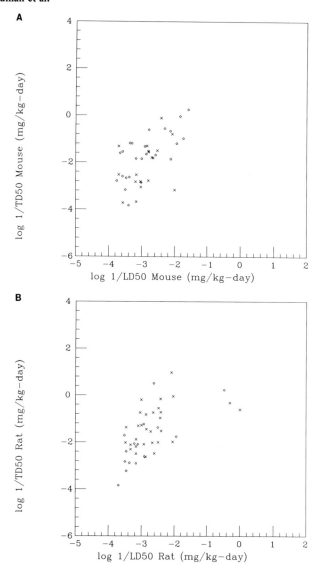

Figure 2. Log-log plot of $1/TD_{50}$ versus $1/LD_{50}$ for NCI/NTP chemicals tested in mice (A) and rats (B). ×, mutagens; ◇, nonmutagens. TD_{50} significant at $P < 0.025$. See text for details.

last sets do not vary significantly between themselves. For the mutagens tested in mice as well as the nonmutagens tested in rats, the increase in variance with decreasing significance-level selection becomes significant (95% confidence) only for comparison

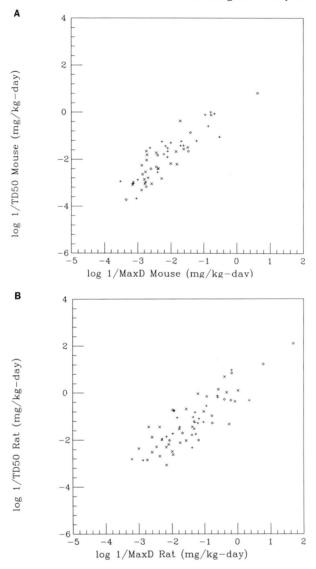

Figure 3. Log-log plot of 1/TD$_{50}$ versus 1/MaxD for Zeiger *Salmonella* mutagens tested in mice (A) and rats (B). +, LED < 10 mg; ×, 10 mg ≤ LED < 100 mg; ◇, LED ≥ 100 mg. TD$_{50}$ significant at *P* < 0.025. See text for details.

of the least stringently selected set (D) with the most stringently selected set (A). For none of the comparisons was there a significant difference (≥90% confidence) in the observed correlation coefficients.

Table 1. Linear Regression of Log($1/TD_{50}$) Versus Log($1/MaxD$) for NCI/NTP and Zeiger Datasets and Log($1/TD_{50}$) Versus Log($1/LD_{50}$) for NCI/NTP Datasets.

Type		TD_{50} significance[a]	Slope	Intercept	r	n	s^2
NCI/NTP carcinogens, MaxD							
Mouse mutagens		A	1.276 ± 0.100	0.882 ± 0.234	0.871	54	0.227
		B	1.189 ± 0.097	0.624 ± 0.226	0.850	60	0.259
		C	1.220 ± 0.093	0.641 ± 0.222	0.851	67	0.262
		D	1.056 ± 0.081	0.220 ± 0.191	0.841	72	0.290
Mouse nonmutagens		A	0.956 ± 0.056	0.131 ± 0.134	0.934	45	0.143
		B	1.009 ± 0.064	0.165 ± 0.155	0.912	53	0.210
		C	1.054 ± 0.062	0.212 ± 0.153	0.913	59	0.221
		D	1.041 ± 0.056	0.101 ± 0.138	0.916	69	0.234
Rat mutagens		A	0.855 ± 0.107	0.017 ± 0.189	0.757	50	0.274
		B	0.915 ± 0.116	0.035 ± 0.209	0.719	60	0.358
		C	0.972 ± 0.112	0.023 ± 0.204	0.740	65	0.358
		D	1.034 ± 0.109	0.094 ± 0.204	0.759	68	0.371
Rat nonmutagens		A	1.022 ± 0.092	0.069 ± 0.216	0.919	25	0.152
		B	0.982 ± 0.081	0.238 ± 0.186	0.919	29	0.190
		C	0.959 ± 0.070	0.381 ± 0.157	0.905	44	0.185
		D	0.956 ± 0.070	0.463 ± 0.158	0.892	50	0.214
NCI/NTP carcinogens, LD_{50}							
Mouse mutagens		B	0.830 ± 0.472	0.254 ± 1.386	0.402	18	0.895
Mouse nonmutagens		B	1.045 ± 0.223	1.340 ± 0.658	0.707	24	0.534
Rat mutagens		B	0.522 ± 0.186	0.054 ± 0.508	0.463	31	0.616
Rat nonmutagens		B	1.054 ± 0.282	1.017 ± 0.857	0.734	14	0.752
Zeiger *Salmonella* mutagens, MaxD							
Mouse	Low LED	B	1.032 ± 0.116	0.423 ± 0.247	0.889	23	0.206
	Medium LED	B	1.096 ± 0.182	0.416 ± 0.453	0.788	24	0.271
	High LED	B	1.105 ± 0.119	0.296 ± 0.273	0.967	8	0.151
	All	B	1.083 ± 0.078	0.423 ± 0.180	0.887	55	0.222
Rat	Low LED	B	0.874 ± 0.140	0.045 ± 0.235	0.800	24	0.294
	Medium LED	B	0.952 ± 0.140	0.046 ± 0.261	0.806	27	0.410
	High LED	B	1.052 ± 0.165	0.233 ± 0.205	0.887	13	0.373
	All	B	0.969 ± 0.077	0.137 ± 0.130	0.848	64	0.343

Abbreviations: LD, lethal dose; MaxD, maximum dose administered; n, the number of chemicals; NCI/NTP, National Cancer Institute/National Toxicology Program; r, the observed correlation coefficient; s^2, the sample variance (standard deviation squared); TD, tumor dose.

[a] TD_{50} statistical significance criteria: A, $P < 0.01$; B, $P < 0.025$; C, $P < 0.05$; D, $P < 0.1$.

Pseudo single-dose experiments and simulations

Linear regression was performed for each experimental dataset; the sample variances are given in Table 3, along with the observed correlation coefficients. There is no significant difference ($\geq 90\%$ confidence) between any pair of mutagen/nonmutagen variances obtained in the pseudo single-dose experiments, in contrast to the complete experiments (Table 2). The mutagen/nonmutagen comparison of observed correlation coefficients revealed significant differences for all mouse datasets (A, 99% confidence; B and C, 95% confidence; D, 90% confidence) and for rat datasets B, C, and D (95% confidence). Again, we suggest that the comparison of sample variances is a more meaningful indicator of the strength of the relationship between TD_{50} and MaxD; the failure

Table 2. Comparison of Slopes, Sample Variances and Observed Correlation Coefficients for the Linear Regression of $Log(1/TD_{50})$ Versus $Log(1/MaxD)$ (a and c) or $Log(1/LD_{50})$ (b), for Mutagens and Nonmutagens (a and b) and Low/Medium/High LEDs (c).

Comparison			TD_{50} significance[a]	Slopes differ?	Variances differ?	Correlation coefficients differ?
(a) NCI/NTP carcinogens, MaxD						
Mutagen/Nonmutagen	Mouse	A		Yes[b]	Yes[c]	Yes[e]
		B		No	No	No
		C		No	No	No
		D		No	No	Yes[f]
	Rat	A		No	Yes[c]	Yes[f]
		B		No	Yes[d]	Yes[g]
		C		No	Yes[d]	Yes[g]
		D		No	Yes[d]	Yes[f]
(b) NCI/NTP carcinogens, LD_{50}						
Mutagen/Nonmutagen	Mouse	B		No	No	No
	Rat	B		Yes[b]	No	No
(c) Zeiger *Salmonella* mutagens, MaxD						
Low/Medium LED	Mouse	B		No	No	No
Low/High LED		B		No	No	No
Medium/High LED		B		No	No	Yes[f]
Low/Medium LED	Rat	B		No	No	No
Low/High LED		B		No	No	No
Medium/High LED		B		No	No	No

Abbreviations: LD, lethal dose; LED, lowest effective dose; MaxD, maximum dose administered; NCI/NTP, National Cancer Institute/National Toxicology Program; TD, tumor dose.

[a] Statistical significance criteria for A, B, C, and D as in Table 1.

[b] Probability is <0.5% that the two-dataset combination has the same slope as the dataset consisting of mutagens alone.

[c] Probability of falsely rejecting $H_0:(s_1^2 = s_2^2)$ is <10%.

[d] Probability of falsely rejecting $H_0:(s_1^2 = s_2^2)$ is <5%.

[e] Probability of falsely rejecting $H_0:(r_1 = r_2)$ is <10%.

[f] Probability of falsely rejecting $H_0:(r_1 = r_2)$ is <5%.

[g] Probability of falsely rejecting $H_0:(r_1 = r_2)$ is <1%.

of the pseudo single-dose experiments to replicate mutagen/nonmutagen differences found with the complete experiments indicates that the former are a poor surrogate for the latter.

Simulations were performed five times for each dataset, and the sample variances and observed correlation coefficients were averaged over these five independent simulations. For two datasets (mouse mutagens set D and mouse nonmutagens set A), the simulation was performed 100 times, and the sample variances and correlation coefficients were averaged accordingly and compared with the 5× averages, in order to check that the first five random number seeds were not atypical. The 5× averaged (or 100× averaged, for these two datasets) sample variances and observed correlation coefficients for the simulations are shown in Table 4, along with results of the comparison of simulated and experimental pseudo single-dose experiments.

In every case except for rat mutagens set D, the simulated sample variance is greater than the experimental sample variance. Only for mouse mutagens sets A and B

Table 3. Comparison of Sample Variances and Observed Correlation Coefficients for the Linear Regression of Log(1/TD$_{50}$) on Log(1/MaxD) for Mutagens (s_m^2 and r_m) and Nonmutagens (s_{nm}^2 and r_{nm}), Pseudo Single-dose NCI/NTP Data.

Pseudo single-dose dataset (Mutagen/Nonmutagen)[a]		s_m^2/s_{nm}^2	r_m/r_{nm}	Variances differ?[b]	Correlation coefficient differ?
Mouse dataset	A	0.127/0.130	0.839/0.949	No	Yes[c]
	B	0.177/0.182	0.828/0.923	No	Yes[d]
	C	0.191/0.183	0.803/0.916	No	Yes[d]
	D	0.200/0.187	0.865/0.924	No	Yes[e]
Rat dataset	A	0.160/0.108	0.893/0.925	No	No
	B	0.218/0.839	0.1420/0.935	No	Yes[d]
	C	0.225/0.156	0.822/0.923	No	Yes[d]
	D	0.268/0.195	0.781/0.906	No	Yes[d]

Note: The number of chemicals in each dataset is the same as for the corresponding complete dataset for mutagens or nonmutagens listed in Table 1.

Abbreviations: MaxD, maximum dose administered; NCI/NTP, National Cancer Institute/National Toxicology Program; TD, tumor dose.

[a] Data sets A, B, C, and D defined by statistical-significance criteria as in Table 1.

[b] Probability that H$_0$:(s_m^2 = s_{nm}^2) is true is ≥10% in every case.

[c] Probability of falsely rejecting H$_0$:(r_m = r_{nm}) is <1%.

[d] Probability of falsely rejecting H$_0$:(r_m = r_{nm}) is <5%.

[e] Probability of falsely rejecting H$_0$:(r_m= r_{nm}) is <10%.

and nonmutagens set A is the difference statistically significant at the 95% confidence level. For rat mutagens set A and for rat nonmutagens sets A and C, the difference is significant at the 90% level. No significant differences in observed correlation coefficients were found (≥90% confidence).

Discussion

Distribution of mutagens versus nonmutagens

Only for the most stringently selected mouse dataset ($P < 0.01$) were the data consistent with different 1/TD$_{50}$ versus 1/MaxD distributions: both slope and intercept are significantly larger for the mutagens than for the nonmutagens. Examination of the data (Fig. 1A) shows that the difference appears when 1/MaxD > 10^{-2} (MaxD < 100 mg/kg-day), where the mutagens tend to have a higher carcinogenic potency relative to MaxD than do nonmutagens. The four chemicals with the lowest MaxDs, which presumably are the most toxic (reserpine, dieldrin, heptachlor, and aldrin), are all nonmutagens. For the chemicals with MaxD > 100 mg/kg-day, there is no apparent difference in the distributions.

Sample variances of mutagens versus nonmutagens

For the data based on MaxD, in the most stringently selected mouse dataset and in all the rat datasets the difference in sample variances between mutagens and nonmuta-

Table 4. Comparison of Sample Variances and Observed Correlation Coefficients for the Linear Regression of Log(1/TD$_{50}$) Versus Log(1/MaxD) for Experimental ($s_e{}^2$ and r_e) and Simulated ($s_s{}^2$ and r_s) Pseudo Single-dose NCI/NTP Data.

Pseudo single-dose dataset (Simulated/Experimental)[a]		$s_s{}^2/s_e{}^2$	r_s/r_e	Variances differ?	Coefficient coefficients differ?
Mouse mutagens dataset	A	0.237/0.127	0.803/0.839	Yes[b]	No
	B	0.274/0.177	0.798/0.828	Yes[b]	No
	C	0.248/0.191	0.812/0.803	No	No
	D	0.242/0.200	0.848/0.865	No	No
Mouse nonmutagens dataset	A	0.245/0.130	0.901/0.949	Yes[b]	No
	B	0.244/0.182	0.908/0.923	No	No
	C	0.249/0.183	0.892/0.916	No	No
	D	0.249/0.187	0.902/0.924	No	No
Rat mutagens dataset	A	0.237/0.160	0.838/0.893	Yes[c]	No
	B	0.251/0.218	0.808/0.839	No	No
	C	0.251/0.225	0.818/0.822	No	No
	D	0.241/0.268	0.816/0.781	No	No
Rat nonmutagens dataset	A	0.208/0.108	0.899/0.925	Yes[c]	No
	B	0.215/0.142	0.915/0.935	No	No
	C	0.237/0.156	0.879/0.923	Yes[c]	No
	D	0.253/0.195	0.874/0.906	No	No

Note: The number of chemicals is the same for each pair of experimental and simulated datasets as for the corresponding complete dataset listed in Table 1.

Abbreviations: MaxD, maximum dose administered; NCI/NTP, National Cancer Institute/National Toxicology Program; TD, tumor dose.

[a] Datasets A, B, C, and D defined by statistical-significance criteria as in Table 1.
[b] Probability of falsely rejecting H_0:($s_s{}^2 = s_s{}^2$) is <5%.
[c] Probability of falsely rejecting H_0:($s_s{}^2 = s_s{}^2$) is <10%.

gens is significant at the 90% confidence level or better. The mutagens demonstrate a larger variance than nonmutagens, and this difference is more significant (95% confidence) for three of the rat datasets (B, C, and D). This suggests that for mutagens, the TD$_{50}$ is less tied to the MaxD than it is for nonmutagens, which would follow if some mutagens are inducing neoplasms by mechanisms other than those mediated by toxicity, or if combined genotoxic and toxic mechanisms are prevalent. This would not be unanticipated, but the fact that it occurs to a larger extent for the less stringently selected rat data is puzzling. We do not understand this phenomenon, but perhaps it suggests that rat mutagens with potencies that are low relative to the MTD are more likely than those with higher relative potency to produce tumors by means of genotoxic mechanisms.

Simulation of sample variance

Significant differences between sample variances were found for the comparison of simulated and experimental pseudo single-dose data. No such differences between correlation coefficients were found for this comparison. Recall, however, that for comparison of mutagens and nonmutagens in the complete datasets, a difference in correlation coefficient always accompanies a difference in sample variance (Table 2); the fact that this is not observed for the comparison of simulated and experimental pseudo single-dose data is therefore disturbing. It is possible that the differences in sample variance might be a spurious result of the absence of selection criteria in the simulation. Unfortunately, this finding sheds no light on the more interesting question of whether simulation of the complete experiments would reveal a similar lack of difference in sample variances. Based on the sample-variance differences between mutagens and nonmutagens in the complete sets, we suggest that simulation of the complete data would show that the simulated sample variance is larger than the experimental sample variance, at least for nonmutagens with TD_{50} values significant at $P < 0.01$.

The pseudo single-dose model described here, which is equivalent to that analyzed by Bernstein et al. (2), does not approximate the actual distribution of $1/TD_{50}$ versus $1/MaxD$ closely enough to be useful for examining artifacts in the apparent correlation of these two variables. Both simulated and actual pseudo single-dose experiments fail to account for the significantly different sample variances for mutagens and nonmutagens that arise when the complete experiments are considered. This may be because differences in tumor response between mutagens and nonmutagens appear in the sub-MaxD dose groups more often than in the MaxD dose group. For both mutagens and nonmutagens, at the MaxD the tumor response might be converging toward the same dependence on toxicity.

Conclusions

In the linear regression of $1/TD_{50}$ on $1/MaxD$, the sample variance for mutagens is slightly or in some cases significantly elevated relative to nonmutagens. The fact that there exists a significant difference depending on mutagenicity, which is an unrelated variable, suggests that at least a portion of the correlation is nonspurious. Our work provides evidence that the Bernstein et al. pseudo single-dose simulation (2) is not detailed enough for describing the actual relationship between TD_{50} and MaxD; we are engaged, therefore, in a more complete simulation using Monte Carlo methodology (Shlyakhter, Goodman, and Wilson, unpublished data). However, we have not ruled out the possibility, especially for mutagens, that there is little more (or no more) quantitative information to be gained from the relationship between carcinogenic potency and MTD than is already contained in (a) the statistical significance level at which the potency is chosen, and (b) the fact that chemicals producing a 100% level of tumors at the MTD are rare. In this we concur with much of what Bernstein et al. (2) and Rieth and Starr (22) have previously concluded. The carcinogenic potency is more strongly associated with the MTD for nonmutagens than for mutagens. But differences between sample variances for mutagens and nonmutagens are small, and probably not very useful for predictive purposes, overall. Our findings are consistent with the premise that, even for most mutagens, at high doses carcinogenicity is associated mechanistically with toxicity.

The implications of our findings are far from obvious. Although often assumed, it is by no means certain that most mutagens and other genotoxic agents induce cancer in humans by means of genotoxic mechanisms. Most epidemiologic evidence for chemical carcinogenesis in humans comes from industrial or medical exposures in which the dose levels were high, approaching the MTD in many cases. Thus, toxicity could have been a real factor in these cases as well. The best-studied agent known to cause human cancer is tobacco smoke, which produces acute toxic effects in the lungs and respiratory system at all levels of usage. It may be argued that the target-tissue dose level is high for the duration of inhalation, regardless of how few or how many cigarettes are smoked per day. For this reason, toxic effects cannot be ruled out as a contributing cause or even as the main cause of smoking-related carcinogenesis, despite the fact that tobacco smoke contains potent mutagens. Our results are in line with the suggestion that toxic effects are as important or more important than mutagenic events not only in the production of tumors in the rodent bioassay, but in the etiology of environmentally associated human cancer as well. We therefore agree with Benigni (25) that division of carcinogens into the categories "primary" (genotoxic) and "secondary" (nongenotoxic) would seem, for the present, an unsuitable basis for risk assessment.

Acknowledgments

This work has been supported by gifts to Harvard University from a number of sources: Monsanto, Gillette, Bristol-Myers, and Rohm & Haas. Richard Wilson acknowledges support from the FDA by an Interagency Personnel Agreement.

Notes

Data sets, including chemical names, are available from G. Goodman upon request.

References

1. Zeise L, Wilson R, Crouch E. Use of acute toxicity to estimate carcinogenic risk. Risk Anal 4:187–199, 1984.
2. Bernstein L, Gold LS, Ames BN, Pike MC, Hoel DG. Some tautologous aspects of the comparison of carcinogenic potency in rats and mice. Fundam Appl Toxicol 5:79–86, 1985.
3. Zeise L, Crouch EAC, Wilson R. Reply to comments: On the relationship of toxicity and carcinogenicity. Risk Anal 5:265–270, 1985.
4. Zeise L, Crouch EAC, Wilson R. A possible relationship between toxicity and carcinogenicity. J Am Coll Toxicol 5:137–151, 1986.
5. Crouch E, Wilson R, Zeise L. Tautology or not tautology? J Toxicol Environ Health 20:1–10, 1987.
6. Ames BN, Magaw R, Gold LS. Ranking possible carcinogenic hazards. Science 236:271–280, 1987.
7. Ames BN. Mutagenesis and carcinogenesis: Endogenous and exogenous factors. Environ Mol Mutagen 14:66–77, 1989.
8. Fischer SM, Floyd RA, Copeland ES. Oxy radicals in carcinogenesis—A Chemical Pathology Study Section Workshop. Cancer Res 48:3882–3887, 1988.
9. Gold LS, Sawyer CB, Magaw R, Backman GM, de Veciana M, Levinson R, Hooper NK, Havender WR, Bernstein L, Peto R, Pike MC, Ames BN. A carcinogenic potency database of the standardized results of animal bioassays. Environ Health Perspect 58:9–319, 1984.
10. Gold LS, de Veciana M, Backman GM, Magaw R, Lopipero P, Smith M, Blumenthal M, Levinson R, Bernstein L, Ames BN. Chronological supplement to the Carcinogenic Potency Database: Standardized results of animal bioassays published through December 1982. Environ Health Perspect 67:161–200, 1986.
11. Gold LS, Slone TH, Backman GM, Magaw R, Da Costa M, Lopipero P, Blumenthal M, Ames BN. Second chronological supplement to the Carcinogenic Potency Database: Standardized results of animal bioassays published through December 1984 and by the National Toxicology Program through May 1986. Environ Health Perspect 74:237–329, 1987.
12. Gold LS, Bernstein L, Magaw R, Slone TH. Interspecies extrapolation in carcinogenesis: Prediction

between rats and mice. Environ Health Perspect 81:211–219, 1989.

13. Farber E. The multistep nature of cancer development. Cancer Res 44:4217–4223, 1984.

14. Cohen SM, Ellwein LB. Cell growth dynamics in long-term bladder carcinogenesis. Toxicol Lett 43:151–173, 1988.

15. Ashby J, Tennant RW. Chemical structure, *Salmonella* mutagenicity and extent of carcinogenicity as indicators of genotoxic carcinogenesis among 222 chemicals tested in rodents by the U.S. NCI/NTP. Mutat Res 204:17–115, 1988.

16. International Agency for Research on Cancer. Genetic and Related Effects. IARC Monographs on the Evaluation of Carcinogenic Risk to Humans, Suppl 6. Lyons: World Health Organization, 1987.

17. Haworth S, Lawlor T, Mortelmans K, Speck W, Zeiger E. *Salmonella* mutagenicity test results for 250 chemicals. Environ Mutagen 5 (Suppl. 1):2–142, 1983.

18. Dunkel VC, Zeiger E, Brusick D, McCoy E, McGregor D, Mortelmans K, Rosenkranz HS, Simmon VF. Reproducibility of microbial mutagenicity assays: II. Testing of carcinogens and noncarcinogens in *Salmonella typhimurium* and *Escherichia coli*. Environ Mutagen 7 (Suppl. 5):1–248, 1985.

19. Zeiger E, Anderson B, Haworth S, Lawlor T, Mortelmans K. *Salmonella* mutagenicity tests: IV. Results from the testing of 300 chemicals. Environ Mol Mutagen 11 (Suppl. 12):1–158, 1988.

20. Sweet D (ed): Registry of Toxic Effects of Chemical Substances (RTECS), 1985-86 edition. Washington, DC: U.S. Government Printing Office, 1987.

21. Weisberg S. Applied Linear Regression. New York: John Wiley & Sons, 1980.

22. Rieth JP, Starr TB. Experimental design constraints on carcinogenic potency estimates. J Toxicol Environ Health 27:287–296, 1989.

23. Peto R, Pike M, Bernstein L, Gold LS, Ames BN. The TD50: A proposed general convention for the numerical description of the carcinogenic potency of chemicals in chronic-exposure animal experiments. Environ Health Perspect 58:1–8, 1984.

24. Sawyer C, Peto R, Bernstein L, Pike MC. Calculation of carcinogenic potency from long-term animal carcinogenesis experiments. Biometrics 40:27–40, 1984.

25. Benigni R. Rodent tumor profiles, *Salmonella* mutagenicity and risk assessment. Mutat Res, in press.

Chemically Induced Cell Proliferation:
Implications for Risk Assessment, pages 517-532
©1991 Wiley-Liss, Inc.

Chemicals, Cell Proliferation, Risk Estimation, and Multistage Carcinogenesis

Henry C. Pitot, Yvonne P. Dragan, Mark J. Neveu, Tahir A. Rizvi, James R. Hully, and Harold A. Campbell

The rate, duration, and characteristics of cell replication are significant if not critical factors in the development of neoplasia. The role(s) played by cell proliferation during the process of carcinogenesis may be quite subtle; cell division in individual organs that is induced by administering specific chemicals may be a factor in this process, particularly when the chemicals provoke the development of neoplasia through mechanisms that do not structurally alter the genome. The role of cell proliferation must also be reconciled with the multistage nature of carcinogenesis. This study presents one possible relationship of cell proliferation to the initiation and promotion stages of hepatocarcinogenesis in the rat.

Cell proliferation in multistage hepatocarcinogenesis

Although this discussion is concerned primarily with cell proliferation and multistage hepatocarcinogenesis, the conclusions drawn may have ramifications in other multistage carcinogenesis models such as mouse epidermis (1), cultured Syrian hamster embryo cells (2,3), rat kidney (4–6), and rat bladder (7–9).

Initiation. The characteristics of the initiation and other stages of rat hepatocarcinogenesis have been previously described (10). A slightly modified, somewhat restrictive definition of this first stage is: the intracellular process that occurs when a chemical, physical, or biologic agent irreversibly alters heritable cell structure(s). This reaction gives a cell the potential to develop into a clone of preneoplastic or neoplastic cells during the stages of promotion or progression, respectively.

This definition is based on the interpretation of initiation as a process that is analogous to a genomic DNA mutation. Although carcinogenesis cannot be universally correlated with mutagenesis (11–13), specific chemical classes in which virtually all members exhibit mutagenicity under appropriate circumstances do show a higher correlation (14). Furthermore, the necessity for one or several cycles of DNA synthesis to occur in the presence of the initiating agent in order for this stage to be "fixed" is analogous to mutation fixation in microorganisms (15). DNA synthesis must occur in the presence of the carcinogenic agent for initiation to ensue (16–18) in hepatocarcinogenesis and in other systems (19,20). In addition, Rabes (21) has described the importance of the time point in the cell's cycle at which the initiating event occurs, as it relates to the chemical's metabolism to its ultimate form and the repair of the DNA adduct. While cell division during initiation is critically important, so also is the generalization that tissues with relatively high proliferation rates, whose cells are not rapidly eliminated from the organism, are most susceptible to carcinogenesis. These include epithelial tissues of the skin, lung, colon, bone marrow, and genital tissues. In addition, there is a strong correlation between the susceptibility of fetal tissue to carcinogenesis and those periods of gestation that have the highest rate of tissue growth (22).

Extensive experimentation, including the data described above, indicates that cell proliferation and DNA synthesis are required to complete the initiation process. Recent studies by Columbano and his associates (23) have demonstrated that chemical mitogens do not induce initiation in the liver. While it is not clear what mechanism is responsible for this apparent lack of initiation, these authors suggested that cells stimulated to divide in the presence of mitogens may be destined to undergo apoptosis once the mitogen is removed; therefore, such cells would not survive. Those cells undergoing DNA synthesis during compensatory hyperplasia are not always destined to undergo apoptosis; thus, once initiated, they may either remain dormant or develop into clones of preneoplastic cells.

Another aspect of cell replication that is especially important in hepato-carcinogenesis is the ploidy of the target cells at initiation. Although almost two-thirds of hepatocytes in rat liver are tetraploid in the adult state (24), several studies have now demonstrated that the majority of altered hepatic foci (25,26), as well as hepatocellular nodules and carcinomas (27), are diploid; this suggests that the diploid hepatocyte population is the most susceptible to initiation. Once initiated, such cells may be incapable of polyploidization as they replicate (28).

Promotion. Cell proliferation is absolutely critical for promotion, a stage that is characterized by the clonal expansion of initiated cells (10). Equally important is operational reversibility, a factor that deemphasizes the significance of DNA damage during this stage. The promotion stage has been defined as: the natural history of neoplastic development that is characterized by (1) the reversible expansion of the initiated cell population and (2) the reversible alteration of genetic expression (29).

The reversibility of both the clonal expansion and gene expression of initiated cells has been discussed extensively in other publications (10,29,30). However, the mechanisms of reversibility in both processes play a significant role in our understanding of tumor promotion. The ability of several promoting agents to alter gene expression and increase cell replication appears to be mediated by receptor mechanisms, as exemplified by the two most potent promoting agents, 12-O-tetradecanoylphorbol-13-acetate (TPA) (31) and its congeners (32), and 2,3,7,8-tetrachlorodibenzo-p-dioxin (TCDD) (33,34). When cell division ceases upon removal of the promoting agent, cells in the promotion stage during hepatocarcinogenesis either die and are eliminated by the process of apoptosis (35) or differentiate (remodel) into normal-appearing hepatocytes (36).

Alterations in gene expression and cell proliferation during the promotion stage in hepatocarcinogenesis. A distinct advantage of the multistage hepatocarcinogenesis model in the rat is the capability to score and quantitate the clonal expansions of individual initiated cells, called altered hepatic foci (AHF) (37). Such focal lesions may be identified by characteristics determined with the light microscope (37) or with a variety of enzymatic, immunohistochemical, and molecular biologic markers. Studies from this laboratory (38) have demonstrated the phenotypic distribution of AHF in livers of animals initiated with diethylnitrosamine (DEN) and promoted with pheno-barbital (PB) through the use of three enzymatic markers, γ-glutamyltranspeptidase (GGT), canalicular ATPase (ATP), and glucose-6-phosphatase (G6P). Under these conditions, a predominance (75%) of the AHF exhibited GGT expression. When PB promotion was omitted, each of the markers scored an approximately equal fraction of AHF. Later studies (39) with TCDD as a promoting agent resulted in AHF with the same phenotypic distribution as was observed with PB. A possible explanation for the difference in the efficiency of GGT as a marker of AHF between rats given PB or TCDD and those animals given neither agent was proposed by Sirica et al. (40). These investigators demonstrated that PB administration caused an increase in GGT activity within individual AHF and nodules in the liver. In contrast, when PB was removed from the diet, the number of AHF and the total volume of the liver occupied by AHF decreased dramatically within a few days. The phenotypic distribution of these three markers was the same as that observed with animals maintained on the promoting agent (41). Readministration of the promoting agent to animals withdrawn for various periods resulted in a rapid reappearance of AHF (42). The stability of AHF phenotypic distribution in the presence of a specific promoting agent has also been described by others (43).

More recent studies from our laboratory with other promoting agents (Fig. 1, A–D) have revealed that several of these agents promoted AHF with phenotypic distributions distinct from one another and from the distributions seen with PB. As shown in this figure, which includes the placental isozyme of glutathione S-transferase (GST-P) as a fourth marker, PB promotion induced focal lesions scored predominantly by GST-P and GGT. Careful examination of these and other data (44) demonstrated that these two markers together score virtually all of the focal lesions revealed by the four markers used in experiments with PB promotion. Two other agents recently shown to be effective promoters in hepatocarcinogenesis—the commercial dye C.I. Solvent Yellow 14 and the acyclic chlorinated hydrocarbon chlorendic acid (45)—produce AHF with phenotypic distributions different from those observed for PB and TCDD or for the antiestrogen tamoxifen. These AHF are detected primarily by their increased expression of GST-P; GGT is an inefficient marker in this case. In contrast, the antiestrogen tamoxifen promoted focal lesions that were scored predominantly by G6P and to a lesser extent by GGT.

These distinctive AHF phenotypic distributions with different promoting agents may result from the reversible alteration of the expression of specific genes such as GGT within the AHF, caused by the transcriptional activation by that particular promoting agent. This mechanism has not yet been fully explored, but recent studies by Yeldandi et al. (46) suggest that the phenotypic expression induced by promotion with a peroxisome proliferator is not altered by replacement of this promoting agent with 2-acetylaminofluorene. In contrast, Ito and his associates (47) have presented data indicating that peroxisome proliferators that exhibit tumor-promoting activity will inhibit the expression of GST-P within AHF; this suggests that these agents exert some degree of gene regulation in preneoplastic lesions. GST-P (48) and GGT (48,49) are inefficient markers for the class of promoting agents that induce the formation of peroxisomes, findings that may relate to the fact that the same agents inhibit both GGT

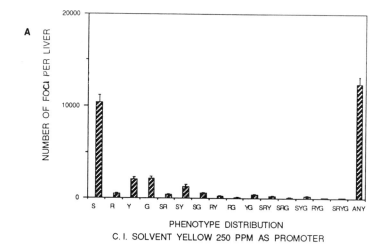

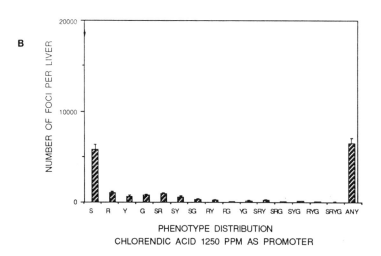

Figure 1. Phenotypic distribution of the number of altered hepatic foci in female rats treated with C.I. Solvent Yellow 14 (A), chlorendic acid (B), PB (C), or tamoxifen (D). As previously described (44), S denotes the placental isozyme of GST-P, R denotes GGT, Y denotes the canalicular ATP, and G denotes GGP. T = standard error of mean.

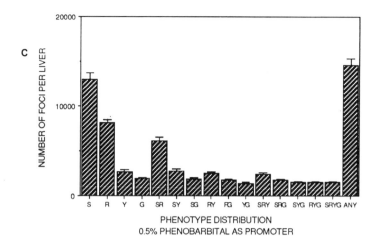

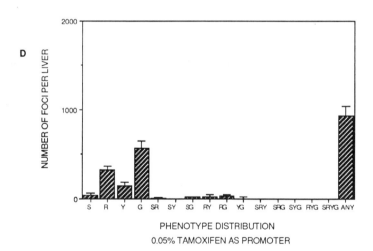

(50) and GST-P expression (51). Peroxisome proliferators thus provide another example of a different phenotypic distribution resulting from promotion with a specific class of chemicals.

An alternative hypothesis might be that a promoting agent may stimulate the proliferation of only a subset of initiated cells characterized by a specific programmed phenotype. As Figure 1 shows, we found a smaller number of AHF resulting from initiation with DEN when agents other than PB or TCDD were tested for promoter activity. In addition, the peroxisome proliferators induced a large number of quite small AHF scored by GST-P and GGT in addition to large AHF and neoplasms expressing ATP and G6P, but not GST-P or GGT. The concept of selective promotion of specific initiated cell populations has been previously proposed by Columbano et al. (52) on the basis of selection protocols such as those pioneered by Solt and Farber (53). Clearly, various promoting agents alter gene expression within clones of initiated hepatocytes and stimulate cell proliferation of such clones in a manner that may, in some circumstances, cause the selective proliferation of certain populations of initiated cells with specific phenotypes. One may speculate that such a selection may be related to a receptor mechanism and that receptors for specific promoting agents are present in only some initiated cells. The above data thus indicate that regulating cell proliferation in initiated cells and their progeny by administering promoting agents during hepatocarcinogenesis is apparently more complicated than originally thought.

Marker gene expression and cell proliferation during the promotion stage. The relationship of cell proliferation to the expression and phenotypic distribution is of considerable importance in our understanding of its relationship to other factors during promotion. The "phenotypic complexity," defined as the number of genes whose expression differs from the norm (43), is related to cell proliferation because AHF with greater degrees of phenotypic complexity also exhibit higher levels of DNA synthesis and, presumably, cell proliferation (54,55). These studies were conducted while animals were given PB continuously, a regimen that causes a slight inhibition of the proliferation of hepatocytes surrounding AHF, but no inhibition of cells within the AHF (56). This action of PB on nonfocal hepatocytes is distinctly different from the stimulation of hepatocyte hyperplasia seen shortly after PB administration begins; the latter is inhibited by the blockade of the α-$_1$ adrenergic receptor (57).

Although the markers in Figure 1 have not correlated closely with DNA synthesis or cell proliferation, others, such as G6P dehydrogenase, may be more directly related to the process of cell proliferation (58). Another class of markers closely related to cell proliferation are, in most instances, the products of proto-oncogene expression. Fausto and his associates (59) reported that the expression of c-Ki-*ras*, c-Ha-*ras*, and c-*myc* increased significantly following a carcinogenic regimen, i.e., a choline-deficient diet containing 0.1% ethionine for only 2 weeks. No changes were seen in c-*src* expression in this study. Similarly, Corral et al. (60) found an increase in c-*fos* expression after only 8 days of feeding DEN. The increased expression of other cellular oncogenes, including c-*jun* (61), c-*erb*A (62), and N-*myc* (63), has also reportedly occurred under similar circumstances in hepatocarcinogenesis. However, most or all of these genes also exhibit significant increases in expression during induced or naturally occurring cell proliferation of hepatocytes during fetal liver development (59), during induced hepatic regeneration (64), and in primary culture (65-67). PB treatment of liver-derived cells in culture stimulated the expression of c-Ki-*ras*, c-*fos*, and c-*myc* (68), but did not change their expression in vivo (69).

Whereas these studies were performed with nonneoplastic hepatocytes, investigations of AHF and hepatic nodules have not given such consistent results. Beer et al. (70) demonstrated an increase in expression of the proto-oncogene c-*raf* in almost all neoplastic nodules and hepatomas investigated. In this instance, the changes in c-*raf* expression did not correlate with cell proliferation as judged by the expression of H-4 histone, a measure of S-phase activity. Other studies (71-73) with protocols involving toxic DEN doses for initiation resulted in AHF and nodules, with the majority exhibiting increased expression of c-Ha-*ras* (71) and c-*myc* (72,73). In contrast, in studies from our laboratory in which animals were initiated with a nontoxic dose of DEN and promoted with PB (38), the vast majority of AHF exhibited a decreased expression of several proto-oncogenes including c-*myc*, c-Ha-*ras*, and a c-*fos*–like gene product (74). Therefore, as has been indicated previously (30), increased expression of proto-oncogenes in AHF may reflect not simply an increased rate of cell proliferation, but cellular changes characteristic of the terminal stage of progression (75). Cells whose phenotype diverges most extensively from their normal cell of origin exhibit relatively higher rates of cell proliferation may reflect changes characteristic of promotion and possess a greater potential for progression.

Recent studies have demonstrated that a more ubiquitous marker for AHF than those previously reported is a deficiency in the expression of the gap junction protein, connexin 32, previously known as the 27-kd gap junction protein (76). Earlier studies from this laboratory (70) reported a decreased expression of connexin 32 in nodules and hepatomas. A more recent study (76) has shown a marked reduction in the connexin 32 protein within AHF in livers that have been initiated and promoted with a variety of agents. However, the expression of this marker within individual cells and within AHF is not directly related to DNA synthesis (Fig. 2). Expression of connexin 32, as determined by the number of gap junctions per cell, is extremely low within the majority of AHF while most of the cells are in or have recently completed the S phase of the cell cycle. In centrolobular cells, there is also a decrease in the expression of connexin 32; these cells exhibit a very low incidence of labeling with [^{3}H]Tdr. Hepatocytes in the portal areas exhibit essentially the normal expression of connexin 32, and the labeling pattern is increased only slightly over that in the centrolobular areas. Thus, although overall connexin 32 expression is decreased (70) in a normal liver, creating a regenerative process, the promoting agent PB inhibits expression of the connexin 32 gene in the centrolobular areas without affecting it in the periportal areas. Thus, as shown in Figure 2, there is no obvious relationship between the expression of this gene, DNA synthesis, and cell proliferation. Furthermore, if one removes PB from the diet, within a short time almost all AHF develop essentially normal expression of the connexin 32 gene (76).

Cell proliferation and altered gene expression are essential characteristics of promotion. However, the data reviewed here indicate that in most instances these two processes are not directly correlated except in the expression of those genes critical to or regulated by cell division.

Progression. Our knowledge of the progression stage in hepatocarcinogenesis and in other histogenetic neoplasms is not so advanced as our knowledge of initiation and promotion. However, a number of the characteristics of progression have been described (75), including malignant neoplasia, the end point of this stage, and karyotypic instability, which involves obvious changes in the genome. Such changes are accompanied by alterations in the regulation (77) and the time of DNA synthesis (78) during hepatocarcinogenesis. Furthermore, while promoting agents may enhance cell proliferation in the early stages of progression (30,75), they do not directly influence lesions that have already progressed (79). Therefore, as in the promotion stage, cell proliferation is necessary for expressing the progression stage; however, the mechanisms

Uncoupling Cx32 Expression From DNA Synthesis by Phenobarbital

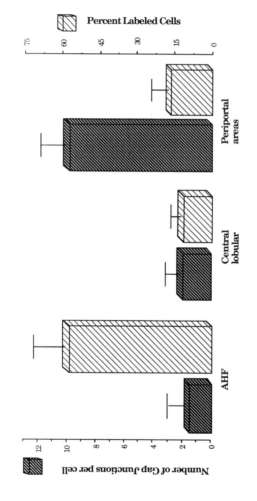

Figure 2. The effect of PB administration after DEN initiation of female rats on the number of gap junctions per cell in relation to the percentage of cells labeled with [3H]Tdr. Female rats were initiated with DEN (15 mg/kg) after a 70% partial hepatectomy (38) while on a semipurified AIN-76 diet. Two weeks after initiation, 0.1% PB was added to the diet and fed to animals for 8 months. [3H]Tdr was administered with an Alzet mini-pump for a period of 8 days prior to sacrifice. Determination of the number of gap junctions per cell was carried out as previously described (76), and autoradiography to determine thymidine labeling was done by standard techniques (cf. 54).

responsible for the alterations in cell proliferation and genome structure during this stage still elude us.

Quantitation of cell proliferation during initiation and promotion in relation to risk estimation

Proliferation of a stable cell population is a necessary prerequisite for the initiation stage. However, some initiating agents offer greater potential for the development of this stage. Until the advent of clearly defined and quantifiable multistage carcinogenesis models, it was not possible to determine this potential with any accuracy. This is now possible in multistage hepatocarcinogenesis in the rodent through the technique of quantitative stereology (80). By using this technique to determine the total number of AHF within the liver, one can assess on a molar basis an agent's effectiveness to initiate hepatocytes. We have performed this analysis on a number of chemicals and have defined a parameter, the Initiation Index (81), which is analogous to determining the number of colonies on a plate. The Initiation Index is defined as:

$$\text{Initiation Index} = \text{Number of AHF induced} \times \text{liver}^{-1} \times [\text{mmol/kg body wt}]^{-1}$$

This parameter differs by several orders of magnitude from that established to assess the effectiveness of complete carcinogens as initiating agents (81).

More germane to this discussion, however, is the assessment of each chemical agent's potential for promotion. Using quantitative stereology, one may determine not only the number of AHF within the entire liver, but also the volume of the liver occupied by the total AHF population. This is calculated as a percentage of the total liver volume and is a reflection of the total number of cells within the AHF. The Promotion Index is defined as:

$$\text{Promotion Index} = V_f/V_c \times 1/\text{mmol per week}$$

V_f is the total volume fraction (percentage) occupied by AHF in the livers of rats treated with the promoting agent after initiation, and V_c is the total volume of AHF in control animals that have only been initiated. A range of promotion indices, given in Table 1,

Table 1. Comparison of the calculated promotion index of seven agents that act as tumor promoters in the rat model of hepatocarcinogenesis.[+]

Compound	Promotion index
2,3,7,8-Tetrachlorodibenzo-p-dioxin	28,000,000
Ethinyl estradiol	93,000
Mestranol	54,000
1'-OH-Safrole	950
Tamoxifen	700
Phenobarbital	140
WY 14,643	60

[+] Adapted from Dragan et al. (82).

indicates that these various agents' potential for promotion ranges over almost six orders of magnitude. Furthermore, these promotion indices reflect the agents' effectiveness in stimulating the proliferation of preneoplastic hepatocytes that are the progeny of initiated cells. In this way the relative potency of promoting agents can be directly related to their effectiveness in stimulating proliferation of preneoplastic hepatocytes, although it has not yet been possible to relate these parameters to proliferation of normal hepatocytes.

Modeling of multistage hepatocarcinogenesis as an aid to risk assessment of chemical carcinogens

One goal of biology, toxicology, and pathology is the mathematical-statistical formulation of models that describe the mechanisms of normal and disease processes. However, as described by several scientists (83-85), no mathematical-statistical model of a biologic process has faithfully described the mechanisms of an entire biologic phenomenon, especially for the field of carcinogenesis (86), where many models have been proposed in the past. Recent advances in our understanding of the mechanisms of carcinogenesis as a multistage process have allowed, at least potentially, for a closer congruence between models representative of carcinogenesis and the actual development of cancer.

A model that most directly reflects the multistage nature of neoplastic development is that proposed by Moolgavkar and his associates (84). Since the model seen in Figure 3 simulates the three stages in the development of neoplasia, it thus should be possible to utilize the quantitative parameters derived from biologic experiments to test this model.

In a recent publication (87), such an exercise was conducted with only the stages of initiation and promotion, in which the numbers of intermediate cells (Fig. 3) were determined by the relationship:

$$I(t) \sim \mu_1 \mu_2 \int X(s) \exp[(\alpha_2 - \beta_2)(t-s)] ds \ (1)$$

where $I(t)$ = incidence function at time t
$X(s)$ = the number of normal susceptible cells at time (age)s
μ_1 = the rate of the "first event" (initiation)
α_2 = the rate of division of "intermediate cells" (cells in the stage of promotion)
β_2 = rates of "differentiation" and "death" of "intermediate cells" (apoptosis and/or differentiation of cells in the stage of promotion).

Each of these parameters may be determined experimentally or obtained from the literature to test whether the calculated number of intermediate cells reflects with reasonable accuracy the numbers used in the experiment. Such an analysis of previously reported data (88) provides the expected relationships seen in Figure 4, in which the observed numbers agree with the expected numbers of cells in AHF for the first four time points of the experiment. At 12 months of promotion, however, the model greatly overpredicts the number of cells. This suggests that the net growth rate of AHF decreases with prolonged promotion. Since the parameter $(\alpha_2-\beta_2)$ was estimated from the volume percentage determined experimentally (88), a more accurate determination of the individual components of this parameter might provide a closer fit throughout the entire curve. In any event, it is clear that the biologic model can be reasonably expressed in mathematic terms. Such relationships can potentially be used to predict the effectiveness of chemical agents as initiators and/or promoters at the present time, and may allow one to model the stage of progression in the future with further refinements of the techniques.

Thus, the relationships determined in multistage hepatocarcinogenesis may allow one to make predictions concerning the potency of specific promoting agents and, in the future, of complete carcinogens; this will be accomplished on the basis of dose-response relationships with only the input of the mathematic model. Further study of the role of cell proliferation in these processes and its expression may, through careful quantitation and appropriate modeling, lead not only to a better understanding of the carcinogenic process itself, but also to better predictions of the potency of individual chemical carcinogens and their potential risk to the human population.

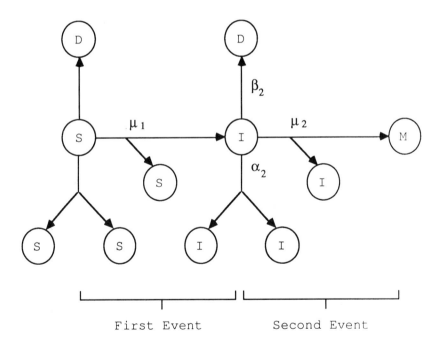

Figure 3. A Moolgavkar representation of multistage carcinogenesis. S = normal stem cells, I = intermediate (one-hit) cell, D = differentiated or deceased cell, M = malignant cell; μ_1 = rate of first event occurrence, μ_2 = rate of second event occurrence, α_2 = rate of division of intermediate cells (cells in the stage of promotion), β_2 = rate of differentiation and cell death in the promotion stage. Adapted from Moolgavkar (84).

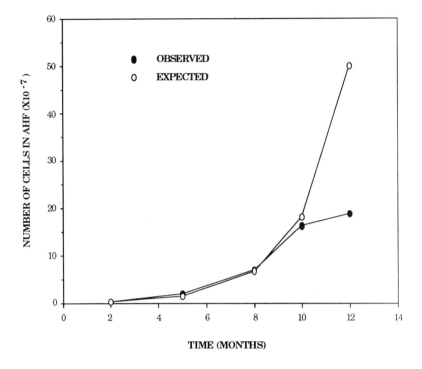

Figure 4. Observed and expected numbers of cells in AHF, where expectations are calculated from parameters described in the original reference (87). These parameters were estimated from "best"-fit of the model to the first four data points (i.e., 2,5,8, and 10 months), in which there is excellent agreement between expected and observed data. There is no indication of a decrease in $(\alpha_2-\beta_2)$ (see Fig. 3) except at 12 months. See the original reference (87) for further details.

References

1. Boutwell RK. Some biological aspects of skin carcinogenesis. Prog Exp Tumor Res 4:207–250, 1964.
2. DiPaolo JA, DeMarinis AJ, Evans CH, Doniger J. Expression of initiated and promoted stages of irradiation carcinogenesis in vitro. Cancer Lett 14:243–249, 1981.
3. Crawford BD, Barrett JC, Ts'o PO. Neoplastic conversion of preneoplastic Syrian hamster cells: rate estimation by fluctuation analysis. Mol Cell Biol 3:931–945, 1983.
4. Shirai T, Ohshima M, Masuda A, Tamano S, Ito N. Promotion of 2-(ethylnitrosamine)ethanol-induced renal carcinogenesis in rats by nephrotoxic compounds: positive responses with folic acid, base lead acetate, and N-(3,5-dichlorophenyl)succinimide but not with 2,3-dibromo-1-propanol phosphate. J Natl Cancer Inst 72:477–482, 1984.
5. Short BG, Steinhagen WH, Swenberg JA. Promoting effects of unleaded gasoline and 2,2,4-trimethylpentane on the development of atypical cell foci and renal tubular cell tumors in rats exposed to N-ethyl-N-hydroxyethylnitrosamine. Cancer Res 49:6369–6378, 1989.
6. Rosenberg MR, Novicki DL, Jirtle RL, Novotny A, Michalopoulos G. Promoting effect of nicotinamide on the development of renal tubular cell tumors in rats initiated with diethylnitrosamine. Cancer Res 45:809–814, 1985.

7. Hicks RM. Multistage carcinogenesis in the urinary bladder. Brit Med Bull 36:39–46, 1980.
8. Cohen SM. Promotion in urinary bladder carcinogenesis. Environ Health Perspect 50:51–59, 1983.
9. Ito N, Fukushima S. Promotion of urinary bladder carcinogenesis in experimental animals. Exp Pathol 36:1–15, 1989.
10. Pitot HC, Beer D, Hendrich S. Multistage carcinogenesis: the phenomenon underlying the theories. In: Theories of Carcinogenesis, O. Iversen (ed), Washington: Hemisphere Press, 1988, pp. 159–177.
11. Bartsch H, Terracini B, Malaveille C, Tomatis L, Wahrendorf J, Brun G, Dodet B. Quantitative comparison of carcinogenicity, mutagenicity, and electrophilicity of 10 direct-acting alkylating agents and of the initial O^6:7-alkylguanine ratio in DNA with carcinogenic potency in rodents. Mutat Res 110:181–219, 1983.
12. Elmore E, Kakunaga T, Barrett JC. Comparison of spontaneous mutation rates of normal and chemically transformed human skin fibroblasts. Cancer Res 43:1650–1655, 1983.
13. Piegorsch WW, Hoel DG. Exploring relationships between mutagenic and carcinogenic potencies. Mutat Res 196:161–175, 1988.
14. Jones CA, Huberman E. The relationship between the carcinogenicity and mutagenicity of nitrosamines in a hepatocyte-mediated mutagenicity assay. In: Genotoxicology of N-Nitroso Compounds, T. K. Rao, W. Lijinsky, and J. L. Epler (eds), New York: Plenum Publishing Corp, 1984, pp. 119–127.
15. Hartman PE. Bacterial mutagenesis: review of new insights. Environ Mol Mutagen 2:3–16, 1980.
16. Warwick GP. Effect of the cell cycle on carcinogenesis. Fed Proc 30:1760–1765, 1971.
17. Columbano A, Rajalakshmi S, Sarma DSR. Requirement of cell proliferation for the initiation of liver carcinogenesis as assayed by three different procedures. Cancer Res 41:2079–2083, 1981.
18. Kaufmann WK, Rice JM, Wenk ML, Devor D, Kaufman DG. Cell cycle-dependent initiation of hepatocarcinogenesis in rats by methyl(acetoxymethyl)nitrosamine. Cancer Res 47:1263–1266, 1987.
19. Kakunaga T. The role of cell division in the malignant transformation of mouse cells treated with 3-methylcholanthrene. Cancer Res 35:1637–1642, 1975.
20. Hennings H, Michael D, Patterson E. Croton oil enhancement of skin tumor initiation by N-methyl-N'-nitro-N-nitrosoguanidine: possible role of DNA replication (40126). Proc Soc Exp Biol Med 158:1–4, 1978.
21. Rabes HM. DNA adducts and cell cycle. J Cancer Res Clin Oncol 112:189–195, 1986.
22. Kondo S. Carcinogenesis in relation to the stem-cell-mutation hypothesis. Differentiation 24:1–8, 1983.
23. Ledda-Columbano GM, Columbano A, Curto M, Ennas MG, Coni P, Sarma DSR, Pani P. Further evidence that mitogen-induced cell proliferation does not support the formation of enzyme-altered islands in rat liver by carcinogens. Carcinogenesis 10:847–850, 1989.
24. Carriere R. The growth of liver parenchymal nuclei and its endocrine regulation. Int Rev Cytol 25:201–276, 1969.
25. Sarafoff M, Rabes HM, Dörmer P. Correlations between ploidy and initiation probability determined by DNA cytophotometry in individual altered hepatic foci. Carcinogenesis 7:1191–1196, 1986.
26. Sargent L, Xu Y-H, Sattler GL, Meisner L, Pitot HC. Ploidy and karyotype of hepatocytes isolated from enzyme-altered foci in two different protocols of multistage hepatocarcinogenesis in the rat. Carcinogenesis 10:387–391, 1989.
27. Saeter G, Schwarze PE, Nesland JM, Juul N, Pettersen EO, Seglen PO. The polyploidizing growth pattern of normal rat liver is replaced by divisional, diploid growth in hepatocellular nodules and carcinomas. Carcinogenesis 9:939–945, 1988.
28. Styles JA, Kelly M, Elcombe CR. A cytological comparison between regeneration, hyperplasia, and early neoplasia in the rat liver. Carcinogenesis 8:391–399, 1987.
29. Pitot HC. Principles of carcinogenesis: chemical. In: Cancer—Principles and Practice of Oncology, Vol. 1, 3rd Ed., V. T. DeVita, Jr., S. Hellman, and S. A. Rosenberg (eds), Philadelphia: J. B. Lippincott Co., 1989, pp. 116–135.
30. Pitot HC. Characterization of the stage of progression in hepatocarcinogenesis in the rat. In: Boundaries between Promotion and Progression, O. Sudilovsky, L. Liotta, and H. C. Pitot (eds), New York: Plenum Press, in press.
31. Ashendel CL. The phorbol ester receptor: a phospholipid-regulated protein kinase. Biochim Biophys Acta 822:219–242, 1985.
32. Itai A, Kato Y, Tomioka N, Iitaka Y, Endo Y, Hasegawa M, Shudo K, Fujiki H, Sakai S-I. A receptor model for tumor promoters: rational superposition of teleocidins and phorbol esters. Proc Natl Acad Sci USA 85:3688-3692, 1988.

33. Safe S, Bandiera S, Sawyer T, Zmudzka B, Mason G, Romkes M, Denomme MA, Sparling J, Okey AB, Fujita T. Effects of structure on binding to the 2,3,7,8-TCDD receptor protein and AHH induction—halogenated biphenyls. Environ Health Perspect 61:21–33, 1985.

34. Poland A, Glover E. 2,3,7,8-Tetrachlorodibenzo-p-dioxin: segregation of toxicity with the Ah locus. Mol Pharmacol 17:86–94, 1980.

35. Bursch W, Lauer B, Timmermann-Trosiener I, Barthel G, Schuppler J, Schulte-Herrmann R. Controlled death (apoptosis) of normal and putative preneoplastic cells in rat liver following withdrawal of tumor promoters. Carcinogenesis 5:453–458, 1984.

36. Enomoto K, Farber E. Kinetics of phenotypic maturation of remodeling of hyperplastic nodules during liver carcinogenesis. Cancer Res 42:2330–2335, 1982.

37. Pitot HC. Altered hepatic foci: their role in murine hepatocarcinogenesis. Annu Rev Pharmacol Toxicol 30:465–500, 1990.

38. Pitot HC, Barsness L, Goldsworthy T, Kitagawa T. Biochemical characterization of stages of hepato-carcinogenesis after a single dose of diethylnitrosamine. Nature 271:456–458, 1978.

39. Pitot HC, Goldsworthy T, Campbell HA, Poland A. Quantitative evaluation of the promotion by 2,3,7,8-tetrachlorodibenzo-p-dioxin of hepatocarcinogenesis from diethylnitrosamine. Cancer Res 40:3616–3620, 1980.

40. Sirica AE, Jicinsky JK, Heyer EK. Effect of chronic phenobarbital administration on the γ-glutamyl transpeptidase activity of hyperplastic liver lesions induced in rats by the Solt/Farber initiation:selection process of hepatocarcinogenesis. Carcinogenesis 5:1737–1740, 1984.

41. Glauert HP, Schwarz M, Pitot HC. The phenotypic stability of altered hepatic foci: effect of the short-term withdrawal of phenobarbital and of the long-term feeding of purified diets after the withdrawal of phenobarbital. Carcinogenesis 7:117–121, 1986.

42. Hendrich S, Glauert HP, Pitot HC. The phenotypic stability of altered hepatic foci: effects of withdrawal and subsequent readministration of phenobarbital. Carcinogenesis 7:2041–2045, 1986.

43. Peraino C, Staffeldt EF, Carnes BA, Ludeman VA, Blomquist JA, Vesselinovitch SD. Characterization of histochemically detectable altered hepatocyte foci and their relationship to hepatic tumorigenesis in rats treated once with diethylnitrosamine or benzo[a]pyrene within one day after birth. Cancer Res 44:3340–3347, 1984.

44. Xu Y-h, Campbell HA, Sattler GL, Hendrich S, Maronpot R, Sato K, Pitot HC. Quantitative stereological analysis of the effect of age and sex on multistage hepatocarcinogenesis in the rat using four cytochemical markers. Cancer Res 50:472–479, 1990.

45. Maronpot RR, Pitot HC, Peraino C. Use of rat liver altered focus models for testing chemicals that have completed two-year carcinogenicity studies. Toxicol Pathol 17:651–662, 1989.

46. Yeldandi AV, Subbarao V, Rajan A, Reddy JK, Rao MS. b-Glutamyltranspeptidase-negative phenotypic property of preneoplastic and neoplastic liver lesions induced by ciprofibrate does not change following 2-acetylaminofluorene administration. Carcinogenesis 10:797–799, 1989.

47. Hosokawa S, Tatematsu M, Aoki T, Nakanowatari J, Igarashi T, Ito N. Modulation of diethylnitrosamine-initiated placental glutathione S-transferase positive preneoplastic and neoplastic lesions by clofibrate, a hepatic peroxisome proliferator. Carcinogenesis 10:2237–2241, 1989.

48. Rao MS, Reddy JK. Peroxisome proliferation and hepatocarcinogenesis. Carcinogenesis 8:631–636, 1987.

49. Glauert HP, Beer D, Rao MS, Schwarz M, Xu Y-D, Goldsworthy TL, Coloma J, Pitot HC. Induction of altered hepatic foci in rats by the administration of hypolipidemic peroxisome proliferators alone or following a single dose of diethylnitrosamine. Cancer Res 46:4601–4606, 1986.

50. Furukawa K, Numoto S, Furuya K, Furukawa NT, Williams GM. Effects of the hepatocarcinogen nafenopin, a peroxisome proliferator, on the activities of rat liver glutathione-requiring enzymes and catalase in comparison to the action of phenobarbital. Cancer Res 45:5011–5019, 1985.

51. Awasthi YC, Singh SV, Goel SK, Reddy JK. Irreversible inhibition of hepatic glutathione S-transferase by ciprofibrate, a peroxisome proliferator. Biochem Biophys Res Commun 123:1012–1018, 1984.

52. Columbano A, Ledda GM, Rao PM, Rajalakshmi S, Sarma DSR. Initiation of experimental liver carcinogenesis by chemicals: are the carcinogen altered hepatocytes stimulated to grow into foci by different selection procedures identical? In: Chemical Carcinogenesis, C. Nicolini (ed), New York: Plenum Publishing Corporation, 1982, pp. 167–178.

53. Solt D, Farber E. New principle for the analysis of chemical carcinogenesis. Nature 263:701–703, 1976.

54. Pugh TD, Goldfarb S. Quantitative histochemical and autoradiographic studies of hepatocarcinogenesis in rats fed 2-acetylaminofluorene followed by phenobarbital. Cancer Res 38:4450–4457, 1978.

55. Estadella MD, Pujol MJ, Domingo J. Enzyme pattern and growth rate of liver preneoplastic clones during carcinogenesis by diethylnitrosamine. Oncology 41:276–279, 1984.
56. Tatematsu M, Aoki T, Kagawa M, Mera Y, Ito N. Reciprocal relationship between development of glutathione S-transferase positive liver foci and proliferation of surrounding hepatocytes in rats. Carcinogenesis 9:221–225, 1988.
57. Tsai W-H, Cruise JL, Michalopoulos GK. Blockade of α-1 adrenergic receptor inhibits hepatic DNA synthesis stimulated by tumor promoters. Carcinogenesis 10:73–78, 1989.
58. Moore MA, Nakamura T, Shirai T, Ichihara A, Ito N. Immunohistochemical demonstration of increased glucose-6-phosphate dehydrogenase in preneoplastic and neoplastic lesions induced by propylnitrosamines in F344 rats and Syrian hamsters. Jpn J Cancer Res (Gann) 77:131–138, 1986.
59. Yaswen P, Goyette M, Shank PR, Fausto N. Expression of c-Ki-ras, c-Ha-ras, and c-myc in specific cell types during hepatocarcinogenesis. Mol Cell Biol 5:780–786, 1985.
60. Corral M, Tichonicky L, Guguen-Guillouzo C, Corcos D, Raymondjean M, Paris B, Kruh J, Defer N. Expression of c-fos oncogene during hepatocarcinogenesis, liver regeneration and in synchronized HTC cells. Exp Cell Res 160:427–434, 1985.
61. Sakai M, Okuda A, Hatayama I, Sato K, Nishi S, Muramatsu M. Structure and expression of the rat c-jun messenger RNA: tissue distribution and increase during chemical hepatocarcinogenesis. Cancer Res 49:5633–5637, 1989.
62. Himeno Y, Fukuda Y, Hatanaka M, Imura H. Expression of oncogenes during rat chemical hepato-tumorigenesis promoted by estrogen. Jpn J Cancer Res 80:737–742, 1989.
63. Corral M, Paris B, Guguen-Guillouzo C, Corcos D, Kruh J, Defer N. Increased expression of the n-myc gene during normal and neoplastic rat liver growth. Exp Cell Res 174:107–115, 1988.
64. Fausto N, Shank PR. Oncogene expression in liver regeneration and hepatocarcinogenesis. Hepatology 3:1016–1023, 1983.
65. Ikeda T, Sawada N, Fujinaga K, Minase T, Mori M. c-H-ras gene is expressed at the G1 phase in primary cultures of hepatocytes. Exp Cell Res 185:292–296, 1989.
66. Sawada N. Hepatocytes from old rats retain responsiveness of c-myc expression to EGF in primary culture but do not enter S phase. Exp Cell Res 181:584–588, 1989.
67. Kruijer W, Skelly H, Botteri F, van der Putten H, Barber JR, Verma IM, Leffert HL. Proto-oncogene expression in regenerating liver is simulated in cultures of primary adult rat hepatocytes. J Biol Chem 261:7929–7933, 1986.
68. Lafarge-Frayssinet C, Frayssinet C. Overexpression of proto-oncogenes: ki-ras, fos and myc in rat liver cells treated in vitro by two liver tumor promoters: phenobarbital and biliverdin. Cancer Lett 44:191–198, 1989.
69. Hsieh LL, Peraino C, Weinstein IB. Expression of endogenous retrovirus-like sequences and cellular oncogenes during phenobarbital treatment and regeneration in rat liver. Cancer Res 48:265–269, 1988.
70. Beer DG, Neveu MJ, Paul DL, Rapp UR, Pitot HC. Expression of the c-raf proto-oncogene, γ-glutamyltranspeptidase, and gap junction protein in rat liver neoplasms. Cancer Res 48:1610–1617, 1988.
71. Galand P, Jacobovitz D, Alexandre K. Immunohistochemical detection of c-Ha-ras oncogene p21 product in pre-neoplastic and neoplastic lesions during hepatocarcinogenesis in rats. Int J Cancer 41:155–161, 1988.
72. Nagy P, Evarts RP, Marsden E, Roach J, Thorgeirsson SS. Cellular distribution of c-myc transcripts during chemical hepatocarcinogenesis in rats. Cancer Res 48:5522–5527, 1988.
73. Ito S, Watanabe T, Abe K, Yanaihara N, Tateno C, Okuno Y, Yoshitake A, Miyamoto J. Immunohisto-chemical demonstration of the c-myc oncogene product in rat chemical hepatocarcinogenesis. Biomed Res 9:177–180, 1988.
74. Pitot HC, Neveu MJ, Hully JR, Sargent L. Gene activation and deactivation during multistage hepatocarcinogenesis in the rat. In: Chemical Carcinogenesis: Modulating Factors in Multistage Carcinogenesis, F. Feo, P. Pani, A. Columbano, and R. Garcea (eds), New York: Plenum Press, in press.
75. Pitot HC. Progression: the terminal stage in carcinogenesis. Jpn J Cancer Res 80:599–607, 1989.
76. Neveu MJ, Hully JR, Paul DL, Pitot HC. Reversible alteration in the expression of the gap junctional protein, connexin 32, during tumor promotion in rat liver. Cancer Commun 2:21–31, 1990.
77. Barbason H, Betz EH. Liver cell control after discontinuation of DENA feeding in hepatocarcinogenesis. Eur J Cancer Clin Oncol 17:149–154, 1981.
78. Post J, Hoffman J. The replication time and pattern of carcinogen-induced hepatoma cells. J Cell Biol 22:341–350, 1964.

532 / Pitot et al.

79. Hayes MA, Lee G, Tatematsu M, Farber E. Influences of diethylnitrosamine on longevity of surrounding hepatocytes and progression of transplanted persistent nodules during phenobarbital promotion of hepatocarcinogenesis. Int J Cancer 40:58–63, 1987.

80. Campbell HA, Xu Y-D, Hanigan MH, Pitot HC. Application of quantitative stereology to the evaluation of phenotypically heterogeneous enzyme-altered foci in the rat liver. J Natl Cancer Inst 76:751–767, 1986.

81. Pitot HC, Goldsworthy TL, Moran S, Kennan W, Glauert HP, Maronpot RR, Campbell HA. A method to quantitate the relative initiating and promoting potencies of hepatocarcinogenic agents in their dose-response relationships to altered hepatic foci. Carcinogenesis 8:1491–1499, 1987.

82. Dragan YP, Xu Y-D, Pitot HC. Tumor promotion as a target for estrogen/anti-estrogen effects in rat hepatocarcinogenesis. Prev Med, in press.

83. Whittemore AS. Quantitative theories of oncogenesis. Adv Cancer Res 27:55–88, 1978.

84. Moolgavkar SH. Carcinogenesis modeling: from molecular biology to epidemiology. Annu Rev Public Health 7:151–169, 1986.

85. Alavanja M, Aron J, Brown C, Chandler J. Cancer risk-assessment models: anticipated contributions from biochemical epidemiology. J Natl Cancer Inst 78:633–643, 1987.

86. Chu KC. A nonmathematical view of mathematical models for cancer. J Chron Dis 40:163S–170S, 1987.

87. Pitot HC, Neveu MJ, Hully JR, Rizvi TA, Campbell H. Multistage hepatocarcinogenesis in the rat as a basis for models of risk assessment of carcinogenesis. In: Scientific Issues in Quantitative Cancer Risk Assessment, S. Moolgavkar (ed), Boston: Birkhauser Boston, Inc., 1990, pp. 69–96.

88. Rizvi TA, Kennan W, Xu Y-H, Pitot HC. The effects of dose and duration of administration on the promotion index of phenobarbital in multistage hepatocarcinogenesis in the rat. APMIS 2,96:262–268, 1988.

Index

2–Acetylaminofluorene (AAF)
    animal mitogenic testing, 11
    bladder tumor promotion and, 352–353
    hepatocyte proliferation and, 392–393
    65–kDa protein expression and, 92
    liver DNA synthesis and, 62
4–Acetylaminofluorene (4–AAF),
    mitogenicity of, 259
Acoustic neuromas, trauma and, 30
Additive hyperplasia, definition of, 254
Adenocarcinomas, 27, 46
Adenomas, colinic, 399–400
Adenomatous hyperplasias, 46
AF2
    forestomach lesion reversibility, 46–47
    stomach carcinogenicity of, 43–44
AHF. *See* Altered hepatic foci
Alcohol, cancer and, 28
Allylamine
    aortic smooth muscle cell proliferation,
        431–436
    characterization of, 431
    phosphoinoside metabolism in smooth
        muscle and, 431–436
Allyl isothiocyanate, clastogenicity of, 7
Altered hepatic foci
    DEN–initiated, 93–101
    estimation of, 526–528
    peroxisome proliferators and, 522
    during promotion stage of
        hepatocarcinogenesis, 518–519
Ames test, 461, 463
D–Amino acid oxidase, 79
Aminotriazole, thyroid cell proliferation
    and, 174, 178–182
Angiotensin II, 230
Angiotensin III, 230

Animal cancer tests, mitogenesis and,
    11–12
Anthralin, epithelial hyperplasia and, 36
Anti–LC[1–30], 213
Antioxidants
    carcinogenicity studies of, 43, 46–51
    early stomach lesions induced by, 46
    stomach carcinogenicity of, 46
    two–stage stomach carcinogenesis and,
        48–51; *see also specific*
        antioxidants
Anti–pre[266–278], 213
AOM (azoxymethane), 401
Apoptosis
    cell proliferation and, 238
    definition of, 254
    markers of, 239
    in normal liver, 238–239
    in preneoplastic foci in liver, 239–240
    radiation exposure and, 159, 161
    in tumors, 240
Arsenicals, epithelial hyperplasia and, 36
Asbestos, 10, 29, 77
Atherogenesis, monoclonal theory of, 436
Atherosclerosis
    occupational and environmental
        exposures and, 430–431
    pathogenesis of, 429
    risk factors, 430
ATPase, 519
Atypical cell foci, kidney carcinogenesis
    and, 361–363
Augmentative hepatomegaly, 232–233
Autoimmune deficiency syndrome–related
    lymphoma, 26
Autoradiography, 266–267
Azoxymethane (AOM), 401

533